Timeline for Application/Admission

This should be considered a general guide for applicants. It is important that an applicant considering medical school consult with his or her prehealth advisor to devise a schedule that works for the individual.

COLLEGE YEAR 1	• Fall semester
	  o Meet prehealth advisor and investigate prehealth advisory program
	  o As applicable, ensure that prehealth advisor receives course directors' evaluations
	  o Successfully complete first-semester required premedical coursework and other degree requirements
	• Spring semester
	  o Visit "Considering a Career in Medicine" Web site (www.aamc.org/students/considering)
	  o Identify summer employment/volunteer medically related opportunities
	  o Successfully complete second-semester required premedical coursework and other degree requirements
	  o Ensure that prehealth advisor receives course directors' evaluations

SUMMER 1	• Complete summer employment/volunteer medically related experience • Attend summer school, if necessary

COLLEGE YEAR 2	• Fall semester
	  o Check in with prehealth advisor and participate in prehealth activities
	  o Investigate available volunteer/paid medically related clinical or research activities
	  o Successfully complete first-semester required premedical coursework and other degree requirements
	  o Ensure that prehealth advisor receives course directors' evaluations
	• Spring semester
	  o Check in with prehealth advisor and participate in prehealth activities
	  o Participate in volunteer/paid medically related clinical or research activities
	  o Identify summer employment/volunteer medically related opportunities
	  o Successfully complete second-semester required premedical coursework and other degree requirements
	  o Ensure that prehealth advisor receives course directors' evaluations

SUMMER 2	• Complete summer employment/volunteer medically related experience • Participate in a summer health careers program, if available • Attend summer school, if necessary

COLLEGE YEAR 3	• Fall semester
	  o Check in with prehealth advisor and participate in prehealth activities
	  o Continue participation in volunteer/paid medically related activities
	  o Investigate:
	    • Medical education options in MSAR and (www.aamc.org/members/listings/msalphaae.htm)
	    • Medical College Admission Test (MCAT) Web site (www.aamc.org/mcat)
	    • Information about the Medical College Admission Test (MCAT) and American Medical College Application Service (AMCAS) fee assistance on the AAMC Fee Assistance Program Web site (www.aamc.org/fap), as appropriate
	    • AAMC's "Applying to Medical School" Web site (www.aamc.org/students/applying/start.htm)
	    • As applicable, information for students from groups underrepresented in medicine on the AAMC Minorities in Medicine Web site (www.aamc.org/students/minorities/start.htm)
	  o Begin preparation for spring MCAT administration
	  o Successfully complete first-semester required premedical coursework and other degree requirements
	  o Ensure that prehealth advisor receives course directors' evaluations
	• Spring semester
	  o Consult regularly with prehealth advisor regarding:
	    • Schedule for completion of school-specific requirements for advisor/committee evaluation
	    • Advice about medical education options
	  o Continue participation in volunteer/paid medically related activities
	  o Prepare for spring MCAT administration
	  o Continue review of medical education options

continued...

continued from page one

COLLEGE YEAR 3	o Take spring MCAT
	o Investigate information about the:
	• AMCAS Web site (☞ www.aamc.org/amcas)
	• Texas Medical and Dental Schools Application Service (TMDSAS) Web site (☞ www.utsystem.edu/tmdsas/)
	• Ontario Medical School Application Service (OMSAS) (☞ www.ouac.on.ca/)
	• American Association of Colleges of Osteopathic Medicine (AACOM) (☞ www.aacom.org/)
	• American Association of Colleges of Osteopathic Medicine Application Service (AACOMAS) (☞ https://aacomas.aacom.org/)
	o Investigate:
	• As applicable, AAMC Curriculum Directory Web site (☞ http://services.aamc.org/currdir) for information about medical school curricula and joint, dual, and combined-degree programs
	o Successfully complete second-semester required premedical coursework and other degree requirements
	o Ensure that prehealth advisor receives course directors' evaluations
SUMMER 3	• Participate in a summer health careers program, if available
	• Complete AMCAS application
	• Take summer MCAT
	• Attend summer school, if necessary
	• Investigate:
	o AAMC *Recommendations Concerning Medical School Acceptance Procedures for First-Year Entering Students* document (☞ www.aamc.org/students/applying/policies)
	o *Applicant Responsibilities* document (☞ www.aamc.org/students/applying/policies)
COLLEGE YEAR 4	• Fall semester
	o Complete supplementary application materials for schools applied to
	o Consult regularly with prehealth advisor regarding:
	• Completion of school-specific requirements for advisor/committee evaluation
	• Status of application/admission process at medical schools applied to
	o Continue participation in volunteer/paid medically related activities
	o Interview at medical schools
	o Continue review of medical education options
	o Investigate:
	▪ Financial aid planning process with AAMC (MD)[2]: *Monetary Decisions for Medical Doctors* online program (☞ www.aamc.org/md2)
	▪ Financial aid forms required by school of interest with the AAMC *Financial Aid Forms Required by Medical Schools* searchable database (http://services.aamc.org/msar_reports/)
	o Successfully complete first-semester elective science and non-science coursework and other degree requirements
	o Ensure that prehealth advisor receives course directors' evaluations
	• Spring semester
	o Make interim and final decisions about medical school choice
	o Immediately notify medical schools that you will not be attending
	o Ensure that all IRS forms are submitted as early as possible
	o Successfully complete second-semester elective science and non-science coursework and other degree requirements
	o Graduate
SUMMER 4	o Prepare for medical school enrollment: purchase books and equipment and make appropriate living arrangements
	o Relax and prepare for medical school
	o Attend orientation programs and matriculate in to medical school

ASSOCIATION OF AMERICAN MEDICAL COLLEGES

Medical School Admission Requirements
United States and Canada   2005-2006
The ONLY Guide Fully Authorized by ALL Medical Schools

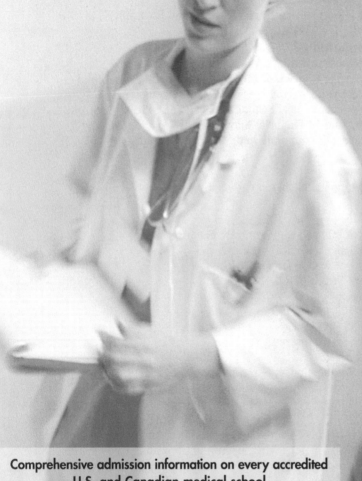

Comprehensive admission information on every accredited
U.S. and Canadian medical school

Find the most up-to-date information on:

Application deadlines and procedures
•
Acceptance rates
Tuition and student fees

from every accredited U.S. and Canadian medical school

www.aamc.org/students

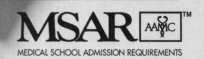

MSAR
MEDICAL SCHOOL ADMISSION REQUIREMENTS

Medical School Admission Requirements, 2005–2006, United States and Canada

AAMC Staff

Content Coordinator
Tami Levin

Staff Associate
La'Verne Alexander

Staff Assistant
Elita Goggins

Content Specialist
Robert F. Sabalis, Ph.D., Associate Vice President for Student Affairs and Programs

Consultants
Gwen Garrison, Ph.D., Director, Student and Applicant Studies
H. Collins Mikesell, Senior Research Associate for the Division of Medical School Services and Studies
Ellen Julian, Ph.D., Assistant Vice President and Director, Medical College Admission Test
Barbara Gordon, Assistant Vice President, Medical School Application Services
Paula Craw, Director, Student Financial Services
Lily May Johnson, Manager, Division of Community and Minority Programs

Revised annually; new edition available in early spring.

To order additional copies of this publication, please contact:
Association of American Medical Colleges
Section for Publication Orders
2450 N Street, NW
Washington, DC 20037
Phone: 202-828-0416
Fax: 202-828-1123
Web site: www.aamc.org

Price: $25.00, plus $7 shipping (single copy)

ISBN 1-57754-030-1

Printed in the United States of America

Group on Student Affairs (GSA) Steering Committee, 2003–2004

CHAIR
Richard Wheeler, M.D.
University of Arkansas, College of Medicine

CHAIR ELECT
Peter J. Katsufrakis, M.D.
University of Southern California, Keck School of Medicine

GSA VICE CHAIR
Patricia J. Metting, Ph.D.
Medical College of Ohio

CHAIR, GSA-MAS
James L. Phillips, M.D.
Baylor College of Medicine

CHAIR, CENTRAL REGION
Paul C. Bunger, Ph.D.
University of South Dakota, School of Medicine

CHAIR, SOUTHERN REGION
Mason P. Thompson, M.D.
Medical College of Georgia, School of Medicine

CHAIR, NORTHEAST REGION
Clara A. Callahan, M.D.
Jefferson Medical College of Thomas Jefferson University

CHAIR, WESTERN REGION
Peter J. Katsufrakis, M.D.
University of Southern California, Keck School of Medicine

CHAIR, COMMITTEE ON ADMISSIONS
Mark A. Notestine, Ph.D.
Ohio State University, College of Medicine and Public Health

CHAIR, COMMITTEE ON STUDENT AFFAIRS
Geoffrey H. Young, Ph.D.
University of Medicine and Dentistry of New Jersey
Robert Wood Johnson Medical School

CHAIR, COMMITTEE ON STUDENT FIINANCIAL ASSISTANCE
Stacey R. McCorison
Duke University, School of Medicine

CHAIR, COMMITTEE ON STUDENT RECORDS
Jean Lantz
University of Iowa, Carver College of Medicine

COUNCIL OF DEANS LIAISON
Robert C. Talley, M.D.
University of South Dakota, School of Medicine

CHAIR, ORGANIZATION OF STUDENT REPRESENTATIVES
Yvette Martin
Mayo Clinic College of Medicine

NATIONAL ASSOCIATION OF ADVISORS FOR THE HEALTH PROFESSIONS
A. Kenneth Moore, Ph.D.
Seattle Pacific University, Department of Biology

Association of American Medical Colleges

The Association of American Medical Colleges (AAMC) has as its purpose the advancement of medical education and the nation's health. In pursuing this purpose, the Association works with many national and international organizations, institutions, and individuals interested in strengthening the quality of medical education at all levels, searching for biomedical knowledge, and applying these tools to providing effective health care.

As an educational association representing members with similar purposes, the primary role of the AAMC is to assist those members by providing services at the national level that will facilitate the accomplishment of their missions. Such activities include collecting data and conducting studies on issues of major concern, evaluating the quality of educational programs through the accreditation process, providing consultation and technical assistance to institutions as needs are identified, synthesizing the opinions of an informed membership for consideration at the national level, and improving communication among those concerned with medical education and the nation's health. Other activities of the Association reflect the expressed concerns and priorities of the officers and governing bodies.

The AAMC represents all 126 accredited U.S. medical schools; the 16 accredited Canadian medical schools; some 400 major teaching hospitals, including 56 affiliated health systems and 66 Veterans Affairs medical centers; 94 academic and professional societies representing 88,000 faculty members; the nation's 67,000 medical students and 103,000 residents; and more than 650 individuals interested in medical education.

In addition to the activities listed above, the AAMC is responsible for the Medical College Admission Test (MCAT®) and the American Medical College Application Service (AMCAS®) and provides detailed admissions information to the medical schools and to undergraduate premedical advisors.

Important Notice

The information in this book is based on the most recent data provided by member medical schools prior to publication at the request of the Association of American Medical Colleges (AAMC). This material has been edited and in some instances condensed to meet space limitations. In compiling this edition, the AAMC made every reasonable effort to assure the accuracy and timeliness of the information, and, except where noted, the information was updated as of February 2004. All information contained herein, however, especially figures on tuition and expenses, is subject to change and is non-binding for medical schools listed or the AAMC. All medical schools listed in this edition, as with other educational institutions, are also subject to federal and state laws prohibiting discrimination on the basis of race, color, religion, sex, age, handicap, or national origin. Such laws include Title VI of the Civil Rights Act of 1964, Title IX of the Education Amendments of 1972, Section 504 of the Rehabilitation Act of 1973, and the Age Discrimination Act of 1975, as amended. For the most current and complete information regarding costs, official policies, procedures, and other matters, individual schools should be contacted.

In applying to U.S. or Canadian medical schools, applicants need not go through any commercial agencies. The AAMC neither endorses nor has any relationship with commercial agencies.

All URLs in this book can be found at ☞www.aamc.org/msar.

AAMC POSITION ON EQUAL OPPORTUNITY

The Association strongly reaffirms the principle of equal opportunity for individuals who are qualified for education and training in, and the practice of, the health professions, without regard to sex, race, creed, color, national origin, age, or handicap. In pursuit of this principle and policy, the AAMC:

1. Requests member institutions to continue to monitor their admission policies and practices to ensure equal opportunity of admission to their educational and training programs.

2. Requests member institutions to continue to undertake and to reinforce programs of affirmative action to increase the numbers and proportions of students in the health professions from groups that are presently underrepresented in those professions.

Further, recognizing that the underrepresentation of some groups in health professions educational and training programs is but a symptom of broad social and economic problems, the AAMC:

1. Actively supports the organized study of the basic causes of underrepresentation and possible cures.

2. Actively supports the initiation of new programs, and the broadening of existing programs, which are designed to overcome these problems. These programs include, but are not limited to, those designed to afford women the opportunity to fulfill their educational-professional goals and their cultural roles without sacrifice to either, programs designed to eliminate economic barriers to education in the health professions, and programs designed to develop increased interest in careers in the health professions on the part of members of underrepresented groups at the secondary school and college levels.

Contents

List of Tables and Charts

Alphabetical Listing of Medical Schools

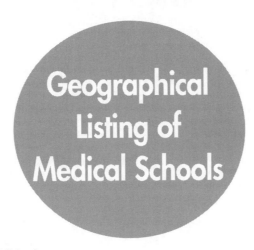

Geographical Listing of Medical Schools

Chapter 11 • U.S. Medical Schools

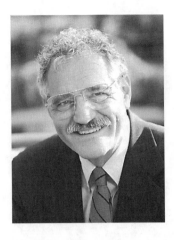

Let me be the first to congratulate you on your decision to pursue a career in medicine. Undoubtedly, this is one of the most important decisions you will make during your lifetime. In my own opinion, admittedly biased by my own gratifying experiences as a physician, no other profession offers as many challenges, as many chances to be of service to others, and as many opportunities for a satisfying and rewarding career.

As you begin to contemplate the "when, where, and how" of applying to medical school, this year's *Medical School Admission Requirements* will be of invaluable help. In addition to the annual updates from all U.S. and Canadian medical schools, this edition contains a wonderful chronology of events in the life of medical students, from prerequisites, to the "pre-application" phase, to graduation, and beyond. Throughout, you will find helpful pointers to the Web sites of the Association of American Medical Colleges (AAMC) and other organizations where up-to-date information on a variety of programs will help you find your way.

I can't imagine a more exciting time to begin medical school. Just think of what you have to look forward to. Tomorrow's doctors will be at the forefront of the most dramatic developments in medical science in all of history. They will be armed with unimaginably powerful tools to relieve human suffering and prevent the ravages of disease. They will help shape technological improvements that will revolutionize both the way doctors conduct research and the way they diagnose and treat patients. And they will be in a position to help reshape the way the healthcare delivery system provides affordable services of high quality to everyone who needs them.

Despite this wealth of opportunity, I know that many aspiring medical school applicants are advised by some well-meaning friends and family members not to pursue their dream of becoming doctors. It seems to me that those who proffer such advice are overly influenced by the current anxieties about rising medical care costs, malpractice concerns, and the prospects for a major restructuring of the way health care is organized and financed. What they fail to take into account, however, is a fundamental truth about the human condition: people get sick and, when they do, they need help. And that's what medicine is all about. Caring for and about people has always been the essence of the medical profession and the principal reason students choose to study medicine.

Medical School Admission Requirements may be your first contact with the AAMC and its family of services for applicants to medical school, as well as for students and residents. I hope your relationship with AAMC is long and fruitful, and that this new edition will be of help as you take the first steps toward a career in medicine. Please accept my best wishes for success.

Jordan J. Cohen

Jordan J. Cohen, M.D.
President
Association of American Medical Colleges (AAMC)

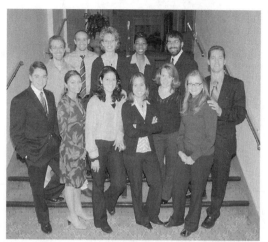

Organization of Student Representatives

Congratulations on considering a career in medicine. Your decision thus far demonstrates your enthusiasm for improving humanity's health and well-being, a core principle of the medical profession.

Now begins your path toward becoming a part of this challenging yet rewarding profession. The medical school admission process can seem overwhelming at times and the choices seem endless – Which medical school is the best match for your learning style? What career path are you interested in? Would your future career benefit from enrollment in a dual degree program? Since only you can answer these questions, the best way to approach this process is to be as informed as possible.

Utilizing the many resources available, such as this guide, will equip you with the tools to make the best and most informed decision for you. The AAMC updates this guide annually, so you can be confident that you have the most reliable and timely information available as you make these critical decisions.

Furthermore, you should consult your mentors, advisors, peers, and medical school faculty and staff in your quest for answers to your questions. They can provide you with perspective, guidance, and encouragement since the process can be lengthy. Additionally, an often overlooked resource is your medical school interviews. Take these opportunities to learn about the life of a medical student at each institution such as what support and extracurricular opportunities are available. Ultimately, by utilizing these diverse sources of information, you will be empowered to make decisions that will enrich your life for years to come.

You have already taken the first steps toward a rich and fulfilling life in medicine. At times this process may seem demanding, but keep in perspective that the medical school admission process and the variety of choices that you have are designed to help you shape your educational experience and future career.

Please accept my best wishes as you pursue the goal of becoming an outstanding physician.

Sincerely,

Yvette N. Martin
M.D.-Ph.D. Student
Mayo Medical and Mayo Graduate School
2003-2004 Chair, Organization of Student Representations, AAMC

CHAPTER 1

Medicine as a Career

For those interested in a career in medicine, the choices are almost innumerable.

From clinical practice to surgery, to public health, to military medicine, to biomedical research – medicine is an inclusive profession that offers incredibly varied opportunities to its physician ranks. Ideally, all physicians aspire to be:

- altruistic, compassionate, and truthful in their relationships with patients, patients' family members, and professional colleagues
- knowledgeable about the scientific basis of medicine and the normal and abnormal functioning of the body
- skillful in communicating with and caring for patients
- dutiful in working with others to promote the health of individual patients and the broader community

Which Path Is Right for You?

Men and women bring to the profession of medicine a broad range of personal interests, educational backgrounds, and occupational histories, as well as unique sets of skills, abilities, and philosophies. Aspiring physicians seek to achieve lofty but attainable professional goals in a variety of specialties and clinical settings:

- The satisfaction of enduring patient relationships is the draw of family medicine or internal medicine, where the "art" of medicine flourishes in every encounter with each patient. Others with a commitment to social justice and the well-being of a community, and an interest in fulfilling the health care needs of the underserved and disadvantaged, can meet these challenges in urban and rural clinics, in community medicine and public health, or as medical missionaries.

- An investigative bent and the desire to expand the boundaries of medical knowledge are traits of those in the nation's private and public laboratories and research institutions. Physicians interested in communicating their colleagues' laboratory-derived discoveries and in interpreting their impact on society flourish as medical editors, journalists, or experts in medical ethics.

- Careers in general surgery often suit those physicians with a desire for immediate and direct feedback about the results of their interventions. Plastic and reconstructive surgery draws others with artistic skills, excellent eye-hand coordination, and aesthetic interests.

- Those interested in mind-body interactions and the emotional lives of their patients might find a home in neurology or psychiatry. Others interested in our national defense or the challenges inherent in emergency situations use their skills as flight surgeons, in aerospace medicine, or in military medicine.

- The economic and public policy aspects of health care guide some physicians to lead think tanks and health-related associations and organizations, and to serve in the legislative and executive branches of government. The more visceral aspects of medicine draw some to work with crime and accident victims as emergency medicine physicians or trauma surgeons; others work with patients with bone and joint problems in orthopedic surgery.

*All URLs mentioned in this chapter can be found at ➣ www.aamc.org/msar

- For those fascinated by the issues facing groups of patients with age-defined illnesses and problems — from the risks of infancy and early childhood to the challenges of later life — fulfillment may come as pediatricians and geriatricians. Others prefer to pursue detailed knowledge about the intricacies of a single body organ or system, such as that required of ophthalmologists, dermatologists, or neurosurgeons.

- Assisting couples in overcoming complex fertility and gestational problems is the hallmark of the specialties of reproductive endocrinology and obstetrics and gynecology. Those with a long-range interest in reducing the incidence of birth defects and inherited syndromes might find their calling in the field of medical genetics.

- The detection, prevention, and eradication of injury and disease in groups and populations, both here and abroad, draw people to preventive medicine and epidemiology at such organizations as the Centers for Disease Control and Prevention or the World Health Organization. Those same interests at the local level can be fulfilled in forensic pathology, in coroners' and medical examiners' offices, or in state or county health departments.

As you can see, the possibilities are almost endless.

No matter what your personal interests or needs may be, medicine encourages and permits you to find your niche. Should your interests, abilities, or needs change with time and experience, medicine — because of its emphasis on lifelong learning and its periodic requirements for demonstrating competence — affords ongoing opportunities for refining your skills and reorienting your practice.

Career Guidance and Decision-Making

Medical schools in the United States recognize the critical role they play in helping medical students to assess their personal values and interests, identify career options, determine their personal "fit" with those options, and make well-informed decisions about specialty choice. This recognition is reflected in the Careers in Medicine program, created by the AAMC in collaboration with its 125 member medical schools. The four-phase career decision-making format used in this program is similar to that used by premedical students in deciding on medicine as a career, and in deciding which medical schools would be an appropriate match.

In Phase 1 of Careers in Medicine, Personal Career Assessment, medical students explore who they are, what activities they enjoy, the values that underlie their lives and work, and the nature of their relationships with other people. During Phase 2, Career Exploration, tools are provided for exploring specialties and other career options. Phase 3, Decision-Making, focuses on comparing the personal information obtained in Phase 1 with the specialty and career options gleaned in Phase 2. Finally, in Phase 4, Implementation, plans are laid for application to residency training programs and related activities, such as personal statements and interviews.

The process of career assessment, planning, decision-making, and implementation is dynamic and ongoing. Consider familiarizing yourself with the Careers in Medicine program at ⌁ www.aamc.org/students/cim as you work on plans for medical education and for application to medical school.

Combined, Dual, and Joint Degree Programs

The U.S. medical education system is designed to support the process of identifying and achieving your place in medicine. During both the four years of medical school — known as undergraduate medical education — and in the residency and fellowship training that follows (graduate medical education), opportunities abound for specialized education and training. At medical schools and residency training programs across the country, students and residents are enrolled in combined, dual, and joint degree programs that prepare them well for future careers. Federally funded Medical Scientist Training Programs (MSTPs) assist students in obtaining both an M.D. and Ph.D. degree in areas related to medical research, and in working with mentors to prepare for careers as academic physicians and clinician-scientists.

Medical schools on university campuses provide dual M.D./graduate and professional degree programs in a variety of academic disciplines, including the basic sciences, business administration, computer science, education, law, and public health. Graduates of such programs may pursue careers as National Institutes of Health scientists, medical school faculty members, hospital administrators, health care entrepreneurs, medical informatics and diagnostic experts, or forensic scientists and medical examiners; they also become authorities in epidemiology, public health, and preventive medicine.

Information about combined college/M.D. programs for high school students can be found in Chapter 10 and on the AAMC Curriculum Directory Web site at ✑http://services.aamc.org/currdir/. Information about combined, dual, and joint M.D./graduate and professional degree programs (e.g., M.Ed., M.P.H., J.D., M.B.A., and various Ph.D. specializations) can be found in a database that is searchable by school and program type, also found at the AAMC Curriculum Directory Web site. The information in the Curriculum Directory is provided, and periodically updated, by medical school personnel through the AAMC Curriculum Management and Information Tool (CurrMIT).

Characteristics of U.S. and Canadian Medical Schools

The missions of the 126 accredited U.S. and 16 accredited Canadian allopathic schools vary as widely as the motivations of individual medical students. (Allopathic medical schools grant the M.D. degree, while osteopathic medical schools grant the D.O. degree.) Each U.S. medical school is periodically required to document that it has met strict accreditation standards set by the Liaison Committee on Medical Education (LCME, ✑www.lcme.org), the joint accrediting body of the American Medical Association (AMA, ✑www.ama-assn.org), located in Chicago, and the AAMC (✑www.aamc.org), located in Washington, D.C. Canadian medical schools are jointly accredited by the LCME and the Committee on Accreditation of Canadian Medical Schools of the Association of Canadian Medical Colleges (✑www.acmc.ca/comitt_acred.htm).

Fundamental elements of medical education are shared by all schools: the acquisition of basic science knowledge and elementary clinical skills during the first component of the curriculum, and acquisition of more advanced clinical skills under the supervision of attending physician faculty members during the second component of the curriculum. Medical schools also vary on many important characteristics: institutional mission, curricular emphasis and structure, class size and applicant pool, cost, and ownership and hospital affiliations.

What Kind of School for You?

As applicants embark on their journey toward a medical career, consideration of the type of medical school is important. Some medical school curricula emphasize the education and training of primary care physicians, usually meaning general pediatricians, general internists, and family physicians (although obstetrician/gynecologists and others who are the first point of contact for patients are also sometimes included). Some medical schools emphasize the education and training of physicians who will serve the needs of rural patients. Still other schools emphasize research skills and investigative activities on the part of medical students, with their graduates going on to careers in academic medicine and basic and clinical research. Some schools were founded by state legislatures with a curricular emphasis on the needs of a particular patient population, such as older patients.

A number of schools provide educational opportunities on multiple campuses. In some, students complete their first two years in classrooms and laboratories on a central campus, then disperse to separate clinical campuses to complete core and elective clinical experiences in their final two years. In other institutions, the opposite occurs.

Entering class sizes at U.S. medical schools range from 37 to 313 people. Applicant pools at U.S. schools also vary greatly; some public medical schools in smaller states have small pools, with first-year classes selected primarily from state residents. Other private schools select new entrants from national pools of several thousand applicants, with little regard to state of legal residence.

Public or Private?

Medical schools generally fall into two categories as a function of their funding sources: public and private. Public medical schools usually receive substantial amounts of operating revenue from state or federal government, while private schools usually generate revenue from other sources, including endowments and tuition. The annual cost of attending state-supported medical schools is often less than that of private schools, especially for state residents, because educational costs are underwritten with tax revenues. This tuition differential, however, usually disappears for students who are not state residents; tuition at public medical schools for non-residents often equals that of private institutions.

Some medical schools, both public and private, own and manage their own hospitals, outpatient facilities, and health care systems. Others, sometimes referred to as community-based schools, establish ongoing affiliations with existing inpatient and ambulatory care facilities in their surrounding communities, where students complete the clinical components of their education under the supervision of faculty members.

While all medical schools were established to educate future physicians, they can differ substantially in their educational programs. This and other information about U.S. and Canadian medical schools is presented in greater detail in the school profile pages that begin on page 109. Complete information can also be found on each school's Web site ⬳ www.aamc.org/members/listings/msalphaae.htm and in institutional academic bulletins, brochures, and related publications.

CHAPTER

2

The Process of Medical Education

The path to medical practice consists of five phases:

- undergraduate premedical education (college)
- undergraduate medical education (medical school)
- graduate medical education (residency and fellowship training)
- licensure and certification
- continuing medical education

None of these educational elements stands alone; the successful completion of each component is a building block, laying a strong, broad foundation for the practice of medicine.

Undergraduate Premedical Education

For future physicians, college provides opportunities for excelling in the natural sciences, the social sciences, and the humanities; for fostering inquiry and problem-solving skills; for honing communication and interpersonal skills; and for developing intellectual discipline. College begins to prepare students for the academic and personal rigors of a medical education. There they learn to appreciate the continuum of human experience — to value the unique doctor-patient relationship and to recognize the impact of culture and family dynamics on human development.

Medicine is practiced in a social context. Physicians must be able to communicate effectively with people from a variety of backgrounds and life experiences. Medical school admission committees seek to enroll students who bring diverse talents and interests to medicine; their goal is to identify students whose personal and career aspirations are compatible with society's health care needs, whether coping with the AIDS epidemic, responding to bioterrorism, or caring for the medically underserved.

Undergraduate Medical Education

Curricula at Canadian and U.S. medical schools have common elements, although they vary in educational approaches. All medical schools share the goals of preparing students in the art and science of medicine, and providing them with the background necessary to enter a three- to seven-year-long period of graduate medical education. A significant amount of information about medical school curricula and institutional characteristics can be found in the AAMC databases at ✑ http://services.aamc.org/currdir.

Each medical school's faculty establishes standards for students' academic performance, personal and professional conduct, and promotion and graduation. Many schools have developed comprehensive learning objectives for their educational programs, along with detailed descriptions of how students will be assessed at various stages. Faculty members determine whether students have met curricular learning objectives by requiring them to demonstrate mastery of both course content and clinical skills — through written tests, oral examinations, and laboratory exercises — and by observing their clinical acumen. Many schools require students to complete local and national standardized examinations before they can progress to further clinical training. The frequency and methods of evaluation vary from school to school.

Over the past decade medical schools have revised their educational programs, moving from more passive approaches to learning to more active ones. Modes of learning such as lectures have been de-emphasized; learning opportunities now often promote self-assessment, problem-solving, integration of the basic and clinical sciences, and collaboration with faculty and peers. Increasingly, schools are also requiring students to complete year-end and overall comprehensive examinations prior to promotion and graduation.

Grading procedures at medical schools vary. Many have pass/fail or honors/pass/fail grading systems, while others continue to use letter grades. Whatever the assessment structure, students' knowledge and skills are carefully scrutinized on a periodic basis by members of the faculty. Recently, attempts have been made to differentiate the assessment of academic achievement from that of personal and professional behavior, with complementary evaluations during each classroom and clinical experience. In the clinical environment, one-on-one relationships between faculty members and students permit close observation and feedback.

At three percent, the rate of attrition at U.S. medical schools is relatively low. Students who are deficient in certain areas often have opportunities for remediation and assistance. Nevertheless, all medical school faculties reserve the right to dismiss any student whose academic or personal characteristics are incompatible with a physician's professional responsibilities.

THE FIRST TWO YEARS. Initially, students learn those basic sciences essential to medicine. The normal structure and function of human systems are taught through gross and microscopic anatomy, biochemistry, behavioral science, physiology, and neuroscience. Subsequently, the educational focus shifts to abnormalities of structure and function, disease, and general therapeutic principles through exposure to microbiology, immunology, pathology, and pharmacology. Throughout the first two years, the clinical significance of basic science material is continuously stressed.

In addition to the core scientific work, students are exposed to a wide variety of topics:

- nutrition
- medical ethics
- genetics
- laboratory medicine
- health care delivery systems
- substance abuse
- human values
- research
- preventive medicine
- community health
- geriatrics
- human sexuality

Lecture-style teaching methods no longer dominate the classroom; small-group learning, multi-disciplinary clinical conferences, and problem-based approaches all have a place in the first two years. These experiences can be with actual patients and with people trained to simulate pathological conditions, known as standardized patients.

By the end of these two years, students have learned the scientific underpinnings of medicine. They also have learned the basics of interviewing and obtaining historical data from patients, as well as conducting physical examinations. Students are now prepared to make the transition to the clinical environment on a full-time basis.

THE SECOND TWO YEARS. The second period of undergraduate medical education consists of a series of required clinical rotations, or clerkships, usually lasting from 4 to 12 weeks, during which medical students work with patients and their families in inpatient and outpatient settings. Here, they function under the supervision of physician faculty members – known as attending physicians – and residents, and work with other members of the clinical team, including nurses, social workers, psychologists, pharmacists, and technical staff. The pattern, length, and number of rotations differ from school to school, but core clinical training usually includes clerkships in internal medicine, obstetrics/gynecology, pediatrics, psychiatry, and surgery. Depending on the school, required clerkships can also include family medicine, primary care, neurology, or a community or rural medicine preceptorship.

During clinical clerkships, students are assigned to an outpatient clinic or inpatient hospital unit where they assume responsibility for "working-up" a number of patients each week, that is, collecting relevant data and information from them and presenting findings to a faculty member for diagnosis and treatment planning. Students also participate in the ongoing clinical care of patients assigned to a medical team. Ideally, students follow their patients over time, either during hospitalizations or through the course of outpatient treatment. When appropriate, students also relate to patients' family members – providing information, answering questions, and preparing them for the outcome of patients' care.

During these clinical education experiences, students learn to apply their basic science knowledge and clinical skills in diagnosing and treating patients' illnesses and injuries. They learn clinical decision-making and patient management skills. They interact daily with faculty members, whether at the bedside, during inpatient team discussions ("rounds"), on patient visits, or in case-based lectures and small-group discussions.

ELECTIVES. Most medical schools provide curricular opportunities for students to pursue special interests through supplemental educational experiences known as electives, which are offered in the basic, behavioral, and clinical sciences, and in basic and clinical research. Electives are usually available during the final year of medical school. Students can complete electives on their own campuses, at other medical schools, through federal and state agencies (such as the Institute of Medicine, the Indian Health Service, and the Centers for Disease Control and Prevention), in international settings, and through external non-academic service organizations.

Clinical electives include opportunities in the entire range of medical and surgical specialties and subspecialties. Students seek these experiences for several reasons: to acquaint themselves with additional career options, to enrich their educational experience, and to expose themselves to areas of specialization that are one-time opportunities.

RESIDENCY OR SPECIALTY. During the fourth year of medical school, students also make decisions about medical specialties and apply to graduate training programs (residencies) through the National Resident Matching Program (NRMP, ⌘www.nrmp.org). The NRMP is a Web-based program that matches applicants' preferences for residency positions with program directors' preferences for applicants.

Graduate Medical Education

The third phase of medical training prepares physicians for independent practice in a medical specialty. Residency programs focus on the acquisition of detailed factual knowledge and the development of clinical skills and professional competencies in a particular specialty. These programs are based in hospitals or other health care institutions and, in most specialties, utilize both inpatient and outpatient settings for teaching purposes. Residency programs are accredited by the Accreditation Council for Graduate Medical Education (⌘www.acgme.org) and its associated Residency Review Committees. Residents, also known as house officers or house staff, typically complete educational requirements for certification through a specialty board recognized by the American Board of Medical Specialties (⌘www.abms.org). Information about medical specialties and subspecialties can also be found at ⌘www.aamc.org/students/cim.

For medical students who decide to practice in a medical or surgical specialty, the requirements of that specialty's certifying board will influence the choice of the first-postgraduate-year (PGY1) program. Family medicine, internal medicine, pediatrics, and general surgery encourage students to enter PGY1 programs in that specialty directly, and to continue in these programs until they have completed all specialty board requirements. Satisfactory completion of three years of training in family practice, internal medicine, or pediatrics or five years of training in general surgery generally qualifies an individual to take the board certification examinations in that specialty.

Students seeking careers in other medical or surgical specialties (e.g., anesthesiology, dermatology, psychiatry, and radiology) are first exposed to a broad range of clinical experiences during their PGY1 year. Usually these students complete this first residency training clinical year in internal medicine or in a diversified "transitional year" program, with the expectation that they will enter a program in the specialty of their choice in the second postgraduate year (PGY2). In some cases, the year of broad clinical exposure may be in the same institution where subsequent subspecialty training occurs. In other instances, specialty training must be completed elsewhere.

Education and training in a medical or surgical subspecialty (e.g., cardiology, pulmonology, geriatrics, hematology/oncology, and cardiothoracic surgery) take place for varying periods of time after completion of the appropriate preparatory residency training. These trainees are sometimes referred to as fellows, although resident or resident physician is the current term of art.

Licensure and Certification

The fourth phase of medical training involves licensure to practice medicine and certification in a specialty. Medical practice is regulated by each individual state or jurisdiction. Each state has statutes known as medical practice acts that describe the practice of medicine and identify a public agency to license physicians and regulate medical practice. These agencies protect the public from potentially unprofessional or incompetent physicians.

All states require applicants for a medical license to document that they have both completed educational and training programs and achieved passing scores on licensure examinations approved by the relevant state agency or board. In 1990, the Federation of State Medical Boards (⌖ www.fsmb.org) and the National Board of Medical Examiners (⌖ www.nbme.org) established the United States Medical Licensing Examination, or USMLE, (⌖ www.usmle.org), a single, three-step licensing examination utilized by all U.S. licensing jurisdictions.

USMLE Step 1 assesses whether the examinee can understand and apply important concepts of the sciences basic to the practice of medicine, with special emphasis on principles and mechanisms underlying health, disease, and modes of therapy. Step 1 ensures mastery of the sciences that provide a foundation for the safe and competent practice of medicine in the present, and the scientific principles required for the maintenance of competence through lifelong learning.

Beginning in June 2004, USMLE Step 2 will consist of two components: Clinical Knowledge and Clinical Skills. USMLE Step 2 assesses the examinee's ability to apply medical knowledge, skills, and understanding of clinical science essential for the provision of patient care under supervision, and includes emphasis on health promotion and disease prevention. Step 2 ensures that due attention is devoted to principles of clinical sciences and basic patient-centered skills that provide the foundation for the safe and competent practice of medicine.

USMLE Step 3 assesses whether the examinee can apply medical knowledge and understanding of biomedical and clinical science essential for the unsupervised practice of medicine, with an emphasis on patient management in ambulatory settings. Step 3 provides a final assessment of a physician's ability to assume independent responsibility for delivering general medical care.

In addition to receiving a license from a public regulatory agency, physicians are strongly encouraged to voluntarily apply for certification in a medical or surgical specialty from one of the 24 approved boards of the American Board of Medical Specialties. Through comprehensive examinations, these specialty boards determine if candidates have been appropriately prepared in accordance with established educational standards. Those who have satisfied all board requirements are certified and are known as "diplomates" of the specialty board; periodic recertification is offered at intervals of 7 to 10 years.

Continuing Medical Education

The fifth and final phase of medical training is continuing medical education, or CME. Physicians continue the educational process in the specific medical specialty in which they completed residency training; CME reflects the commitment to life-long learning that is a hallmark of the medical profession. By attending CME programs regularly, practicing physicians maintain their clinical competence over time and enhance their knowledge and skills. The Accreditation Council for Continuing Medical Education (⌖ www.accme.org) provides a system of voluntary accreditation for providers of continuing medical education programs.

CHAPTER

Undergraduate Premedical Preparation

During college, the successful premedical student completes several important tasks; he or she:

- selects a personally challenging major
- completes required premedical courses in a timely fashion
- establishes an ongoing relationship with an informed advisor
- participates in a variety of extracurricular experiences
- masters both course content and academic skills
- balances intellectual development with social and interpersonal growth

Academic Preparation

CHOICE OF MAJOR. Medical schools recognize the importance of a strong foundation in the natural sciences – biology, chemistry, physics, and mathematics – and most schools have established minimum course requirements for admission. These courses usually represent about one-third of the credit hours needed for graduation. This approach deliberately leaves room for applicants from a broad spectrum of college majors, including those in the humanities and social sciences. No medical school requires a specific major of its applicants or matriculants. Admission committee members know that medical students can develop the essential skills of acquiring, synthesizing, applying, and communicating information through a wide variety of academic disciplines.

Nevertheless, many premedical students choose to major in science. Ideally, they do so because they are fascinated by science and perceive that such a major can be the foundation for a variety of career options. Choosing science based primarily on enhancing one's chances for admission to medical school is not in a student's long-term best interest. Medical school admission committees seek students whose intellectual curiosity leads them to a variety of disciplines and whose intellectual maturity assures that their efforts are persistent and disciplined.

SCIENCE PREPARATION. The study and practice of medicine are based on modern concepts in biology, chemistry, and physics, and on an appreciation of the scientific method. Hence, mastery of these basic scientific principles is expected of all entering medical students. Medical schools generally require successful completion of one academic year (two semesters or three quarters) of biology and physics and one academic year each of general and organic chemistry. These courses should be academically rigorous and acceptable for students majoring in those areas. All science courses should include adequate laboratory experiences.

Although only a few medical schools require applicants to complete a specific course in mathematics, all schools appreciate mathematical competence as a strong foundation for understanding the basic sciences. In addition, a working knowledge of statistics helps medical students and physicians to become critical evaluators of the medical literature; familiarity with computers is helpful during the educational experience, as well as in medical practice. Thus, many medical schools recommend coursework in mathematics, statistics, and computer science.

Advanced science coursework is not typically required by medical schools. Students may choose to take upper-level science courses because of their own interests or undergraduate major requirements. Taking additional science courses that duplicate the basic science material in the first two years of medical school is not recommended. In fact, practicing physicians often recommend that, during their college years, premedical students take advantage of what might be their last opportunity for the study of non-science areas (music,

*All URLs mentioned in this chapter can be found at ✐ www.aamc.org/msar

art, history, and literature) that might become avocational interests later in life. Table 3-A gives an overview of the most common courses required by medical schools.

AP AND CLEP CREDIT. Premedical students intending to apply college credit earned through Advanced Placement (AP) and College Level Examination Placement (CLEP) to meet premedical requirements should be aware that some medical schools restrict such use of this credit. In most cases, the restrictions involve the official reporting of AP and CLEP credit on the college transcript, establishing an upper limit of such credit toward courses required for admission, or requiring additional upper-level courses in the science areas where credit was received. Premedical students should carefully review Chapter 11 and pertinent medical school Web sites and publications for additional information.

ADVANCED WORK. Medical schools encourage honors, independent study, and research work by premedical students. These activities demonstrate in-depth, sustained scholarly exploration, as well as the presence of life-long learning skills, that are essential to a career in the medical profession.

Development of Personal Attributes

Academic or scientific accomplishment alone is not sufficient to be admitted to the medical profession. Intellectual capacity is obviously important, but it is not enough; the most critical aspect of practicing medicine is the physician-patient relationship.

In a publication that outlines learning objectives for all medical students, the AAMC reported that, while physicians are certainly expected to be knowledgeable and skillful, they are also expected to be altruistic and dutiful. The required knowledge and skills are developed in part through the college and medical school educational processes. Dedication to duty and altruism are nurtured through experience – with family, with friends, and with people in need.

In the report *Medical School Objectives Program: Learning Objectives for Medical Student Education: Guidelines for Medical Schools* (✎ www.aamc.org/meded/msop/start.htm), dutifulness is defined as:

- an appreciation of the complex non-biological determinants of poor health

- an awareness of community and public health issues

- the ability to identify risk factors for disease

- a commitment to the early identification and treatment of disease

- an acceptance of the responsibility for making scientifically based medical decisions and for advocating for the care of the underserved

- an understanding of basic issues in health care financing and delivery

Altruism is defined as involving:

- ethical decision-making
- compassion, respect, honesty, and integrity
- collaborative work with other team members
- advocating for one's patients
- sensitivity to potential conflicts of interest
- the capacity to recognize one's limits
- the commitment to continuously improve one's knowledge and abilities

These basic elements of the "art" of medicine, along with other important characteristics such as motivation, persistence, and communication and interpersonal skills, evolve over time. Experience in a health-care setting, caring for an ill or elderly family member, participating in basic or clinical science research efforts, working as an emergency medical technician, "shadowing" a physician, or providing emotional support to people in a rape crisis center, emergency room, or social service agency — these kinds of service activities are recommended to those considering medicine as a career.

By participating in such activities, premedical students learn about the medical profession and about themselves. They learn about their tolerance for stress, their ability to communicate and empathize with people of different backgrounds and cultures, their problem-solving skills, and their willingness to put others' needs before their own. They also come to better understand the nature of medical practice and the daily demands placed upon physicians and their family members. After learning these important lessons, they can decide whether medicine is an appropriate career choice.

Finally, premedical students should know how these experiences are assessed by medical school admission committees. At least three criteria are used: length of time, depth of experience, and lessons learned. Short-term experiences such as day-long blood drives are less enlightening than semester or year-long commitments. Passive activities such as observation are less instructive than those requiring active participation. Most important, admission committees want to know what students derived from these experiences. Applicants should be prepared to respond to these kinds of questions about their clinical or research experiences.

For the enrolled medical student, the satisfaction derived from these experiences is often the motivation that helps them to "pull through" the challenging demands of medical school, which affect even the best students.

Premedical Advising

Students investigating a career in medicine — no matter where they are in the process — can get extremely valuable advice from their campus prehealth advisor. Depending on the individual school, prehealth advisors function on either a full- or part-time basis. They can be a faculty member (often in a science department), a staff member in the office of an academic dean or the career center, the director of an advising office for pre-professional students, or a physician in part-time practice. Ideally, prehealth advisors are knowledgeable and supportive, as well as well-informed about medical education programs, both locally and nationally. Advisors belong to organizations such as the National Association of Advisors for the Health Professions (☞ www.naahp.org) that assist them in their work. They provide both information and guidance to interested students and, at times, even challenge students to consider new options or reconsider their decisions.

Prehealth advisors help premedical students to:

- identify college courses that satisfy premedical requirements
- determine an appropriate sequence for completing those courses
- find tutorial assistance, if needed
- plan academic schedules to accommodate both premedical coursework and other educational objectives, including a study program abroad, a dual major, or a senior honors thesis
- find paid or volunteer clinical/research experiences
- strengthen the medical school application
- prepare for interviews and standardized tests
- arrange for letters of evaluation and recommendation
- determine the most appropriate career paths based on individual assets, liabilities, values, and life goals

Premedical students usually meet with prehealth advisors when they:

- enter into a premedical curriculum
- join a prehealth student society
- switch majors or courses of study
- need information about medical school admission requirements
- prepare to apply to medical school
- seek clinical or research experiences
- require advice about resolving academic problems
- want to discuss future career paths
- plan a postbaccalaureate premedical program or coursework
- prepare for health profession school admission tests
- need letters of evaluation or recommendation

SERVICES PROVIDED BY A PREHEALTH ADVISOR. Advisors' services typically vary according to the advisor's employment status, the number of premedical students served, and the philosophy and organization of the institution. Students should contact their school's advisor to determine what services are available; they generally fall into five categories:

- *Academics.* Advisors are well informed about premedical coursework on their campuses and about developing suitable academic programs for prehealth students. They collaborate with campus academic staff in designing study, reading skill, and test preparation workshops, and in offering tutoring programs. Advisors publicize regional and national programs of interest to their students.

- *Clinical and research experiences.* Advisors often work with advisory groups composed of college and medical school teaching and research faculty and community clinicians. These groups help identify part-time jobs, volunteer positions, and opportunities for independent study credit in local laboratories and offices.

- *Assistance to student organizations.* Advisors often advise the organizations and academic societies that serve prehealth students. These groups plan programs, identify funding sources, and arrange for campus visits from admissions and financial aid personnel, as well as medical school alumni.

- *Advising and support.* Advisors help students pursue realistic individual goals and maximize their potential. They meet with students individually and provide group opportunities for students to meet each other and to meet community representatives from various health professions. Advisors establish peer advising and mentoring programs. They are sensitive to the needs of students, including their financial needs, their being part of a group underrepresented in medicine, or their being first in their families to attend college.

- *Sharing resources.* Prehealth advisors disseminate information and publications from relevant organizations, including the AAMC and the National Association of Advisors for the Health Professions. They provide computer access to Web-based health careers programs and those on educational financing. They distribute information about local, regional, and national research and service opportunities. They stock a library of publications related to medical school and medical education, including *Medical School Admission Requirements.*

THE PREHEALTH COMMITTEE LETTER OF RECOMMENDATION. One important service provided by the advisor to prehealth students, and frequently to alumni, is the prehealth committee letter of recommendation. This is usually a composite letter written on behalf of an applicant to medical schools by the college or university's prehealth committee. The prehealth advisor may be a committee member or the chair, and is usually the liaison between students and the committee, facilitating letter writing and the distribution of letters to schools.

This letter presents an overview of the student's academic strengths, exposure to health care and medical research environments, contributions to the campus and community, and personal attributes such as maturity and altruism. The letter may also address any extenuating circumstances about the student's poor performance during a course or semester, or provide perspective on problems the student may have encountered. The letter can also explain school-specific courses and programs in which the student has participated.

Some undergraduate institutions do not provide composite letters of recommendation. Instead, they collect individual letters during the student's enrollment and distribute them at the appropriate time to the medical schools where the student has applied. Students should inquire about the specific services that their institution's prehealth advisor provides.

FINDING A PREHEALTH ADVISOR. Students who have difficulty identifying an advisor on their campus should contact the National Association of Advisors for the Health Professions (NAAHP) on the Web at ⬡www.naahp.org. If a student's school does not have a prehealth advisor, volunteer advisors at other institutions can be identified. The NAAHP also offers publications to help students prepare for medical school. You can contact the NAAHP at the following address:

National Association of Advisors for the Health Professions
P.O. Box 1518, Champaign, IL 61824-1518
(217) 355-0063 ▪ Fax (217) 355-1287
naahpinc@aol.com

Special Programs

The majority of medical school applicants are seniors in college. However, numerous schools offer special programs to accommodate "non-traditional" medical students:

COMBINED COLLEGE/MEDICAL SCHOOL PROGRAMS. These programs begin after high school and combine undergraduate and medical school curricula. About 5 percent of medical students begin their medical education in these programs, which vary by school. Most include the typical eight years of premedical and medical study, although some programs permit students to complete both college and medical school in six to seven years. Several programs are limited to state residents, and many require prospective medical students to be enrolled at specific undergraduate institutions. Additional information can be found in Chapter 10.

DEFERRED ENTRY. Many medical schools consider requests from accepted applicants who want to defer matriculation, usually for a year, to take advantage of a special opportunity or for other personal reasons. Most schools require a written application and review requests on an individual basis. Some schools require deferred applicants to sign an agreement to attend that school the following year; others will hold a place in the next entering class until a mutually agreed upon date, even if the applicant seeks admission to other schools for the next year. Interested applicants should obtain additional information from individual medical schools; the school-specific pages in Chapter 11 also provide relevant information.

POSTBACCALAUREATE PREMEDICAL PROGRAMS. Not all medical school applicants are college seniors; some are college graduates. Some embarked on other careers after college, but then decided to apply to medical school. If these graduates were not science majors, they must complete required premedical coursework through postbaccalaureate premedical programs, which exist at colleges and universities across the country, both public and private. The programs range from formal, one- and two-year programs for full-time students to more informal part-time ones; some specialize in applicants changing careers, while others focus on those attempting to enhance prior academic performance. A searchable database of postbaccalaureate premedical programs can be found on the AAMC Student Hub at ⬡http://services.aamc.org/postbac.

CHAPTER

The Application Process

The annual medical school application process begins each spring, as applicants use one of three different processes for applying to U.S. medical schools:

- the American Medical College Application Service (AMCAS) for the 117 U.S. schools that participated in AMCAS for the 2004 entering class (www.aamc.org/amcas) (There are 120 schools and programs participating in AMCAS for the 2005 entering class.)
- the Texas Medical and Dental Schools Application Service (TMDSAS) for the six public allopathic medical schools in Texas; more information can be found at www.utsystem.edu/tmdsas
  - school-specific application forms for two medical schools with their own individual application processes

Individual schools often supplement AMCAS and TMDSAS application materials with their own forms and materials, known as "supplemental application materials."

Application Procedures

AMCAS, TMDSAS, and individual schools manage their application processes and the procedures by which applicant information is made available to medical school admission committee members. The authority and responsibility for selecting individuals who will be admitted to a medical school rest with each school's faculty. Acting through its standing admission committee, the faculty develops and approves criteria for admission. The administrative responsibility for receiving and processing applications rests with admissions officers and members of their staff. The responsibility for reviewing applicant information, interviewing candidates, and making decisions about admitting candidates rests with admission committee members.

COMPOSITION OF THE ADMISSION COMMITTEE. Medical school admission committees typically include representatives from the faculties of both basic science and clinical departments. Membership also frequently includes faculty from other colleges and schools in the university, community physicians, other community members, and medical students.

APPLICATION PROCESSING. Applications are screened and categorized by admissions office staff according to criteria established by the admission committee. Depending on the school, supplemental application materials (including letters of recommendation, an essay, legal residency and other school forms, and a fee) may be requested from all or some applicants, or only from those that meet specific criteria.

As applications are completed, applicants that interest schools most are contacted by admissions office staff, and arrangements are made for campus visits and interviews with admission committee members. At some institutions, meetings with off-campus interviewers, including practicing physicians located near an applicant's home or school, may be required. As the process continues, other applicants may also be contacted and interviewed.

Applicants are typically interviewed by more than one committee member, either individually or in a group. After completion of the interview process, interviewers' evaluations are correlated with all other application materials and presented to the admission committee. Final decisions about admission are usually made by the committee acting as a whole.

*All URLs mentioned in this chapter can be found at www.aamc.org/msar

All applicants, whether they are interviewed or not, are informed of the admission committee's decision according to the school's individual schedule. Committee decisions can range from an offer of immediate acceptance, to the placement of the applicant in a "hold" category or on an alternate list, to non-acceptance. As the admission cycle continues, acceptances are offered until the required number of matriculants have been identified for that year's entering class.

EARLY DECISION PROGRAM OR REGULAR APPLICATION? One of an applicant's first decisions is whether to apply to a medical school through the Early Decision Program (EDP) or the regular application process. The fact that candidates applying through the EDP are informed about the outcome of their application at a participating school by October 1 affords candidates sufficient time to apply to other schools through the regular process if they are not accepted through the EDP.

The decision to apply through the EDP should be made carefully. While criteria for accepting EDP applicants vary among schools, a frequent criterion is that applicants show extraordinary credentials for admission. Applicants considering an EDP application should contact the medical school admissions office for information.

EDP applicants must agree:

- not to apply through the EDP if they have already submitted an initial or secondary (AMCAS or non-AMCAS) application to the M.D. degree program at a U.S. allopathic medical school for the current entering class

- to apply to only one AMCAS medical school through the EDP

- not to submit additional (AMCAS or non-AMCAS) applications until they have received notification of non-acceptance through the EDP, or they have been formally released from the EDP commitment, or the October 1 EDP notification deadline has passed

- to attend the school if offered an EDP acceptance

All EDP applicants accepted by a medical school must adhere to the tenets of the program; any violation will result in an investigation by AMCAS.

With regard to the EDP, medical schools agree to:

- notify each EDP applicant of the admission decision by October 1

- defer each EDP applicant to the regular applicant pool in those instances when an EDP non-acceptance decision is made

TIMING OF THE APPLICATION PROCESS. Each medical school establishes annual deadlines for receipt of both initial and complete application materials, including supplemental application materials, at the school. These dates are published in medical school bulletins and application materials, on school Web sites, and in Chapter 11. (They range from mid-October to mid-December for receipt of initial application materials at AMCAS-participating schools and November 1 for TMDSAS-participating schools, with varying dates for school-specific applications.) Deadlines for receipt of completed applications at medical schools also vary. Applicants should be aware of all deadline dates for schools to which they are applying.

The deadline for receipt by AMCAS of the application, fee, and official transcripts for EDP applicants is August 1. (Contact the admissions office or see Chapter 11 for early decision application deadlines at schools that do not participate in AMCAS.) All supplemental application materials must be received at the EDP school by the school's deadline date. EDP candidates may be interviewed by admission committees in late August or September so that final decisions can be made and communicated to EDP candidates by October 1.

Admission committees generally interview candidates for regular admission during the fall, winter, and spring months. Most regular admission offers are made during the winter months. Medical schools collectively agree to issue, by March 30 of the matriculation year, a number of acceptances at least equal to the size of the first-year entering class. Applicants are therefore encouraged to submit their applications as early in the application process as possible. They are also responsible for ensuring that all required materials are received by the relevant application service and individual medical school in a timely fashion. Medical schools are not responsible for notifying applicants if parts of their application file are missing.

NOTIFICATION OF ACCEPTANCE. For the past four decades, AAMC-member medical schools, regardless of the type of application system used, have agreed to observe a set of acceptance procedures for first-year entering students, commonly referred to as the "traffic rules." Observing these recommendations (see Page 48 or ✎ www.aamc.org/students/applying/policies) ensures that applicants and schools know, usually by June, who will be matriculating at each school in the fall. The deadline for notification of EDP admission decisions is October 1. The earliest and latest dates for notification of regular applicants' acceptance, and the time allowed for applicants to respond to acceptance offers, are indicated in each school's entry in Chapter 11. The "traffic rules" also recommend that school deposits required of accepted applicants not exceed $100, and be refundable until May 15. The deposit amount and refund policy for each school are also indicated in Chapter 11.

APPLICANT RESPONSIBILITIES. Just as medical schools agree to a set of "traffic rules" in the application and admission process, applicants are also expected to observe a set of procedures (see Page 50 or ✎ www.aamc.org/students/applying/policies), thus ensuring an orderly and timely selection process for other applicants and for schools.

Schools' and applicants' observance of these procedures helps to ensure that applicants are afforded timely notification of the outcome of their medical school applications and timely access to available first-year positions and that schools are protected from having unfilled positions in their entering classes.

Falsifications, omissions, or discrepancies in application materials or irregular behavior during administration of the MCAT will be investigated in accordance with AAMC investigation policies.

The Medical College Admission Test

The Medical College Admission Test (MCAT) is a standardized examination designed to assist medical school admission committees in assessing applicants' academic preparation, achievement in science, and written communication skills, and in predicting which applicants will perform adequately in the rigorous medical school curriculum. The MCAT consists of multiple-choice questions and a writing assessment.

The MCAT provides admission committees with standardized measures of performance for all examinees. The test battery was developed with input from medical school admissions officers, premedical faculty members, medical educators, practicing physicians, AAMC staff, and a group of testing experts under contract to the AAMC.

The MCAT is also designed to encourage those interested in medicine to pursue broad undergraduate study in the natural and social sciences and in the humanities. The MCAT assesses facility with scientific problem-solving, critical thinking skills, and writing ability, as well as the understanding of scientific concepts and principles identified as required for the study of medicine.

The four sections of the MCAT are Physical Sciences, Verbal Reasoning, Biological Sciences, and Writing Sample:

- *Physical Sciences and Biological Sciences.* These sections are constructed to assess material covered in introductory undergraduate courses in biology; chemistry, including inorganic chemistry and organic chemistry; and general, non-calculus physics. Both sections consist entirely of science problems and may include data presented in graphs, tables, and charts. Both sections are designed to evaluate knowledge of basic concepts, facility with scientific problem-solving, and the ability to interpret data presented in a tabular or graphic format.

- *Verbal Reasoning.* This section is designed to assess applicants' abilities to comprehend, reason, and think critically. It draws upon material from the humanities, social sciences, and natural sciences. Subject-matter knowledge is not evaluated; content information necessary to answer test questions is presented in each passage. In preparation for this section, examinees are encouraged to familiarize themselves with the practice of critical thinking and the use of reasoning skills in these disciplines.

- *Writing Sample.* The essay topics that constitute this section are designed to provide examinees with an opportunity to demonstrate writing and analytical skills. Examinees are allotted 30 minutes to write an essay on a first assigned topic, then another 30 minutes to write an essay on a second assigned topic; each requires an expository response. Essay topics do not pertain to the technical content of biology, chemistry, physics, or mathematics; the medical school application process; reasons for desiring a career in medicine; social or cultural issues not part of the general experience of MCAT examinees; religious issues; or emotionally charged subjects.

MCAT SCORING. Four scores are reported, one for each MCAT section. Scores for the Verbal Reasoning, Physical Sciences, and Biological Sciences sections are presented on a numerical scale, ranging from a low of 1 to a high of 15. Scores for the Writing Sample section are presented on an alphabetical scale, ranging from a low of J to a high of T. A total score is also reported, which is the sum of the Verbal Reasoning, Biological Sciences, and Physical Sciences sections, along with the Writing Sample score: for example, 31S.

The MCAT is administered and scored by the MCAT Program Office at the direction of the AAMC. Information about the specific content of the examination, its organization, and the scoring system appears on the MCAT Web site at ☞ www.aamc.org/mcat.

SCORE REPORTING. Payment of the MCAT examination fee includes the reporting of test scores to AMCAS, other application services, and individual medical schools. Once MCAT scores are available (approximately 60 days after the examination date), they can be sent to institutions using the online system at ☞ www.aamc.org/mcat. In 2003, the concept of a "score report" was replaced with an online "MCAT Testing History (THx) System," where all of an examinee's testing history is reported to institutions rather than specific sets of scores. All 2003 and later MCAT scores will automatically be released to AMCAS and included in the MCAT THx System (formerly known as Additional Score Reports or ASR).

No longer do applicants need to specify on test day the non-AMCAS schools to which their MCAT scores should be sent. Instead, applicants may use the online MCAT THx System to specify the non-AMCAS schools and application services to which their MCAT testing history should be sent. This service is free for scores after 1990 that have been electronically requested via the MCAT THx System. Since all THx reports are paperless, they will be sent to recipients electronically. To request MCAT scores prior to 1991, complete the request form available at ☞ www.aamc.org/mcat.

Examinees will be able to view their most recent MCAT scores, as soon as they are available to the AAMC, online at ☞ www.aamc.org/mcat.

MCAT examinees are encouraged to request, at the time of registration, that their scores be sent directly to their premedical advisors, which is also a free service.

TEST DATES. The MCAT is administered twice a year, on a Saturday in April and a Saturday in August; 2004 testing dates are April 17 and August 14. Potential applicants are advised to take the MCAT about 18 months prior to their expected entry into medical school. There is no provision for make-up examinations, but, where possible, special Sunday test centers can be arranged for examinees who present, in advance, evidence of unavoidable conflicts that prevent them from taking the examination on a regularly scheduled date. Examinees pay an additional fee for these special arrangements. Only those persons who intend to apply to a school of allopathic, osteopathic, podiatric, or veterinary medicine are permitted to take the MCAT; any other potential examinees must receive special permission prior to taking the examination.

Many medical schools prefer that applicants take the MCAT in April because of the short time between the availability of the August scores and school application deadlines. Taking the MCAT in April also ensures the timely completion and review of an applicant's file by medical school admission committees. Furthermore, in most cases, very little course content that would be helpful to a student on the MCAT would be covered at a college or university between the April and August MCAT administrations, except for those instances when introductory science courses are taught during the intervening summer months. For students enrolled in such summer courses, an August MCAT administration may be preferable.

FEES AND REGISTRATION. The examination fee is $190 for each of the 2004 MCAT administrations. Registration for the 2004 MCAT is available only online at ☞ www.aamc.org/mcat and begins in early January. Prior to registering for the MCAT, students must familiarize themselves with the information in the publication *2004 MCAT Essentials*, available on the MCAT Web site.

PREPARATION FOR THE MCAT. The MCAT is a "high stakes" examination; scores are carefully evaluated by medical school admission committees. The MCAT is also a test of achievement, not aptitude; the MCAT measures mastery of what one has learned rather than one's potential for learning. For these reasons, examinees should prepare for the MCAT by completing the usual premedical biology, general and organic chemistry, and physics coursework (see Chapter 3) prior to taking the MCAT for the first time. The MCAT should not be taken "blind" or for "diagnostic" reasons; the MCAT Practice Tests can be used for preparation. If some time has elapsed since the completion of premedical courses, review of course material prior to taking the MCAT is highly recommended. Potential examinees with ongoing challenges in reading speed or comprehension are advised to address and resolve those issues prior to taking the examination. Campus academic advising or academic skills staff are often well informed about these and related issues.

MCAT PUBLICATIONS. The AAMC publishes a variety of materials, including a series of official MCAT Practice Tests. These tests are composed of previously administered MCAT items and provide prospective examinees with an accurate estimate of their likely MCAT scores, given their level of preparation at the time they take the practice test. The MCAT Practice Tests are updated periodically to reflect the most current content, format, and scoring of the MCAT and are available in both Web and paper formats. Solutions to the items are provided, as well as examples of scored Writing Sample (WS) essays.

MCAT Practice Online provides hundreds of MCAT items, including several full-length practice tests. Features include automated scoring, integrated solutions, diagnostic reports, customized item selection, daily test-taking tips, discussion boards, paper test scoring, and enhanced printing options. Free access to a single full-length MCAT with all the features of MCAT Practice Online is available at ✐ www.e-mcat.com. MCAT publications are available for purchase online through the MCAT Web site (✐ www.aamc.org/mcat).

The MCAT Web site also contains free publications with detailed information about the format and content of the examination and outlines the problem-solving, critical thinking, and communication skills tested by the MCAT.

RETAKING THE MCAT. Applicants who are not satisfied with their MCAT scores should confer with their premedical advisor about whether retaking the test is advised. Legitimate reasons for retaking the MCAT include:

- a significant discrepancy between college grades and MCAT scores

- having taken the examination prematurely (i.e., without adequate preparation or prior to completion of all relevant premedical coursework)

- serious illness at the time of the examination

- a recommendation from a medical school admissions officer or admission committee member that the MCAT be retaken

Application procedures for retaking the examination are identical to those for initial testing. The MCAT may be taken three times before additional documentation from the examinee is required.

TESTING UNDER SPECIAL CONDITIONS. Potential examinees with a disability of sufficient severity to meet the definition of the Americans with Disabilities Act (ADA) may request an appropriate accommodation. Examples of accommodations include a reader, a person to record answers, a separate testing room, extra testing time, or large-print examination test books and answer documents. Information about the documentation that must accompany applications for test accommodations and application deadline dates is available at ✐ www.aamc.org/mcat.

American Medical College Application Service (AMCAS)

The American Medical College Application Service (AMCAS) is a non-profit, centralized application processing service for applicants to the first-year entering classes at participating U.S. medical schools. AMCAS policies and procedures are developed in consultation with representatives of participating medical schools. AMCAS benefits both schools and applicants by collecting, verifying, and processing application data and MCAT scores on behalf of participating medical schools and transmitting those data to them.

AMCAS also assists admission committees by providing rosters and statistical reports regarding the national and individual medical school applicant pools, as well as aggregate data about accepted applicants at medical schools across the nation. AMCAS data are used by the AAMC in various research efforts regarding the medical school applicant and matriculant pools.

AMCAS does not render admission decisions or advise applicants as to the medical schools to which they should apply. Each medical school, through its admission committee and its admissions officer, is completely autonomous in its admission decisions.

For the 2005 entering class, 120 U.S. medical schools and programs will participate in AMCAS. The eight U.S. medical schools that will not participate in AMCAS for the 2005 entering class include:

- University of Missouri-Kansas City School of Medicine

- University of North Dakota School of Medicine and Health Sciences

- Texas A&M University System Health Science Center College of Medicine

- Texas Tech University Health Sciences Center School of Medicine

- University of Texas Southwestern Medical Center in Dallas Southwestern Medical School*

- University of Texas Medical School at Galveston

- University of Texas Medical School at Houston

- University of Texas Medical School at San Antonio

The most current listing of participating schools and programs is available at ✍ www.aamc.org/students/amcas/participatingschools.htm.

THE AMCAS APPLICATION. The AMCAS application is available via the AMCAS Web site (✍ www.aamc.org/amcas). On the AMCAS Web site, applicants will find links to key steps in starting an application, an application worksheet that previews the application content, an application timeline, important FAQs, and other resources to assist them with the application, such as an instruction booklet in PDF.

The AMCAS application permits applicants to complete, certify, and submit their AMCAS application via the AMCAS Web site. The AMCAS application is accessible 24 hours a day, beginning on or about May 1, 2004, for the 2005 entering class.

AAMC REGISTRATION. The AAMC has a global registration system. Applicants who have previously registered for the MCAT THx System, Fee Assistance Program, AMCAS, or other AAMC services, have already selected an AAMC username and password and been assigned an AAMC ID; they should use the same access information to enter the AMCAS application. Those who have not recently registered for AAMC services must complete the AMCAS registration form, select a username and password, and be assigned an AAMC ID. The AAMC secure username, login, and password sequence ensures the confidentiality of their application information.

TRANSCRIPT REQUIREMENTS AND DEADLINES. Applicants must request that an official transcript be forwarded to AMCAS by the registrar of every postsecondary school at which they have ever been registered.

AMCAS provides a "transcript request form" that expedites the cataloguing and processing of transcripts. To generate a transcript request form, the applicant must complete the Identifying Information and Schools Attended sections of the AMCAS application and follow the directions for printing the transcript request form. Prior to submitting this form to the registrar's office, the form should be carefully reviewed to ensure that the information is accurate and the registrar's address is current. Simultaneously, applicants are encouraged to request personal copies of each transcript for completing the Academic Record section of their AMCAS applications.

Transcripts are required from every junior college, community college, trade school, or professional school within the United States, Canada, or U.S. territories, regardless of whether or not credit was earned. This requirement applies also to college courses taken while in high school. Transcripts submitted to AMCAS for prior years' applications cannot be used to verify coursework and grades for an application to the 2005 entering class.

Application materials and official transcripts for the Early Decision Program (EDP) must be received by AMCAS by August 2, 2004. For regular applicants, all official transcripts must be received no later than two weeks following the deadline date for application materials. Refer to the AMCAS online instruction booklet or help text for detailed information about official transcript requirements and deadlines at ✍ www.aamc.org/amcas. AMCAS begins accepting official transcripts on or about May 1, 2004.

COMPLETING THE AMCAS APPLICATION. The application is divided into different sections, which may be completed during multiple sittings. Extensive on-screen instructions and help text are provided. Payment is also received online. Applicants are encouraged to print their application after submitting it to AMCAS. To ensure that the submission process was completed, applicants should check the Date Submitted field in the upper left-hand corner of the first page of the application. The date submitted field should have been modified from "N/A" to the current date.

APPLICANT MONITORING RESPONSIBILITIES. AMCAS provides an "audit page" (dynamic welcome page) detailing the status of each application. Applicants are responsible for checking this page and addressing identified errors and omissions. Applicants are also expected to thoroughly review changes made by AMCAS during the verification correction process and alert AMCAS to any issues regarding these changes.

The M.D./Ph.D. program associated with the University of Texas Southwestern Medical Center in Dallas will participate in AMCAS for the 2004 entering class. Please refer to Chapter 11 for more information.

Applicants may change certain information on their application and apply to additional medical schools, using their username, login, and password sequence, after their initial application has been submitted; each add/change requires the applicant to recertify and resubmit the application.

PROCESSING OF APPLICATIONS. Regardless of the number of AMCAS schools to which an individual applies, only one application should be submitted to AMCAS. After receipt of the service fee and an official transcript from each postsecondary school where the applicant has been registered, AMCAS staff members then assemble the application file, verify the Academic Record portion of the application, and forward the application to all designated medical schools. AMCAS also distributes MCAT scores, provided that the applicant has released those scores to AMCAS. All 2003 and later MCAT scores are automatically included in an applicant's AMCAS application. Scores from MCAT administrations in years prior to 2003 are provided to AMCAS only if the applicant has released those scores to AMCAS.

AAMC Fee Assistance Program (FAP)

The AAMC Fee Assistance Program (FAP) provides applicants a one-time fee assistance application for both MCAT registration and the AMCAS application.

The FAP is provided to assist individuals with **extreme** financial limitations whose inability to afford the full MCAT registration fee or the AMCAS application fee would prevent them from taking the MCAT or applying to medical school. Eligibility policies and operating procedures for the FAP are established annually by the AAMC. The FAP is not related to any governmental or financial aid program. Because the FAP does not distinguish between dependent and independent student status, all FAP applicants must provide parental financial data. Once provisional approval has been granted online, qualified applicants must submit documentation for themselves and their parents, in the form of W-2 forms, tax return forms, financial aid award letters, and documentation of non-taxable income for the prior year's income. If an applicant's FAP application is not approved, then no documentation is necessary.

Once an FAP application has been fully approved, the fee assistance may be applied to any subsequently submitted MCAT registration or AMCAS application during that calendar year. The FAP approval is not retroactive. FAP benefits include:

- reduction of the MCAT registration fee from $190 to $85 for test administrations in 2004

- waiver of the application fee for submitting the completed AMCAS application to up to 10 medical schools; beyond the 10 free applications, applicants pay $30 for each additional school

The FAP application becomes available in January. However, persons planning to apply should note that FAP documentation should be received by the AAMC by the following dates:

- February 20, 2004 for the April 17, 2004 MCAT administration

- June 18, 2004 for the August 14, 2004 MCAT administration

- three weeks prior to the first medical school application deadline (of all schools applied to) for AMCAS 2005

Any individual who has submitted an FAP application must wait to be informed about the FAP decision before submitting an MCAT registration or AMCAS application.

Eligibility for the FAP is limited to five funded years.

Additional information about the FAP, including instructions, the application, and information about relevant deadline dates, is available at ☞ www.aamc.org/fap.

CHAPTER

5

Applicant and Accepted Applicant Data

In 2002-2003, 34,786 persons applied to the 126 U.S. medical schools. By the fall of 2003, 17,539 applicants had been offered an acceptance to at least one medical school, and 16,538 accepted applicants matriculated. These accepted applicants possessed a wide range of MCAT scores and undergraduate grade point averages, and a wide variety of personal characteristics and life experiences. Both male and female applicants were distributed across numerous racial and ethnic groups. A small number applied through the Early Decision Program, but the majority used regular application processes.

This chapter contains graphic representations of relevant data for the entire applicant pool, as well as for accepted and non-accepted applicants, for the 2003 entering class. All data presented in this chapter are accurate as of November 6, 2003 [Source: AAMC Data Warehouse; Applicant Matriculant File]. In the following charts:

- "All Applicants" means all applicants to the 2003 entering class

- "Accepted Applicants" means those applicants accepted to at least one medical school

- "Not Accepted" applicants means those applicants not accepted to any medical school

A small number of accepted applicants chose not to matriculate in 2003.

By familiarizing themselves with this information and comparing themselves with applicants for the 2003 entering class, potential applicants can determine their relative standing on a variety of admission-related factors and can, with their advisors' help, make decisions that are right for them. Extensive information about medical school applicants and matriculants can also be found online at ➱ www.aamc.org/data/facts.

Performance on the MCAT

Charts 5-A – 5-E present information about the performance of applicants on the MCAT:

- Chart 5-A shows that applicants achieved Verbal Reasoning (VR) scores at each score from 1 to 14; the largest number achieved a VR score of 9. Accepted applicants' scores ranged from 1 to 14, although very few had VR scores below 5 (just under 75). The VR score at which the number of accepted applicants exceeded the number not accepted was 9.

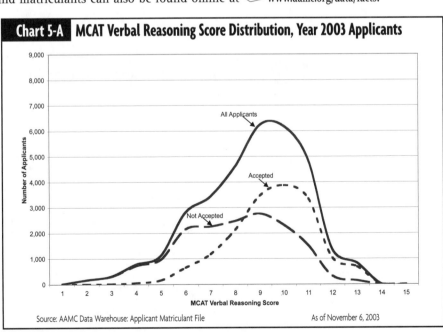

Chart 5-A MCAT Verbal Reasoning Score Distribution, Year 2003 Applicants

Source: AAMC Data Warehouse: Applicant Matriculant File   As of November 6, 2003

*All URLs mentioned in this chapter can be found at ➱ www.aamc.org/msar

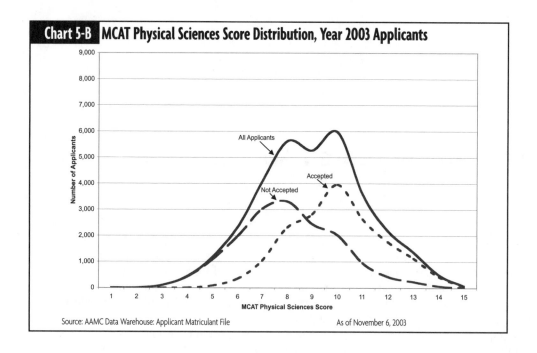

Chart 5-B | MCAT Physical Sciences Score Distribution, Year 2003 Applicants

Source: AAMC Data Warehouse: Applicant Matriculant File
As of November 6, 2003

- Chart 5-B shows that applicants achieved Physical Sciences (PS) scores at each score from 1 to 15; the largest number achieved a PS score of 10, with slightly fewer applicants scoring an 8. Accepted applicants' scores ranged from 3 to 15; fewer than 90 accepted applicants achieved a score of 5 or below. Accepted applicants exceeded not accepted applicants at a PS score of 9.

- Chart 5-C shows that applicants achieved Writing Sample (WS) scores at each score from J to T; the largest number achieved a WS score of Q. Accepted applicants' scores ranged from J to T; the number with scores of K and below was about 200. At a score of O, the number of applicants accepted and not accepted is approximately equal.

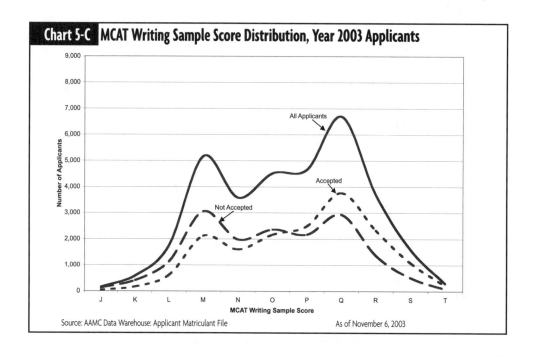

Chart 5-C | MCAT Writing Sample Score Distribution, Year 2003 Applicants

Source: AAMC Data Warehouse: Applicant Matriculant File
As of November 6, 2003

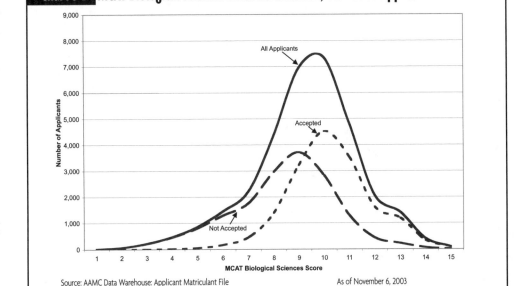

Chart 5-D | MCAT Biological Sciences Score Distribution, Year 2003 Applicants

All Applicants

Accepted

Not Accepted

Number of Applicants

MCAT Biological Sciences Score

Source: AAMC Data Warehouse: Applicant Matriculant File   As of November 6, 2003

- Chart 5-D shows that applicants achieved Biological Sciences (BS) scores at each score from 1 to 15; the largest number achieved a BS score of 10. Accepted applicants' scores ranged from 3 to 15; about 60 scored 5 or below. Accepted applicants exceeded not accepted applicants at a score of 10.

- Chart 5-E – which shows total scores on the numerically scored sections of Verbal Reasoning, Physical Sciences, and Biological Sciences – reveals that applicants achieved total scores from 5 to 43; the largest number achieved a total score of 28. Accepted applicants achieved total scores from 11 to 43; the number of accepted applicants with total scores of 17 and below (an average of almost 6 on each section) was 60. Accepted applicants exceeded not accepted applicants at a total score of 27.

No score on a single MCAT section and no total MCAT score "guarantees" admission to medical school. Charts 5-A, 5-B, and 5-D reveal that, while applicants with VR, PS, and BS scores of 10 and above are more likely to be accepted, a significant number of applicants with such scores were not accepted. The same holds true for the Writing Sample section; a score of P and above is a likely, though not definite, barometer for acceptance. Finally, Chart 5-E shows that a substantial number of applicants with total MCAT scores of 27 and above were not accepted. These findings reveal the importance of factors other than MCAT performance – including undergraduate academic performance and a variety of personal characteristics and experiences – in the medical student selection process.

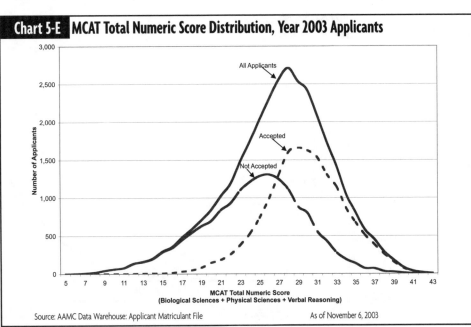

Chart 5-E | MCAT Total Numeric Score Distribution, Year 2003 Applicants

All Applicants

Accepted

Not Accepted

Number of Applicants

MCAT Total Numeric Score
(Biological Sciences + Physical Sciences + Verbal Reasoning)

Source: AAMC Data Warehouse: Applicant Matriculant File   As of November 6, 2003

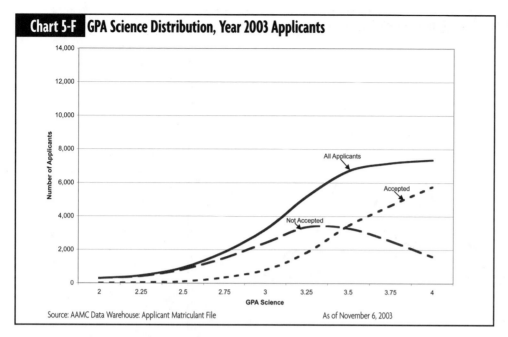

Chart 5-F | GPA Science Distribution, Year 2003 Applicants

Source: AAMC Data Warehouse: Applicant Matriculant File   As of November 6, 2003

Undergraduate Grade Point Average

Charts 5-F — 5-H present information about the undergraduate academic performance of applicants:

- Chart 5-F: undergraduate science GPA (Biology, Chemistry, Physics, and Mathematics)
- Chart 5-G: undergraduate non-science GPA
- Chart 5-H: undergraduate total GPA

Chart 5-F shows that the undergraduate science GPAs of all applicants were on a continuum from 2.0 to 4.0, on a 4.0 scale; most were between 3.75 and 4.0. Accepted applicants also had undergraduate science GPAs across the entire range, but few had GPAs of 2.50 or below (just over 150). The undergraduate science GPA at which accepted applicants exceeded those not accepted was between 3.25 and 3.50.

Chart 5-G shows applicants' undergraduate non-science GPAs along the continuum from 2.0 to 4.0, with most between 3.75 and 4.0. Accepted applicants' undergraduate non-science GPAs crossed the entire GPA range, but only about 125 had a GPA of 2.75 or below. At 3.50-3.75, accepted applicants exceeded not accepted applicants.

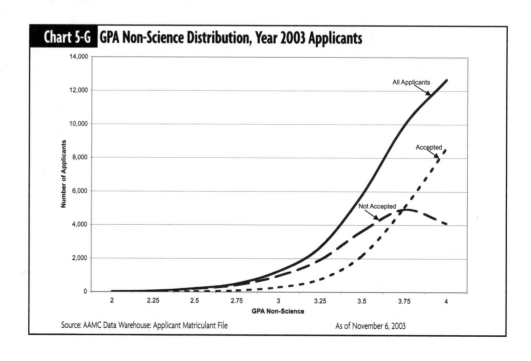

Chart 5-G | GPA Non-Science Distribution, Year 2003 Applicants

Source: AAMC Data Warehouse: Applicant Matriculant File   As of November 6, 2003

Chart 5-H **GPA Total Distribution, Year 2003 Applicants**

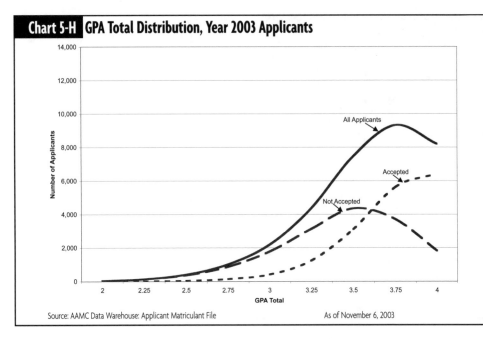

Source: AAMC Data Warehouse: Applicant Matriculant File   As of November 6, 2003

As shown in Chart 5-H, all applicants had total undergraduate GPAs from 2.0 to 4.0, and most were in the range of 3.50-3.75. Accepted applicants could be found across the entire GPA range, but only about 185 possessed undergraduate total GPAs of 2.75 or below. Accepted applicants exceeded not accepted applicants at an undergraduate total GPA of between 3.50 and 3.75.

As is the case with MCAT data, GPA data in Charts 5-F – 5-H show

that no undergraduate GPA assures admission to medical school. While applicants with undergraduate science, non-science, and overall GPAs in the range of 3.25-3.50, 3.50-3.75, and 3.50-3.75, respectively, were more likely to be accepted to medical school, a significant number of such applicants were not accepted. Again, these findings underscore the importance of a wide variety of personal characteristics and experiential variables in the medical student selection process.

Undergraduate Major

Chart 5-I presents information about the undergraduate majors of all medical school applicants from the 1992-2003 entering classes. Over the past decade, approximately three-fifths of applicants reported undergraduate biological science majors, while the remainder reported a variety of majors, including the humanities, mathematics, physical sciences, social sciences, other health sciences, and a broad "other" category. The proportion of these majors has remained relatively constant over time, despite annual fluctuations in the applicant pool.

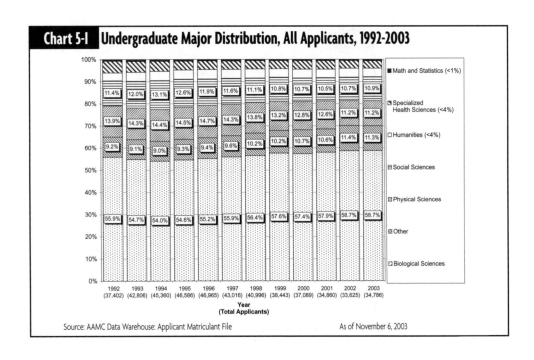

Chart 5-I **Undergraduate Major Distribution, All Applicants, 1992-2003**

Source: AAMC Data Warehouse: Applicant Matriculant File   As of November 6, 2003

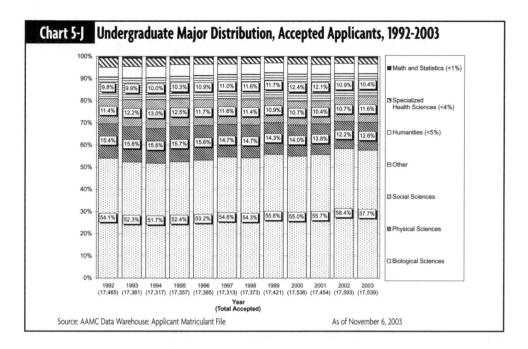

Chart 5-J | **Undergraduate Major Distribution, Accepted Applicants, 1992-2003**

Source: AAMC Data Warehouse: Applicant Matriculant File   As of November 6, 2003

Chart 5-J presents similar information about the undergraduate majors of applicants accepted to the 1992-2003 entering classes. Comparisons of the majors of the total applicant pool with those of accepted applicants reveal acceptance rates, for various science-related majors, ranging from 40.0 percent for applicants with specialized health science majors, to 49.5 percent for biological science majors, to 56.7 percent for physical science majors. Among all undergraduate majors, the rate of acceptance was highest for math and statistics majors at 57.7 percent, but interpretation of this finding is limited by the fact that math and statistics majors made up less than one percent of all applicants to the 2003 entering class.

Gender

Chart 5-K presents information about the number and gender of the entire applicant pool and accepted applicants for the 1992-2003 entering classes. The largest annual applicant pool during the past decade was for the 1996 entering class; since that year, it gradually declined until 2003, when there was a slight increase (3.5 percent) in applicants. The number of male applicants to the 2003 entering class increased slightly from the number of male applicants to the previous year's entering class, but was still smaller than it had been for any other entering class since 1992. The number of female applicants for the 2003 class repre-

sented a significant increase over the number of female applicants to the previous year's entering class, but was still smaller than it had been for any of the entering classes from 1993 through 1998. However, the number of accepted applicants has remained fairly constant for 10 years, from a low of 17,313 in 1997 to a high of 17,593 in 2002. The number of accepted men

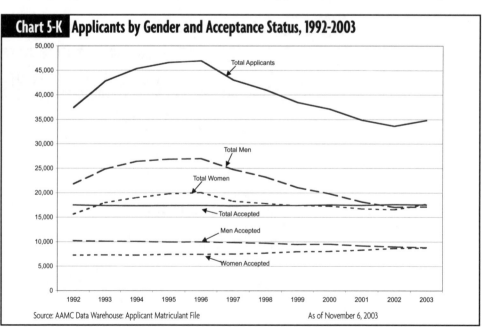

Chart 5-K | **Applicants by Gender and Acceptance Status, 1992-2003**

Source: AAMC Data Warehouse: Applicant Matriculant File   As of November 6, 2003

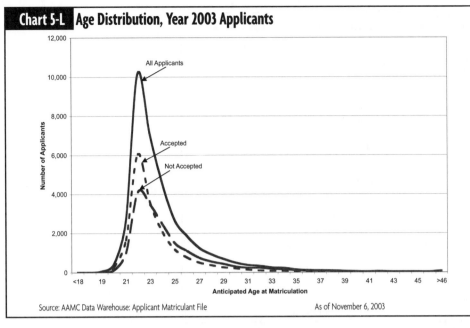

Chart 5-L Age Distribution, Year 2003 Applicants

All Applicants

Accepted

Not Accepted

Number of Applicants

Anticipated Age at Matriculation

Source: AAMC Data Warehouse: Applicant Matriculant File

As of November 6, 2003

has fluctuated from a high of 10,208 in 1992 to a low of 8,807 in 2003. The number of accepted women has increased, with small fluctuations, from a low of 7,255 in the 1994 entering class to a high of 8,732 in 2002.

The significant gaps between male and female applicants for the 1992 entering class (6,166) and the 1993 entering class (6,892) have disappeared; in fact, 558 more women than men applied to the 2003 entering class. During the same time span, the gaps between accepted male and female applicants also dropped. Accepted male applicants outnumbered accepted female applicants by 2,951 for the 1992 entering class, but only by 75 for the 2003 entering class. The national ratio of male to female applicants was 49.2 : 50.8 percent for the 2003 entering class, the first time that the number of female applicants was greater than the number of male applicants to medical school.

Age

Chart 5-L shows that the age distribution for all applicants to the 2003 entering class was broad, with six applicants under 18 at the time of anticipated matriculation, and six applicants aged 55 and over. The largest contingent of applicants, 31,073, was between 21 and 28 at the time of anticipated matriculation; the rest of the applicant pool were either under 21 (504) or over 28 (3,209) when they applied. Chart 5-L illustrates a similar finding for accepted applicants. Accepted applicants for the 2003 entering class were between 17 and 53 years of age at the time of expected matriculation.

Type of Application

Chart 5-M presents information about application outcomes for Early Decision Program (EDP) and regular applicants to the 2003 entering class: 97.1 percent were regular applicants and 2.9 percent EDP applicants. Of all applicants, 48.6 percent were accepted to at least one medical school through the regular application process; 1.6 percent were accepted to one medical school through EDP prior to October 1; and 0.2 percent were accepted to at least one medical school after not being accepted before October 1 through EDP. Conversely, 48.5 percent of regular applicants and 1.1 percent of EDP applicants were not accepted to any medical school for 2003.

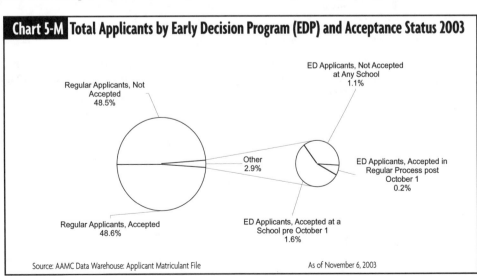

Chart 5-M Total Applicants by Early Decision Program (EDP) and Acceptance Status 2003

ED Applicants, Not Accepted at Any School
1.1%

Regular Applicants, Not Accepted
48.5%

Other
2.9%

ED Applicants, Accepted in Regular Process post October 1
0.2%

Regular Applicants, Accepted
48.6%

ED Applicants, Accepted at a School pre October 1
1.6%

Source: AAMC Data Warehouse: Applicant Matriculant File

As of November 6, 2003

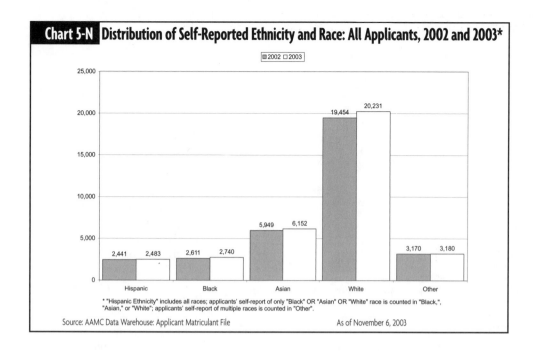

Chart 5-N Distribution of Self-Reported Ethnicity and Race: All Applicants, 2002 and 2003*

■2002 □2003

* "Hispanic Ethnicity" includes all races; applicants' self-report of only "Black" OR "Asian" OR "White" race is counted in "Black,", "Asian," or "White"; applicants' self-report of multiple races is counted in "Other".

Source: AAMC Data Warehouse: Applicant Matriculant File   As of November 6, 2003

Race and Ethnicity

In accordance with the requirements of the U.S. Office of Management and Budget Directive 15, data about race and ethnicity were collected differently by AMCAS for applicants to the 2002 and 2003 entering classes than they were for applicants to prior entering classes. For that reason, this section presents applicant data beginning with 2002 only. Additional applicant data regarding race and ethnicity for prior years are presented on the AAMC Web site at ⌐ www.aamc.org/data/facts.

Chart 5-N shows applicant self-reported race and ethnicity data for all applicants to the 2002 and 2003 entering classes. Chart 5-O shows applicant self-reported race and ethnicity data for all accepted applicants to the 2002 and 2003 entering classes.

The following changes occurred in the self-reported racial and ethnic make-up of the applicant pool from 2002 to 2003:

- The number of self-described white applicants in 2002 was 19,454; the number of white applicants in 2003 was 20,231, an increase of 4 percent.

- The number of self-described Asian applicants in 2002 was 5,949; the number of Asian applicants in 2003 was 6,152, an increase of 3.4 percent.

- The number of self-described black applicants in 2002 was 2,611; the number of black applicants in 2003 was 2,740, an increase of 4.9 percent.

- The number of self-described Hispanic applicants in 2002 was 2,441; the number of Hispanic applicants in 2003 was 2,483, an increase of 1.7 percent.

- The number of applicants in 2002 whose self-description of their race or ethnicity was in some other category was 3,170; the number of applicants in this cohort in 2003 was 3,180, an increase of less than 1 percent from 2002.

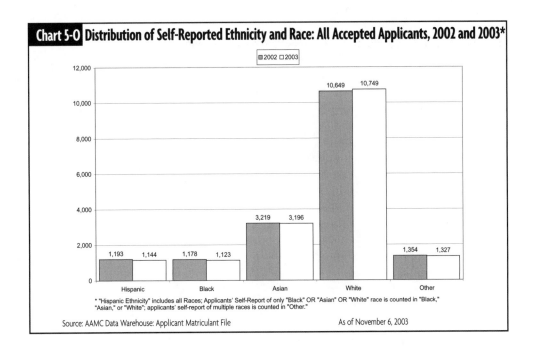

Chart 5-O Distribution of Self-Reported Ethnicity and Race: All Accepted Applicants, 2002 and 2003*

■ 2002 □ 2003

	Hispanic	Black	Asian	White	Other
2002	1,193	1,178	3,219	10,649	1,354
2003	1,144	1,123	3,196	10,749	1,327

* "Hispanic Ethnicity" includes all Races; Applicants' Self-Report of only "Black" OR "Asian" OR "White" race is counted in "Black," "Asian," or "White"; applicants' self-report of multiple races is counted in "Other."

Source: AAMC Data Warehouse: Applicant Matriculant File   As of November 6, 2003

Simultaneously, the following changes occurred among those applicants accepted to the 2002 and 2003 entering classes:

- The number of self-described white accepted applicants in 2002 was 10,649; the number of white accepted applicants in 2003 was 10,749, an increase of less than one percent.

- The number of self-described Asian accepted applicants in 2002 was 3,219; the number of accepted Asian applicants in 2003 was 3,196, a decrease of less than 1 percent.

- The number of self-described black accepted applicants in 2002 was 1,178; the number of accepted black applicants in 2003 was 1,123, a decrease of 4.7 percent.

- The number of self-described Hispanic accepted applicants in 2002 was 1,193; the number of Hispanic accepted applicants in 2003 was 1,144, a decrease of 4.1 percent.

- The number of accepted applicants in 2002 whose self-description of their race or ethnicity was in some other category was 1,354; the number of accepted applicants in this cohort in 2003 was 1,327, a decrease of two percent from 2002.

Additional information of interest to applicants from groups underrepresented in medicine is available in Chapter 6.

CHAPTER

Increasing Diversity in Medical School

The mission of the Association of American Medical Colleges (AAMC) is to improve the nation's health through the advancement of medical schools and teaching hospitals. This mission addresses three main areas: medical education, health care, and research. To help fulfill its mission, the AAMC views diversity as a key component because of the educational and health-care benefits that can come from having students, faculty, physicians, and researchers with different backgrounds, experiences, and views learning and working together. Diversity is a broad term that can encompass gender, place of birth or upbringing, life experiences, work experiences, point of view, areas of interest, and sexual orientation, as well as race and ethnicity. The AAMC supports diversity in its broadest sense and recognizes that it is up to individual medical schools to determine how to embrace diversity

Within this general context, the AAMC has worked consistently for more than 30 years on increasing the number of medical students who are from racial and ethnic populations that are underrepresented in the medical profession relative to their numbers in the general population. (For more information about the AAMC's definition about "underrepresented in medicine," see ✑ www.aamc.org/meded/urm.) In particular, the AAMC's Division of Community and Minority Programs (DCMP) promotes diversity and equity by coordinating medical education programs and services and working with constituent medical schools. The AAMC, medical schools, colleges and universities, and various foundations have initiated and supported a number of education-pipeline enrichment programs and resources for students who are interested in careers in medicine. The examples that are listed below, while open to all students, are sensitive to the challenges and needs of individuals from racial and ethnic groups that are underrepresented in medicine.

ENRICHMENT PROGRAMS. Medical schools nationally have programs and resources specifically designed to assist in preparing and recruiting students for medical education. Some of these programs are held during the school year, while others take place during the summer. Some are designed for high school students, others for college students, and still others for post-baccalaureate students. The AAMC is affiliated with two such opportunities:

- The *Annual Minority Workshop and Recruitment Fair* for high school and college students is held each fall during the AAMC's annual meeting. Representatives from all 125 U.S. medical schools are invited, and students have the opportunity to talk with them about medical school preparation, enrichment programs, admission policies and procedures, financial aid, and more. The dates and locations of upcoming AAMC annual meetings can be found at ✑ www.aamc.org/meetings/annual/start.htm.

- The *Summer Medical Education Program (SMEP)* is a free, six-week, residential summer program that provides college students (and some post-baccalaureate students) with intensive, personalized medical school preparation. SMEP is funded by The Robert Wood Johnson Foundation and is offered at 11 U.S. medical schools around the country. The AAMC's DCMP serves as the national program office. Additional information can be found at ✑ www.aamc.org/smep.

PRE-MEDICAL SCHOOL PROGRAMS AT UNDERGRADUATE COLLEGES. Prehealth advisors at undergraduate colleges can provide pertinent information on medical school admission or refer students to appropriate contacts. Premedical advisors also are knowledgeable about programs and resources that students from groups underrepresented in medicine are likely to find useful.

MINORITY STUDENT OPPORTUNITIES IN UNITED STATES MEDICAL SCHOOLS (MSOUSMS). DCMP produces a biennial publication (in even-numbered years) that provides information supplied by individual medical schools about student recruitment, admission, and other topics related to increasing student diversity.

Table 6-A Matriculants by Medical School and Race and Ethnicity 2003*

State	School Name	Mexican American	Cuban	Puerto Rican	Other Hispanic	Non-Hispanic	Chinese	Asian Indian	Pakistani	Filipino	Japanese	Korean	Vietnamese	Other Asian	Native American (incl. AK)	Black	Native Hawaiian/OPI	White	Other Race	Unduplicated Total
AL	Alabama	1	0	0	0	158	3	13	1	2	1	2	1	6	2	6	0	128	0	160
	South Alabama	0	0	1	1	63	0	0	1	1	0	2	0	0	0	6	0	57	0	64
AR	Arkansas	1	1	0	2	136	2	2	0	1	0	0	1	2	3	5	0	127	2	140
AZ	Arizona	5	0	1	3	102	3	4	1	0	2	0	0	3	2	3	0	94	10	110
CA	Drew/UCLA Joint Program	4	0	0	2	19	1	0	0	7	1	0	0	0	1	9	0	5	5	24
	Loma Linda	3	0	3	5	140	14	6	0	7	1	13	1	5	0	8	1	98	9	165
	Southern Cal-Keck	7	1	0	4	147	18	8	0	8	0	9	5	6	1	2	0	95	12	160
	Stanford	12	0	0	2	72	14	8	1	1	0	4	0	5	1	2	0	39	9	87
	UC Berkeley/SF Joint Prog	0	0	0	0	12	3	8	0	0	2	0	0	5	0	0	0	8	1	12
	UC Davis	5	1	0	4	84	16	4	0	3	5	3	4	7	0	2	0	47	13	93
	UC Irvine	6	0	0	4	82	11	8	0	0	5	0	0	8	0	2	0	59	7	92
	UC San Diego	5	1	0	6	111	21	13	0	0	5	6	8	5	0	2	3	59	7	121
	UC San Francisco	8	0	0	9	123	17	11	0	2	3	2	3	5	4	11	0	54	14	141
	UCLA-Geffen	11	0	0	11	121	22	11	1	3	2	9	1	8	1	10	1	80	25	144
CO	Colorado	5	0	0	7	118	6	1	0	1	0	1	1	3	0	7	0	108	5	130
CT	Connecticut	1	0	2	2	63	5	4	1	0	0	2	0	3	0	5	0	50	1	73
	Yale	2	2	1	7	82	7	13	2	0	2	2	0	2	0	5	0	60	7	99
DC	George Washington	4	1	1	3	155	3	19	4	1	2	7	0	3	2	12	0	111	12	165
	Georgetown	0	2	0	6	159	6	7	0	2	5	4	5	2	0	8	0	132	8	170
	Howard	0	0	0	1	98	1	2	1	2	0	0	0	0	0	90	0	5	1	110
FL	Florida	0	3	0	6	106	2	11	0	0	0	0	2	4	0	6	0	86	6	115
	Florida State	0	5	1	1	40	1	6	0	2	0	3	0	1	0	4	1	32	1	46
	Miami	0	18	1	12	111	5	19	1	2	0	3	0	1	0	4	0	97	10	141
	South Florida	0	3	3	7	103	2	10	3	0	0	2	3	2	5	9	0	82	8	115
GA	Emory	0	2	0	1	106	3	9	0	0	0	3	2	3	0	7	0	83	1	113
	Georgia	0	0	0	2	178	3	9	2	0	0	3	1	1	3	16	0	146	4	180
	Mercer	0	1	0	0	59	3	5	0	0	0	0	0	2	0	2	0	54	0	60
	Morehouse	0	0	1	0	51	3	5	0	0	0	0	0	2	0	32	0	13	1	52
HI	Hawaii-Burns	0	0	0	4	58	17	0	0	11	23	2	0	10	1	0	6	24	1	62
IA	Iowa-Carver	7	0	1	1	133	4	2	0	1	2	0	2	1	1	5	0	126	6	142
IL	Chicago Med-Finch	3	0	4	4	167	20	26	2	5	1	10	7	6	0	3	0	91	11	184
	Chicago-Pritzker	1	2	1	4	94	18	6	0	4	3	6	6	1	1	10	0	73	5	104
	Illinois	23	4	3	6	279	18	56	5	5	1	22	3	9	2	26	1	154	26	313
	Loyola-Stritch	2	0	0	0	138	6	5	1	4	2	3	0	3	2	3	2	121	3	140
	Northwestern-Feinberg	0	2	0	7	153	21	21	0	3	2	4	0	7	2	14	2	84	8	170
	Rush	3	0	0	7	116	7	21	4	2	0	4	2	7	0	5	0	70	8	120
	Southern Illinois	0	0	0	2	70	0	4	2	2	1	0	0	0	0	5	0	60	0	72
IN	Indiana	5	0	0	3	269	7	13	0	0	3	4	1	4	3	8	0	240	8	280
KS	Kansas	4	0	0	5	167	6	5	1	0	0	1	5	3	7	13	0	136	8	175
KY	Kentucky	0	0	0	1	92	1	5	0	3	0	0	0	2	0	6	0	75	1	95
	Louisville	0	0	0	0	149	1	6	0	9	0	1	1	2	0	14	0	122	2	149
LA	LSU New Orleans	1	1	0	0	165	2	6	2	0	0	2	4	0	0	18	0	132	8	167
	LSU Shreveport	1	0	0	0	98	3	1	0	4	0	2	3	0	0	2	1	91	5	101
	Tulane	2	2	0	8	134	3	13	0	2	0	0	0	2	3	8	0	115	5	153
MA	Boston	4	0	4	2	143	18	24	2	4	1	6	1	5	1	19	0	74	6	155
	Harvard	10	0	1	4	138	10	16	2	0	1	2	0	5	4	26	1	87	11	165
	Massachusetts	1	0	1	2	96	5	6	0	0	0	2	3	1	0	0	1	84	0	100
	Tufts	4	0	2	4	161	17	15	1	2	2	10	5	10	0	6	0	101	5	170
MD	Johns Hopkins	2	0	2	4	101	8	12	0	0	0	1	3	4	0	14	1	68	4	114
	Maryland	1	0	0	1	145	16	11	1	3	0	10	0	2	0	25	0	84	6	150
	Uniformed Services-Hebert	5	0	2	1	159	4	1	1	9	2	7	5	2	2	4	2	141	4	167
MI	Michigan	6	0	1	1	161	14	22	4	0	2	10	0	6	2	12	0	100	9	170
	Michigan State	6	0	0	5	95	7	6	0	4	0	2	0	0	0	7	0	74	9	106
	Wayne State	2	0	0	0	252	6	16	3	2	1	5	0	5	1	32	0	185	14	257
MN	Mayo	1	0	1	1	41	3	2	0	0	2	0	1	0	3	4	1	32	2	44
	Minnesota Duluth	2	0	0	0	50	0	0	1	1	1	1	0	0	2	0	0	49	0	53
	Minnesota Twin Cities	3	0	0	4	155	11	1	3	1	1	3	0	4	4	2	1	141	7	165
MO	Missouri Columbia	2	0	0	3	92	3	4	0	0	0	0	0	23	1	4	0	84	0	96
	Missouri Kansas City	2	0	0	0	85	0	3	2	3	0	0	4	5	1	5	1	44	0	85
	St Louis	2	0	1	2	152	11	22	2	2	4	1	0	2	1	5	0	105	5	158
	Washington U St Louis	2	0	1	3	114	13	15	1	0	0	0	0	0	0	7	0	76	8	122
MS	Mississippi	0	0	0	1	99	3	2	0	0	0	0	0	0	1	6	0	90	0	100
NC	Duke	2	0	0	0	89	7	10	0	0	0	3	1	1	4	13	0	58	1	100
	East Carolina-Brody	0	0	0	0	72	7	5	0	0	0	3	0	0	2	16	0	46	4	72
	North Carolina	0	0	2	1	159	3	11	1	0	1	2	4	2	1	21	0	121	4	160
	Wake Forest	1	0	0	1	101	7	4	1	0	2	2	4	0	0	9	0	76	3	108
ND	North Dakota	1	0	0	1	59	0	0	0	0	0	0	0	1	6	1	0	56	0	61

Table 6-A Matriculants by Medical School and Race and Ethnicity 2003* continued

State	School Name	Mexican American	Cuban	Puerto Rican	Other Hispanic	Non-Hispanic	Chinese	Asian Indian	Pakistani	Filipino	Japanese	Korean	Vietnamese	Other Asian	Native American (incl. AK)	Black	Native Hawaiian/OPI	White	Other Race	Unduplicated Total
NE	Creighton	2	0	0	3	114	1	7	0	2	1	0	5	2	2	3	0	93	5	120
	Nebraska	3	0	0	0	113	0	4	0	2	0	1	1	0	1	3	0	103	2	116
NH	Dartmouth	0	0	0	1	74	6	2	0	0	0	0	0	4	1	5	0	57	1	78
NJ	UMDNJ New Jersey	4	4	3	13	147	8	21	2	3	1	11	1	4	0	23	0	89	16	170
	UMDNJ-RW Johnson	1	1	3	3	149	10	31	2	5	1	4	1	7	0	19	0	70	8	156
NM	New Mexico	11	0	0	6	58	3	0	0	0	2	0	2	2	3	0	0	60	9	75
NV	Nevada	0	0	0	4	48	1	1	0	1	0	0	2	1	4	2	0	42	6	52
NY	Albany	2	0	1	4	122	4	21	2	1	1	3	1	3	0	3	0	83	6	133
	Buffalo	0	0	1	2	135	9	14	1	1	0	2	1	1	0	8	0	97	10	138
	Columbia	2	0	3	5	134	9	9	0	0	0	4	0	2	0	17	2	98	8	149
	Cornell-Weill	3	0	2	5	94	12	17	1	2	1	9	2	4	0	14	0	61	4	101
	Einstein	1	1	5	12	165	10	6	0	2	0	6	2	5	0	12	0	108	14	180
	Mount Sinai	5	1	1	1	91	10	6	2	6	2	10	2	8	0	7	0	69	15	117
	New York Medical	1	0	3	6	185	11	25	2	6	3	2	0	2	0	10	0	111	3	189
	New York University	2	2	3	6	146	11	13	1	0	2	9	0	2	0	10	1	105	10	160
	Rochester	0	0	0	6	99	13	13	1	0	2	2	0	6	2	20	0	66	5	100
	SUNY Downstate	2	1	1	10	167	19	19	3	4	1	8	2	6	2	20	1	101	11	180
	SUNY Upstate	0	1	2	2	144	4	18	0	1	1	0	0	6	2	4	0	109	4	149
	Stony Brook	0	1	2	7	93	7	14	0	1	0	6	0	6	0	9	0	53	9	102
OH	Case Western	1	0	1	0	143	8	11	0	3	1	5	2	4	0	25	0	90	3	146
	Cincinnati	3	0	0	3	156	3	15	2	4	1	2	1	1	1	10	0	125	5	161
	MC Ohio	0	0	0	3	149	7	16	5	0	0	2	1	3	1	1	0	120	3	156
	Northeastern Ohio	0	0	0	1	101	1	24	3	2	2	2	1	11	4	3	0	63	2	101
	Ohio State	5	0	3	3	198	13	17	3	2	0	0	0	2	0	14	0	144	6	211
	Wright State	2	0	0	3	86	8	8	0	1	0	1	0	5	0	10	0	69	1	91
OK	Oklahoma	3	0	1	2	137	4	7	4	2	2	0	4	0	10	2	0	113	5	142
OR	Oregon	0	0	0	5	104	5	2	0	0	1	1	3	2	3	4	0	91	2	107
PA	Drexel	2	1	0	5	242	20	42	8	5	2	5	7	10	1	5	2	147	15	250
	Jefferson	1	1	2	1	217	21	21	1	0	1	7	2	4	2	3	0	170	4	229
	Penn State	0	0	1	1	121	6	10	0	0	1	2	1	2	1	12	0	89	4	125
	Pennsylvania	4	0	1	5	134	13	20	0	2	2	3	2	2	0	15	0	103	4	147
	Pittsburgh	0	0	1	0	144	13	13	0	1	2	7	1	5	2	7	0	99	7	145
	Temple	3	0	3	2	171	19	20	0	1	0	4	1	5	0	15	1	116	26	177
PR	Caribe	0	4	50	9	4	0	0	0	0	0	0	0	0	0	5	0	36	19	62
	Ponce	0	6	46	10	7	0	0	1	1	0	0	0	0	0	5	0	48	30	66
	Puerto Rico	0	3	114	2	0	1	0	0	0	1	0	0	0	3	12	0	86	1	115
RI	Brown	0	0	0	1	60	2	5	1	0	1	1	1	3	1	1	0	12	1	65
SC	MU South Carolina	0	0	1	0	141	2	5	1	0	0	0	0	3	1	14	0	119	1	143
	South Carolina	0	0	1	1	79	0	4	1	2	0	1	0	1	1	5	0	68	0	80
SD	South Dakota	0	0	0	0	50	1	0	1	0	0	0	0	0	0	0	1	49	0	50
TN	East Tennessee-Quillen	0	0	0	0	60	0	2	0	0	0	1	0	2	1	5	0	51	3	60
	Meharry	0	0	2	4	72	0	3	1	1	0	0	0	1	1	62	1	6	3	80
	Tennessee	1	0	0	0	148	3	9	0	0	0	2	1	5	0	16	0	116	1	150
	Vanderbilt	0	0	0	0	98	9	4	0	1	0	3	4	4	2	9	0	67	7	104
TX	Baylor	8	0	0	3	157	20	26	2	1	0	3	4	9	0	14	0	96	4	168
	Texas A & M	4	0	0	2	63	2	4	2	0	0	2	7	9	0	3	0	36	5	70
	Texas Tech	8	0	0	5	114	8	7	3	5	0	2	10	3	2	2	1	84	16	127
	UT Galveston	19	1	2	8	168	2	16	0	3	0	0	6	3	2	18	1	125	15	203
	UT Houston	16	0	1	5	178	11	11	1	2	0	4	6	2	3	10	1	157	13	202
	UT San Antonio	25	1	0	6	175	11	19	0	2	1	6	7	5	0	14	0	139	14	205
	UT Southwestern	20	0	0	1	189	20	18	1	0	2	7	1	3	1	14	1	133	2	217
UT	Utah	1	1	1	1	97	2	0	0	0	6	0	0	1	1	3	0	91	2	102
VA	Eastern Virginia	0	1	0	2	107	2	10	0	5	0	1	1	4	0	8	0	79	3	110
	Virginia	0	0	0	3	136	10	9	0	3	2	4	4	3	0	8	0	106	2	140
	Virginia Commonwealth	0	0	0	1	183	5	30	3	3	0	5	4	0	1	14	1	115	6	184
VT	Vermont	0	0	1	0	99	5	6	0	1	1	3	5	3	1	1	1	74	5	100
WA	U Washington	2	0	0	0	175	5	3	0	6	3	4	4	6	3	4	2	156	8	178
WI	MC Wisconsin	4	1	0	2	195	6	17	1	3	2	4	1	3	2	7	0	159	7	205
	Wisconsin	5	0	0	0	143	5	9	0	0	0	3	1	1	0	7	0	120	7	150
WV	Marshall-Edwards	0	0	0	0	53	0	2	0	2	0	0	1	1	0	1	0	47	2	53
	West Virginia	0	0	1	1	108	5	5	3	5	0	0	0	1	0	0	0	99	2	109
Totals		366	85	306	392	15,240	848	1,301	126	203	149	387	237	394	168	1,203	42	11,285	800	16,538

Source: AAMC: Data Warehouse: Applicant Matriculant File as of 11/06/2003. Hispanic ethnicities are alone or in combination with some other Hispanic ethnicity and include any race. Ethnicity counts include U.S. Citizens and permanent residents only. Race counts include U.S. citizens and permanent residents only, are alone or in combination with some other race, and include both Hispanic and non-Hispanic ethnicity. The total represents an unduplicated count and also includes matriculants for whom we have no race data or who are foreign.

Information on enrichment programs offered by medical schools also is listed on a school-by-school basis. MSOUSMS is designed to be used in conjunction with *Medical School Admission Requirements*. Details about the content of MSOUSMS and ordering information can be found at ☞ www.aamc.org/students/minorities/resources/msousms.htm.

FEE ASSISTANCE PROGRAM (FAP). The AAMC's FAP helps students with extreme financial limitations whose inability to pay the full Medical College Admissions Test (MCAT) registration fee or the American Medical College Application Service (AMCAS) fee would prevent them taking the examination or applying to medical school. Details about the FAP can be found at ☞ www.aamc.org/fap.

MEDICAL MINORITY APPLICANT REGISTRY (MED-MAR). Students applying to medical school who are from groups that are underrepresented in medicine or who are economically disadvantaged are given the opportunity to register for Med-MAR at the time they take the Medical College Admission Test (MCAT). The Med-MAR program then circulates basic biographical information about the examinee and the examinee's MCAT scores to all U.S. medical schools. Confidential Med-MAR data files are circulated to schools twice a year, usually in July (following the April MCAT) and November (following the August MCAT). Details about the registry can be found at ☞ www.aamc.org/students/minorities/resources/medmar.htm.

FINANCIAL ASSISTANCE FOR MEDICAL SCHOOL. Any individual with an interest in a medical career should not rule out medical school solely because of financial status. Public and private medical schools work hard to offer a variety of financial aid plans to their accepted and enrolled students. Students applying to medical schools should discuss possibilities for financial assistance with the financial aid officers of the medical schools that interest them, as well as discuss how best to plan their educational financing. General information about financing a medical education also can be found in Chapter 9 of this publication and at ☞ www.aamc.org/students/minorities/scholarships.htm.

PROGRAMS AT MEDICAL SCHOOLS. Once students enroll in medical school, academic and personal support programs are available to them. These programs assist students from various backgrounds to successfully complete their medical studies, with the ultimate goal of increasing racial and ethnic diversity among physicians entering careers in patient care, teaching, and research, and eliminating racial and ethnic disparities in health care and health status. The staff members at each medical school who are primarily responsible for these programs are identified in the school-by-school entries in Chapter 11 of this publication.

DATA ABOUT RACE AND ETHNICITY IN MEDICINE. The AAMC has a great deal of information on medical education, including detailed data about medical students from an array of racial and ethnic groups:

- AAMC information about recent matriculant data for each medical school is contained in this publication in Table 6-A, *Matriculants by Medical School and Race and Ethnicity, 2003.*

- Chapter 5 includes a section on the self-reported racial and ethnic identification of medical school applicants and accepted applicants for the 2002 and 2003 entering classes.

- Additional data about medical school applicants, matriculants, and graduates are available on the AAMC Web site at ☞ www.aamc.org/data/facts/start.htm.

- Data on medical school faculty—including information on faculty by race and ethnicity—can be found at ☞ www.aamc.org/facultyroster/reports.htm.

- The publication *Facts & Figures* provides race and ethnicity data on medical school applicants, accepted applicants, matriculants, enrollment, graduates, and faculty, along with detailed tables; the full text of *Facts & Figures* can be accessed from ☞ www.aamc.org/students/minorities/start.htm.

Note: A wide variety of information and hyperlinks of interest to applicants and students from various racial and ethnic backgrounds is available in the "Minorities in Medicine" section of the AAMC Web site at ☞ www.aamc.org/students/minorities/start.htm.

CHAPTER

Selection

Decisions about the admission of applicants to medical school are based upon multiple criteria, developed by the faculty of each medical school, and are related to the school's specific mission and goals. In general, all schools admit applicants who, on the basis of materials presented during the application process, have documented that they possess the personal characteristics desired in future physicians, the ability to successfully complete the academically rigorous curriculum, and the potential to fulfill the institution's goals.

Personal Characteristics

Candidates' personal attributes and experiences are very important factors in selection decisions. All admission committees seek information about the following qualities in an applicant's personal statement, in evaluations and letters of recommendation from premedical advisors and others who know the applicant well, and in personal interviews:

- psychological maturity
- character and integrity
- self-discipline
- judgment
- compassion and empathy
- communication skills
- concern for helping others
- intellectual curiosity and enthusiasm
- motivation and persistence
- reliability and dependability
- resilience
- accountability
- leadership skills
- experience with, and knowledge of, medicine

Some medical schools supplement these with other characteristics, such as research experience and potential, commitment to caring for the underserved and disadvantaged, volunteer experiences, and knowledge about health care delivery systems. Applicants should address these areas in a focused manner in their personal statements, discussing their decision to pursue a medical career, relevant extracurricular and occupational accomplishments, altruistic efforts, and personal experiences. The quality, rather than quantity, of these experiences should be emphasized.

Letters of Evaluation and Recommendation

Medical schools usually ask applicants to indicate who will submit letters of evaluation and recommendation on their behalf. Schools typically require at least one letter from the premedical advisor or committee at the undergraduate school where the applicant completed required premedical coursework. Additional letters are usually sought from college faculty members and other advisors who have both personal knowledge of the applicant's accomplishments and an ability to objectively assess the applicant's abilities, interests, and plans. Admission committee members give less weight to subjective recommendations from friends, family, and political figures. If an applicant had significant employment or military experience during or after college, letters from employers, supervisors, and commanding officers are also appropriate.

An applicant's personal and professional conduct is a crucial factor in admission decisions. Therefore, applicants are expected to disclose any disciplinary action taken against them by an institution of higher learning for violation of institutional regulations or codes of conduct; such information is also often reported in the premedical advisor's or committee's letter. Applicants are also expected to report any legal action taken against them for violating the law and to submit a straightforward explanation of the circumstances and penalties. Applicants should also discuss, as appropriate, lessons learned and implications of the incident for their personal growth.

AMCAS requires an applicant to disclose any felony convictions on the AMCAS application. Failure to disclose or falsification of any official college or legal action is taken very seriously by both AMCAS and medical schools, and can prompt an official AMCAS investigation that may result in the withdrawal of an admission offer.

Academic Ability

Admission committees seek to enroll students who have acquired the academic skills and knowledge necessary to progress successfully through the medical curriculum and who can be active learners throughout their medical careers. Committee members rely on an applicant's academic record and MCAT scores in evaluating academic ability. The former measures an applicant's academic competitiveness over time; the latter provides objective information about the applicant's knowledge base compared with others in the national applicant pool.

ACADEMIC HISTORY. Given the challenges inherent in a medical education, an applicant's academic history allows admission committee members to determine whether the applicant's study skills, persistence, course of study, and grades predict success in medical school. The Academic Record on the AMCAS application, containing verified and standardized grades from college transcripts, is carefully reviewed by committee members to determine the:

- grades earned in each course and laboratory
- number of credit hours carried in each academic period
- distribution of coursework among the biological, physical, and social sciences and the humanities
- need for remediation of unsatisfactory academic work
- frequency of Incomplete grades and course withdrawals
- number of years taken to complete degree program

Although each medical school establishes its own admission criteria, schools usually prefer applicants who completed their college degrees in a timely manner, carried respectable course loads, balanced science and humanities coursework, and earned consistent 3.0-4.0 grades (on a 4.0 scale). Chapter 5 contains information about the range of science, non-science, and overall grade point averages of all applicants for the 2003 entering class.

In assessing an applicant's academic work, admission committees also consider the characteristics of the academic institution. Coursework at colleges known for rigorous academic standards get greater weight. Because medical schools vary on accepting high school AP and CLEP credits, the admission policies of individual schools in Chapter 11 should be carefully reviewed. Additional information can be achieved on a school's Web site, in its academic bulletin, or from discussions with admissions office personnel.

An applicant who earned less-than-competitive grades in a given course or academic period should not simply decide to forgo a career in medicine. With the help of a premedical advisor and with additional work completed more competitively, an applicant with prior academic problems may still be able to generate a successful application. Just as in medical care and practice, the ability to persist successfully in the face of initial adversity may be perceived as an important attribute in the application and admission process.

MCAT SCORES. Scores on the MCAT can provide supplementary information about a candidate's academic ability and potential. Each medical school decides how MCAT scores are factored into determining an applicant's ability to accomplish the academic work. Some schools average multiple MCAT scores, some accept the highest score in each section from multiple MCAT administrations, while others emphasize the most recent set of MCAT scores. Chapter 11 presents school-specific policies about the oldest MCAT scores considered for admission. In addition, the data in Chapter 11 indicate that the range of MCAT scores deemed acceptable for admission varies among schools.

MCAT scores may receive greater attention from admission committees when a candidate's academic record is marginal, or when committee members are not familiar with the candidate's undergraduate institution. In addition, a comparison of grades with MCAT scores can provide committee members with more information than either provides on its own.

Since an applicant's academic ability is a critical selection factor for medical schools, assessing it typically includes a review of both grades and scores on the four sections of the MCAT. Evaluating the academic preparation and ability of applicants who are not recent college graduates usually includes, in addition to the overall college record, a review of achievement in postbaccalaureate courses. Similarly, the academic abilities of candidates from groups underrepresented in medicine and socioeconomically disadvantaged groups require special attention; additional information can be found in Chapter 6 and in the AAMC publication *Minority Student Opportunities in United States Medical Schools* (✍ www.aamc.org/students/minorities/resources/msousms.htm).

Interviews

Medical school policies for granting and scheduling admission committee interviews vary. Some public schools grant an interview to all candidates who are state residents, while other schools invite candidates only after an extensive screening and prioritizing process. In some instances, the interview is a final step in the assessment process for applicants already deemed to be highly attractive candidates. In other instances, the interview process occurs before any preliminary decision-making by the admission committee. Almost always, an interview is required before a final admission decision is made.

Information about a school's interview policies and procedures is generally provided to applicants in the initial stages of the selection process. Questions and requests for clarification should be directed to staff in the school's admissions office.

Applicant interviews are usually held on the medical school campus. Sometimes an applicant will be asked to interview with a graduate of the school or with a physician in the applicant's area. Some schools have designated interviewers in different geographic regions to minimize time and expense for applicants, but many schools do not offer these off-campus opportunities.

At some schools, interviews are held with individual admission committee members; at others, group interviews are the norm. Some interviewers have prior access to the applicant's information, including grades, MCAT scores, and letters of evaluation, but other interviewers do not, and they focus instead on the candidate's experiential attributes. The interview can be an excellent opportunity for applicants to visit a campus; view the basic science and clinical facilities; meet faculty, staff, and students; and have their questions answered by members of the faculty and staff who are knowledgeable about the school and its programs.

The interview provides candidates opportunities to discuss their personal histories and motivation for a medical career, as well as any aspects of their application that merit special attention or explanation. Candidates should be prepared to discuss all aspects of their application, including their interest in the specific institution. Applicants should be forthright, open, and informative. Most admission committee members are experienced interviewers who want to learn about the "real" person; applicants should not try to "game" the interview or paint a picture they believe the interviewer wants to see. For those applicants who are apprehensive about the process, practice interviews with a trusted advisor or friend can help them to present themselves in the best possible light.

AAMC Policies and Procedures For Investigating Reported Violations of Admission and Enrollment Standards

Purpose

Two significant responsibilities of the Association of American Medical Colleges (AAMC) are to promote integrity in the processes associated with entry into medical school or a graduate medical education program, and to encourage high standards during the course of enrollment. These policies and procedures have been developed to advance these purposes by addressing cases that arise in the following areas, while ensuring the rights of all concerned parties.

Policies

APPLICATION CASES

The AAMC requires applicants to present accurate and current information at the time application materials are submitted and during all phases of the admission process for entry into medical school or a graduate medical education program. It is the policy of the AAMC to investigate discrepancies in credentials, attempts to subvert the admission process, and any other irregular matter that occurs in connection with application activities.

TESTING CASES

The AAMC requires candidates for examination to present accurate and current information at the time registration materials are submitted and to adhere to all Test Center Regulations and Procedures as outlined in the MCAT Announcement. It is the policy of the AAMC to investigate discrepancies, attempts to subvert eligibility requirements, violations of Test Center Regulations, and irregular behavior exhibited during the administration of the MCAT or other tests affiliated with the AAMC.

This investigation is distinct from a Score Validity Inquiry by the MCAT Program pertaining to the legitimacy of test scores as accurate representations of the individual's performance levels.

OTHER CASES

The AAMC may investigate and/or facilitate the reporting of certain cases that occur subsequent to an individual's enrollment in medical school. Such cases include, but are not limited to, academic and ethical violations and criminal activities. In addition, reports documenting cases submitted by other educational agencies may be disseminated by the AAMC to legitimately interested parties after notice and opportunity to comment are afforded the subject of the reports.

REPORTING OF CASES

The AAMC will prepare and issue a report documenting the nature of a confirmed case and any attachments provided by the individual in accordance with the procedures outlined below. *With the issuance of a report, the AAMC makes no judgment as to the culpability of any person with respect to matters reported and does not assess the suitability of an individual to study or practice medicine.* Rather, the AAMC strives to communicate complete and accurate information to legitimately interested parties. Evaluation of this information is the responsibility of the recipient of the report.

continued...

Procedures

INVESTIGATION PROCEEDINGS

The subject of any case is informed of the existence of the investigation and is offered an opportunity to respond to the allegations. The individual is also provided with the opportunity to review a draft of any report proposed for distribution prior to issuance. Unless otherwise requested, the final report will include any explanation or justification provided by the individual during the course of the investigation.

A pending investigation may interrupt the processing of application or registration materials of questionable validity. Such action by the AAMC, however, does not relieve the individual of the responsibility for the payment of normal processing fees.

ARBITRATION

The AAMC offers the option and reserves the right to request arbitration should the individual conclude that a draft report inaccurately characterizes the matter under investigation or when an agreement between parties on the content and language of the report cannot be reached. Such arbitration must be requested prior to the conclusion of an investigation and the issuance of a final report.

Arbitration is conducted by a neutral arbitrator selected by the Washington, D.C., office of the American Arbitration Association. The arbitrator acts solely on the basis of a written record submitted by both parties and no hearing or oral arguments are held. The arbitrator will have final authority to conclude whether: (1) the report should be distributed as written or (2) the report should be modified in accordance with the arbitrator's directions before distribution or (3) no report should be distributed. In addition, the arbitrator determines which party is responsible for the arbitration fee. All other costs associated with arbitration are borne by the party incurring them.

REPORT RECIPIENTS

The report in final form will be issued to all medical schools or residency programs to which the individual has applied or matriculated during the current cycle and medical schools and residency programs to which the applicant applies or matriculates in the future. If, at the time of the investigation, the individual is enrolled in a medical school or graduate medical education program, the report will be forwarded to the current institution of attendance and will be distributed in response to all future application or matriculation activity.

In addition to its members, the AAMC provides services to other educational institutions. For example, the MCAT examination is used by a variety of health profession and graduate programs in addition to medicine. The report in final form is therefore subject to issuance in response to application or matriculation at such institutions of which the AAMC has knowledge.

Reports may contain information relevant to academic or disciplinary proceedings, criminal investigations, and decisions relative to entry into graduate medical education programs and professional licensure. It is the position of the AAMC to cooperate with duly constituted agencies by responding to official requests for such reports.

CHAPTER

Acceptance

Medical schools make admission offers to applicants during the months before the medical school fall semester – as early as September of the year prior to matriculation for Early Decision Program (EDP) applicants, and as late as the first day of class for regular applicants. This process can sometimes become complex, especially when an applicant is admitted to more than one school. Both schools and applicants have rights and responsibilities in this process.

All AAMC-member medical schools agree to observe a set of recommendations on medical school acceptance procedures for first-year entering students (☞ www.aamc.org/students/applying/policies), commonly known as the "traffic rules." Applicants should be familiar with them, as they ensure that application and acceptance processes are timely and fair for all concerned. These recommendations:

- contain important dates applicants should know
- reserve the right of applicants to hold places at multiple schools without losing an acceptance deposit, usually until May 15
- indicate policies for schools to follow after May 15 regarding applicants holding multiple places
- set forth prohibitions about a medical school's offering admission to applicants who have already enrolled in, or begun orientation programs at, a medical school

Individual schools' acceptance policies are contained in Chapter 11, although applicants are encouraged to contact the schools that are of interest to them, as well.

Applicants also have responsibilities (☞ www.aamc.org/students/applying/policies). During the application process for the 2003 entering class, 7,518 applicants were accepted to two or more medical schools. Although multiple family, personal, and financial factors affect applicants' ultimate decisions about which school to attend, they are strongly encouraged to hold only one medical school acceptance at a time. Once applicants make a final decision, they are obliged to withdraw applications promptly from other schools. When possible, applicants holding multiple acceptances should accept their first-choice offer and withdraw from other schools. If a subsequent admission offer is received, applicants can accept the new offer and withdraw from the school at which they were originally accepted.

Citizenship and Residency

CITIZENSHIP. The 2003 entering class at U.S. medical schools included 209 students who were not U.S. citizens or who were not permitted to reside permanently in this country by the U.S. Immigration and Naturalization Service. This relatively small number of international matriculants results from several factors:

- Many public medical schools limit enrollment to state residents.
- State residency statutes require that applicants be either U.S. citizens or permanent residents.
- Many private medical schools require international applicants to document their ability to independently finance a medical education.
- Many countries impose severe restrictions on exportation of currency.
- Federal financial aid sources generally require either U.S. citizenship or permanent residency.

*All URLs mentioned in this chapter can be found at ☞ www.aamc.org/msar

- Many medical schools require completion of premedical coursework at a U.S. college or university.

- Medical schools require documentation of English language proficiency, either from an American undergraduate college or the official agency in the applicant's home country. Information about the Test of English as a Foreign Language can be found at ⌒ www.toefl.org.

Private medical schools are more likely to accept international students than public schools. However, they frequently require the international matriculant to show evidence of a U.S. bank account containing sufficient resources to cover tuition and expenses for one or two years of medical education. International applicants should be aware of these issues and be prepared to meet all special requirements.

STATE RESIDENCY. State-supported medical schools generally give preference for admission and transfer to state residents. Some states have additional requirements regarding county or regional residence. Requirements are established by state legislatures and are usually available from school officials or on the school's or state's Web site. For students who are financially independent of their parents, documentation of state residency typically involves:

- payment of state resident income taxes

- voter registration in the state

- physical residence in the state for a prescribed period of time

- possession of a state driver's license

- motor vehicle registration in the state

For students who are financial dependents, the state of residence is usually the same as that of their parents. A school's state residency definitions for the purpose of in-state tuition and fee eligibility may differ from definitions for other purposes, such as voting.

An applicant can usually have official state residency in only one state at a time. Because of the relationship between state of residence and probability of admission, applicants are strongly encouraged to clarify their official residency status with preferred schools before initiating a formal application.

State residents enrolled in public schools customarily pay much lower tuition than nonresidents. Some private schools also show preference for state residents for at least some of their places because the school receives state government support. Some states without a public medical school participate in special interstate and regional agreements to provide their residents access to a medical education. Registrars and residency officers, located either on the medical school or parent institution's campus, can assist applicants with state residency issues.

Individual school entries in Chapter 11 present data about resident and nonresident applicants and matriculants. Nationally, 64.0 percent of the 2003 matriculants attended schools in their home states; 82.9 percent of students in public schools and 36.6 percent in private schools were state residents. Public schools are unlikely to admit nonresidents unless they have exceptionally strong credentials or strong ties to the state through prior residency, employment, education, or family members.

Special Regional Opportunities for Applicants

Five interstate agreements provide special opportunities for residents of certain states:

- The Western Interstate Commission for Higher Education (WICHE) supports the Professional Student Exchange Program, enabling students from Montana and Wyoming, after certification by their states, to attend a participating medical school and to pay in-state tuition at a public school or reduced tuition at a private one. The student's home state pays a fee to the admitting medical school to help cover costs. Additional information can be found at ⌒ www.wiche.edu/sep/psep/index.asp, or from:

  Professional Student Exchange Program, WICHE
  P.O. Box 9752, 2520 55th Street, Boulder, CO 80301-9752
  (303) 541-0200
  info-sep@wiche.edu

- The 30-year-old WWAMI (Washington, Wyoming, Alaska, Montana, and Idaho) program of decentralized medical education affords a medical education to students from the five states. WWAMI students complete their first year at participating institutions in their home states and their second year at the University of Washington in Seattle. Clerkship options are available for third- and fourth-year students in community settings throughout the five-state region. Additional information is available at ✑ www.washington.edu/medical/som/wwami/index.html, or from:

  > Office of Admissions, A-300 Health Sciences Center
  > Box 356340, Seattle, WA 98195-6340
  > (206) 543-7212
  > askuwsom@u.washington.edu

- Under the auspices of the Southern Region Education Board, some students from Alabama, North Carolina, and Tennessee, who have been accepted at Meharry Medical College, can pay reduced tuition at that school. Some Georgia students are eligible for similar arrangements at Emory University School of Medicine, Mercer University School of Medicine, and Morehouse School of Medicine. For more information, see the SREB Web site at ✑ www.sreb.org, or contact SREB:

  > Southern Regional Education Board
  > 592 10th St. N.W., Atlanta, GA 30318
  > (404) 875-9211
  > acm-rep@sreb.org

- The Finance Authority of Maine's (FAME) Maine Access to Medical Education Program — through relationships with Dartmouth Medical School and the University of Vermont College of Medicine — ensures preference each year for several first-year places for Maine residents certified as eligible by the state. FAME seeks applicants who are most likely to practice primary care in underserved areas of the state. The program pays the school a fee for each student. Although tuition and fees are not reduced, students do receive priority for need-based loans of $5,000 to $20,000 annually.

  Students must commit to completing at least two primary care clinical rotations in Maine: one at a Maine Family Practice residency program during the third year and one at a rural ambulatory care site in the fourth year. Applicants should know that the state of Maine will encourage them to select primary care specialties and to practice in the state. Maine's Advisory Committee on Medical Education reviews all applications, but individual medical schools make final admission decisions. Additional information can be found at ✑ www.famemaine.com, or from:

  > Maine Access to Medical Education Program, Finance Authority of Maine
  > 5 Community Drive, P.O. Box 949, Augusta, ME 04332-0949
  > (800) 228-3734, x306
  > or (207) 623-3263

- The Delaware Institute of Medical Education and Research provides payment to Jefferson Medical College of Thomas Jefferson University to reserve at least 20 admissions each year for Delaware residents. To be eligible, applicants must meet the premedical academic requirements of Jefferson Medical College and apply through the American Medical College Application Service (AMCAS). Applicants' undergraduate degrees can be from any accredited U.S. college or university. Additional information is available at ✑ www.state.de.us/dhcc/dimer.htm, or from:

  > Delaware Institute of Medical Education and Research
  > The Delaware Higher Education Commission, Carvel State Office Building
  > 820 North French Street, Wilmington, DE 19801
  > (302) 577-3240, (800) 292-7935

Deferring Entry into Medical School

An accepted applicant may encounter a special, one-time opportunity that is too attractive to pass up, or be invited to spend an additional year in an ongoing research project, or want to live abroad. In recent years, most medical schools have developed delayed matriculation programs that allow applicants to pursue these opportunities without giving up their medical school slots.

These deferred-entry programs usually require a written request, and some schools may ask for a report at the end of the deferral period. Delays of matriculation are usually granted for one year, although some schools may defer for longer periods of time. Some schools require delayed matriculants to sign an agreement to not apply to other medical schools in the interim. Deferred matriculants will receive instructions from the school granting the deferral about requirements for another application for the year of actual matriculation. The number of deferrals may be limited and there may be a deadline date for such applications. Interested applicants should seek specific information from schools that interest them. The school-specific pages in Chapter 11 also contain information about deferred entrance.

Multiple Acceptances and Final Decisions

Applicants fortunate enough to receive multiple admission offers should not delay their fellow applicants by holding those acceptances for an extended time. Decisions should be made and schools notified as promptly as possible. In early May, AMCAS shares acceptance information with all medical schools. By mid-May, the AAMC expects that all medical schools will have notified accepted applicants of their financial aid awards and that accepted applicants will have decided which school to attend. May 15 is the deadline for acceptance deposit refunds and for applicants' final decisions about medical schools; after May 15, schools can require applicants to choose the school that they will attend. Under no circumstances should applicants be required to withdraw from other schools' waiting lists as a condition of accepting a medical school place. Ultimately, decisions about where to attend belong to applicants, not schools.

Orientation Programs

Most medical schools hold orientation programs for entering students just prior to the start of the first term. These programs familiarize students with their new environment; provide opportunities to meet fellow students, staff and faculty; facilitate book and equipment purchases; and start to acculturate students to medicine's professional codes and responsibilities.

Once these orientation periods have begun, students can no longer accept admission offers from other schools, and they should withdraw their names from all waiting lists at other schools.

AAMC Recommendations for Medical School Admission Officers

The following recommendations are promulgated by the Association of American Medical Colleges (AAMC) to ensure that applicants are afforded timely notification of the outcome of their medical school applications and timely access to available first-year positions and that schools are protected from having unfilled positions in their entering classes. These recommendations are being distributed for the information of prospective medical students, their advisors, and personnel at the medical schools to which they have applied.

The AAMC recommends that:
1. Each school:

    a.   Publish annually, amend publicly, and adhere to its application, acceptance, and admission procedures.

    b.   Utilizing an application service abide by all conditions of its participation agreement with that application service.

2. Each school:

    a.   Between August 1 and March 15 notify the AAMC Section for Medical School Application Services of all admission actions within four weeks of those actions being taken.

    b.   Between March 16 and the first day of class, notify the AAMC Section for Medical School Application Services of all admission actions within seven days of those actions being taken.

continued...

AAMC Recommendations for Medical School Admission Officers continued

3. Each school notify all applicants — other than combined college/M.D., Early Decision Program (EDP), and deferred matriculation applicants — of acceptance to medical school only after October 15 of each admission cycle. It may be appropriate to communicate notifications of decisions other than acceptance to medical school to applicants prior to October 15.

4. By March 30 of the matriculation year, each school have issued a number of offers of acceptance at least equal to the expected number of students in its first-year entering class and have reported those acceptance actions to the AAMC Section for Medical School Application Services.

5. Prior to May 15 of the matriculation year (April 15 for schools whose first day of class is on or before July 30), each school permit ALL applicants (except for EDP applicants) — including those applying to M.D./Ph.D. programs and those to whom merit or other special scholarships have been awarded:

    a. A minimum two-week time period for their response to the acceptance offer.

    b. To hold acceptance offers from any other schools without penalty.

6. After May 15 of the matriculation year (April 15 for schools whose first day of class is on or before July 30), each school implement school-specific procedures for accepted applicants who, without adequate explanation, continue to hold one or more places at other schools. These procedures:

    a. May require applicants to:

        i. Respond to acceptance offers in less than two weeks.

        ii. Submit a statement of intent, a deposit, or both.

    b. Should recognize the problems of applicants with multiple acceptance offers, applicants who have not yet received an acceptance offer, and applicants who have not yet been informed about financial aid opportunities at schools to which they have been accepted.

    c. Should permit accepted applicants to remain on other schools' waiting lists and to withdraw if they later receive an acceptance offer from a preferred school.

7. Each school's acceptance deposit not exceed $100 and be refundable until May 15 (except for EDP applicants). If the applicant enrolls at the school, the school is encouraged to credit the deposit toward tuition.

8. After June 1, any school that plans to make an acceptance offer to an applicant already known to have been accepted by another school for that entering class ensure that the other school is advised of this offer at the time that the offer is made. This notification should be made immediately by telephone and promptly thereafter by written correspondence delivered by regular or electronic methods. Schools should communicate fully with each other with respect to anticipated late roster changes in order to minimize inter-school miscommunication and misunderstanding, as well as the possibility of unintended vacant positions in a school's first-year entering class.

9. No school make an acceptance offer, either verbal or written, to any individual who has enrolled in, or begun an orientation program immediately prior to enrollment at, a U.S. or Canadian school. Enrollment is defined as being officially matriculated as a member of the school's first-year entering class.

10. Each school treat all letters of recommendation submitted in support of an application as confidential, except in those states with applicable laws to the contrary. The contents of a letter of recommendation should not be revealed to an applicant at any time.

Approved: AAMC Executive Committee, October 3, 2003

AAMC Recommendations for Medical School Applicants

The following recommendations are promulgated by the Association of American Medical Colleges (AAMC) to ensure that applicants are afforded timely notification of the outcome of their medical school applications and timely access to available first-year positions and that schools are protected from having unfilled positions in their entering classes. These recommendations are being distributed for the information of prospective medical students, their advisors, and personnel at the medical schools to which they have applied.

The AAMC recommends that:

1. Each applicant be familiar with, understand, and comply with the application, acceptance, and admission procedures at each school to which the applicant has applied, as well with as these Recommendations.

2. Each applicant provide accurate and truthful information in all aspects of the application, acceptance, and admission processes for each school to which the applicant has applied.

3. Each applicant submit all application documents (e.g., primary and secondary application forms, transcript[s], letters of evaluation/recommendation, fees) to each school in a timely manner and no later than the school's published deadline date.

4. Each applicant promptly notify all relevant medical school application services and all medical schools with independent application processes of any change, permanent or temporary, in contact information (e.g., mailing address, telephone number, e-mail address).

5. Any applicant who will be unavailable for an extended period of time (e.g., during foreign travel, vacation, holidays) during the application/admission process:
   a. Provide instructions regarding his or her application and the authority to respond to offers of acceptance to a parent or other responsible individual in the applicant's absence.
   b. Inform all schools at which the applicant remains under consideration of this individual's name and contact information.

6. Each applicant respond promptly to a school's invitation for interview. Any applicant who cannot appear for a previously scheduled interview should notify the school immediately of the cancellation of the appointment in the manner requested by the school.

7. Each applicant in need of financial aid initiate, as early as possible, the steps necessary to determine eligibility, including the early filing of appropriate need analysis forms and the encouragement of parents, when necessary, to file required income tax forms.

8. In fairness to other applicants, when an applicant has made a decision, prior to May 15, not to attend a medical school that has made an offer of acceptance, the applicant promptly withdraw his or her application from that (those) other school(s) by written correspondence delivered by regular or electronic methods.

9. By May 15 of the matriculation year (April 15 for schools whose first day of class is on or before July 30), each applicant who has received an offer of acceptance from more than one school choose the specific school at which the applicant prefers to enroll and withdraw his or her application, by written correspondence delivered by regular or electronic methods, from all other schools from which acceptance offers have been received.

10. Immediately upon enrollment in, or initiation of an orientation program immediately prior to enrollment at, a U.S. or Canadian school, each applicant withdraw his or her application from consideration at all other schools at which he or she remains under consideration.

Approved: AAMC Executive Committee, October 3, 2003

CHAPTER

9

Financing a Medical Education

After being accepted to medical school, prospective students must finalize plans for covering the significant costs of a medical education, including tuition, fees, books, equipment, living expenses, medical and disability insurance, and transportation. Two major skills are involved: the ability to develop realistic and proactive financing plans, and the ability to manage educational debt. Several factors impact students' financial decisions:

- Medical school tuition and fees have increased significantly over the past decade.

- Primary financial responsibility rests with students and their families.

- Student loans are the most common form of financial assistance.

- Most medical students are unable to supplement their income with employment.

- Students with a history of credit problems may not qualify for the private loans that often supplement federal borrowing.

- Credit card and other consumer debt obligations cannot be met with student financial aid.

- Available financial assistance is finite, especially for living expenses.

- Criteria for financial aid awards differ from school to school.

- Funding and eligibility requirements for federal financial aid programs are subject to change at any time.

Information about the financial aid forms required by each medical school can be found in the searchable database on the AAMC Web site at: ☞ http://services.aamc.org/msar_reports/

TABLE 9-A

Tuition and Student Fees for 2003–2004 First-Year Students in U.S. Medical Schools (in Dollars)

Categories of Students	Private Schools			Public Schools		
	Range	Median	Average	Range	Median	Average
Resident	$10,500–$40,459	$33,965	$32,588	$4,922–$26,422	$16,332	$16,155
Nonresident	$22,500–$40,459	$34,550	$34,169	$12,392–$69,174	$32,662	$33,635

Figures based on data provided summer 2003. This table excludes Uniformed Services University of the Health Sciences, a public institution that does not charge tuition or student fees.

(MD)² : Monetary Decisions for Medical Doctors

(MD)² : Monetary Decisions for Medical Doctors is a comprehensive, Web-based program (☞ www.aamc.org/md2) developed by the AAMC to assist premedical and medical students in their financial planning. Divided into three sections – The Premedical School Years, The Medical School Years, and The Residency and Early Practice Years – (MD)² provides information tailored to the specific needs of students

TABLE 9-B
Federal Loan Programs for Students

Characteristic	Primary Care Loan	Federal Perkins	Federal Subsidized Stafford	Federal Unsubsidized Stafford
Lender	Medical school financial aid office on behalf of the Department of Health and Human Services	Medical school financial aid office on behalf of the federal government	Bank or other lending institution, the federal government or an eligible institution	Bank or other lending institution, the federal government or an eligible institution
Based on need	Note[1]	Yes	Yes	No
Citizenship requirement	U.S. citizen, U.S. national, or U.S. permanent resident	U.S. citizen, U.S. national, or U.S. permanent resident	U.S. citizen, U.S. national, or U.S. permanent resident	U.S. citizen, U.S. national, or U.S. permanent resident
Borrowing limits	Up to cost of attendance (Third- and fourth-year students may receive additional funds to repay previous educational loans received while attending medical school)	$6,000/year $40,000 aggregate undergraduate and graduate	$8,500 annual maximum; $65,500 cumulative maximum including premed and medical borrowing[2]	$38,500 less subsidized Stafford annual maximum; $189,125 less subsidized Stafford cumulative maximum premed and medical borrowing[2]
Interest rate	Note[3]	5%	In school, grace, and deferment: 91-day Treasury bill rate plus 1.7%, not to exceed 8.25%. In repayment: 91-day Treasury bill rate plus 2.3%, not to exceed 8.25%.	In school, grace, and deferment: 91-day Treasury bill rate plus 1.7%, not to exceed 8.25%. In repayment: 91-day Treasury bill rate plus 2.3%, not to exceed 8.25%.
Borrower is responsible for interest during:				
School	No	No	No	Yes
Deferments	No	No	No	Yes
Grace period	No	No	No	Yes

[1]Yes; in addition, borrower must agree upon signing loan agreement to enter and complete a primary care residency and practice in a primary care field until the loan is repaid in full. Family resource information is required for consideration.

[2]Both annual and cumulative maximums are subject to change, pending congressional action.

[3]Five percent; however, rate is recomputed at 18% from the date of noncompliance should borrower fail to meet primary care requirements (for primary care loans made on or after November 13, 1998).

during different phases of their education. Information covered includes credit and consumer debt, types of financial aid, and the application process, along with relevant reference materials.

Planning for the Financing of a Medical Education

In 2002, graduating medical students reported an average educational debt of $109,457. Tuition and expenses vary from school to school; entries in Chapter 11 provide information about individual schools' tuition and fee schedules. Since most students rely on loans to pay for medical school, they should be aware of two general borrowing concepts:

TABLE 9-B (continued)
Federal Loan Programs for Students

Characteristic	Primary Care Loan	Federal Perkins	Federal Subsidized Stafford	Federal Unsubsidized Stafford
Grace period	1 year after graduation	9 months after graduation	6 months after graduation	6 months after graduation
Deferments	During school and primary care residency; check your promissory note or ask your financial aid officer	During school and up to three years of demonstrated economic hardship; check your promissory note or ask your financial aid officer	During school and up to three years of demonstrated economic hardship; check your promissory note or ask your financial aid officer	During school and up to three years of demonstrated economic hardship; check your promissory note or ask your financial aid officer
Repayment requirements	Minimum: $40/month ; 10 to 25 years to repay; not eligible for loan consolidation	Minimum: $40/month including interest; maximum 10 years to repay; eligible for loan consolidation	Minimum: $50/month; level, graduated, income-based, and extended repayment options available; eligible for loan consolidation	Minimum: $50/month; level, graduated, income-based, and extended repayment options available; eligible for loan consolidation
Prepayment penalties	None	None	None	None
Allowable cancellations	Death or total and permanent disability	Death or total and permanent disability	Death or total and permanent disability	Death or total and permanent disability

CHAPTER

9

- Borrowing encumbers future income. When taking an educational loan, the student is obligating future income to pay it off, which means that income will not be available for opening a practice, purchasing a home, buying a car, or starting a family. Some financial analysts estimate that three dollars of future income are needed to pay off every dollar of current borrowing. Medical students should be aware of the implications of borrowing.

- The borrower must decide whether the value of a medical degree is approximately equal to the future income necessary to satisfy educational loans. While borrowing for educational purposes is an investment in one's future, it has an impact on personal and professional lifestyle. Only the individual student can assess whether the potential return is worth the initial investment.

Debt Management

Learning to manage money takes constant practice. Formulating and living within a budget are essential elements in managing debt. Skilled budgeting can result in less borrowing now and more disposable income later. Several practices are key to good budgeting:

- Have a spending plan. Prepare a strategy for allocating resources and anticipating periodic expenses, such as car insurance premiums, and unexpected emergencies, such as medical bills.

- Use credit prudently. Possessing one low-interest, low-fee credit card and paying the full balance monthly are highly recommended. Timely payments enhance personal credit ratings and prevent late fees.

- Use financial windfalls wisely. Use the rule of "thirds" for unexpected gifts or tax refunds: one-third to savings, one-third to pay down debt, and one-third to spending.

- Calculate ownership costs. Owning a house or car involves insurance and maintenance costs as well as mortgage and loan payments.

- Plug spending leaks. Even minor expenditures such as restaurant meals, if they are incurred daily or weekly, add up over time.

- Limit careless shopping. Impulse buying can ruin even the best financial plan. Shop with a list and buy only when specific items are needed.

- Save whenever possible. Saving even a small amount each week can quickly add up.

- Practice delayed gratification. Answering these questions can pare down spending: Is this a want or a need? Must I have it now? Can I pay less elsewhere? Can I borrow or rent it instead?

- Live on less. Even the essential expenses of housing, transportation, and food can be reduced by living with a roommate, carpooling, using public transportation, or preparing meals at home.

In addition to good budgeting, debt management also requires good record keeping. The borrower is responsible for maintaining records on monies owed, terms and conditions of each loan, the agencies that service loans, deadline dates, and deferment policies. Copies of application forms and promissory notes should be kept in a safe place. Many loan programs and financial institutions help in this process by providing access to information on their Web sites. Carefully tracking due dates and deadlines is also beneficial.

Borrowers are also responsible for keeping loan providers and servicers notified of changes in name, contact information, and enrollment status. Borrowers who fail to maintain contact with lenders risk becoming delinquent in their loan payments or defaulting on their loans. Either situation can cause long-term consequences to the borrower's credit rating and can endanger future borrowing.

The AAMC MEDLOANS Program sponsors a nationally known debt management program available on its Web site at ✎ www.aamc.org/debthelp. Information about various types of loan assistance, including subsidized and unsubsidized loans, interest rates, capitalization, grace period and deferment provisions, forbearance provisions, repayment options, and consolidation can be found there, as well as information about the consequences of delinquency and default.

Financial Aid Philosophy

Financial aid provides assistance for postsecondary education and opportunities for students to attend schools of their choice. The philosophy of financial aid is that a student's family bears primary responsibility, to the extent possible, for paying educational expenses. From undergraduate to graduate and professional education, there is a decided shift in who bears the main responsibility for paying educational expenses, as explained below.

Eligibility for financial aid is generally determined by answering three questions:

1. **How much does it cost?** The answer varies by school and by year in school. Cost is composed of three components: tuition and fees; books, supplies, and equipment; and living expenses. These are frequently referred to as the "cost of attendance" or the "student financial aid budget." The cost of attendance by school year should be available from each medical school's financial aid officer.

2. **What are the student's resources?** The amount that a student's family can contribute to a medical education is called the "expected family contribution." It is determined through a need-analysis formula at the time of the financial aid application, which ensures that all students are compared equitably. Unlike most undergraduates, graduate and professional students are considered financially independent in determining the expected family contribution for most types of federal financial aid; both income and assets are taken into account. However, eligibility for some types of federal aid requires reporting of family financial information, even though the student is technically considered independent. This is also the

case at some institutions in determining eligibility for institutional grants, scholarships, and school-based loans. In theory, this approach ensures that certain types of aid are awarded to those with the greatest need. When school officials request financial information of parents or family members, they are assessing ability, rather than willingness, to pay. In applying for aid, applicants and students should work closely with medical school financial aid officers.

3. **What additional resources are needed?** The financial aid officer compares the student's expected family contribution and other resources with the institution's total cost of attendance to determine how much assistance is needed for the academic year. The student then receives an award letter that describes the actual package of financial aid from all available sources.

General Eligibility Criteria

Financial aid programs usually require that the applicant or student is:
- a U.S. citizen or permanent resident
- making satisfactory academic progress
- in compliance with Selective Service registration requirements
- not in default on other loans

An applicant or student who has defaulted on prior loans will not qualify for most federal programs and may thus be prevented from attending medical school, as the federal government is the most substantial source of financial aid. Some educational financing programs may also require a service commitment as a condition of assistance.

Types of Financial Aid

In general, there are two types of financial assistance available to medical students:
- **Grants and Scholarships.** The type and amount of this support vary by school and may include state and institutional funds. Grants and scholarships do not have to be repaid, but their availability may be very limited. The medical school financial aid officer is the best source of information on what is available and how to qualify.

- **Loans.** Most medical student funding is in the form of loans, and details on various programs are available from the financial aid officer. There are two types: subsidized and unsubsidized. Subsidized loans carry no interest cost to borrowers during the in-school period, grace period, and any deferment periods and hence are the most desirable. Unsubsidized loans accrue interest from the date of disbursement; the borrower is responsible for interest and it will eventually be capitalized (added back to the loan principal). While borrowers are not required to pay interest on unsubsidized loans during school enrollment, grace, and any deferment periods, they will eventually be responsible for the interest costs. Private loans, used to supplement other types of aid including federal loans, are examples of unsubsidized loans. Borrowers should seek out private loans very carefully.

While medical students may also be able to work or receive funding through work-study programs offered by parent colleges or universities, participation in these programs is not the norm.

Credit Issues

Students must not only show a cost of attendance that supports their borrowing from private loan programs; they must also be "credit ready," meaning they have either a positive credit history or no credit history at all. Students with a history of late payments on consumer obligations are likely to find themselves excluded from private loans until they can resolve credit problems.

Some medical schools require a credit history as a part of the financial aid application; applicants are advised to request their credit report prior to applying for aid. If problems are identified, the student may be able to resolve them before the financial aid application process gets underway. Alternately, the student may choose to defer matriculation until these problems can be resolved and expunged from the credit record. Many medical schools will grant a delay of matriculation to an accepted applicant who needs to address credit problems. Even prospective students with excellent credit histories, but with significant consumer debt, may encounter difficulty in financing medical school.

In all instances, applicants are strongly advised to make early contact with the financial aid officer at medical schools of interest to them to discuss financial aid eligibility and, if necessary, resolve out outstanding credit problems.

AAMC MEDLOANS Program

The MEDLOANS Program, sponsored and managed by the AAMC, has provided more than $2 billion to medical students over the past 19 years. MEDLOANS provides a comprehensive package of student loans, including the Federal Stafford Loan, the private Alternative Loan Program (ALP), MEDEX for fourth-year students needing loans for residency interview and travel expenses, and the MEDLOANS Consolidation Loan. MEDLOANS offers:

- **Rewards for responsible repayment behavior.** MEDLOANS rewards borrowers with interest rate reductions and account credits or cash option for making payments on time. See the accompanying chart for more details on MEDLOANS 2004-2005 terms and conditions.

- **Life-of-loan servicing.** MEDLOANS borrowers receive specialized telephone customer service regarding their loan portfolios. MEDLOANS guarantees one servicer throughout the life of the loan, which helps avoid unnecessary paperwork and confusion during residency and repayment years. Repayment plan options include standard, graduated, or income-sensitive plans, as well as loan consolidation. Terms and conditions are available at ☞ www.aamc.org/MEDLOANS/.

- **Debt management assistance.** MEDLOANS borrowers have access to the MEDLOANS Electronic Loan Portfolio (ELP) debt management software created specifically for medical students. They receive copies of the MEDLOANS Borrower Notebooks, which feature loan terms and conditions, budgeting materials, and a convenient centralized place for storage of loan promissory notes and records. Easy Web access to student loan portfolios is available for up-to-date information on loan disbursements and balances.

MEDLOANS is interested in helping students who need financial aid, but a student's first contact for financial aid should be the medical school financial aid officer. Up-to-date information (including current terms and conditions) is available at ☞ www.aamc.org/MEDLOANS or from MEDLOANS Customer Assistance, (800) 858-5050.

Service Commitment Programs

Service commitment programs – awards available through the U.S. Army, Navy, and Air Force, federal agencies, and some state agencies – provide financial assistance to enrolled medical students in return for physician services after completion of medical training. These programs are not need- or cost-based or, strictly speaking, a form of financial aid.

- **The Armed Forces Health Professions Scholarship Program.** These programs offer full support to students enrolled in civilian medical schools in exchange for service, after residency training, in the branch (Army, Navy, or Air Force) that provided the support. Applications are handled by military recruiters and are very competitive. Additional information is provided in Table 9-D.

- **The National Health Service Corps (NHSC).** The National Health Service Corps (NHSC) is a part of the federal Health Resources and Services Administration's (HRSA) Bureau of Health Professions. The NHSC's mission is to improve the health of the nation's underserved populations by assisting communities to recruit and retain community-responsive, culturally competent primary care clinicians. The NHSC offers a variety of programs to dedicated students and clinicians interested in pursuing careers in primary care to the underserved, including the NHSC's Scholarship and Loan Repayment programs. Both programs offer financial support in exchange for the opportunity to practice in the nation's most needy communities. The NHSC Scholarship Program is available to qualifying students upon matriculation. Information on the NHSC Scholarship and Loan Repayment opportunities, as well as all NHSC opportunities to serve the underserved, can be found at ☞ http://nhsc.bhpr.hrsa.gov/ or obtained by calling 1-800-221-9393; in the AAMC's State and Other Loan Repayment/Forgiveness and Scholarship Programs, available online at ☞ www.aamc.org/students/financing/repayment; from school financial aid officers; and from on-campus faculty NHSC "Ambassadors" in health professions schools across the country. A listing of Ambassadors can be found on the NHSC Web site or obtained by calling 1-800-221-9393.

TABLE 9-C MEDLOANS 2004–2005 Terms and Conditions

	Federal Stafford Loans Subsidized and Unsubsidized	Alternative Loan Program (ALP)
Eligibility	Be enrolled in an eligible school at least 1/2 time. Meet other eligibility criteria in the federal Stafford loan promissory note.	Meet established credit criteria. Be currently enrolled at an approved school. All outstanding student loans in good standing.
Loan limits	Annual $38,500 Aggregate Limits $189,125 *Unsubsidized loan limit is less any subsidized loan amount. (Subsidized limit: $8,500).	Minimum: $500 Annual maximum: Cost of education minus other financial aid. Aggregate maximum: $220,000 (total educational indebtedness from all sources)
Interest rates	**In-school, grace and deferment:** Bond-equivalent rate for 91-day T-bill plus 1.7%, not to exceed 8.25%. **In Repayment:** Bond-equivalent rate for 91-day T-bill plus 2.3%, not to exceed 8.25%.	**Prior to repayment:** Variable, adjusted monthly to the Prime Rate +0% **In repayment:** Variable, adjusted quarterly to the Prime Rate +1.25%. See Borrower Benefits for further details.
Subsidy & capitalization	No interest on the subsidized Stafford while in school, grace and deferment. For unsubsidized Stafford loans, accrued interest capitalizes **ONCE** at repayment (following uninterrupted periods of grace and deferment).	Interest may be deferred during school and during the three-year residency grace period. Unpaid interest is capitalized when repayment begins.
Fees	Guarantee fee: .50% for new Stafford Loans guaranteed beginning April 1, 2004. 1% for new Stafford Loans guaranteed beginning Nov. 1, 2004. Origination fee: 3% Fees subtracted from loan proceeds.	0% at loan origination. **At repayment:** Based on a borrower's credit analysis at repayment and voluntary payments made during residency. Supplemental fee will be lower if minimum $50 payments are made in residency.

Repayment	Begins following six-month grace period after leaving school or dropping to less than half time status. Deferment and forbearance options for residency.
	
	Borrowers have a maximum of 10 years to repay. Additional options and years to repay available through:
	
	    Standard Repayment
	    Graduated Repayment
	    Income Sensitive Repayment
	    Flex Repay
		Begins three years after graduation, or nine months after enrollment status drops to less than half time.
		
		Borrowers have a maximum of 20 years to repay.
		
		    Standard Repayment
		    Alternative Repayment Terms

Borrower benefits	**MEDLOANS Healthier Returns℠ Program** Receive an immediate loan credit or cash option equal to 3.5% of your original principal balance. Just graduate, enroll in Sallie Mae's Manage Your Loans℠, and agree to receive account information at a valid e-mail address. **MEDLOANS Stafford Cash Back™ Program** Make your first 33 scheduled payments on time and receive a 4.5% credit of original principal balance of eligible Stafford loans. A check for this credit may also be requested. Just enroll in Sallie Mae's Manage Your Loans℠ and agree to receive account information at a valid e-mail address.	The ALP Repayment Rate of Prime Rate +1.25% is available to those borrowers participating in the MEDLOANS Direct Repay Plan and the MEDLOANS Rewards® Program; otherwise the rate is Prime Rate +2.0%. **MEDLOANS Direct Repay Plan** Pay electronically and receive a 0.25 percentage point interest rate reduction. **MEDLOANS Rewards Program** Maintain a schedule of on time monthly payments and receive a 0.50 percentage point interest rate reduction.

CHAPTER

9

- **State Loan Forgiveness or Repayment Programs.** State programs are frequently available to students and graduates in return for a commitment to serve in the state's areas of need. Most often available to residents and practicing physicians, these programs are sometimes open to enrolled medical students. Information can again be found in the searchable database on the AAMC Web site at ➣ www.aamc.org/students/financing/repayment, and from school financial aid officers.

TABLE 9-D
Armed Forces Health Professions Loan Repayment Scholarship Programs

	Source of Grant		
Characteristic	Air Force	Army	Navy
Provider	USAF Recruiting HPSP Central Office 550 D Street West, Suite 1 Randolph AFB, TX 78150-4527 1 (800) 443-4690 www.airforce.com	U.S. Army Recruiting Command Attn: RCRO-HS-MC 1307 Third Avenue Fort Knox, KY 40121-2726 1 (800) USA-ARMY; www.goarmy.com	Headquarters, Navy Recruiting Command 801 N. Randolph Street Arlington, VA 22203-1991 www.navy.com/healthcare/ physicians
Based on need	No	No	No
Citizenship requirement	U.S. citizen only	U.S. citizen only	U.S. citizen only
Service commitment	Yes	Yes	Yes
Nature of commitment	One year of service for each year of support	One year of service for each year of support	One year of service for each year of support (minimum three-year obligation)
Level of support	Full tuition, monthly living stipend, book and supply allowance	Full tuition, monthly living stipend, book and supply allowance	Full tuition, monthly living stipend, book and supply allowance

10

Information on Combined College/M.D. Programs for High School Students

About one quarter of U.S. medical schools offer combined college/M.D. programs for high school students; these programs range in length from six to nine years. The first two to four years of the curriculum consist of undergraduate courses, including required premedical courses; the remaining years are devoted to the medical school curriculum. Graduates receive both a bachelor's degree from the undergraduate institution and an M.D. degree from the medical school.

The purposes of these programs vary by institution:
- to permit highly qualified students to plan and complete a broad liberal arts education before initiating medical studies
- to attract highly capable students to the sponsoring medical school
- to enhance diversity among enrolled medical students
- to reduce the total number of years for completing the M.D. degree
- to educate physicians likely to practice in particular geographic areas or to work with underserved populations
- to reduce costs of a medical education
- to prepare physician-scientists and future leaders in health policy

Potential applicants should familiarize themselves with the mission and goal statement of each combined degree program in which they are interested in order to ensure a match between their educational and professionals goals and those of the program.

These programs typically represent relationships between a medical school and one or more undergraduate colleges located in the same geographic region. They are sometimes part of the same university system, or they can be independent institutions.

Admission is open to highly qualified, mature high school students who are committed to a future career in medicine. State-supported schools generally admit few out-of-state applicants to their combined college/M.D. programs; private schools tend to have greater flexibility.

While academic requirements vary the among schools sponsoring these programs, they typically include biology, chemistry, physics, English, mathematics, and social science courses. Calculus and foreign-language courses are also frequently required; a computer science course is sometimes recommended. Admission to the medical curriculum may occur immediately or after a student completes a prescribed number of semesters with a minimum grade point average (GPA). In some programs, students are not required to take the MCAT, while in others, a minimum MCAT score is required.

Progressing through the program from the undergraduate to the medical curriculum is usually contingent on a student's achieving specific criteria in terms of standardized test scores and GPAs and meeting the school's expectations regarding personal and professional behavior.

High school students interested in a combined college/M.D. program should consult their high school guidance counselor to ensure that they are enrolled in a challenging college preparatory curriculum that incorporates specific courses required for admission to the program.

The program descriptions that follow were compiled from responses to a questionnaire sent to all medical schools sponsoring programs of interest to high school students. For medical school tuitions for the 2004-2005 entering class, refer to the school entries in Chapter 11. For additional information, contact each school directly.

The following abbreviations are used in the school entries in this chapter:

ACT - American College Testing Program
CEEB - College Entrance Examination Board
FAFSA - Free Application for Federal Student Aid
GPA - Grade Point Average
MCAT - Medical College Admission Test
SAT - Scholastic Aptitude Test
USMLE - United States Medical Licensing Examination

List of Medical Schools Offering Combined College/
M.D. Programs for High School Students
2005–2006

Alabama

University of Alabama School of Medicine
University of South Alabama College of Medicine

California

University of California, Riverside, and David Geffen School of Medicine at University of California, Los Angeles
University of California, San Diego, School of Medicine
University of Southern California College of Letters, Arts, and Sciences and Keck School of Medicine

Connecticut

University of Connecticut and University of Connecticut School of Medicine

District of Columbia

The George Washington University School of Medicine and Health Sciences and The Columbian School of Arts and Sciences
Howard University

Florida

University of Florida College of Medicine
University of Miami

Illinois

Rosalind Franklin University of Medicine and Science/Chicago Medical School and Illinois Institute of Technology
Northwestern University Feinberg School of Medicine
University of Illinois at Chicago College of Medicine

Massachusetts

Boston University

Michigan

Michigan State University College of Human Medicine
Wayne State University School of Medicine

Missouri

Saint Louis University School of Medicine
University of Missouri—Columbia School of Medicine
University of Missouri—Kansas City School of Medicine

New Jersey

University of Medicine and Dentistry of New Jersey—New Jersey Medical School
Rutgers University and University of Medicine and Dentistry of New Jersey—
    Robert Wood Johnson Medical School

New York

Brooklyn College and State University of New York Downstate Medical Center College of Medicine
New York University
Rensselaer Polytechnic Institute and Albany Medical College
Siena College and Albany Medical College
Sophie Davis School of Biomedical Education/City University of New York
Stony Brook University and Stony Brook University School of Medicine
SUNY Upstate Medical University/Wilkes University/GUTHRIE-Robert Packer Hospital
Union College and Albany Medical College
University of Rochester School of Medicine and Dentistry

Ohio
Case Western Reserve University
Northeastern Ohio Universities College of Medicine
The Ohio State University College of Medicine and Public Health
University of Cincinnati College of Medicine

Pennsylvania
Drexel University and Drexel University College of Medicine
Lehigh University and Drexel University College of Medicine
Pennsylvania State University and Jefferson Medical College of Thomas Jefferson University
Temple University School of Medicine
Villanova University and Drexel University College of Medicine

Rhode Island
Brown University

Tennessee
East Tennessee State University
Fisk University and Meharry Medical College

Texas
Rice University and Baylor College of Medicine
University of Texas Medical School at San Antonio

Virginia
Eastern Virginia Medical School
Virginia Commonwealth University

Wisconsin
University of Wisconsin Medical School

CHAPTER

10

Number of Years Required by Undergraduate and U.S. Medical Schools
to Complete the Combined College/M.D. Program
2005–2006

6 Years

University of Missouri—Kansas City School of Medicine

Rensselaer Polytechnic Institute and Albany Medical College

6-7 Years

University of Miami

Northeastern Ohio Universities College of Medicine

Pennsylvania State University and Jefferson Medical College of Thomas Jefferson University

7 Years

University of California, Riverside, and David Geffen School of Medicine at University of California, Los Angeles

The George Washington University School of Medicine and Health Sciences and The Columbian School of Arts and Sciences

University of Florida College of Medicine

Northwestern University Feinberg School of Medicine

Boston University*

University of Medicine and Dentistry of New Jersey—New Jersey Medical School

Sophie Davis School of Biomedical Education/City University of New York

Union College and Albany Medical College

The Ohio State University College of Medicine and Public Health

Drexel University and Drexel University College of Medicine

Lehigh University and Drexel University College of Medicine

Villanova University and Drexel University College of Medicine

Fisk University and Meharry Medical College

University of Texas Medical School at San Antonio

University of Wisconsin Medical School†

8 Years

University of Alabama School of Medicine

University of South Alabama College of Medicine

University of California, San Diego, School of Medicine

University of Southern California College of Letters, Arts, and Sciences and Keck School of Medicine

University of Connecticut and University of Connecticut School of Medicine

Howard University

Rosalind Franklin University of Medicine and Science/Chicago Medical School and Illinois Institute of Technology

University of Illinois at Chicago College of Medicine

Michigan State University College of Human Medicine

Wayne State University School of Medicine

Saint Louis University School of Medicine

University of Missouri—Columbia School of Medicine

Rutgers University and University of Medicine and Dentistry of New Jersey—Robert Wood Johnson Medical School

Brooklyn College and State University of New York Downstate Medical Center College of Medicine

New York University

Siena College and Albany Medical College

Stony Brook and Stony Brook School of Medicine

SUNY Upstate Medical University/Wilkes University/GUTHRIE-Robert Packer Hospital

University of Rochester School of Medicine and Dentistry

Case Western Reserve University

University of Cincinnati College of Medicine

Temple University School of Medicine

Brown University

East Tennessee State University

Rice University and Baylor College of Medicine

Eastern Virginia Medical College

Virginia Commonwealth University

9 Years

University of Cincinnati College of Medicine (College of Engineering—undergraduate)

*with an 8-year option

†7- to 9-year program

University of Alabama School of Medicine

Birmingham, Alabama

Address Inquiries To:

UAB Office of Undergraduate Admissions
HUC 260
University of Alabama School of Medicine
1530 3rd Avenue, S.
Birmingham, Alabama 35294-1150
(205) 934-8221
Web site: www.uab.edu/emsap

Purpose

The UAB Early Medical School Acceptance Program (EMSAP) is designed to give exceptional high school graduates an opportunity to take advantage of the best resources of the undergraduate and medical programs through a mentored relationship with medical school faculty.

Requirements for Entrance

Students are selected in their senior year of high school. Both residents and nonresidents of Alabama are eligible to apply to the program. Applicants must submit the following: two letters of recommendation from high school administrators, counselors, or teachers describing their suitability for a career in medicine and a brief essay incorporating information about themselves and their career objectives and expectations for contributing to society. Applicants must meet the requirements for freshman admission.

Selection Factors

Applicants must have a minimum ACT score of 30, an SAT I score of 1320, and a minimum academic GPA of 3.5. Selected applicants are invited for a required interview.

Curriculum

This eight-year program leads to a baccalaureate degree awarded by the University of Alabama, Birmingham (UAB), and to the M.D. degree granted by the University of Alabama School of Medicine. Students must meet the regular undergraduate course requirements for the University of Alabama. Students must take the MCAT, and receive a minimal total score of 25, maintain an overall GPA of 3.6 and science GPA of 3.5, and receive their baccalaureate degree, in order to transition to admission to the medical school phase of the program. After the second year of medical school, the student must pass the USMLE Step 1 in order to be promoted and graduate. Passing of USMLE Step 2 is required in order to graduate from the medical school.

Expenses

In 2003-2004 the annual undergraduate tuition for residents was $3,474 and $8,694 for nonresidents.

Financial Aid

UAB awards comprehensive federal, state, institutional, and private financial aid on the basis of merit, financial need, or both. Each year the university offers more than 1500 scholarships, including approximately $1.5 million in merit-based awards.

Applicants are automatically considered for all academic scholarships when accepted to the university. Academic scholarships are awarded on a first come-first served basis, so applicants are encouraged to apply early.

APPLICATION AND ACCEPTANCE POLICIES

Filing of application:
  Earliest date: September 1, 2004
  Latest date: January 1, 2005
Application fee: None
Acceptance notice:
  Earliest date: Mid-February 2005
  Latest date: Late February 2005
Applicant's response to acceptance offer:
  Maximum time: March 15, 2005
Deposit to hold place in class: None
Starting date: Mid-August

INFORMATION ON 2003–2004 ENTERING CLASS

Number of	In-State	Out-of-State	Total
Applicants	80	22	102
Applicants Interviewed	25	3	28
New Entrants	10	0	10
Total number of students enrolled in program: 30			

University of South Alabama
College of Medicine

Mobile, Alabama

Address Inquiries To:

Office of Admissions
University of South Alabama
Administrative Building
Room 182
Mobile, Alabama 36688-0002
(334) 460-6141 or (800) 872-5247
Web site: www.usouthal.edu

Purpose

Candidates selected for the program will receive early acceptance from the University of South Alabama and its College of Medicine. Students participating in the program are expected to enter the University of South Alabama College of Medicine in the fall after completion of the baccalaureate degree.

Requirements for Entrance

Students in the senior year of high school or recently graduated individuals who have not yet entered college are eligible to apply for the program. Both residents and nonresidents of Alabama may apply.

Selection Factors

Candidates must have a minimum high school GPA of 3.5 as computed by the University of South Alabama and must present a minimum enhanced composite ACT score of 32 (or comparable SAT score). Candidates must also have demonstrated leadership qualities, community service, communication skills, and motivation for the study of medicine.

Curriculum

The curriculum will include core requirements for the selected baccalaureate program and prerequisites for matriculation in medical school. Students in the program must maintain a minimum overall GPA of 3.5 and a minimum GPA of 3.4 in the sciences (biology, chemistry, physics) and mathematics. All required courses must be taken at the University of South Alabama unless otherwise approved in advance by the student's undergraduate program director and the associate dean of the College of Medicine.

Students will be required to participate in CP-200 (Career Planning; Clinical Observation) for a minimum of four quarters. Students will be given the opportunity to participate in a special summer premedical clerkship. These activities will be planned to give participants a broad exposure to medical education.

Students will be required to take the MCAT for admission to the College of Medicine and will be required to achieve a score above the national average. A formal assessment, including an interview, will be conducted after the student has completed 96 quarter hours of work. At this time, students' academic performance and continued interest in a medical career will be assessed.

Expenses

The 2003–2004 annual tuition for students at the University of South Alabama was $3,500 for residents and $7,000 for nonresidents. Medical school tuition for residents was $10,500 and $21,000 for nonresidents.

Financial Aid

Information can be obtained from the Office of Financial Aid, Administration Building, Room 260, University of South Alabama, Mobile, Alabama 36688-0002; or phone (251) 460-6231; or at ✑www.finaid2.usouthal.edu.

APPLICATION AND ACCEPTANCE POLICIES

Filing of application:
  Earliest date: Rolling applications
  Latest date: December 1, 2004
Application fee: $25
Acceptance notice:
  Earliest date: April 1, 2005
  Latest date: Until program is filled
Applicant's response to acceptance offer:
  Maximum time: 2 weeks
Deposit to hold place in class: None
Starting date: August 15, 2005

INFORMATION ON 2003–2004 ENTERING CLASS

Number of	In-State	Out-of-State	Total
Applicants	80	48	128
Applicants Interviewed	30	15	45
New Entrants	10	5	15
Total number of students enrolled in program: 60			

University of California, Riverside, and David Geffen School of Medicine at University of California, Los Angeles

Riverside, California

Address Inquiries To:

Student Affairs Officer
Division of Biomedical Sciences
University of California, Riverside
Riverside, California 92521-0121
(909) 787-4334
Web site: www.biomed.ucr.edu

Purpose

The University of California, Riverside/University of California, Los Angeles (UCR/UCLA) Thomas Haider Program in Biomedical Sciences offers the first two years of medical school at the University of California, Riverside, exclusively to 24 UCR undergraduates per year. Students complete their medical school training at the David Geffen School of Medicine at UCLA.

Requirements for Entrance

The 24 medical students are selected exclusively from UCR students pursuing bachelor's degrees in any major who have attended UCR for a minimum of two years prior to matriculation into Year 1 of medical school. Transfer students from community colleges, as well as students who have been full-time UCR students for six quarters of continuous enrollment (excluding summer sessions), are eligible to apply. For admission to UCR, students must meet the standard requirements of the University of California. Admissions requirements for the Haider Program are identical to those of the David Geffen School of Medicine at UCLA.

Selection Factors

Admission to the Program in Biomedical Sciences and to the David Geffen School of Medicine at UCLA depends on the student's undergraduate science, non-science, and overall GPAs at UCR, results of the MCAT, letters of recommendation, and required interviews. Additional selection criteria will be employed during the admissions process that are compatible with the mission of the Program in Biomedical Sciences: "To prepare graduates for distinguished medical careers in service to the people of California, with emphasis upon the needs of the underserved, inland, and rural populations."

In the 2003-2004 class entering the UCLA School of Medicine from Riverside's combined-degree program, the 24 students had an average undergraduate GPA of 3.8, an average MCAT of 9.6, and an average combined SAT score of 1328.

Curriculum

While most successful applicants will have their bachelor's degrees before matriculation, exceptional students can enter medical school following their junior year. These students must meet the minimum academic requirements for admission into the David Geffen School of Medicine at UCLA. They will either become eligible to enter medical school directly with senior status as undergraduates, or for the Early Decision Program and can spend an additional year prior to matriculation pursuing interests related to the goals of the program.

Expenses

For California residents, there is no tuition for undergraduate work, but fees amount to $5,952.75 per year. Cost for out-of-state undergraduate students total $20,163.75, including fees. For Years 1 and 2 of medical school, California residents pay fees of $15,746.50 annually; nonresidents pay $27,992.50.

Financial Aid

Sources of aid are scholarships, grants, work-study, and student loans. Applicants can receive more information from the Financial Aid Office, University of California, Riverside, Riverside, California 92521.

APPLICATION AND ACCEPTANCE POLICIES FOR UNDERGRADUATE PORTION AT RIVERSIDE

Filing of application:
   Earliest date: November 1, 2004
   Latest date: November 30, 2004
Application fee: $40
Acceptance notice:
   Earliest date: March 1, 2005
   Latest date: n/a
Applicant's response to acceptance offer:
   Latest date: May 1, 2005
Deposit to hold place in class: $100; nonrefundable
Starting date: August 1, 2005

INFORMATION ON 2003–2004 ENTERING CLASS UCLA SCHOOL OF MEDICINE FROM THE COMBINED-DEGREE PROGRAM AT RIVERSIDE

Number of	In-State	Out-of-State	Total
Applicants	n/a	n/a	57
Applicants Interviewed	n/a	n/a	57
New Entrants	n/a	n/a	24
Total number of students enrolled in program: n/a			

CHAPTER

10

University of California, San Diego, School of Medicine

La Jolla, California

Address Inquiries To:
Yvonne Coleman
Director of Medical Scholars Program
University of California, San Diego, School of Medicine
Office of Admissions, 0621
9500 Gilman Drive
La Jolla, California 92093-0621
(858) 534-3880; 534-5282 (FAX)
Web site:
http://meded.ucsd.edu/admissions/med_scholar.html

Purpose

The Medical Scholars Program was established to encourage the recruitment of unusually talented high school students, who would then be attracted to both the University of California, San Diego, (UCSD) undergraduate and medical schools, and to promote the goal of increasing diversity on both campuses.

Requirements for Entrance

Students are selected for this program during their senior year of high school. The program is open to California residents only. Applicants must meet course requirements for UCSD undergraduate admission. They must take either the SAT or ACT and achieve a minimum score of 1500 on the SAT or 32 on the ACT.

Selection Factors

To be eligible for consideration, applicants must have a minimum high school GPA of 4.0 and 1500 on the SAT. The average high school grade-point average for the 2003–2004 entering class was 4.29. Applicants must also demonstrate strong extracurricular involvement, particularly in community service and leadership. Letters of recommendation and an essay are additional considerations. An interview is required. The MCAT is not required.

Curriculum

This program leads to a baccalaureate degree granted by the University of California, San Diego, and to the M.D. degree granted by the UCSD School of Medicine. It takes eight years to fulfill the requirements for both degrees. The specific course requirements for the baccalaureate degree include a minimum of 6 quarters in either humanities or social sciences, and 15 quarters in the natural and physical sciences. Students must take Step 1 of the USMLE after the second year of medical school. Passing Steps 1 and 2 of the USMLE is required in order to be promoted and graduate.

Expenses

In 2003–2004 undergraduate student fees were $6,104.50, and medical school fees were $16,677.50.

Financial Aid

Sources of financial aid include scholarships, grants, loans, and work-study. Additional information is available through the undergraduate financial aid office: Building 201, University Center, La Jolla, California 92093-0013 or at ✎ www.ucsd.edu/finaid.

APPLICATION AND ACCEPTANCE POLICIES

Filing of application:
   Earliest date: February 1, 2004
   Latest date: March 31, 2004
Application fee: None
Acceptance notice:
   Earliest date: April 1, 2005
   Latest date: April 30, 2005
Applicant's response to acceptance offer:
   Maximum time: 1 week
Deposit to hold place in class: None
Starting date: September 2005

INFORMATION ON 2003–2004 ENTERING CLASS

Number of	In-State	Out-of-State	Total
Applicants	215	n/a	215
Applicants Interviewed	23	n/a	23
New Entrants	8	n/a	8
Total number of students enrolled in program: 26			

University of Southern California College of Letters, Arts, and Sciences and Keck School of Medicine

Los Angeles, California

Address Inquiries To:

Office of Admission
College of Letters, Arts, and Sciences
University of Southern California
Los Angeles, California 90089-0152
(213) 740-5930; 740-1338 (FAX)
E-mail: colladm@usc.edu
Web site: http//college.usc.edu/bamd

Purpose

The goal of this program is to encourage bright and motivated students to expand the breadth of their education through a diverse liberal arts education. Students accepted into this program have the opportunity to study a wide variety of disciplines beyond the course of the standard premedical curriculum. It is the hope of the university to graduate physicians who are educated in medical science, arts, and the humanities.

Requirements for Entrance

Students are selected for this program in the senior year of high school. Both residents and nonresidents of California and international students are eligible to apply. There are no specific high school course requirements, but applicants are required to take either the SAT or ACT.

Selection Factors

Academic factors considered include grades and standardized test scores. Participation in extracurricular activities and demonstrated leadership and community service are valued. Students who enrolled in 2003 had a mean high school GPA of 4.28 and a mean SAT score of 1470. An interview is required and is granted by invitation following careful evaluation of an applicant's file.

Curriculum

This program leads to a baccalaureate degree awarded by the University of Southern California, and the M.D. degree granted by the University of Southern California Keck School of Medicine.

This is not an accelerated program; all students must complete four years of undergraduate education and four years of medical school.

Students must complete requirements for the bachelor's degree and may pursue any major offered in the university that is compatible with the requirements of the program. There are specific requirements for the bachelor's degree, which include the humanities and social, natural, and physical sciences.

Advancement to the medical school phase of the program is based on acceptable academic performance and MCAT scores as defined by the program. The MCAT is required and must be taken by the spring of the junior year. Students must take USMLE Steps 1 and 2, and pass Step 1 of the USMLE in order to graduate.

Expenses

In 2003–2004, undergraduate tuition for residents and nonresidents was $28,692. The medical school tuition was $35,928.

Financial Aid

Sources of aid include scholarships, grants, work-study programs, and loans. Contact the Office of Financial Aid, University of Southern California, Los Angeles, California 90089-0912; or call (213) 740-1111; or visit ✎ www.usc.edu/dept/fao, for additional information.

APPLICATION AND ACCEPTANCE POLICIES

Filing of application:
  Earliest date: August 1, 2004
  Latest date: December 10, 2004
Application fee: None
Acceptance notice:
  Earliest date: n/a
  Latest date: April 1, 2005
Applicant's response to acceptance offer:
  Maximum time: 1 month
Deposit to hold place in class: $300; nonrefundable
Starting date: August 2005

INFORMATION ON 2003–2004 ENTERING CLASS

Number of	In-State	Out-of-State	Total
Applicants	139	349	488
Applicants Interviewed	60	40	100
New Entrants	17	10	27

Total number of students enrolled in program: 133

CHAPTER

10

University of Connecticut and University of Connecticut School of Medicine

Storrs, Connecticut

Address Inquiries To:

Office of Undergraduate Admissions
Special Programs in Medicine and Dental Medicine
University of Connecticut
2131 Hillside Road, U-88
Storrs, Connecticut 06269-3088
(860) 486-3137; 486-1476 (FAX)
Web site: www.uconn.edu

Purpose

This program offers gifted and talented high school students, who are focused on a career in medicine, the opportunity to combine a broad-based liberal arts program with a medical education. This program links undergraduate preparation with four years of medical education, resulting in dual degrees: a B.A. or B.S. and M.D.

Requirements for Entrance

Students are selected for this program during the senior year of high school. Both residents and nonresidents of Connecticut are eligible to apply. Applicants must take either the SAT I or ACT.

Selection Factors

To be considered for this program, the student should have the following: a high school class ranking in the top 5 percent; an overall high school grade-point average of 3.5 (4.0 scale); an SAT combined score of 1300 or an ACT composite score of 30; a completed regular undergraduate admission application and a supplemental application for the program in medicine by the January 1 postmark deadline; and an interview at the School of Medicine.

In addition, recommendations from teachers/advisors, as well as maturity, curricular activities, and commitment to the health profession, are considered.

Upon completion of undergraduate preparation, to matriculate in the School of Medicine, the student must meet additional criteria that include: maintaining a college 3.5 cumulative grade-point average (4.0 scale); ordinarily obtaining an MCAT score of 30+ (with a minimum score of 28), with section scores of 7 or greater; participating in clinical, research, and community service activities; and favorable interviews during the senior undergraduate year.

For more information on the medical school program, please contact Dr. Keat Sanford, assistant dean for medical school admissions, at (860) 679-3874 or sanford@nso1.uchc.edu.

Curriculum

Students must complete requirements for a baccalaureate degree from the University of Connecticut. Requirements include courses in the humanities and social sciences. The curriculum typically takes eight years to complete; Years 1 through 4 in the liberal arts and sciences, and Years 5 through 8 in the school of medicine.

The MCAT is required for admission to the medical school phase of the program. Students are required to pass Step 1 of the USMLE for promotion and Steps 1 and 2 of the USMLE in order to graduate.

Expenses

The undergraduate tuition for 2003-2004 was $5,442 for residents of Connecticut and $14,560 for nonresidents, plus fees. The medical school tuition for residents and nonresidents was $12,000 and $27,300, respectively.

Financial Aid

All enrolled candidates will be automatically considered for merit scholarships. A full range of financial aid options based on student financial need is available, as well. Candidates for need-based aid must submit the Free Application for Federal Student Aid (FAFSA) by March 1.

For more information about student aid programs, contact the University of Connecticut's Student Financial Aid Services at (860) 486-2819, write to U-4116, Storrs, Connecticut 06269, or visit the UConn homepage at www.uconn.edu.

APPLICATION AND ACCEPTANCE POLICIES

Filing of application:
  Earliest date: September 1, 2004
  Latest date: March 1, 2005
Application fee: $50
Acceptance notice:
  Earliest date: March 15, 2005
  Latest date: Until fall
Applicant's response to acceptance offer:
  Latest date: May 1, 2005
Deposit to hold place in class: $150; nonrefundable
Starting date: August 2005

INFORMATION ON 2003–2004 ENTERING CLASS

Number of	In-State	Out-of-State	Total
Applicants	102	96	198
Applicants Interviewed	14	11	25
New Entrants	4	0	4
Total number of students enrolled in program: 16			

68

Medical School Admission Requirements, 2005-2006

The George Washington University School of Medicine and Health Sciences and The Columbian College of Arts and Sciences

Washington, D.C.

Address Inquiries To:

Office of Admissions
The George Washington University
2121 "I" Street, N.W., Suite 201
Washington, D.C. 20052
(800) 447-3765
Web site: gwired.gwu.edu/adm
E-mail: gwadm@gwu.edu

Purpose

This program is designed to afford highly motivated and talented students the opportunity to prepare for a career in medicine and explore their academic interests beyond the required premedical coursework. The baccalaureate degree can be awarded after Year 4 (the first year of medical school) or received before entrance to the M.D. program. The School of Medicine and clinical facilities are on the campus of the university.

Requirements for Entrance

Students are selected in their senior year of high school. There are no residency requirements. In addition to meeting the requirements for freshman admission, applicants are also required to submit the results of the SAT II in writing, mathematics, and a science. Some experience within the health care field is expected.

Selection Factors

Academic factors considered in selecting applicants include strength of academic program, grades in high school, class rank, and standardized test scores. The average SAT score of the entering class for 2003-2004 was 1484. In addition to academic factors, extracurricular and health-related activities, community service, and letters of recommendation are reviewed. An interview is required. The interview is by invitation only.

Curriculum

This seven-year program leads to the baccalaureate degree granted by The George Washington University Columbian College of Arts and Sciences and the M.D. degree granted by The George Washington University School of Medicine and Health Sciences. The course requirements for the baccalaureate degree in the humanities and social sciences vary, but students *must* complete a minimum of 32 semester hours in the natural and physical sciences. The MCAT is not required for promotion to the medical school program.

A seminar offering health care information is a bridge between the B.A. and M.D. programs. The medicine portion of the curriculum includes a course, *Practice of Medicine*, which involves clinical apprenticeships, group-mentor teams, and problem-based learning groups. Students begin to work with patients in the first semester of Year 1 of the medical school phase of the program. A new state-of-the-art hospital opened in the summer of 2002.

Students are required to pass Steps 1 and 2 of the USMLE.

Expenses

Students in the program pay a special rate, which remains constant for all seven years of the program. Significant scholarship money is awarded annually.

Financial aid

Information may be obtained from The George Washington University, Office of Student Financial Assistance, 2121 "I" Street, N.W., #310, Washington, D.C. 20052. (1-800-222-6242)

APPLICATION AND ACCEPTANCE POLICIES

Filing of application:
 Earliest date: September 2004
 Latest date: December 1, 2004 (Part I);
  January 15, 2005 (Part II and Supplemental)
Application fee: $60
Acceptance notice:
 Earliest date: April, 2005
 Latest date: n/a
Applicant's response to acceptance offer:
 Latest date: May 1, 2005
Deposit to hold place in class: $800; nonrefundable
Starting date: August 2005

INFORMATION ON 2003–2004 ENTERING CLASS

Number of	In-State	Out-of-State	Total
Applicants	n/a	n/a	371
Applicants Interviewed	n/a	n/a	60
New Entrants	n/a	n/a	n/a
Total number of students enrolled in program: 22			

CHAPTER

10

Howard University

Washington, D.C.

Address Inquiries To:

Dr. G. Aboko-Cole, *Director*
Center for Preprofessional Education
College of Arts and Sciences
P.O. Box 473
Administration Building
Howard University
Washington, D.C. 20059
(202) 238-2363

Reprinted from Medical School Admission Requirements, 2004-2005

Purpose

The goal of this combined-degree program is to encourage talented undergraduate students to choose medicine as a career and to retain these excellent students in the Howard University College of Medicine.

Requirements for Entrance

Students can be selected for this program during the senior year of high school or during the first year of college. There are no state residence requirements. Applicants are expected to have completed the following courses by the time they graduate from high school: at least two years of a foreign language; at least one year each of biology, chemistry, and physics; two years of mathematics; and four years of English, including literature. They must take either the SAT or the ACT Assessment.

Selection Factors

The academic factors considered in offering admission to an applicant are rank in high school class, GPA, and test scores. Applicants are expected to be in the top 5 percent of their high school class. In the 2002–2003 entering class, the average GPA was 3.7 and the average SAT combined score was 1300. ACT Assessment cumulative scores ranged from 25 to 29. Personal qualities considered include self-esteem, realistic self-appraisal, a realistic assessment of the medical profession, leadership, and superior writing skills. An interview is required.

Curriculum

This program leads to a bachelor's degree awarded by the College of Arts and Sciences at Howard University and the M.D. degree granted by the College of Medicine, also at Howard University.

Students must complete work for a baccalaureate degree. They are expected to complete at least 40 semester hours of humanities and social sciences to fulfill general education requirements and at least 46 semester hours of natural and physical sciences. Students meet with the director (the advisor) of the Center for Preprofessional Education to design a curriculum tailored to their individual needs. The specific course selection must have the advisor's approval. Students are encouraged to select a major of personal interest.

The curricula for both degrees are completed in six years. In the first two years, the curriculum focuses on work toward the bachelor's degree and premedical requirements, and in the last four years the focus is on studies related to medicine. Students in this program must take the MCAT in April of the second year. The results of this test and the GPA are major factors in gaining admission to the medical school phase of the combined degree program. Students are also expected to take Steps 1 and 2 of the USMLE while at Howard University College of Medicine, and they must pass these examinations for graduation.

Expenses

In 2002–2003, the annual undergraduate tuition for students in the College of Arts and Sciences was $5,160 per semester; ($10,320 a year). There are also student fees, which are subject to change.

Financial Aid

Information can be obtained from the Office of Financial Aid, Howard University, Johnson Administration Building, 2400 - 6th Street, N.W., Washington, D.C. 20059.

APPLICATION AND ACCEPTANCE POLICIES

Filing of application:
  Earliest date: n/a
  Latest date: Rolling admission
Application fee: $45
Acceptance notice:
  Earliest date: n/a
  Latest date: n/a
Applicant's response to acceptance offer:
  n/a
Deposit to hold place in class: $150; nonrefundable
Starting date: Late August 2004

INFORMATION ON 2002–2003 ENTERING CLASS

Number of	In-State	Out-of-State	Total
Applicants	n/a	n/a	40
Applicants Interviewed	n/a	n/a	20
New Entrants	n/a	n/a	10
Total number of students enrolled in program: 10			

University of Florida College of Medicine

Gainesville, Florida

Address Inquiries To:

Robyn Sheppard
Medical Selection Committee
University of Florida College of Medicine
P.O. Box 100216
Gainesville, Florida 32610
(352) 392-4569; 846-0622 (FAX)
Web site: www.med.ufl.edu

Purpose

The Junior Honors Medical Program is for undergraduate students who have chosen a career in the medical profession and who have demonstrated superior scholastic ability and personal development during their first two academic years.

Requirements for Entrance

Students are selected for this program during the sophomore year of college. Admission is open to all possible candidates who are Florida residents. There are no specific high school course requirements; however, admissions tests such as SAT achievement tests are required.

Selection Factors

The academic factors considered in offering admission to an applicant are sophomore standing, GPA, and completion of grades in prerequisite courses. The MCAT is currently not required. Selected applicants are invited for a required interview.

Curriculum

The most frequent major for the baccalaureate degree is interdisciplinary biomedical sciences. It is awarded at the University of Florida College of Liberal Arts and Sciences. Requirements are evaluated by the CLAS Advisement Center. The Doctor of Medicine degree is awarded at the University of Florida College of Medicine. It takes seven years to complete requirements for both degrees.

All courses in the first two years are liberal arts courses. In Year 3, half of the curriculum is in the liberal arts and half in medicine. In Years 4 through 7, all courses are in medicine.

Year	Percent Liberal Arts	Percent Medicine
1	100	0
2	100	0
3	50	50
4	0	100
5	0	100
6	0	100
7	0	100

Expenses

Undergraduate and medical school tuition in 2003–2004 was $58.45 per credit hour for state residents, plus fees.

Financial Aid

Several sources of financial aid are available to students, including college scholarships and loans, federal Stafford loans, and state National Merit and Robert Byrd Scholarships, if eligible. For more information, contact Office of Financial Aid, P.O. Box 100216 HSC, Gainesville, Florida 32610, (352) 392-7800, or E-mail eparris@ufl.edu.

APPLICATION AND ACCEPTANCE POLICIES

Filing of application:
    Earliest date: January 15, 2004
    Latest date: February 1, 2004
Application fee: None
Acceptance notice:
    Earliest date: May 15, 2005
    Latest date: August 15, 2005
Applicant's response to acceptance offer:
    Maximum time: 2 weeks
Deposit to hold place in class: None
Starting date: August 2005

INFORMATION ON 2003–2004 ENTERING CLASS

Number of	In-State	Out-of-State	Total
Applicants	83	4	87
Applicants Interviewed	28	0	28
New Entrants	12	0	12
Total number of students enrolled in program: 12			

CHAPTER

10

University of Miami

Miami, Florida

Address Inquiries To:

Office of Admissions
University of Miami
P.O. Box 248025
Coral Gables, FL 33124
(305) 284-4323
Web sites: www.miami.edu
www.miami.edu/medical-admissions

Purpose

The Honors Program in Medicine (HPM) offers exceptionally motivated and talented high school students who have reached a mature and independent decision to study medicine, an opportunity to earn the B.S. and M.D. degrees in either six or seven years.

Requirements for Entrance

Applicants must be U.S. citizens or permanent residents. Both residents and nonresidents of Florida are considered for admission. Applicants must be in their last year of high school at the time of application. Applicants must have a minimum combined score of 1360 on the SAT or a composite score of 31 on the ACT, and take the SAT II Subject Tests in English, mathematics, and science (no minimum score required). All must have completed eight semesters of English and mathematics and two semesters each of biology and chemistry by the time of graduation from high school.

Selection Factors

Academic factors taken into account include scores on standardized tests, the quality of the high school curriculum (including the number and nature of Advanced Placement courses), and the amount of university-level work already completed. Of equal importance to academic achievements are personal factors such as maturity of thought and action, common sense, empathy, interpersonal skills, appropriate freedom from parental influence, and social cognizance. Most important, the applicant must have made a practical decision to study medicine based on self-initiated patient-contact experiences. "Skipping" grades or graduating early from high school confers no advantage.

Curriculum

The first two years are spent on the Coral Gables campus taking required science and humanities courses and focusing almost exclusively on work related to the bachelor's degree. The undergraduate portion of the curriculum may be extended to three years if the student is in good academic standing and has established a clear plan of academic and personal growth. HPM students major most frequently in biology, followed by biochemistry. All HPM students must have a 3.2 science GPA and a 3.4 cumulative GPA and take the MCAT before starting medical school. MCAT scores do not factor into subsequent promotion to medical school but are used as one indicator of the student's preparedness to study medicine. The medical curriculum is four years long. HPM students usually qualify for the B.S. degree after successfully completing the first year of medical school.

Expenses

In 2003–2004, tuition for the undergraduate portion of the HPM program was $24,810. Tuition at the School of Medicine was $28,050 ($36,740 for nonresidents), and fees were $140.

Financial Aid

Scholarships, work-study, loans, and state tuition grants are sources of financial assistance. Information on undergraduate financial aid is available from the Office of Admissions on the Coral Gables campus.

APPLICATION AND ACCEPTANCE POLICIES

Filing of application:
  Earliest date: October 15, 2004
  Latest date for receipt of all materials: January 15, 2005
Application fee: $50
Acceptance notice:
  All decisions are made on April 1, 2005
Applicant's response to acceptance offer:
  Maximum time: 1 month
Deposit to hold place in class (applied to tuition): $300; nonrefundable
Starting date: August 2005

INFORMATION ON 2003–2004 ENTERING CLASS

Number of	In-State	Out-of-State	Total
Applicants	n/a	n/a	139
Applicants Interviewed	n/a	n/a	126
New Entrants	n/a	n/a	26
Total number of students enrolled in the program: 114			

Rosalind Franklin University of Medicine and Science/ Chicago Medical School and Illinois Institute of Technology

Chicago, Illinois

Address Inquiries To:

Office of Admission
Illinois Institute of Technology
B.S./M.D. Program
Rosalind Franklin University of Medicine and Science
10 West 33rd Street • Chicago, Illinois 60616
(312) 567-3025; outside Chicago, (800) 448-2329
Web sites: www.iit.edu • www.finchcms.edu
On-line application: www.iit.edu/~apply

Purpose

The honors program allows superior students to earn both an Accreditation Board for Engineering and Technology (ABET)-accredited Bachelor of Science degree in biomedical chemical, electrical, mechanical engineering, molecular biochemistry and biophysics, computer science, and the M.D. degree in eight years. The goal is to produce graduates who understand the intricacies of technology applied to medicine and who will be future innovators in improving medical diagnoses and treatment for their patients.

Requirements for Entrance

Students are selected for this program during their senior year of high school. The program is open to U.S. citizens and permanent residents. Applicants are expected to have completed the following courses by the time of graduation from high school: four years of mathematics (through calculus) and three years of life sciences (chemistry, biology, and physics). Applicants must take either the SAT or the ACT Assessment.

Students must eventually take the MCAT, but scores are not a factor in admission to the medical school.

Selection Factors

Academic factors considered in offering admission to an applicant include high school class rank, GPA, curriculum, essay, and letters of recommendation. In the 2003–2004 entering class, the average score on the ACT was 33 and on the SAT was 1440; the average high school grade-point average was 4.0. An interview is required. Students should also demonstrate an interest in engineering and medicine through medical-related research, hospital volunteer work, or participation in engineering and medically-related organizations.

Curriculum

This program leads to a baccalaureate degree granted by the Illinois Institute of Technology (IIT) and to the M.D. degree granted by the Rosalind Franklin University of Medicine and Science/Chicago Medical School. The most frequent majors for a baccalaureate degree are molecular biochemistry and biophysics, followed by biomedical engineering. Continuation on to medical school is contingent upon maintaining a 3.3 GPA, earning no course grade below a C, and displaying ethical behavior appropriate for a future physician. Students enter medical school in the fifth year. Students are required to pass Steps 1 and 2 of the USMLE before graduation.

Expenses

In 2003–2004, the undergraduate tuition was $19,775. The medical school tuition was $36,740, plus $100 in yearly fees. Tuition is subject to change at both institutions.

Financial Aid

Sources of financial aid include university grants, work-study, loans, and merit scholarships. For more information, contact Undergraduate Admissions at (312) 567-3025 or (800) 448-2329 (outside Chicago); ✎ www.iit.edu, or admission@iit.edu.

APPLICATION AND ACCEPTANCE POLICIES

Filing of application:
  Earliest date: n/a
  Latest date: January 15, 2005
Application fee: $30
Acceptance notice:
  Earliest date: n/a
  Latest date: April, 2005
Applicant's response to acceptance offer:
  Latest date: May 1, 2005
Deposit to hold place in class: $200; nonrefundable
Starting date: August 16, 2005

INFORMATION ON 2003-2004 ENTERING CLASS

Number of	In-State	Out-of-State	Total
Applicants	n/a	n/a	300
Applicants Interviewed	n/a	n/a	60
New Entrants	n/a	n/a	20
Total number of students enrolled in the program: 70			

Northwestern University Feinberg School of Medicine

Chicago, Illinois

Address Inquiries To:

Office of Admission and Financial Aid
Northwestern University
1801 Hinman Avenue
Evanston, Illinois 60204-3060
(312) 908-8915; 908-0855 (FAX)
Website: www.med.northwestern.edu/hpmd
E-mail: ug-admission@northwestern.edu

Purpose

The Honors Program in Medical Education (HPME), one of the oldest in the nation, provides highly motivated and gifted students an individualized undergraduate curriculum that shortens premedical preparation and assures entry into medical school.

Requirements for Entrance

Students are selected for this program during the senior year of high school. Both residents and nonresidents of Illinois are eligible to apply. Applicants must meet the following high school course requirements: English, eight semesters; mathematics, including differential and integral calculus, eight semesters; chemistry, two semesters; physics, two semesters; biology, two semesters; and foreign language, four semesters. They must take either the SAT I or the ACT Assessment plus the SAT II Subject Tests in mathematics IIC, chemistry, and writing.

Selection Factors

Academic factors considered in selecting applicants include class rank, grades in high school, and scores on college entrance tests. Average test scores of students in the 2003–2004 entering class were: SAT Verbal, 759; SAT Mathematics, 777; CEEB Achievement Tests–Writing, 752; Mathematics IIC, 786; Chemistry, 763. Nonacademic factors considered are motivation, concern for others, maturity, and involvement in extracurricular activities. An interview is required.

Curriculum

The degrees offered in the honors program are a baccalaureate degree (B.S. in medicine, B.S. in biomedical engineering, B.S. in communication, or B.A.) and the M.D., all from Northwestern University.

Students must complete requirements for a baccalaureate degree in addition to the required science courses (inorganic and organic chemistry, calculus-based physics, biological science sequence). The majority of students in the Weinberg College of Arts & Science major in biological sciences but have many other options within the college. Students in the McCormick School of Engineering & Applied Sciences major in biomedical engineering, taking the basic and advanced engineering courses, in addition to non-science courses. The program in the School of Communication includes special courses in communication sciences and disorders.

The curriculum usually takes seven years to complete. In Years 1 through 3, the curriculum consists entirely of courses in the liberal arts and sciences, engineering, or speech. In Years 4 through 7, the curriculum focuses on medicine. The MCAT is not required. Students must take Step 1 of the USMLE, but passing that examination is not a requirement for graduation from the medical school.

Expenses

In 2003–2004 tuition for the B.S. degree was $28,404 per year, plus annual fees of $1,326. Medical school tuition was $34,998, plus annual fees of $2,060.

Financial Aid

Sources of aid include Northwestern University and federal, state, and private programs. Undergraduate applicants can receive more information from the Office of Admission and Financial Aid, 1801 Hinman Avenue, Evanston, Illinois 60204–3060; or phone (847) 491-7271. Information about medical school financial aid can be obtained from Financial Aid Professional Schools, Abbott Hall, 710 Superior Street, Chicago, Illinois 60611.

APPLICATION AND ACCEPTANCE POLICIES

Filing of application:
  Earliest date: n/a
  Latest date: January 1, 2005
      of applicant's senior year of high school
Application fee: $60
Acceptance notice:
  Earliest date: April 1, 2005
  Latest date: n/a
Applicant's response to acceptance offer:
  Latest date: May 1, 2005
Deposit to hold place in class: $400; nonrefundable
Starting date: September 14, 2005

INFORMATION ON 2003–2004 ENTERING CLASS

Number of	In-State	Out-of-State	Total
Applicants	n/a	n/a	509
Applicants Interviewed	n/a	n/a	135
New Entrants	n/a	n/a	44

Total number of students enrolled in program: 172

University of Illinois at Chicago College of Medicine

Chicago, Illinois

Address Inquiries To:

Special Projects Unit
Office of Admissions and Records
University of Illinois at Chicago
P.O. Box 6020
Chicago, Illinois 60680-6020
(312) 996-8365; 413-7628 (FAX)
Web site: www.uic.edu

Purpose

The Guaranteed Professional Program Admissions (GPPA) program is a combined effort of the UIC (University of Chicago) Honors College on the undergraduate campus and the College of Medicine. This program is offered only to Illinois resident high school seniors. The GPPA guarantees incoming freshmen a seat in the College of Medicine (provided they qualify upon completion of their undergraduate studies at UIC).

Requirements for Entrance

Students are selected for this program during the senior year of high school. There are no specific high school course requirements.

Selection Factors

The academic factors considered in offering admission to an applicant are rank in high school class, grade-point average, and test scores. Applicants must be in the top 15 percent of their high school class. Applicants must have a minimum ACT composite score of 28, or a minimum SAT score of 1240.

This program is limited to Illinois residents. In addition to academic factors, extracurricular health-related activities and letters of recommendations are required. Selected applicants are invited for a required interview.

Curriculum

Students in this program are required to complete a baccalaureate degree at the University of Illinois at Chicago (UIC). Students are free to choose any of UIC's majors in eight undergraduate colleges. The most popular major is biology, followed by chemistry and biochemistry. The Doctor of Medicine degree is awarded at the University of Illinois College of Medicine. It takes at least seven years to fulfill the requirements for both degrees.

Students admitted to the program are required to take the MCAT during their junior year. Students must earn an average score of at least 10, with no section score below 9. Students must maintain a 4.5/5.0 cumulative grade-point average. From freshman year to junior year, students must take a total of four courses that will introduce them to various aspects of the medical profession. Once enrolled in the College of Medicine, students in the program are bound by the policies in force at the time of their entry.

Expenses

The undergraduate tuition for 2003-2004 was $4,898 for nonresidents, plus annual student fees of $1,906. The medical school tuition was $20,874 for residents, $48,310 for nonresidents, plus annual student fees of $1,906.

Financial Aid

For information about undergraduate financial aid, contact: Financial Aid Office, 1200 W. Harrison Avenue, 1800 SSB, Chicago, Illinois 60607, (312) 996-3126.

Financial aid available to medical students includes federal, state, and institutional loan programs, as well as need-based scholarships and other scholarships.

APPLICATION AND ACCEPTANCE POLICIES

Filing of application:
　Earliest date: September 15, 2004
　Latest date: December 15, 2004
Application fee: $40
Acceptance notice:
　Earliest date: March 15, 2005
　Latest date: March 31, 2005
Applicant's response to acceptance offer:
　Maximum time: 1 $1/2$ months
Deposit to hold place in class: None
Starting date: August 2005

INFORMATION ON 2003-2004 ENTERING CLASS

Number of	In-State	Out-of-State	Total
Applicants	287	n/a	287
Applicants Interviewed	100	n/a	100
New Entrants	42	n/a	42
Total number of students enrolled in program: 164			

CHAPTER
10

Boston University

Boston, Massachusetts

Address Inquiries To:

Office of Undergraduate Admissions
Boston University
121 Bay State Road
Boston, Massachusetts 02215
(617) 353-2300; 353-9695 (FAX)
Web site: www.bu.edu/admissions/discover/accelerate.html

Purpose

This combined-degree program, one of the oldest in the nation, provides an undergraduate premedical preparation that also emphasizes the humanities and social sciences and affords a quality medical education even though the overall period of study is shortened.

Requirements for Entrance

Students are selected for the program at Boston University during the senior year of high school (or after high school if they have not been enrolled in any other degree-granting program). There are no state residence requirements. Students who are completing their high school graduation requirements in three years in order to graduate early are not eligible for this program. Applicants are expected to have completed the following courses by the time they graduate from high school: four years each of English and mathematics (one year of calculus is required); three years of a foreign language; and one year each of biology, chemistry (AP chemistry is *strongly* recommended), and physics. They must take the SAT II Subject Exams in writing, mathematics IIC, and chemistry. The SAT II Subject Exam in a foreign language is recommended.

Selection Factors

The academic factors taken into account in offering admission to an applicant include the following: the high school GPA, the SAT I or ACT score, scores on the SAT II Subject Exams, rank in high school class, and the nature of the applicant's high school curriculum. In the 2003–2004 entering class, the average high school GPA was an unweighted 3.90 on a 4.0 scale, and rank in class was in the top two percent. The average combined SAT score was 1490. SAT II Subject Exam scores in chemistry averaged 715. The scores on the SAT II Subject Exams in Math IIC averaged 760 and in Writing averaged 730. Personal characteristics sought in applicants are motivation, maturity, and an understanding of a career in medicine. An interview with College of Arts and Sciences and School of Medicine faculty is required.

Curriculum

This program leads to a baccalaureate degree granted by the College of Arts and Sciences at Boston University and to the M.D. degree awarded by Boston University School of Medicine.

Students must complete work for the baccalaureate degree with a major in medical sciences and a minor concentration in a division of the College of Arts and Sciences. Students must also satisfy the course distribution and language requirements of the College. Requirements for this degree include nine one-semester courses in the natural and physical sciences and two one-semester courses in the humanities, mathematics and computer science, and social sciences. The program is seven years in length, with an eight-year option.

Students must meet GPA and MCAT requirements of the program. They are also required to take Step 1 of the USMLE during the medical school portion of the program. Taking Step 2 of the USMLE is not a requirement for graduation but is strongly recommended.

Expenses

In 2003–2004, undergraduate tuition was $28,512 per year for residents and nonresidents, plus $394 for student fees. Medical school tuition was $36,530 for residents and nonresidents.

Financial Aid

The usual sources of financial aid are available to students during the undergraduate portion of this program. Once in the medical school, students can qualify for need-based, low-interest, and government-sponsored loans. More information about aid can be obtained from the Office of Financial Assistance, Boston University, 881 Commonwealth Avenue, Boston, Massachusetts 02215; or phone (617) 353-2965.

APPLICATION AND ACCEPTANCE POLICIES

Filing of application:
  Earliest date: September 1, 2004
  Latest date: December 1, 2004
Application fee: $70; $60 online
Acceptance notice:
  Earliest date: March 15, 2005
  Latest date: April 15, 2005
Applicant's response to acceptance offer:
  Latest date: May 1, 2005
Deposit to hold place in class: $500; nonrefundable
Starting date: n/a

INFORMATION ON 2003–2004 ENTERING CLASS

Number of	In-State	Out-of-State	Total
Applicants	40	360	400
Applicants Interviewed	8	106	114
New Entrants	0	24	24
Total number of students enrolled in program: n/a			

Michigan State University College of Human Medicine

East Lansing, Michigan

Address Inquiries To:

Margo Smith, M.A.
College of Human Medicine
Office of Admissions
A-239 Life Sciences
Michigan State University
East Lansing, Michigan 48824
(517) 353-9620; 432-0021 (FAX)
Web site: www.chm.msu.edu (click on MD Admissions)

Purpose

The goal of the program is to educate excellent primary care physicians who will establish caring relationships with patients, who will practice in Michigan, especially in underserved rural and inner-city areas, and who will commit to a lifetime of learning and ethical practice.

Requirements for Entrance

Students are selected for this program in the senior year of high school. Both residents and nonresidents of Michigan are eligible to apply. There are no specific high school course requirements, but applicants are required to have an ACT composite score in the range of 29 or higher, or an SAT composite score in the range of 1280 or higher.

Selection Factors

Academic selection factors include class rank in the top 10 percent or a GPA of at least 3.6 achieved in a college preparatory curriculum. Competitive applicants will have strong communication skills, demonstrated leadership, significant work or volunteer experience in the community, and meaningful exposure to the medical setting. Students interested in a career as a primary care physician and students from groups underrepresented in medicine are encouraged to apply. Qualified applicants are invited for a required interview.

In the 2003–2004 entering class, the high school GPA averaged 4.1, and the average mean ACT score was 31; the SAT I score averaged 1417.

Curriculum

Medical Scholars is an enrichment program leading to a baccalaureate degree awarded by Michigan State University and to the M.D. degree granted by Michigan State University College of Human Medicine. It is not an accelerated program; all students must complete requirements for a B.A. or B.S. degree and four years of medical school.

The most frequent majors are biology and human physiology. Premedical course requirements include eight semesters each of humanities, social sciences, natural sciences, and physical sciences.

Medical Scholars complete a liberal arts component that may include a specialization in Health and Humanities. They participate in a research project under the direction of Michigan State University faculty. They complete a year of volunteer community service and at least a year of medical/clinical experience.

Students in this program are not required to take the MCAT for promotion or admission to the medical school. The student must pass Steps 1 and 2 of the USMLE in order to graduate. The USMLE Step 1 is administered at the completion of Year 2.

Expenses

In 2003–2004, undergraduate tuition was $6,266 for residents and $16,170 for nonresidents. Student fees averaged $822 for the year. Medical school tuition for residents was $19,726 and for nonresidents, $43,526. The average cost of student fees was $1,225.

Financial Aid

A number of options are available for aid. These include college work-study, Pell Grants, student aid grants, Supplemental Educational Opportunities Grants, subsidized and Unsubsidized Stafford loans, Parent Loans for Undergraduate Students, and private loans. Applicants can receive more information from Michigan State University, Office of Financial Aid, 252 Student Services, East Lansing, Michigan 48824; (517) 353-5940, 432-1155 (FAX), or E-mail: finaid@msu.edu/med.

APPLICATION AND ACCEPTANCE POLICIES

Filing of application:
  Earliest date: August 15, 2004
  Latest date: November 1, 2004
Application fee: $60
Acceptance notice:
  Earliest date: March 15, 2005
  Latest date: June 15, 2005
Applicant's response to acceptance offer:
  Maximum time: 2 weeks
Deposit to hold place in class: $100; nonrefundable
Starting date: August 2005

INFORMATION ON 2003–2004 ENTERING CLASS

Number of	In-State	Out-of-State	Total
Applicants	157	56	213
Applicants Interviewed	35	11	46
New Entrants	10	0	10
Total number of students enrolled in program: 35			

CHAPTER

10

Wayne State University
School of Medicine

Detroit, Michigan

Address Inquiries To:
Nancy Galster
Program Coordinator, Honors Program
Wayne State University School of Medicine
2100 Undergraduate Library
Detroit, Ml 48202
(313) 577-8523; 577-6425 (FAX)
Web site: www.admissions.wayne.edu

Purpose

The MedStart Program is intended to train medical innovators and creative thinkers. As undergraduates, students are treated as part of the medical community, with an emphasis on mentoring and research.

Requirements for Entrance

Students are selected for this program during their senior year of high school. The program is open to residents of Michigan, along with the four contiguous counties of Ohio (Fulton, Lucas, Ottawa, and Williams). Residents of the District of Columbia may also apply. Although there are no specific high school course requirements, applicants are required to take the ACT.

Selection Factors

To be considered for this program, applicants must have a minimum ACT score of 25 and a high school GPA of at least 3.5. Community service, team activities, leadership, extracurricular activities, and experience in health care are among the personal attributes and experiential factors sought in applicants. An interview is also required.

Once admitted into the program, students are expected to maintain an overall GPA of 3.3 in undergraduate studies. For subsequent admission to Wayne State University School of Medicine, students in this program must complete all prerequisites courses, take the MCAT, and then apply through AMCAS. MCAT scores are not a factor for promotion or admission to the medical school phase.

Curriculum

The Honors Program, eight years in duration, allows students to obtain a baccalaureate degree from Wayne State University and the M.D. degree from Wayne State University School of Medicine.

During the four years of the undergraduate studies, students will spend 100 percent of their time in coursework related to the bachelor's degree. The same amount of time, in the last four years of medical school, will be spent in achieving a medical degree. Students must meet university requirements for the Honors Program and degree completion.

Throughout the eight-year baccalaureate-medical program, monthly seminars are held, which are relevant to medical fields and topics in medicine. Students will have a 10-week paid clinical research experience in the summer following the junior undergraduate year. Mentors from both faculty and students will be provided.

Expenses

In 2003-2004, undergraduate tuition for residents was $4,662 and $10,683 for nonresidents, plus annual fees of $662.40. The tuition for medical school residents was $16,873.20 and $35,114 for nonresidents, in addition to annual fees of $530.

Financial Aid

Information can be obtained from the Office of Scholarships and Financial Aid, Welcome Center, P.O. Box 4230, Detroit, MI 48202, by telephone (313) 577-3378, or visit ✐www.financialaid.wayne.edu.

APPLICATION AND ACCEPTANCE POLICIES

Filing of application:
  Earliest date: December 1, 2004
  Latest date: February 15, 2005
Application fee: $30
Acceptance notice:
  Earliest date: April 1, 2005
  Latest date: n/a
Applicant's response to acceptance offer:
  Latest date: TBD
Deposit to hold place in class: $30; nonrefundable
Starting Date: September 6, 2005

INFORMATION ON 2003–2004 ENTERING CLASS

Number of	In-State	Out-of-State	Total
Applicants	n/a	n/a	n/a
Applicants Interviewed	n/a	n/a	n/a
New Entrants	n/a	n/a	n/a
Total number of students enrolled in program:			
New program; approximately 16 students expected.			

Saint Louis University School of Medicine

St. Louis, Missouri

Address Inquiries To:
Donald O. Schreiweis, Ph.D.
Director, Preprofessional Health Studies
Academic Resources Center
Saint Louis University School of Medicine
3840 Lindell Boulevard, Suite 210
St. Louis, MO 63108-3414
(314) 977-2840; 977-3660 (FAX)
Web site: http://www.slu.edu/colleges/AS/phs/Scholars1.html

Purpose

This combined-degree program awards special recognition to exceptional first year (freshmen) premedical students. It is intended to enhance the educational experience and reduce the stress associated with premedical-medical education.

Requirements for Entrance

Students are selected for this program in their senior year of high school. Both residents and nonresidents of Missouri are eligible to apply to the program. Applicants are required to complete the following courses prior to graduation from high school: one year of biology, one year of chemistry, and three years of mathematics. In addition to meeting these requirements, applicants must take either the ACT (minimum score of 30) or SAT (minimum score of 1320).

Selection Factors

Outstanding academic achievement in high school is a favorable factor in qualifying for the combined-degree program at Saint Louis University. Selected applicants usually rank in the top 10 percent of their high school class. The average high school GPA for the 2003-2004 entering class was 3.88. Admissions essays and recommendations from high school counselors and teachers are also considerable factors for admission to the program. It is required that all candidates achieve a minimum ACT score of 30 or SAT score of 1320. An interview is not required.

Students are required to take the MCAT in April of the junior year (no minimum score required). MCAT scores are not a factor for promotion or admission to the medical school phase of the program.

Curriculum

This eight-year program leads to a baccalaureate degree awarded by Saint Louis University and to an M.D. degree granted by the Saint Louis University School of Medicine. Students are required to pursue a major in the College of Arts and Sciences, clinical lab science in Allied Health, or Biomedical Engineering. The most frequent major is biology, followed by chemistry and psychology. During the first four years of the curriculum, students will spend 100 percent of their time in coursework related to the bachelor's degree, which includes 42 to 46 semester hours of natural and physical science, 3 to 4 semester hours of mathematics, and 12 semester hours of humanities. The remaining four years focus on achieving the M.D. degree.

Expenses

In 2003-2004, the undergraduate tuition for residents and nonresidents was $22,050, plus annual fees of $160.

Financial Aid

Information can be obtained from the Office of Financial Aid/Scholarships, DuBourg Hall 121, Saint Louis University, 221 North Grand Boulevard, St. Louis, MO 63103.

APPLICATION AND ACCEPTANCE POLICIES

No application. Prospective students are invited to this program. The selection process begins December 10, 2004. Applicant must be accepted to an undergraduate freshman class.

INFORMATION ON 2003–2004 ENTERING CLASS

Number of	In-State	Out-of-State	Total
Applicants	74	156	230
Applicants Interviewed	0	0	0
New Entrants	52	37	89

Total number of students enrolled in program: 204

CHAPTER
10

University of Missouri-Columbia School of Medicine

Columbia, Missouri

Address Inquiries To:
Judy Nolke
MA215 Medical Sciences Building
University of Missouri-Columbia
School of Medicine
Columbia, Missouri 65212
(573) 882-9219; 884-2988 (FAX)
Web site: www.muhealth.org/medicine

Purpose

The Conley Scholars Program recruits gifted high school students from Missouri and contiguous states to attend the University of Missouri–Columbia (MU) as undergraduates and to be pre-admitted to the MU School of Medicine.

Requirements for Entrance

Students are selected in their senior year of high school. Both residents of Missouri and contiguous states are eligible to apply to the program. In addition to meeting the requirements for freshman admission, candidates must have a composite ACT score of 30 or SAT of 1300 or higher (Verbal + Mathematics).

Selection Factors

Academic factors that are taken into consideration include rigorous coursework and a high level of achievement. In the 2003-2004 entering class, the average GPA was 3.97 (unweighted on a 4-point scale), and the average ACT Assessment score was 32.2. Selected applicants are invited for a required interview. Additional factors evaluated include school and community activities and tested motivation toward medicine.

Curriculum

This is not an accelerated program; all students must complete four years of undergraduate education and four years of medical school. Students may choose any major, but they must complete the same coursework required of all premedical students. Once their four-year baccalaureate degree program is completed, they may enter medical school at MU or they may choose to attend medical school elsewhere.

Students in this program are not required to take the MCAT for admission to the medical school. After the second year of medical school, students must pass the USMLE Step 1 in order to be promoted and graduate. Passing Step 2 of the USMLE is required in order to graduate from the medical school.

Expenses

In 2003-2004, the annual undergraduate tuition for residents was $5,449, plus $700 in student fees, and for nonresidents was $14,266, with annual student fees of $700. The medical school tuition was $19,572 for residents and $38,358 for nonresidents.

Financial Aid

The sources of financial aid are the same as those for all other enrolled students at the University of Missouri-Columbia. Visit ✍ www.missouri.edu for more information on financial aid.

APPLICATION AND ACCEPTANCE POLICIES

Filing of application:
  Earliest date: n/a
  Latest date: February 1, 2004
Application fee: None
Acceptance notice:
  Earliest date: n/a
  Latest date: May 1, 2005
Applicant's response to acceptance offer:
  Maximum time: n/a
Deposit to hold place in class: None
Starting date: August 2005

INFORMATION ON 2003–2004 ENTERING CLASS

Number of	In-State	Out-of-State	Total
Applicants	69	23	92
Applicants Interviewed	55	15	70
New Entrants	20	8	28
Total number of students enrolled in program: 68			

University of Missouri—Kansas City School of Medicine

Kansas City, Missouri

Address Inquiries To:

Council on Selection
University of Missouri–Kansas City
School of Medicine
2411 Holmes
Kansas City, Missouri 64108–2792
(816) 235-1870; 235-6579 (FAX)
Web site: www.umkc.edu/medicine

Purpose

This combined baccalaureate-M.D. degree program integrates the humanities, social sciences, basic sciences, and clinical medicine throughout the curriculum so that graduates will have the background for lifelong learning in order to meet the needs of their patients, families, and communities.

Requirements for Entrance

The program is primarily designed for high school graduates who are entering college. Residents and nonresidents of Missouri are eligible to apply. An applicant's high school curriculum must include, at a minimum, the following: eight semesters of English; eight semesters of mathematics; six semesters of science, including two semesters of biology and two semesters of chemistry; six semesters of social studies; two semesters of fine arts; and four semesters of a foreign language. One semester of computer science is recommended but not required. Applicants must meet a minimum academic screen based on the ACT composite score and rank in high school class.

Selection Factors

Applicants' academic potential is judged by the quality of high school courses, rank in high school class, and scores on the ACT. In the 2003–2004 entering class, the average test score was in the 90th percentile, and the average rank in class was in the 92nd percentile. Personal qualities include maturity, leadership, stamina, reliability, motivation for medicine, range of interests, interpersonal skills, compassion, and job experience. Qualified applicants are invited for a required interview.

Curriculum

The six-year curriculum leads to a baccalaureate degree granted by the University of Missouri, Kansas City (UMKC) College of Arts and Sciences or the UMKC School of Biological Sciences and the doctor of medicine degree granted by the School of Medicine.

Students must complete requirements for the bachelor's degree. Students have a choice of majors, but most select liberal arts or psychology. Course requirements for the bachelor's degree in liberal arts include 21 semester hours of humanities, 21 semester hours of social sciences, and 50 semester hours of natural and physical sciences.

The curriculum typically takes six years to complete. During the first two years of the curriculum, students spend 75 percent of their time in coursework related to the bachelor's degree. Conversely, in the last four years, students spend 75 percent of their time in courses, clerkships, and electives related to the M.D. degree. Thus, the study of liberal arts, basic sciences, and clinical medicine is integrated throughout the entire curriculum. Students are assigned a faculty advisor (docent), and younger students are paired with older students. During the last four years of the curriculum, students attend a general medicine outpatient clinic for a half-day each week.

Students in this program do not take the MCAT. They must pass Steps 1 and 2 of the USMLE for graduation.

An alternate path is available for extended study.

Expenses

In 2003–2004, estimated tuition for Years 1 and 2 was $22,903 in-state per year and $45,691 out-of-state, plus $1,086 for student fees. Estimated tuition for Years 3 through 6 was $25,094 in-state per year and $50,405 out-of-state, plus $1,086 for student fees.

Financial Aid

Contact the UMKC Financial Aid Office at the Administrative Center, 5115 Oak, Kansas City, Missouri 64110, (816) 235-1154.

APPLICATION AND ACCEPTANCE POLICIES

Filing of application:
    Earliest date: August 1, 2004
    Latest date: November 15, 2004
Application fee: $35 in-state; $50 out-of-state
Acceptance notice:
    Earliest date: April 1, 2005
    Latest date: n/a
Applicant's response to acceptance offer:
    Latest date: May 1, 2005
Deposit to hold place in class: $100;
    refundable before May 15, 2005
Starting date: Mid-August, 2005

INFORMATION ON 2003–2004 ENTERING CLASS

Number of	In-State	Out-of-State	Total
Applicants	258	179	437
Applicants Interviewed	162	48	210
New Entrants	106	18	124
Total number of students enrolled in program: 630			

CHAPTER

10

University of Medicine and Dentistry of New Jersey— New Jersey Medical School

Newark, New Jersey

Address Inquiries To:
Leona Smithson
Office of Admissions
C653 MSB
University of Medicine and Dentistry of New Jersey
New Jersey Medical School
185 South Orange Avenue
P.O. Box 1704
Newark, New Jersey 07101-1790
(973) 972-4631; 972-7986 (FAX)
Web site: http://njms.umdnj.edu

Purpose

New Jersey Medical School has established accelerated baccalaureate/M.D. degree programs in collaboration with eight undergraduate institutions. The goal of these programs is to give highly qualified high school students an opportunity to broaden their premedical preparation without having to compete for admission to medical school.

Requirements for Entrance

The programs are open to all high school seniors who are either U.S. citizens or permanent residents. Application procedures vary slightly among the programs, but SATs are required.

Selection Factors

Applicants should be in the top 5 to 10 percent of their high school class and have a minimum combined SAT score of 1400. Applicants are screened on the basis of academic credentials, letters of recommendation, and an essay. Those who meet screening criteria are invited for an interview at the undergraduate school and at the medical school. The deadline for applications to the undergraduate college is January 7. However, early application is encouraged.

Curriculum

The course of study consists of three years at the undergraduate school, followed by the regular four-year medical program. Students must take the MCAT in their junior year, but scores are not a factor for promotion or admission to the medical school phase. Promotion to the medical school is contingent upon achieving grades of B or better in all premedical courses and maintaining an overall grade point average of at least 3.4 each semester. The baccalaureate degree is awarded by the undergraduate institution upon completion of the first year of medical school. The M.D. degree is awarded by New Jersey Medical School.

Students are required to pass Step 1 of the USMLE for promotion to the fourth year. Passing Step 2 is required for graduation. Eight programs are currently available:

Boston University provides an undergraduate emphasis in liberal arts or humanities. This program is open only to residents of New Jersey. Mailing address: Office of Undergraduate Admissions, Boston University, Commonwealth Avenue, Boston, Massachusetts 02215; E-mail: admissions@bu.edu.

Drew University offers premedical preparation in all sciences and liberal arts subjects. Mailing address: College Admissions, Drew University, Madison, New Jersey 07940; (973) 408-3739; E-mail: cadm@drew. edu.

Montclair State University offers premedical preparation in biology, chemistry, biochemistry, molecular biology, computer science, mathematics, psychology, and anthropology. Mailing address: Dr. Judith Shillcock, Health Professions Committee, Department of Biology, Montclair State University, Upper Montclair, New Jersey 07043.

New Jersey Institute of Technology offers undergraduate study in the Honors Premedical Curriculum within the Engineering Science Program. Mailing address: Dr. David Reibstein, Associate Dean, Honors College, New Jersey Institute of Technology, University Heights, Newark, New Jersey 07102-1982; (973) 642-7664; E-mail: honors@njit.edu.

Rutgers University–Newark Campus offers premedical preparation in the sciences. Mailing address: James Flowers, Admissions Counselor, Office of Admissions, Rutgers University, 249 University Avenue, Newark, NJ 17102; (973) 353-5205, ext. 12.

Stevens Institute of Technology offers premedical preparation in chemical biology. Mailing address: Edwina W. Fleming, Director of Honors Admissions Programs, Stevens Institute of Technology, Castle Point–on–the–Hudson, Hoboken, New Jersey 07030; (201) 216-5193; E-mail: efleming@stevens-tech.edu.

The College of New Jersey offers preparation in biology, chemistry, history, philosophy, and psychology. Mailing address: Dr. Dennis Shevlin, Chair, Medical Careers Committee, The College of New Jersey, P.O. Box 7718, Ewing, NJ 08628-0718; (609) 771-2021.

The Richard Stockton College of New Jersey offers preparation in chemistry, biology, physics, and liberal arts. Mailing address: Dr. Ralph Werner, Assistant Professor, The Richard Stockton College of New Jersey, Jimmie Leeds Road, Pomona, New Jersey 08240-0088; (609) 642-7664; E-mail: admissions@stockton.edu.

Application is made through the undergraduate institutions listed above.

Total number of students enrolled in program: 102

Rutgers University and University of Medicine and Dentistry of New Jersey—Robert Wood Johnson Medical School

Piscataway, New Jersey

Address Inquiries To:

Bachelor/Medical Degree Program
Health Professions Office
Nelson Biological Laboratory
Rutgers University
604 Allison Road
Piscataway, New Jersey 08854-8082
(732) 445-5667; 445-6341 (FAX)
Web site: http://lifesci.rutgers.edu/~hpo
E-mail: hpo@biology.rutgers.edu

Purpose

The program permits the early identification and admission of quality medical students. It also integrates medical studies with liberal arts study.

Requirements for Entrance

Applicants must be students at Rutgers University and are selected for this program at the end of their sophomore year. Residents and nonresidents of New Jersey are considered.

Selection Factors

An applicant's high school and college transcripts and faculty recommendations are taken into account in offering admission. In the 2003–2004 entering class, matriculants had achieved a 3.85 GPA at the end of two years of college. They had an average score of 610 on the SAT Verbal section and 700 on the Mathematics section. Maturity, motivation, and broad interests are personal characteristics sought in applicants. An interview is required. The MCAT is not used.

Curriculum

This program leads to the baccalaureate degree awarded by Rutgers University and to the M.D. degree granted by the University of Medicine and Dentistry of New Jersey–Robert Wood Johnson Medical School. Students must complete requirements for a baccalaureate degree. The most frequent majors for that degree are life sciences, followed by biochemistry.

The program is eight years in duration. As indicated in the curriculum chart to the right, the basic sciences and the liberal arts are studied together during a four-year period.

While in medical school, students must take and pass Steps 1 and 2 of the USMLE.

Expenses

In 2003–2004, residents of New Jersey paid $6,290 per year in undergraduate tuition and $19,776 per year in medical school tuition. In the same year, nonresidents paid $12,804 per year in undergraduate tuition and $30,947 annually in medical school tuition. Annual fees averaged $1,637 for undergraduates and $2,391 for medical students.

Financial Aid

Undergraduates should contact the Office of Financial Aid, Rutgers University, 620 George Street, New Brunswick, New Jersey 08901; (732) 932-7057.

Year	Percent Liberal Arts	Percent Basic Sciences
1	100	0
2	100	0
3	50	50
4	50	50
5	20	80
6	0	100
7	0	100
8	0	100

APPLICATION AND ACCEPTANCE POLICIES

Filing of application:
  Earliest date: April 1, 2004
  Latest date: June 1, 2004
Application fee: None
Acceptance notice:
  Earliest date: July 1, 2004
  Latest date: n/a
Applicant's response to acceptance offer:
  Maximum time: 2 weeks
Deposit to hold place in class: None
Starting date: August 6, 2005

INFORMATION ON 2003–2004 ENTERING CLASS

Number of	In-State	Out-of-State	Total
Applicants	26	2	28
Applicants Interviewed	25	2	27
New Entrants	14	0	14
Total number of students enrolled in program: 23			

CHAPTER

10

Brooklyn College and State University at New York Downstate Medical Center College of Medicine

Brooklyn, New York

Address Inquiries To:

Anthony Sgherza, P.T.A.T.C., Ph.D.
Director, B.A./M.D. Honors Program
2231 Boylan Hall, Brooklyn College
2900 Bedford Avenue, Brooklyn, New York 11210
(718) 951-4706; 677-6185 (FAX)
E-mail: Asgherza@brooklyn.cuny.edu
Web site: http://academic.brooklyn.cuny.edu/

Purpose

The aims of this program are to produce physicians who are humanists, concerned with the caring, as well as curing, dimensions of medicine, and to offer an economically affordable baccalaureate and medical school education.

Requirements for Entrance

Students are selected in their senior year of high school. Preference is given to New York residents. Applicants are expected to have completed the following high school courses: a full year of biology, chemistry, and physics, plus mathematics through trigonometry. Students must have at least a 90 percent CAA (College Admission Average, academic subjects only) and a combined score of at least 1200 on the new SAT scale.

Selection Factors

The academic factors taken into account in offering admission to applicants include the high school GPA, SAT scores, New York State Regents Examination scores, Advanced Placement courses, and CEEB Achievement Tests scores. In the 2003–2004 entering class, most students had a high school average of at least 95, and the median SAT combined score was 1392. Maturity and motivation are personal characteristics sought among applicants. An interview is required.

Curriculum

This program leads to a baccalaureate degree awarded by Brooklyn College and to the M.D. degree granted by the State University of New York Downstate Medical Center College of Medicine.

The baccalaureate program includes eight required semester courses in the natural and physical sciences, seven semester courses in the humanities, and three semester courses in the social sciences. Several of these classes are honors sections specifically for students in the B.A.-M.D. program. The most frequent major is psychology. Students may major in any subject, but non-science majors are encouraged. Students must maintain a 3.5 overall, and 3.5 science, undergraduate GPA to progress to the medical school. Students must take the MCAT before the end of their senior year at Brooklyn College, achieving a score of at least 9 on each of the sections in one test administration.

The program is eight years in length. Students are required to complete three years of community service, as well as a summer clinical internship. The four-year medical school program focuses on the M.D. degree exclusively.

During medical school, students must take and pass Step 1 of the USMLE.

Expenses

In 2003–2004, the undergraduate tuition for state residents was $4,000 per year. The 2003–2004 medical school tuition was $16,800 for state residents. Student fees cost an additional $177 per year at Brooklyn College and $325 per year at the College of Medicine.

Brooklyn College has no dormitory facilities, so students must commute or find lodging in the community. Dormitory space is available during the medical school portion of the program.

Financial Aid

Pell Grants, Stafford loans, work-study, Hearst Scholarships for minority female students, and Presidential Scholarships are available. Applicants can receive more information from the Financial Aid Office at Brooklyn College, Sherwood Johnson, Director, (718) 951-5045.

APPLICATION AND ACCEPTANCE POLICIES

Filing of application:
    Earliest date: September 15, 2004
    Latest date: December 31, 2004
Application fee: None
Acceptance notice:
    Earliest date: April 1, 2005
    Latest date: April 1, 2005
Applicant's response to acceptance offer:
    Latest date: April 15, 2005
Deposit to hold place in class: None
Starting date: August 29, 2005

INFORMATION ON 2003–2004 ENTERING CLASS

Number of	In-State	Out-of-State	Total
Applicants	170	0	170
Applicants Interviewed	69	0	69
New Entrants	16	0	16
Total number of students enrolled in program: 55			

New York University

New York, New York

Address Inquiries To:

Admissions Office
New York University
22 Washington Square North
New York, New York 10011
(212) 998-4500
Web site: www.nyu.edu/ugadmissions/

Purpose

The goal of the B.A.-M.D. program is to train broadly educated physicians who are interested in people and their place in society, and who are excited about the science of medicine.

Requirements for Entrance

Students are selected for this program only during the senior year of high school. There are no state residency requirements. No specific courses are required. Applicants must take the ACT Assessment or SAT I and either three CEEB Achievement Tests or three Advanced Placement Tests (one of which must be English in either case).

Selection Factors

Academic factors considered in offering admission include high school GPA, rank in high school class, and honors or Advanced Placement coursework. The admission's committee looks very closely at each applicant's extracurricular and service activities, writing skills, knowledge of, and enthusiasm for, the medical profession, and general intellectual curiosity. Students with broad interests and diverse backgrounds are sought. Interviews at the College of Arts and Science and the School of Medicine are required.

Curriculum

The B.A.-M.D. program is not an accelerated one. All students must complete four years of undergraduate education and four years of medical school.

Students earn a bachelor's degree, which includes completion of a major and the Morse Academic Plan, the College's integrated general education curriculum in the liberal arts. Students in the combined-degree program are encouraged to pursue any liberal arts major they wish. Additionally, they are required to complete an independent interdisciplinary research project over a period of several semesters. Students are expected to maintain good progress and a satisfactory GPA while in college. They are not required to take the MCAT to advance to the medical school.

Expenses

The annual tuition and fees for the undergraduate portion of the combined-degree program totaled $26,646 in 2003–2004. The medical school portion was $33,500.

Financial Aid

A full range of need-based and merit-based financial aid/scholarships is available to undergraduates. All applicants are automatically considered for merit scholarships, which may include participation in a scholars program. Candidates for financial aid are required to submit the Free Application for Federal Student Aid (FAFSA) by February 15. Applicants can receive more information from the Office of Financial Aid, 25 West 4th Street, New York, New York 10003; or at www.nyu.edu/financialaid/.

APPLICATION AND ACCEPTANCE POLICIES

Filing of application:
  Earliest date: n/a
  Latest date: January 15, 2005
Application fee: $60
Acceptance notice:
  Earliest date: April 1, 2005
  Latest date: n/a
Applicant's response to acceptance offer:
  Latest date: May 1, 2005
Deposit to hold place in class: $200; nonrefundable
Starting date: September 2, 2005

INFORMATION ON 2003–2004 ENTERING CLASS

Number of	In-State	Out-of-State	Total
Applicants	n/a	n/a	751
Applicants Interviewed	n/a	n/a	19
New Entrants	n/a	n/a	6
Total number of students enrolled in program: 16			

CHAPTER

10

Rensselaer Polytechnic Institute and Albany Medical College

Troy, New York

Address Inquiries To:

Dean of Undergraduate Admissions
Rensselaer Polytechnic Institute
110 Eighth Street
Troy, New York 12180-3590
(518) 276-6216
Western Regional Office: (800) 873-9369 or (760) 730-3132
E-mail: admissions@rpi.edu
Web site: http://admissions.rpi.edu/

Purpose

The Accelerated Physician-Scientist Program offers qualified individuals the opportunity to become physicians who are intensively trained in medical research. This innovative approach provides a well-rounded perspective that prepares future practitioners and physician-scientists to perform with confidence and care in a technologically changing environment.

Requirements for Entrance

Students are selected for this program during the senior year of high school. Residents of New York as well as nonresidents of the state are eligible to apply. Applicants are expected to have completed the following courses by the time they graduate from high school: four years of English; one year each of biology, chemistry, and physics; and four years of mathematics (through pre-calculus). They must take the SAT I and the SAT II in mathematics (level IC or level IIC) and writing; and, of the sciences, physics, chemistry, or biology is required. In lieu of these tests, American College Testing (ACT) program scores may be submitted. All tests must be completed by the December testing date prior to the proposed September matriculation.

Selection Factors

Academic factors considered in offering admission to an applicant include the quality and nature of coursework in high school, performance in those courses, rank in high school class, and test scores. The 2003–2004 entering class had an average score of 700 on the SAT Verbal and 740 on the SAT Math. Personal qualities sought in applicants are motivation, maturity, and intellectual capacity necessary to pursue the accelerated course of study. An interview is required.

Curriculum

The program leads to a B.S. degree awarded by Rensselaer Polytechnic Institute and the M.D. degree granted by Albany Medical College.

The curriculum for the B.S. and M.D. degrees usually requires seven years to complete. During the first three years of the program spent at Rensselaer, the curriculum involves 70 percent premedical science courses and 30 percent liberal arts courses. Students take 18 courses in the natural and physical sciences and 8 elective courses in the humanities and social sciences.

The medical college has replaced the traditional two years of basic science and two years of clinical science with an integrated four-year curriculum. Emphasis is placed on the pivotal role of primary care.

Students admitted to the program are not required to take the MCAT for admission to Albany Medical College. Students are expected to take Steps 1 and 2 of the USMLE while at Albany Medical College.

Expenses

The tuition and fees for 2003–2004 were $27,700 at Rensselaer, and $38,860 for state residents at Albany Medical College.

Financial Aid

Sources of financial aid are restricted and include endowed scholarships based on need, merit scholarships, work-study, and student loans through federal and institutional programs. Applicants can receive more information by contacting the Financial Aid Office of Rensselaer Polytechnic Institute at (518) 276-6813 or Albany Medical College at (518) 262-5435.

APPLICATION AND ACCEPTANCE POLICIES

Filing of application:
  Earliest date: September 1, 2004
  Latest date: December 1, 2004
Application fee: $50 (RPI);
  $100 (Albany Medical College)
Acceptance notice:
  Earliest date: March 2005
  Latest date: until class is filled
Applicant's response to acceptance offer:
  Latest date: May 1, 2005
Deposit to hold place in class: $300; nonrefundable
Starting date: August 2005

INFORMATION ON 2003–2004 ENTERING CLASS

Number of	In-State	Out-of-State	Total
Applicants	90	187	277
Applicants Interviewed	37	64	101
New Entrants	8	9	17
Total number of students enrolled in program: 86			

Siena College and Albany Medical College

Loudonville, New York

Address Inquiries To:

Office of Admissions
Siena College
515 Loudon Road
Loudonville, New York 12211-1462
(518) 783-2423; 888-AT-SIENA
Web site: www.siena.edu

Purpose

This program offers an eight-year continuum of education that has a special emphasis on the humanities and on community service while providing a sound understanding of both the natural and social sciences.

Requirements for Entrance

Students are selected for this program during the senior year of high school. Both residents and nonresidents of New York are eligible to apply. Candidates for admission to the Siena/AMC program must have completed at least four years of high school math and science. Typically, successful candidates will have enrolled in, or completed, advanced-level courses by the end of their senior year in high school. A well-rounded background and demonstrated leadership experience are also important. Of equal significance is the student's proven concern for others and for the community. Applicants must take either the SAT I or ACT Assessment. Tests must be completed by the November testing date prior to the proposed September matriculation. Test scores must be received by January 1.

Selection Factors

Academic factors considered in offering admission to an applicant include: required and elective courses taken, grades earned, class standing, SAT I or ACT scores, honors received, letters of recommendation, and unique academic experiences. Of great importance to the admission committee are such factors as extracurricular activities, evidence of intellectual curiosity, and interest in the humanities and in the sciences. Students generally rank among the top 10 percent of their high school class. The 2003–2004 entering class had an average score of 660 on the SAT Verbal and 710 on the SAT Math. An interview is required.

Curriculum

This program offers a coordinated eight-year curriculum of premedical and medical education. The undergraduate phase offers an equal distribution of science and non-science courses. Students graduate in four years with a bachelor of arts degree in biology with a minor in the humanities. The undergraduate phase of the program also includes a required summer of human service in a health-related agency, usually in an urban setting or developing nation. Passage from the undergraduate college to the medical school requires achievement of a 3.40 GPA and a continued interest in the human service dimension of the program. The medical college has replaced the traditional two years of basic science and two years of clinical science with an integrated four-year curriculum. Emphasis is placed on the pivotal role of primary care. The summer between the sophomore and junior years is dedicated to medically related volunteer service, usually in a rural or inner city clinic.

Students are not required to take the MCAT for admission to Albany Medical College. Students are expected to take Steps 1 and 2 of the USMLE.

Expenses

The tuition for 2003–2004 was $18,095 at Siena College, and $38,860 at Albany Medical College.

Financial Aid

Applicants can receive more information by contacting the Siena College Financial Aid Office at (518) 783-2427; or the Albany Medical College Financial Aid Office at (518) 262-5435.

APPLICATION AND ACCEPTANCE POLICIES

Filing of application:
  Earliest date: September 1, 2004
  Latest date: December 15, 2004
Application fee: $40 (Siena);
  $100 (Albany Medical College)
Acceptance notice:
  Earliest date: March 15, 2005
  Latest date: until classes are filled
Applicant's response to acceptance offer:
  Latest date: May 1, 2005
Deposit to hold place in class: $200; nonrefundable
Starting date: September 2005

INFORMATION ON 2003–2004 ENTERING CLASS

Number of	In-State	Out-of-State	Total
Applicants	106	112	218
Applicants Interviewed	25	19	44
New Entrants	10	5	15
Total number of students enrolled in program: 90			

CHAPTER

10

Sophie Davis School of Biomedical Education/ City University of New York

New York, New York

Address Inquiries To:

Sophie Davis School of Biomedical Education
Office of Admission • Harris Hall
138th Street and Convent Avenue
New York, New York 10031
(212) 650-7718; 650-7708 (FAX)
Web site: http://med.cuny.edu

Purpose

The purposes of this combined-degree program are to train primary care physicians who will work in medically underserved urban areas to increase the number of underrepresented minority physicians, to intervene in the disparity of access to high quality pre-college science education, and create a medical school pipeline.

Requirements for Entrance

Students are selected for this program in the senior year of high school. Only residents of New York are eligible to apply. Applicants are expected to have completed the following courses by the time they graduate from high school: two semesters each of chemistry and biology and six to eight semesters of mathematics. They must take the ACT Assessment and SAT tests.

Selection Factors

Academic factors taken into account in offering admission to an applicant are the high school GPA, the SAT scores, the ACT Assessment, and scores on the New York State Regents Examinations. In the 2003–2004 entering class, the high school grades averaged 92, and the subscore on the Mathematics ACT Assessment averaged 27. The SAT Mathematics average was 650, and the SAT Verbal average was 640. Personal qualities sought in applicants include interest in people, concern for others, initiative, and leadership. An interview is required.

Curriculum

This seven-year program leads to a baccalaureate degree granted by the City College of New York (CCNY) and to the M.D. degree awarded by one of six New York medical schools (Albany Medical College, New York Medical College, New York University, SUNY Brooklyn, SUNY Stony Brook University, or SUNY Upstate Syracuse).

During the first five years of the program, students fulfill all requirements for the B.S. degree and study the preclinical portion of the medical school curriculum. After successfully completing the five-year sequence and passing Step 1 of the USMLE, students transfer to one of the participating medical schools in New York for their final two years of clinical training. Students are expected to pass Step 1 of the USMLE to proceed to Years 3 and 4 of medical school. Additionally, students are expected to pass Step 2 of the USMLE to graduate.

Students complete the core liberal arts curriculum of the CCNY during the first two years. At this time they also take courses emphasizing the importance of understanding cultural differences to good medical practice and, through community medicine courses, do field work at various community agencies, including many family practice clinics. The final years of the five-year sequence at CCNY include courses necessary in the first two years of medical school, including basic science courses and several community medicine courses. Students also benefit from counseling and academic support services.

Expenses

In 2003–2004, resident undergraduate tuition per year was $4,000. Student fees were $121.70. A technology fee has been added. Full time students pay an additional $150 per year. Tuition for the final two years of the program varies according to the medical school attended.

Financial Aid

Pell Grants, New York State TAP awards, and NYC Merit Awards are all sources of financial aid. The school generally awards several scholarships to incoming students, including The Lois Pope L.I.F.E. scholarships and the William R. Hearst Endowed Scholarship. Scholarships available later in the program include those from the Alan Seelig Memorial Fund, the Aranow Fund, and the Sophie and Leonard Davis Scholarships. Applicants can contact the Financial Aid Office at (212) 650-5819.

APPLICATION AND ACCEPTANCE POLICIES

Filing of application:
　Earliest date: September, 2004
　Latest date: January 8, 2005
Application fee: None
Acceptance notice: Latest date: April 1, 2005
Applicant's response to acceptance offer:
　Earliest date: n/a
　Latest date: May 1, 2005
Applicant's response to acceptance offer:
　Maximum time: n/a
Deposit to hold place in class: None
Starting date: End of August 2005

INFORMATION ON 2003–2004 ENTERING CLASS

Number of	In-State	Out-of-State	Total
Applicants	n/a	n/a	449
Applicants Interviewed	n/a	n/a	193
New Entrants	n/a	n/a	74
Total number of students enrolled in program: 328			

Stony Brook University and Stony Brook University School of Medicine

Stony Brook, New York

Address Inquiries To:

The Honors College
Scholars for Medicine Program
Stony Brook University
3070 N. Melville Library
Stony Brook, New York 11794-3357
(631) 632-4378; 632-4525 (FAX)
Web site: www.stonybrook.edu/honors

Purpose

The Scholars for Medicine Program offers conditional acceptance to the Stony Brook University School of Medicine to a select number of outstanding and highly motivated students. In addition to acquiring a solid background in the sciences, accepted students have access to a wide array of liberal arts courses offered through the university and its Honors College. Students also have access to medical school programs in research and a series of health–related seminars.

Requirements for Entrance

Students are selected for this program only during the senior year of high school. There are no state residency requirements. No specific courses are required. Applicants must take the ACT or SAT. For non-U.S. citizens, documentation of permanent residency status will be required of accepted students prior to matriculation.

Selection Factors

To be considered for this program, applicants must have a minimum SAT score of 1350 and an unweighted high school GPA of 93. The applicant's high school academic record, standardized test reports, essay, history of interests and activities, and required interview at the School of Medicine are factors taken into account in offering admission.

Curriculum

This eight-year program leads to the baccalaureate and M.D. degrees granted by the Stony Brook University. Students are expected to complete the requirements for any of the baccalaureate degrees awarded by the University. Undergraduate work taken must include courses required by the School of Medicine, including one year each of biology, physics, inorganic chemistry, organic chemistry (all with lab), and English. No specific major is required for the premedical undergraduate phase.

The program provides a seminar series of health-related lectures given by nationally and internationally recognized individuals in health care delivery. In addition, students have an opportunity to engage in cutting-edge research.

Admission to the School of Medicine is contingent upon maintaining a minimum GPA of 3.4. The MCAT is required and the student should attain cumulative scores comparable to the national average of medical school matriculants. The USMLE Steps 1 and 2 are required for promotion and graduation from the School of Medicine.

Expenses

In 2003–2004, the undergraduate tuition for New York State residents was $5,306 and, for nonresidents, $11,256. Student fees were $956.

Financial Aid

Financial aid available to enrolled students includes federal Perkins loans, EOP, federal work-study, federal Pell Grants, Federal Supplemental Educational Opportunity, NY State Tuition Assistance Program (TAP), and NY State Aid for Part-time Students.

Applicants can receive more information by contacting The Office of Financial Aid and Student Employment at Stony Brook University at (631) 632-6840 or visiting the Web site at ✑ http://naples.cc.sunysb.edu/Prov/financial.nsf.

APPLICATION AND ACCEPTANCE POLICIES

Filing of application:
  Earliest date: November 1, 2004
  Latest date: January 15, 2005
Application fee: None
Acceptance notice:
  Earliest date: March 1, 2005
  Latest date: April 5, 2005
Applicant's response to acceptance offer:
  Maximum time: 4 weeks
Deposit to hold place in class: $100; refundable
Starting date: September 2005

INFORMATION ON 2003–2004 ENTERING CLASS

Number of	In-State	Out-of-State	Total
Applicants	125	32	157
Applicants Interviewed	19	4	23
New Entrants	2	0	2
Total number of students enrolled in program: 36			

CHAPTER
10

SUNY Upstate Medical University/Wilkes University GUTHRIE-Robert Packer Hospital

Syracuse, New York

Address Inquiries To:
Eileen Sharp
Coordinator for Health Sciences Professional Programs
Wilkes University
P.O. Box 111
Wilkes-Barre, Pennsylvania 18766
(570) 408-4823
Web site: www.wilkes.edu

Purpose

This cooperative program is motivated by the need for physicians interested in serving in rural and semi-rural health care delivery systems, as well as the interest of each institution in attracting students of superior ability and accomplishment.

Requirements for Entrance

Students apply to the program in their senior year of high school; applicants must be New York State residents. Candidates for admission must have completed the following high school course requirements: four years each of mathematics, English, science, and social science. Applicants must take the ACT Assessment or SAT.

Selection Factors

The following factors are taken into consideration in assessing the applicant for admission: grades, rank in class, SAT (ACT) scores, and extracurricular activities. In the 2003-2004 entering class, the average high school GPA was 95.96, and the average SAT score was 1430. Selected applicants are invited for a required interview.

Curriculum

This eight-year program leads to a baccalaureate degree awarded by Wilkes University and to the M.D. degree granted by the SUNY Upstate Medical University. The most frequent major for the baccalaureate degree is biology, followed by chemistry and biochemistry. The approximate percentage of liberal arts and medical courses in the curriculum each year is as follows: Years 1 through 3, 100 percent liberal arts; Year 4, 50 percent liberal arts and 50 percent medicine; Years 5 through 8, 100 percent medicine. There are no specific humanities course requirements. The M.D. portion of the curriculum does not depart from the "traditional" design.

Upstate accepts a special responsibility to provide physicians to New York's underserved rural communities. A student from a rural setting or one trained there is more likely to subsequently practice there. This BS/MD program attracts students from rural areas who are not likely to otherwise find their way to medical school. Upstate also provides many special opportunities during medical school (Rural Medicine Program, Clinical Campus) to train students in community and rural settings.

Students in this program are not required to take the MCAT for promotion or admission to the medical school. The USMLE Step 1 is required and must be taken prior to clinical rotations. Students must pass Step 1 to be promoted and in order to graduate. USMLE Step 2 is required, but passing is not a factor in graduation from the medical school.

Expenses

In 2003-2004, the annual undergraduate tuition and fees for residents was $19,630. The medical school tuition for residents was $16,840; annual fees were $1,060.

Financial Aid

The sources of available financial aid are grants, scholarships, and student loans. For more information about financial aid, visit ✎ www.wilkes.edu/admissions/finaid/cost/asp, or contact the Financial Aid Office at FinAid@upstate.edu.

APPLICATION AND ACCEPTANCE POLICIES

Filing of application:
    Earliest date: August 1, 2004
    Latest date: December 2004
Application fee: $30 (Wilkes–often waived)
Acceptance notice:
    Earliest date: within 2 weeks
    Latest date: 2 weeks after medical school interview
Applicant's response to acceptance offer:
    Maximum time: 2 weeks
Deposit to hold place in class: $100
    (refundable until May 15 of entry year)
Stating Date: n/a

INFORMATION ON 2003–2004 ENTERING CLASS

Number of	In-State	Out-of-State	Total
Applicants	7	n/a	7
Applicants Interviewed	7	n/a	7
New Entrants	2	n/a	2
Total number of students enrolled in program: 6			

Union College
and Albany Medical College

Schenectady, New York

Address Inquiries To:

Associate Dean of Admissions
Union College
Schenectady, New York 12308
(518) 388-6112; 888-843-6688
E-mail: admissions@union.edu
Web site: www.union.edu/

Purpose

The Leadership in Medicine/Health Management Program is specifically designed for students who want to prepare for the challenge of medical leadership by taking advantage of additional educational opportunities as part of their under-graduate education. In addition to offering the standard coursework required for attaining the degrees of B.S., M.S., or M.B.A. and M.D., the integrated program focuses on three areas essential for future leaders in medicine: health policy and health management, the ethical challenge, and the leadership challenge.

Requirements for Entrance

Students are selected for this program during the senior year of high school. Residents of New York as well as nonres-idents of the state are eligible to apply. Applicants are expected to have completed a challenging curriculum in high school, which must include biology, chemistry and physics. They must take either the ACT Assessment or the SAT I and three SAT IIs (writing, a math, and a science). Tests must be completed by the December testing date prior to the proposed September matriculation.

Selection Factors

Academic factors considered in offering admission to an applicant include the quality and nature of coursework in high school, performance in those courses, rank in high school class, and standardized test scores. In the 2003–2004 entering class, the average score was 700 for SAT Verbal and 730 for SAT Mathematics. Personal qualities sought in applicants include moti-vation, maturity, and personal development. Interviews at Union College and Albany Medical College are required.

Curriculum

This program leads to B.S., M.S., or M.B.A. degrees awarded by Union College and the M.D. granted by Albany Medical College.

At Union College, students take 30 courses (15 science and 15 non-science) and complete an interdepartmental major in the humanities or social sciences. A special bioethics program supplemented by a health services practicum, a term abroad, and a program in health care management at the Union College Graduate Management Institute are also integral parts of the educational experience.

The curriculum for the B.S., M.S., or M.B.A. and M.D. degrees requires eight years to complete. Students take a course in health and human values during the summer before matriculation in the medical school. The medical college has replaced the traditional two years of basic science and two years of clinical science with an integrated four-year curriculum.

Students admitted to the program are not required to take the MCAT for admission to Albany Medical College. Students are expected to take Steps 1 and 2 of the USMLE while at Albany Medical College.

Expenses

The 2003–2004 tuition was $28,608 at Union College and $38,860 at Albany Medical College.

Financial Aid

Sources of financial aid include various programs based on need, student loans through federal and state assistance, work-study, and merit scholarships. For more information contact the Financial Aid Office of Union College at (518) 388-6123 or at Albany Medical College at (518) 262-5435.

APPLICATION AND ACCEPTANCE POLICIES

Filing of application:
  Earliest date: September 1, 2004
  Latest date: December 15, 2004
Application fee: $50 (Union College);
  $100 (Albany Medical College)
Acceptance notice:
  Earliest date: March, 2005
  Latest date: until class is filled
Applicant's response to acceptance offer:
  Latest date: May 1, 2005
Deposit to hold place in class: $400; nonrefundable
Starting date: September 2005

INFORMATION ON 2003–2004 ENTERING CLASS

Number of	In-State	Out-of-State	Total
Applicants	103	139	242
Applicants Interviewed	31	41	72
New Entrants	11	8	19
Total number of students enrolled in program: 101			

University of Rochester School of Medicine and Dentistry

Rochester, New York

Address Inquiries To:

Rochester Early Medical Scholars Coordinator
University of Rochester
Undergraduate Admissions—Box 270251
Rochester, New York 14627-0251
(585) 275-3221 or (888) 822-2256; (585) 461-4595 (FAX)
Web site: www.rochester.edu

Purpose

The Rochester Early Medical Scholars Program (REMS) provides conditional acceptance to the University of Rochester School of Medicine and Dentistry to a group of exceptionally talented and motivated students. REMS allows undergraduates the utmost flexibility in degree programs, mentoring relationships with medical school staff, and early exposure to the medical school curriculum through a series of lectures and seminars.

Requirements for Entrance

Students are selected for this program during their senior year of high school from an international pool. A recommended high school curriculum includes two years of foreign language and four years each of English, social studies, mathematics, and science. A transcript that includes honors or AP courses is preferable. Applicants are expected to take the SAT or ACT Assessment. Achievement tests are highly recommended, especially English composition, Math I or IIC, Biology, or Chemistry.

Selection Factors

Outstanding achievement in a challenging high school curriculum, character, interests, maturity, experience in health care or research settings, and motivation necessary for a career in medicine are required for consideration for entry into the REMS program. Interviews are required. In the 2003–2004 entering class, REMS students had an average SAT Verbal score of 696 and Math score of 724. In order to take their place in the first-year medical school class, REMS students must carry at least a 3.3 overall GPA and a 3.3 premedical course GPA by the end of the sophomore year, and a 3.5 overall GPA by the time of undergraduate graduation.

Curriculum

The eight-year program leads to a baccalaureate degree and the M.D. degree, both granted by the University of Rochester. Students must complete the baccalaureate degree. The most popular major is biology, followed by health and Society, and biomedical engineering. Undergraduates are encouraged to pursue a variety of academic disciplines in addition to completing their premedical course requirements. Completion of a major is required.

The University of Rochester School of Medicine and Dentistry features an exciting newly revised curriculum that emphasizes problem-based learning and early patient contact. See ✍ www.urmc.rochester.edu/smd/admiss/mededu.html for details. The University of Rochester has also pioneered the "biopsychosocial model" of medicine, which stresses approaching the patient as a complete person. The revised curriculum allows early and increased access to patients and close relationships with medical school faculty.

REM students may apply to other University of Rochester combined-degree programs, including M.D.-Ph.D., M.D.-M.P.H., and M.D.-M.B.A. programs. A "Take 5" program, offering a tuition-free fifth undergraduate year, is available to selected REMS students. Summer research programs are available. Extensive international experiences are available at both the undergraduate and medical school levels.

Expenses

Undergraduate tuition in 2003–2004 was $26,900 per year, and annual fees total $12,094. Medical school tuition was $31,500, with annual fees of $2,817.

Financial Aid

University of Rochester scholarships and loans, plus governmental loans, are available. For more information, write the Office of Financial Aid, University of Rochester, Box 270261, Rochester, New York 14627-0261; or phone (585) 275-3226 or (800) 881-8234.

APPLICATION AND ACCEPTANCE POLICIES

Filing of application:
  Earliest date: May 15, 2004
  Latest date: December 15, 2004
Application fee: $50
Acceptance notice:
  Earliest date: March 31, 2005
  Latest date: May 1, 2005
Applicant's response to acceptance offer:
  Maximum time: n/a
Deposit to hold place in class: $400; nonrefundable
Starting date: Early September 2005

INFORMATION ON 2003–2004 ENTERING CLASS

Number of	In-State	Out-of-State	Total
Applicants	173	380	553
Applicants Interviewed	20	16	36
New Entrants	4	1	5
Total number of students enrolled in program: 65			

Case Western Reserve University

Cleveland, Ohio

Address Inquiries To:

Christine DeSalvo
Office of Undergraduate Admission
103 Tomlinson Hall
Case Western Reserve University
10900 Euclid Avenue
Cleveland, Ohio 44106-7055
(216) 368-4450; 368-5111 (FAX)
Web site: http://admission.case.edu/admissions

Purpose

This program is intended to provide college students with a greater sense of freedom and choice in the pursuit of a premedical baccalaureate degree.

Requirements for Entrance

Students are selected for this program during the senior year of high school. Both residents and nonresidents of Ohio are considered for admission. Applicants are expected to have completed the following courses by the time they graduate from high school: one year each of biology, chemistry, and physics and four years of mathematics. They must take either the ACT Assessment or the SAT I and SAT II.

Selection Factors

The applicant's high school academic record, standardized test reports, history of interests and activities, and a required interview are factors taken into account in offering admission. Evidence of strong interpersonal and leadership skills is also sought. In the 2003–2004 entering class, the average combined SAT scores ranged from 1450 to 1540. The average combined ACT score ranged from 30 to 34.

Curriculum

This eight-year program leads to the baccalaureate and M.D. degrees granted by Case Western Reserve University. Students are expected to complete the requirements for any of the baccalaureate degrees awarded by the colleges of the university. They are expected to satisfy all requirements of, and earn a baccalaureate prior to matriculating in, the School of Medicine. The work taken for the baccalaureate must include the studies specifically required of applicants by the School of Medicine including one year of biology, two years of chemistry (including organic chemistry), one year of physics, and freshman expository writing. No specific major concentration is required for the premedical undergraduate phase. To date, the majors most commonly taken have been biology and biochemistry, with anthropology the next most popular major.

The first four years of the program are devoted to study for the baccalaureate and the last four years to the curriculum in medicine. Students in the medical phase are required to pass Step 1 of the USMLE for promotion within the program and to pass Step 2 of the USMLE in order to graduate.

Expenses

In 2003–2004, the tuition for the undergraduate phase of the program was $24,100 per year, plus annual fees. Medical school tuition was $36,500, plus annual fees.

Financial Aid

Sources of aid for the undergraduate phase include merit and need-based aid, college work-study, and university grants and scholarships. For information about aid contact the Office of University Financial Aid at (216) 368-4530.

APPLICATION AND ACCEPTANCE POLICIES

Filing of application:
  Earliest date: n/a
  Latest date: December 15, 2004
Application fee: $35
Acceptance notice:
  Earliest date: n/a
  Latest date: April 15, 2005
Applicant's response to acceptance offer:
  Latest date: May 1, 2005
Deposit to hold place in class: $300; nonrefundable
Starting date: August 23, 2005

INFORMATION ON 2003–2004 ENTERING CLASS

Number of	In-State	Out-of-State	Total
Applicants	143	386	529
Applicants Interviewed	28	42	70
New Entrants	6	9	15
Total students enrolled in program: 60 (approx.)			

Northeastern Ohio Universities College of Medicine

Rootstown, Ohio

Address Inquiries To:
R. Stephen Manuel, *Director of Admission*
Northeastern Ohio Universities
College of Medicine
4209 State Route 44, P.O. Box 95
Rootstown, Ohio 44272-0095
(330) 325-6270; 325-8372 (FAX)
Web site: www.neoucom.edu

Purpose

The mission of the Northeastern Ohio Universities College of Medicine (NEOUCOM) is to graduate qualified physicians oriented to the practice of medicine at the community level, with an emphasis on primary care, including family medicine, internal medicine, pediatrics, and obstetrics-gynecology. All graduates, regardless of specialty, are provided with a strong background in community and public health.

Requirements for Entrance

Students are selected for this program during the senior year of high school. Both residents and nonresidents of Ohio are eligible to apply; strong preference is given to in-state applicants. Applicants are expected to have pursued a solid college preparatory curriculum, including four years of mathematics and four years of science. They must take either the ACT or the SAT.

Selection Factors

The academic factors that are taken into account in offering admission to applicants include standardized test scores, high school GPA and science GPA, extracurricular involvement, medical exposure, coursework, state of legal residence, and interview outcome. In 2003–2004, the mean high school GPA of matriculants was 3.86. The average test score for the ACT was 28, and SAT scores averaged 1282. Career maturity and emotional maturity are among the personal qualities weighed by the admissions committee. An interview is required by invitation only.

Curriculum

Students in this combined-degree program study for a baccalaureate degree granted by Youngstown State University, Kent State University, or the University of Akron, and for the M.D. degree granted by NEOUCOM.

Students must complete requirements for a bachelor's degree with a major in integrated life sciences. The curriculum takes six or seven years to complete. Some of the educational innovations offered include an introduction to clinical medicine course taught at area family practice centers in the first and second medical school years; an integrated infectious disease course that covers the basic microbiological and clinical aspects of disease, as well as methods of treatment and control; and, a one-month primary care preceptorship course in the fourth medical school year. Further, most of the basic science courses are taught in just one year (M1) in contrast to the more traditional two-year sequence.

Students are required to pass USMLE Step 1, as well as Step 2 – Clinical Knowledge (CK) and Step 2 – Clinical Skills (CS) in order to graduate from NEOUCOM.

Expenses

Tuition and fees for Years 1 and 2 for 2003–2004 were determined by each undergraduate university.

Financial Aid

Campus-based financial aid is awarded on the basis of demonstrated need. In general, students apply for this aid by completing the FAFSA (see Part 1) and the NEOUCOM financial aid application, and by submitting copies of federal income tax forms and financial aid transcripts. The awards are made through the Student Aid and Awards Committee after a thorough analysis of the student's financial situation.

Long-term federal educational loans are a major part of the aid program. A limited number of need-based scholarships is available, as well as other limited scholarship funds for disadvantaged and/or minority medical students. About 80 percent of enrolled students receive some form of financial aid. Financial need is not a factor in admission considerations.

APPLICATION AND ACCEPTANCE POLICIES

Filing of application:
  Earliest date: August 15, 2004
  Latest date: December 15, 2004
Application fee: $100
Acceptance notice:
  Earliest date: December 5, 2004
  Latest date: March 19, 2005
Applicant's response to acceptance offer:
  Maximum time: May 1, 2005
Deposit to hold place in class: None
Starting date: June 2005

INFORMATION ON 2003–2004 ENTERING CLASS

Number of	In-State	Out-of-State	Total
Applicants	385	219	604
Applicants Interviewed	213	31	244
New Entrants	98	7	105
Total number of students enrolled in program: 230			

The Ohio State University College of Medicine and Public Health

Columbus, Ohio

Address Inquiries To:

Admissions Office
College of Medicine and Public Health
The Ohio State University
209 Meiling Hall ▪ 370 West 9th Avenue
Columbus, Ohio 43210
(614) 292-7137; 247-7959 (FAX)
Web site: http://medicine.osu.edu/futurestudents/eap.cfm

Purpose

The seven-year Early Admission Pathway provides early entrance into the College of Medicine and Public Health for a select group of National Merit, National Achievement, or National Hispanic finalists entering Ohio State autumn quarter.

Requirements for Entrance

Students are selected in their senior year of high school. Both residents and nonresidents of Ohio are eligible to apply to the program. In addition to meeting the requirements for freshman admission, applicants are required to submit the results of the ACT Assessment or the SAT I.

Selection Factors

The following factors are taken into consideration in assessing applicants for admission: approval for university honors affiliation; selection as a National Merit, National Achievement, or National Hispanic finalist; grade-point average; high school activities; leadership roles; and extracurricular activities. In the 2003-2004 entering class, the average high school GPA was 4.10 (range of 3.77 to 4.50). The average SAT score was 1453 and ACT Assessment score was 31.4.

Curriculum

This seven-year program leads to a baccalaureate degree awarded by the Ohio State University, and to the M.D. degree granted by The Ohio State University College of Medicine and Public Health. The most frequent major for the baccalaureate degree is biology. Students must complete the basic course entry requirements, including one year of biological sciences, one year of general chemistry, one year of organic chemistry with lab, and one year of physics with lab. Students with a cumulative science grade-point average of 3.50 or above by the end of the second year are not required to take the MCAT. The MCAT is required for students earning between a 3.00 and 3.49 average. They must register for, and take, the August MCAT and present a composite score of at least 27, with no sub-score less than 8, to continue in good standing. Students earning less than a 3.00 CPHR or science average at the end of the second year will no longer be eligible for conditional acceptance into the College of Medicine.

Students must submit the AMCAS application and Ohio State secondary application and schedule a final exit interview. During the second year of medical school, students must pass the USMLE Step 1 in order to be promoted to the third year of medical school. Passing Step 2 of the USMLE is required for graduation from the medical school.

Expenses

In 2003-2004, the annual undergraduate tuition was $6,651 for residents and $16,638 for nonresidents. Tuition for the medical school portion was $19,323 for residents and $25,462 for nonresidents. The annual expense associated with all student fees for the program is $12,250.

Financial Aid

The sources of financial aid available are National Merit/Achievement/Hispanic Distinguished Scholarships ($10,164 per year), plus other merit and need-based aid. For more information, contact the Office of Student Financial Aid, The Ohio State University, 517 Lincoln Tower, 1800 Cannon Drive, Columbus, Ohio 43210; (614) 292-0300.

APPLICATION AND ACCEPTANCE POLICIES

Filing of application:
  Earliest date: October 1, 2004
  Latest date: March 1, 2005
Application fee: $40
Acceptance notice:
  Earliest date: April 15, 2005
  Latest date: April 15, 2005
Applicant's response to acceptance offer:
  Latest date: May 1, 2005
Deposit to hold place in class: None
Starting date: September 2005

INFORMATION ON 2003–2004 ENTERING CLASS

Number of	In-State	Out-of-State	Total
Applicants	26	10	36
Applicants Interviewed	22	9	31
New Entrants	14	5	19
Total number of students enrolled in program: 54			

CHAPTER

10

University of Cincinnati College of Medicine

Cincinnati, Ohio

Address Inquiries To:

Jennifer B. Rosichan, M.A.
Director of Dual Admissions
University of Cincinnati
College of Medicine
231 Albert Sabin Way, Room E-251
Cincinnati, Ohio 45267-0552
(513) 558-5581; 558-1165 (FAX)
Web site: www.med.uc.edu/HS2MD

Purpose

The University of Cincinnati College of Medicine has a Dual Admissions Program, which accepts high school seniors into one of five undergraduate Ohio colleges and into the College of Medicine. The College of Medicine has established a partnership with the following Ohio institutions: University of Dayton, John Carroll University, Miami University, Xavier University, University of Cincinnati College of Engineering, and the University of Cincinnati undergraduate campus. Each undergraduate program will invite selected students already accepted into its university to apply for this program. Once accepted to this special program, students will receive an outstanding education while preparing for medical school and developing the qualities and characteristics to become excellent physicians.

Requirements for Entrance

Both residents and nonresidents of Ohio are eligible to apply. Priority will be given to Ohio residents. Each university determines the academic requirements, but the ACT and/or SAT are required.

Selection Factors

In conjunction with the College of Medicine, each undergraduate institution considers an applicant's GPA, standardized test performance, examples of leadership, interpersonal skills, and interest in and motivation for medicine in making admission decisions.

The dual-admission program partnership with Miami University differs from that with the other programs in that students are selected during their first year of college at Miami. The other programs that have partnered with the University of Cincinnati College of Medicine select applicants during their senior year in high school.

Curriculum

The course of study consists of four years at the undergraduate school, followed by four years in the College of Medicine. University of Cincinnati College of Medicine dual-admissions students are required to satisfactorily fulfill graduate requirements at their undergraduate institution. The program with the University of Cincinnati College of Engineering is a nine-year program. Students are strongly urged to complete a baccalaureate degree.

Students must earn a 3.5 cumulative GPA and a 3.40 BCPM GPA by the beginning of the senior undergraduate year.

By the beginning of the senior undergraduate year, students must also earn a 27 composite score on the MCAT, with no less than 9 in biological sciences and no less than an 8 in verbal reasoning or physical sciences.

The student must pass Steps 1 and 2 of the USMLE in order to graduate from the College of Medicine. The USMLE Step 1 is administered at the completion of Year 2.

Expenses

The undergraduate tuition and fees vary with each undergraduate institution. In 2003–2004, medical school tuition and fees were $18,630 for residents and $33,159 for non-residents.

Financial Aid

More information about undergraduate financial aid can be obtained from the undergraduate partners' Office of Admissions.

APPLICATION AND ACCEPTANCE POLICIES

Filing of application:
   Varies with undergraduate university
Application fee: None
Acceptance notice:
   Earliest date: April 1, 2005
   Latest date: n/a
Applicant's response to acceptance offer:
   Latest date: May 1, 2005
Deposit to hold place in class: None
Starting date:
   Varies by undergraduate program

INFORMATION ON 2003–2004 ENTERING CLASS

Number of	In-State	Out-of-State	Total
Applicants	n/a	n/a	n/a
Applicants Interviewed	73	32	105
New Entrants	37	13	50
Total number of students enrolled in program: 215			

Drexel University and Drexel University College of Medicine

Philadelphia, Pennsylvania

Address Inquiries To:

Kristen Schwarze
Admissions Coordinator
Drexel University
3141 Chestnut Street
Philadelphia, PA 19104
(215) 895-2400; 895-5939 (FAX)
Web site: http://www.drexel.edu

Purpose

This combined-degree program provides outstanding high school seniors, who are highly motivated toward the medical profession, an opportunity to combine a strong liberal arts undergraduate program with a medical education in seven years.

Requirements for Entrance

Students are selected for this program during their senior year of high school. Both residents and nonresidents of Pennsylvania are eligible to apply. Prior to graduating from high school, applicants are required to complete one semester of biology, one semester of chemistry, one semester of physics, four years of English, and four years of mathematics. They must take either the SAT or the ACT Assessment.

Selection Factors

The academic factors taken into consideration for admission into the combined-degree program include SAT/ACT scores, high school GPA, and AP and honors courses. The average high school GPA for the 2003-2004 entering class was 4.1, with a mean score of 1445 on the SAT. Medically-related volunteer activities, leadership qualities, and community service are among the personal attributes sought in applicants. An interview is also required.

Once admitted into the program, students are expected to maintain an overall GPA of 3.45 in undergraduate studies; achieve a total minimum MCAT score of 30, or a score of 9 or better on each section of the MCAT; apply through AMCAS in the second year; complete all prerequisite courses; and receive no grade less than a "C" in any course. The MCAT is a factor in admittance and promotion to the medical school phase of the program.

Curriculum

This seven-year program leads to a baccalaureate degree awarded by Drexel University and to the M.D. degree granted by the Drexel University College of Medicine. The most frequent major is biology, followed by chemistry and biomedical engineering. During the first three years of the undergraduate phase, students spend 100 percent of their time in coursework related to the bachelor's degree, which includes 3 semester hours of natural and physical science.

Expenses

In 2003-2004, undergraduate tuition for residents and non-residents was $24,800, plus annual fees of $1,405. The medical school tuition for residents and nonresidents was $33,100, plus annual fees of $1,000.

Financial Aid

Students are required to submit a FAFSA form by March 1st of their senior year in high school. Additional information can be obtained from the Drexel University Financial Aid Office, 3141 Chestnut Street, Philadelphia, Pennsylvania 19104, by phone (215) 895-2537, Email finaid@drexel.edu, or visit ✍ www.drexel.edu/provost/finaid/main_menu.htm.

APPLICATION AND ACCEPTANCE POLICIES

Filing of application:
  Earliest date: Rolling
  Latest date: December 15, 2004
Application fee: $50 (free online)
Acceptance notice:
  Earliest date: March 15, 2005
  Latest date: March 31, 2005
Applicant's response to acceptance offer:
  Latest date: May 1, 2005
Deposit to hold place in class: $200; nonrefundable
Starting date: September 26, 2005

INFORMATION ON 2003–2004 ENTERING CLASS

Number of	In-State	Out-of-State	Total
Applicants	562	704	1,266
Applicants Interviewed	17	32	49
New Entrants	6	10	16
Total number of students enrolled in program: 31			

Lehigh University and Drexel University College of Medicine

Bethlehem, Pennsylvania

Address Inquiries To:

Office of Admissions
Lehigh University
27 Memorial Drive West
Bethlehem, Pennsylvania 18105
(610) 758-3100; 758-4361 (FAX)
Web site: www.lehigh.edu

Purpose

This program is designed to give gifted high school students who are highly motivated for a career in medicine the opportunity to combine a liberal arts program with a medical education. The baccalaureate degree is awarded after Year 4 (the first year of medical school).

Requirements for Entrance

Students are selected for this program during their senior year of high school. Residents and nonresidents of Pennsylvania are considered for this program. Applicants are expected to have completed the following courses by the time they finish high school: four years each of English and mathematics and two years each of history, science, and a foreign language. Applicants are expected to take the SAT; SAT II tests in math, writing, and chemistry are required.

Selection Factors

Generally, a combined SAT score of 1360 (or minimum 31 ACT), a class rank in the top 10 percent of the high school class, and a strong motivation for science are necessary for entrance into this program. Most recent matriculants had a high school GPA of 3.9, an SAT Verbal score of 721, and an SAT Math score of 761. Maturity, stability, scholarship, flexibility, independence, and service to others are personal characteristics sought among applicants. An interview is required. Once admitted to the program, students are expected to maintain an overall grade-point average of 3.45 or better, with no grade less than a "C" in any course. Candidates are required to take the MCAT. It is required that the three numbered scores equal or exceed 9 on the same test. All program requirements must be completed at Lehigh University.

Curriculum

This program, seven years in duration, allows students to obtain a bachelor's degree from Lehigh University and an M.D. degree from Drexel University College of Medicine. Students have the flexibility to pursue additional coursework or study abroad during the undergraduate portion of the program.

Students are not required to complete work for a bachelor's degree; however, specific course requirements for the degree include two semesters of English, three semesters of mathematics, eight semesters of natural and physical sciences, three semesters each of humanities and social sciences, a freshman seminar, a writing intensive, and four elective courses.

All students must pass USMLE Steps 1 and 2 in order to graduate from the medical school.

Expenses

In 2003-2004 tuition at Lehigh University was $27,230 per year.

Financial Aid

Institutional scholarships and loans are available, as well as federal loan programs and armed services scholarships. More financial aid information can be obtained from the Financial Aid Office, Lehigh University, 218 W. Packer Avenue, Bethlehem, Pennsylvania 18015.

APPLICATION AND ACCEPTANCE POLICIES

Filing of application:
  Earliest date: September 1, 2004
  Latest date: November 15, 2004
Application fee: $50
Acceptance notice: April 1, 2005
Applicant's response to acceptance offer:
  Latest date: May 1, 2005
Deposit to hold place in class: $500 nonrefundable
Starting date: August 2005

INFORMATION ON 2003–2004 ENTERING CLASS

Number of	In-State	Out-of-State	Total
Applicants	n/a	n/a	258
Applicants Interviewed	n/a	n/a	71
New Entrants	n/a	n/a	7

Temple University School of Medicine

Philadelphia, Pennsylvania

Address Inquiries To:
Office of Admissions
Temple University School of Medicine
3400 North Broad Street
SFC Suite 305
Philadelphia, PA 19140
(215) 707-3656; 707-6932 (FAX)
Web site: www.medschool.temple.edu

Purpose

The Medical Scholars Program, in conjunction with five undergraduate institutions in Pennsylvania, provides an opportunity for high school seniors to gain a provisional acceptance to Temple University School of Medicine upon achieving an undergraduate degree.

Requirements for Entrance

Students are selected for this program during their senior year of high school. Both residents and nonresidents of Pennsylvania are eligible to apply. Strong preference is given to residents of the Commonwealth of Pennsylvania. Though there are no specific high school course requirements, applicants are expected to have a substantial background in science and mathematics. AP coursework is viewed favorably, and students are required to take the SAT.

Selection Factors

In conjunction with the School of Medicine, each undergraduate institution considers an applicant's GPA, standardized test performance, extracurricular activities (including leadership roles), and interpersonal skills in making admission decisions. Substantial maturity and strong motivation are among the important personal qualities considered by the Admission Committee. The minimum SAT score required is 1270, with most students scoring in excess of 1350. Students are expected to be in the top 1 – 5 percent of their high school graduating class. Academic ability should be demonstrated across a wide variety of courses, including AP science coursework. Selected applicants are required to interview with a representative of the undergraduate institution and a medical school admissions officer.

Contact our partnering undergraduate institutions directly to obtain additional information about the Medical Scholars Program: Duquesne University, (412) 396-6335; Temple University, (215) 204-8669; University of Scranton, (570) 941-7901; Washington and Jefferson College, dtrelka@washjeff.edu; and Widener University, (610) 499-4004.

Curriculum

Students in this eight-year combined-degree program will complete their baccalaureate degree at one of our five partnering universities listed above. The medical degree is granted by Temple University School of Medicine. Students may choose to be a science major, but are free to explore all available options as long as they complete the premedical science requirements. Matriculation to Temple University School of Medicine is conditional upon successful completion of all GPA and MCAT requirements as outlined by each institution's agreement. Educational innovations are unique at each undergraduate institution. All students are required to complete the M.D. program without deviation from the standard curriculum, including passing USMLE Steps 1 and 2.

Expenses

Each undergraduate institution determines tuition and fees. Tuition for the M.D. program for 2003-2004 is $30,020 for Pennsylvania residents and $36,766 for non-residents.

Financial Aid

For information about financial aid, contact the Financial Aid Office of the specific partnering undergraduate institution listed above. Financial aid available to medical students includes grants, scholarships, and student loans. For additional information, visit the web site at: http://www.medschool.temple.edu/Student_Life/Student_Financial_Services.html.

APPLICATION AND ACCEPTANCE POLICIES

The policies vary with each undergraduate institution. Contact the appropriate institution for their dates and deposit information.

INFORMATION ON 2003–2004 ENTERING CLASS

Number of	In-State	Out-of-State	Total
Applicants	n/a	n/a	236
Applicants Interviewed	n/a	n/a	51
New Entrants	n/a	n/a	17
Total number of students enrolled in program: 64			

CHAPTER

10

Pennsylvania State University and Jefferson Medical College of Thomas Jefferson University

University Park, Pennsylvania

Address Inquiries To:

Undergraduate Admissions Office
Pennsylvania State University
201 Shields Building
Box 3000
University Park, Pennsylvania 16804-3000
(814) 865-5471; 863-7590 (FAX)
Web site: www.psu.edu

Purpose

This accelerated, B.S./M.D. premed-med program, which began in 1963 and has graduated over 800 students, is a cooperative effort between Pennsylvania State University, University Park, and Jefferson Medical College of Thomas Jefferson University in Philadelphia. Accepted students can select between either a six- or seven-year schedule, which gives them either two years (with summers) or three years at Pennsylvania State before proceeding to four years at Jefferson.

Requirements for Entrance

Students are selected for this program only during the senior year of high school. Both residents and nonresidents of Pennsylvania are considered for admission, but preference is given to qualified applicants from Pennsylvania. Applicants are expected to have completed the following courses by the time they graduate from high school: four units of English, $1\frac{1}{2}$ units of algebra, one unit of plane geometry, one-half unit of trigonometry, three units of science, and five units of social studies, humanities, and/or the arts.

Selection Factors

To be considered for this program, applicants must be in the top 10 percent of their high school class and offer a minimum combined SAT score of 1450 (recentered). In the 2003–2004 entering class, the average combined score on the SAT was 1510. Motivation, compassion, integrity, dedication, and performance in nonacademic areas are among the personal characteristics sought in applicants. An interview is required.

Special attention is given to the student's progress during each semester while at Pennsylvania State University. Students must take a full course load and maintain a minimum GPA of 3.5 in both science and non-science courses. For subsequent admission to Jefferson Medical College, students in this combined-degree program must take the MCAT prior to matriculation in medical school.

Curriculum

This six-year program leads to a baccalaureate degree granted by Pennsylvania State University and to the M.D. degree awarded by Jefferson Medical College.

Students begin this program in June immediately after high school graduation. They spend two full years on the Pennsylvania State, University Park, campus and then proceed to Jefferson Medical College for the regular four-year curriculum. The B.S. degree from Pennsylvania State University is awarded after successful completion of the second year at Jefferson Medical College, and the M.D. degree is awarded after successful completion of the senior year at Jefferson. Students in the seven-year schedule spend three years at Pennsylvania State, but do not have to attend summer sessions. Their B.S. degree is awarded after year one at Jefferson Medical College.

Expenses

Annual undergraduate tuition at Pennsylvania State University in 2003–2004 was $9,296 for residents of Pennsylvania and $18,918 for nonresidents. Tuition for 2003–2004 at Jefferson Medical College was $34,565 for residents and nonresidents.

Financial Aid

Scholarships, loans, and grants are the sources of financial assistance available. For more information write the Office of Student Financial Aid, Pennsylvania State University, University Park, Pennsylvania 16804-3000; (814) 865-5471.

APPLICATION AND ACCEPTANCE POLICIES

Filing of application:
  Earliest date: August 1, 2004
  Latest date: November 30, 2004
Application fee: $50
Acceptance notice:
  Earliest date: March 15, 2005
  Latest date: n/a
Applicant's response to acceptance offer:
  Latest date: May 1, 2005
Deposit to hold place in class: $300;
  all but $100 refundable
Starting date: June 2005

INFORMATION ON 2003–2004 ENTERING CLASS

Number of	In-State	Out-of-State	Total
Applicants	n/a	n/a	210
Applicants Interviewed	16	69	85
New Entrants	7	17	24
Total number of students enrolled in program: 46			

Villanova University and Drexel University College of Medicine

Villanova, Pennsylvania

Address Inquiries To:

John D. Friede, Ph.D.
Health Professions Advisor
Office of University Admission
Villanova University and
Drexel University College of Medicine
800 Lancaster Avenue
Villanova, PA 19085
(610) 519-4000; 519-6450 (FAX)
Web site: www.villanova.edu

Purpose

This combined-degree program provides outstanding high school seniors, who are highly motivated toward the medical profession, an opportunity to combine a strong liberal arts undergraduate program with medical education in seven years.

Requirements for Entrance

Students are selected for this program in their senior year of high school. Both residents and nonresidents of Pennsylvania are eligible to apply to the program. Applicants are required to complete the following courses prior to graduation from high school: one year of biology, one year of chemistry, one year of physics, four years of English, and four years of mathematics. In addition to meeting these academic requirements, applicants are also required to submit the results of the ACT or SAT (SAT II is recommended).

Selection Factors

The academic factors taken into consideration for admission into the combined-degree program include: SAT scores, high school GPA and class rank, and letters of recommendation. The average high school GPA for the 2003-2004 entering class was 3.75. Extracurricular activities and community service are among the personal attributes sought in applicants. An interview is required.

Once admitted into the program, students are expected to maintain an overall GPA of 3.45, and are required to achieve scores of either a 9 or better on each section of the MCAT, or a combined scores of 30 or better (with no score less than 8 on any section of the MCAT).

Curriculum

Students are required to complete a baccalaureate degree within the first year of medical school. The most frequent major is biology, followed by comprehensive science. This seven-year program leads to a baccalaureate degree awarded by Villanova University and to the M.D. degree granted by the Drexel University College of Medicine. During the undergraduate phase of the program, students will spend 100 percent of their time in coursework related to the bachelor's degree, which includes nine semester hours of natural and physical science, one semester hour of mathematics, and four semester hours of humanities.

Expenses

In 2003-2004, undergraduate tuition for residents and nonresidents was $24,000, plus annual fees of $500. The medical school tuition for residents and nonresidents was $33,100, plus annual fees of $1,000.

Financial Aid

Visit www.finaid.villanova.edu and www.drexed.edu/med/md program/financialplanning.html for information on financial aid.

APPLICATION AND ACCEPTANCE POLICIES

Filing of application:
  Early Decision: September 1, 2004
  Latest date: November 1, 2004
Application fee: $55
Acceptance notice:
  Earliest date: March 15, 2005
  Latest date: March 30, 2005
Applicant's response to acceptance offer:
  Latest date: May 1, 2005
Deposit to hold place in class: $400; nonrefundable
Starting date: August 2005

INFORMATION ON 2003–2004 ENTERING CLASS

Number of	In-State	Out-of-State	Total
Applicants	52	197	249
Applicants Interviewed	6	44	50
New Entrants	0	6	6
Total number of students enrolled in program: 16			

Brown University

Providence, Rhode Island

Address Inquiries To:

College Admission Office
Brown University
Box 1876
Providence, Rhode Island 02912
(401) 863-2378
College Web site: www.brown.edu
PLME Web site: http://bms.brown.edu/plme

Purpose

The Program in Liberal Medical Education (PLME) seeks to graduate physicians who are broadly and liberally educated, and who will view medicine as a socially responsible human service profession. Designed as an eight-year continuum, the PLME combines liberal arts and professional education. Great flexibility is built into the program. Working with PLME advising deans who are physicians, each student develops an individualized educational plan consistent with his or her particular interests. The PLME is the primary route of admission to the Brown Medical School.

Requirements for Entrance

Students are selected for the PLME in the senior year of high school. The Brown Admission Office recommends that applicants should have completed the following courses: four years of English, with significant emphasis on writing; three years of college preparatory mathematics; three years of a foreign language; two years of laboratory science above the freshman level; two years of history, including American history; at least one year of coursework in the arts; and at least one year of elective academic subjects. Prospective science or engineering majors should have taken physics, chemistry, and advanced mathematics. Familiarity with computers is recommended for all applicants. Applicants must take the SAT I and three SAT IIs, or the ACT. (PLME applicants are encouraged to include a science SAT II test.)

Selection Factors

Students are selected on the basis of scholastic accomplishment and promise, intellectual curiosity, emotional maturity, character, motivation, sensitivity, caring, and particularly the degree to which they seem adapted to the special features of the program. In the 2003–2004 entering class, students, on average, were in the top 2 percent of their high school class and had achieved, on average, a score of 710 Verbal and 720 Mathematics on the SAT I. An interview is not required.

Curriculum

The PLME leads to a baccalaureate degree and to the M.D. degree granted by Brown Medical School. Students must complete a baccalaureate degree in the field of their choice. Each student's educational plan is highly individualized. The PLME has introduced several innovations in medical education, including a competency-based curriculum that defines nine abilities and a core knowledge base expected of all graduates.

Expenses

In 2003–2004, the undergraduate tuition at Brown University was $29,200 per year and the medical school tuition was $31,872.

Financial Aid

For undergraduates in the first four years of the PLME, financial aid is awarded by the Financial Aid Office at Brown University as a package. Students are awarded monies via scholarships, work-study, and loans. During the last four years of the PLME, financial aid is administered by the Office of Admissions and Financial Aid of the medical school. Both loans and scholarships are available, although loans are the most common form of assistance.

APPLICATION AND ACCEPTANCE POLICIES

Filing of application:
  Early Decision: November 1, 2004
  Latest date: January 1, 2005
Application fee: $70
Acceptance notice:
  Earliest date: December 15, 2004
  Latest date: Early April, 2005
Applicant's response to acceptance offer:
  Latest date: May 1, 2005
Deposit to hold place in class: None
Starting date: Early September 2005

INFORMATION ON 2003–2004 ENTERING CLASS

Number of	In-State	Out-of-State	Total
Applicants	29	1,295	1,324
Applicants Interviewed	n/a	n/a	n/a
New Entrants	4	57	61

Total number of students enrolled in program: 213

East Tennessee State University

Johnson City, Tennessee

Address Inquiries To:

Dr. Lattie F. Collins
Director, Premedical-Medical Program
Office of Medical Professions Advisement
East Tennessee State University
P.O. Box 70,592
Johnson City, Tennessee 37614-1709
(423) 439-5602; 439-4840 (FAX)
Web site: www.etsu.edu/cas/premed/mpa.htm

Purpose

The Premedical-Medical Program (PMMD Program) at East Tennessee State University is an eight-year coordinated curriculum (four years of undergraduate preparation followed by four years of medical education) leading to the award of both the B.A./B.S. and M.D. degrees. The PMMD Program is designed to (1) identify and accept promising students into medical education early in their college careers; (2) provide a strong liberal arts foundation emphasizing the humanities; (3) eliminate the redundancy of coursework often present in the usual four-year premedical program followed by four years of medical school; and (4) afford students the opportunity for personal growth and maximum benefit from their undergraduate experience by reducing the stress and anxiety associated with the standard medical school application process.

*The PMMD Program is not an accelerated program; eight full years are required from college entry until completion of the M.D. degree. The PMMD Program is not a transfer program; prospective applicants are expected to enter East Tennessee State University as beginning freshmen.

Requirements for Entrance

Students are selected for the PMMD Program at the end of their freshman year on the East Tennessee State University (ETSU) campus, during which they enroll in an approved set of courses. This is not a transfer program; students who have earned more than 14 semester hours of college credit before entering ETSU are not eligible for selection. There are no state residency requirements, but residents of Tennessee will be given preference in the selection process. There are no specific high school course requirements. Applicants must have taken the ACT assessment and/or the SAT.

Selection Factors

Applicants are expected to have graduated in the top 20 percent of their high school classes, and must have scored at or above the 85th percentile for college-bound high school seniors on the ACT and/or SAT. Students must maintain a GPA of 3.3/4.0 or better during their freshman year in order to be considered for admission. The average high school GPA for students admitted to the PMMD Program in summer 2003 was 3.9/4.0, and the average GPA for their freshman year was 3.8/4.0. Their average composite ACT assessment was 28.

Two or more interviews are required. Students are not required to take the MCAT for selection, but are required to take the MCAT and to perform at a satisfactory level prior to beginning the medical school component of the program.

Curriculum

The Premedical-Medical Program leads to a baccalaureate degree in the College of Arts and Sciences and the M.D. degree awarded by the James H. Quillen College of Medicine. All students in this program must complete an undergraduate major or minor in an approved humanities discipline and must participate in a special noncredit seminar on topics of current interest in medicine.

Students are required to pass Step 1 of the USMLE before entering the final year of clerkship studies. Students must pass Step 2 of the USMLE in order to graduate.

Expenses

In 2003–2004, the undergraduate tuition rate was $3,838 per year and the medical school tuition rate was $15,110 per year for Tennessee residents. The corresponding out-of-state tuition rates were $11,770 and $30,800, respectively.

Financial Aid

For more information, contact the Office of Financial Aid, East Tennessee State University, P.O. Box 70,772, Johnson City, Tennessee 37614.

APPLICATION AND ACCEPTANCE POLICIES

Filing of application (end freshman year):
  Earliest date (typical): March 15, 2005
  Latest date (typical): April 1, 2005
Application fee: None
Acceptance notice:
  Earliest date: July 1, 2005
  Latest date: August 1, 2005
Applicant's response to acceptance offer:
  Maximum time: 2 weeks
Deposit to hold place in class: None
Starting date: August 15, 2005

INFORMATION ON 2003–2004 ENTERING CLASS

Number of	In-State	Out-of-State	Total
Applicants	16	4	20
Applicants Interviewed	16	4	20
New Entrants	9	3	12
Total number of students enrolled in program: 20			

CHAPTER

10

Fisk University and Meharry Medical College

Nashville, Tennessee

Address Inquiries To:

Marshana Moore
Senior Admissions Recruiter
Fisk University
Office of Admissions
1000 17th Avenue North
Nashville, Tennessee 37208
(615) 329-8817; (615) 329-8774 (FAX)
Web site: www.fisk.edu

Reprinted from Medical School Admission Requirements, 2003-2004

Purpose

The Joint Program in Biomedical Sciences is designed to address America's need to train bright young students from groups underrepresented in medicines who are dedicated to finding solutions to biomedical problems through research and who will be future health care providers.

Requirements for Entrance

Students are selected at the end of their first semester of undergraduate coursework on the Fisk University campus. There are no specific high school course requirements. Applicants must have taken the ACT assessment and/or the SAT.

Selection Factors

The courses taken and grades earned at Fisk University, plus ACT and/or SAT scores, are considerations for eligibility for this program. Applicants must rank in the top 20 percent of their high school class. Students must take the MCAT prior to admission into the clinical phase of the program, and a satisfactory score is required for medical school admission.

Curriculum

The Joint Program in Biomedical Sciences, seven years in duration, allows students to obtain a baccalaureate degree from Fisk University and the M.D. degree from Meharry Medical College.

Course requirements for the baccalaureate degree include 8 semesters of natural and physical sciences and 12 semesters each in the humanities and social sciences. Students are required to spend two summers in a structured academic enrichment.

Students must take Steps 1 and 2 of the USMLE during the medical school portion of the program. Passing these examinations is a factor in promotion and graduation from medical school.

The most frequent major chosen by students is biology, followed by chemistry.

Expenses

The undergraduate tuition for 2001–2002 was $9,790 for residents and nonresidents, plus $300 in annual fees. Tuition for medical school was $23,208, plus $3,916 in annual fees.

Financial Aid

Applicants and students can apply for institutional scholarships and grants, U.S. Department of Education Title IV Federal Student Aid (work-study and loans), U.S. Department of Health and Human Services Student Aid Programs (loans and scholarships), Southern Regional Education Board Grants, and Tennessee Black Conditional Grants.

Meharry's Office of Student Financial Aid makes available most federal, regional, and state financial aid applications and brochures on numerous funding opportunities. See Meharry's Web site, ☞ www.mmc.edu (index to financial assistance), for sources of financial aid. The Meharry Medical College Library, and local public libraries, have publications on most sources of student financial aid. Applicants can receive more information from the Office of Student Financial Aid, Meharry Medical College, 1005 D.B. Todd Boulevard, Nashville, Tennessee 37208.

APPLICATION AND ACCEPTANCE POLICIES

Filing of application:
 Earliest date: February 1
 Latest date: December 15
Application fee: None
Acceptance notice:
 Earliest date: February 1
 Latest date: March 1
Applicant's response to acceptance offer:
 Maximum time: 1 week
Deposit to hold place in class: None
Starting date: Retroactive second semester,
 undergraduate year 1

INFORMATION ON 2001–2002 ENTERING CLASS

Number of	In-State	Out-of-State	Total
Applicants	n/a	n/a	4
Applicants Interviewed	n/a	n/a	3
New Entrants	n/a	n/a	2
Total number of students enrolled in program: n/a			

104

Rice University and Baylor College of Medicine

Houston, Texas

Address Inquiries To:

Rice University
Office of Admissions—MS-17
P.O. Box 1892
Houston, Texas 77251-1892
(713) 348-7426; (800) 527-6957
(713) 348-5323 (FAX)
E-mail: admi@rice.edu

Purpose

To promote the education of future physicians who are scientifically competent, compassionate, and socially conscious in order to apply insight from extensive study of liberal arts and other disciplines to the study of modern medical science.

Requirements for Entrance

Students are selected for this program during their senior year of high school. Both residents and nonresidents of Texas are considered for admission. Applicants are expected to have had a varied and rigorous high school program with high academic achievement. They must take the SAT I or ACT plus three SAT II subject tests, one of which must be writing.

Selection Factors

The high school academic record, standardized test scores, course selection, extracurricular activities, and letters of recommendation are some of the factors taken into account in offering admission to an applicant. In the 2003–2004 entering class, students averaged above the top 5 percent in their high school class.

Curriculum

This is not an accelerated program; all students must complete four years of undergraduate education and four years of medical school.

Students earn a baccalaureate degree from Rice University, and are awarded the M.D. degree from Baylor College of Medicine. Minimum course requirements for this program include at least two semesters each in the humanities and social sciences and eight semesters in the natural and physical sciences.

The medical part of the curriculum devotes approximately $1\frac{1}{2}$ years to the basic sciences with clinical experience, and $2\frac{1}{2}$ years to clinical science with some basic science coursework.

The MCAT is not required for promotion or admission to the medical school. Students are required to take Step 1 of the USMLE in their second or third years. They are also required to take Step 2 of the USMLE, but passing these examinations is not a graduation requirement.

Expenses

In 2003–2004, the undergraduate tuition for all incoming freshmen was $18,850 per year, plus $811 in student fees. The medical school tuition was $6,550 for residents and $19,650 annually, for nonresidents, plus $2,138 in student fees.

Financial Aid

Sources of aid include academic and athletic scholarships and need-based loans. Applicants can receive more information from the Rice University Admission Office, M.S. 17, 6100 Main Street, Houston, Texas 77035.

APPLICATION AND ACCEPTANCE POLICIES

Filing of application:
  Earliest date: November 1, 2004
  Latest date: December 1, 2004
Application fee: $40
Acceptance notice:
  Earliest date: n/a
  Latest date: Mid-April, 2005
Applicant's response to acceptance offer:
  Latest date: May 1, 2005
Deposit to hold place in class: $100; nonrefundable
Starting date: August 25, 2005

INFORMATION ON 2003–2004 ENTERING CLASS

Number of	In-State	Out-of-State	Total
Applicants	115	122	237
Applicants Interviewed	18	21	38
New Entrants	10	5	15
Total number of students enrolled in program: 62			

CHAPTER

10

University of Texas Medical School at San Antonio

San Antonio, Texas

Address Inquiries To:

David Jones, Ph.D.
Associate Dean for Admissions
University of Texas Medical School at San Antonio
7703 Floyd Curl Drive
Mail Code 7790
San Antonio, TX 78229
(210) 567-6080; 567-6962 (FAX)
Web site: http://som.uthscsa.edu

Purpose

This combined-degree program offers the opportunity to achieve an undergraduate degree in three years, and an M.D. in the remaining four years.

Requirements for Entrance

Students are selected for this program during their senior year of high school. The program is only open to residents of Texas. Though there are no specific high school course requirements, applicants are required to take the SAT and/or ACT.

Selection Factors

Academic factors considered in selecting applicants include strength in science and mathematic coursework. In addition to an impressive academic portfolio, applicants must also demonstrate a sincere interest in medicine, and present letters of recommendation from their high school counselors or teachers. An interview is also required. The mean high school GPA for the 2003-2004 entering class was 94.

Although the MCAT is not a required part of the selection process, it is a factor for admission and promotion to the medical school phase of the program. Students are admitted to medical school based on a sliding scale, attractive MCAT and GPA scores, and a continued commitment to study medicine.

Curriculum

This seven-year-long program grants a baccalaureate degree from University of Texas at Pan America, and an M.D. degree from University of Texas Medical School at San Antonio.

Students will spend 100 percent of their time during the first three years in undergraduate studies. The same amount of time, in the last four years, will be spent in achieving a medical degree. Students are required to take one semester hour each of social science and math, and eight semester hours of natural and physical science.

Expenses

In 2003-2004, undergraduate tuition for residents was $2,300, plus annual fees of $650. The tuition for medical school residents was $6,500 in addition to annual fees of $3,000.

Financial Aid

For information about financial aid, visit ✏ http://student services.uthscsa.edu/fmancialinfo/financialaid.html.

APPLICATION AND ACCEPTANCE POLICIES

Filing of application:
  Earliest date: N/A
  Latest date: February 2, 2004
Application fee: None
Acceptance notice:
  Earliest date: March 1, 2004
  Latest date: March 30, 2004
Applicant's response to acceptance offer:
  Maximum time: Two weeks
Deposit to hold place in class: None
Starting date: April 1, 2005

INFORMATION ON 2001–2002 ENTERING CLASS

Number of	In-State	Out-of-State	Total
Applicants	26	n/a	26
Applicants Interviewed	16	n/a	16
New Entrants	7	n/a	7
Total number of students enrolled in program: 7			

Eastern Virginia Medical School

Norfolk, Virginia

Address Inquiries To:

Office of Admissions
Eastern Virginia Medical School
721 Fairfax Avenue
Norfolk, Virginia 23507-2000
(757) 446-5812; 446-5896 (FAX)
Web site: www.evms.edu

Purpose

Eastern Virginia Medical School currently has combined programs with six colleges and universities—the College of William and Mary, Old Dominion University, Hampton University, Norfolk State University, Hampden-Sydney College, and Virginia Wesleyan College. The purpose of these programs is to enlist outstanding high school and undergraduate students into a track that provides great freedom and choice in the pursuit of a baccalaureate degree.

Requirements for Entrance

Students are selected during their sophomore year of college. Both residents and nonresidents of Virginia are eligible to apply. There are no specific high school course requirements, but students must take the SAT.

Selection Factors

Applicants will be evaluated on their overall high school performance, as well as on their academic performance during their freshman year of college. Selected applicants are invited for an interview.

Curriculum

The eight-year curriculum leads to a baccalaureate degree awarded by the College of William and Mary, Old Dominion University, Hampton University, Norfolk State University, Hampden-Sydney College, or Virginia Wesleyan College. The M.D. degree is granted by Eastern Virginia Medical School. The course requirements for the baccalaureate degree vary at each undergraduate institution, but the most frequent major is biology. This early assurance program does, however, permit the student the opportunity for academic diversity. Students selected who have combined SAT scores greater than 1250 will not be required to take the MCAT. Step 1 of the USMLE must be taken at the completion of the second year of medical school. Students must pass Steps 1 and 2 of the USMLE to complete the program and receive the M.D. degree.

Expenses

In 2003–2004, the annual medical school tuition was $18,975 for state residents and $35,075 for nonresidents. The student fees were $2,966 per year.

Financial Aid

For information about financial aid during the undergraduate phase, contact the Office of Financial Aid at the undergraduate institutions identified. Six programs are available: the College of William and Mary, Randolph A. Coleman, Ph.D., (757) 221-2679; Old Dominion University, Terri Mathews, (757) 683-5201; Hampton University, Harold Marioneaux, D.D.S., Colleges (757) 728-6897; Norfolk State University, Arnetta Sherrod, (757) 823-8512; Hampden-Sydney College, Paul Mueller, Ph.D., (434) 223-6171; and Virginia Wesleyan Colleges, Victor Townsend, Ph.D., (757) 455-3392. For information about financial aid during the medical school phase, contact the Office of Financial Aid at Eastern Virginia Medical School at (757) 446-5813.

CHAPTER
10

APPLICATION AND ACCEPTANCE POLICIES

Information varies at each undergraduate institution.
Application fee: $25–$35

INFORMATION ON 2003–2004 ENTERING CLASS

Number of	In-State	Out-of-State	Total
Applicants	70	47	117
Applicants Interviewed	31	8	39
New Entrants	11	0	11
Total number of students enrolled in program: n/a			

Virginia Commonwealth University

Richmond, Virginia

Address Inquiries To:
Dr. Anne L. Chandler
Associate Director, University Honors Program
Virginia Commonwealth University
P.O. Box 843010
Richmond, Virginia 23284-3010
(804) 828-1803; 827-1669 (FAX)
E-mail: alchandl@vcu.edu
Web site: www.vcu.edu/honors

Purpose

The Guaranteed Admission Program offers academically capable, highly focused students an opportunity to pursue diverse, intellectually challenging programs of study without the pressure of competing further for medical school admission. Close contact with the School of Medicine throughout the undergraduate program aids students in testing their career choice and in preparing for a lifelong commitment to learning in the profession.

Requirements for Entrance

Students are selected during their senior year of high school, and there are no state residency restrictions. All candidates are considered. The specific high school course requirements are as follows: eight semesters of English; six semesters each of social sciences, mathematics, and sciences; a foreign language, or four semesters each of two languages. Also required are standardized admissions tests such as the ACT (composite score at or above 29) or a combined SAT score of 1270 in a single sitting with neither score below 530, and an unweighted GPA of 3.0 (4.0 scale).

Selection Factors

Academic factors considered in offering admission to an applicant include GPA, letters of reference, test scores, well-rounded and rigorous academic preparation, health care-related experience, and written and oral communication skills. The average GPA for the 2003–2004 entering class was 3.77 (unweighted scale of 4.0), and average SAT scores of 1400. Selected applicants are invited for a required interview.

Curriculum

Students are required to complete a baccalaureate degree. The most frequent major is biology; the next most frequent major is chemistry. Both are awarded by Virginia Commonwealth University. Specific course requirements vary, depending upon the major. During the medical school program, there is a longitudinal clinical experience (Foundations of Clinical Medicine) in a community, primary care practice that meets weekly for both of the first two years. Students are required to take Step 1 of the USMLE at the end of their second year. They must also take USMLE Step 2, but passing these examinations is not a promotion or graduation requirement. The Doctor of Medicine degree is also awarded at Virginia Commonwealth University. It takes eight years to fulfill the requirements for both degrees.

Expenses

Tuition for undergraduates in the 2003–2004 academic year was $3,600 for residents and $15,904 for nonresidents. The medical school tuition in 2003–2004 was $18,500 for residents and $34,328 for nonresidents. Annual student fees averaged $1,289 for undergraduates and $1,273 for medical students.

Financial Aid

There are several sources of financial aid available to students—scholarships, loans, grants, and work-study. For more information contact the Virginia Commonwealth University, P.O. Box 842506, Richmond, Virginia 23284-2506; (804) VCU-MONY.

APPLICATION AND ACCEPTANCE POLICIES

Filing of application:
  Earliest date: September 1, 2004
  Latest date: December 15, 2004
Application fee: $30
Acceptance notice:
  Earliest date: April 1, 2005
  Latest date: n/a
Applicant's response to acceptance offer:
  Maximum time: 4 weeks
Deposit to hold place in class: $100; nonrefundable
Starting date: August 2005

INFORMATION ON 2003–2004 ENTERING CLASS

Number of	In-State	Out-of-State	Total
Applicants	38	112	150
Applicants Interviewed	13	37	50
New Entrants	6	13	19
Total number of students enrolled in program: 82			

University of Wisconsin Medical School

Madison, Wisconsin

Address Inquiries To:

Medical Scholars Program
University of Wisconsin Medical School
1300 University Avenue, Room 1110
Madison, Wisconsin 53706
(608) 263-7561; 262-2327 (FAX)
Web site: www.med.wisc.edu/academic
affairs/education/programs/ms/index.asp

Purpose

The Medical Scholars Program provides conditional admission to the University of Wisconsin Medical School for approximately 40 highly qualified Wisconsin high school seniors. Medical scholars are a part of the medical school community and may participate in specially designed basic science and clinical experiences.

Requirements for Entrance

Students are selected for this program during the senior year of high school. Only residents of Wisconsin are eligible to apply. Applicants are expected to have completed the following courses by the time they graduate from high school: eight semesters of mathematics, eight semesters of English, six semesters of science (including at least one semester each of biology, chemistry, and physics), six semesters of social studies, and four semesters of a foreign language. They must take either the SAT or the ACT Assessment.

Selection Factors

To be eligible for application, students must have attained a minimum academic GPA of 3.8 (including English, mathematics, science, social studies, and foreign language courses in grades 9 through 11), or be ranked in the top 5 percent of their high school class, or have a minimum combined SAT score of 1300 or a minimum composite score of 30 on the ACT Assessment. In the 2003–2004 entering class, the average GPA was 3.97, the average SAT combined score was 1430, and the average composite score on the ACT Assessment was 33. An interview may be required.

Curriculum

This program, usually seven to nine years in duration, permits students to obtain a bachelor's degree from the University of Wisconsin–Madison and the M.D. degree from the University of Wisconsin Medical School.

Students are expected to complete work for the bachelor's degree. Requirements for that degree vary according to the major chosen, but all include coursework in the humanities, social sciences, and natural and physical sciences. The most frequent major chosen by students in this program is molecular biology, followed by zoology.

Educational innovations offered include: (a) a wide range of experiences in medical science research and exposure to clinical medicine allowing students to integrate undergraduate and medical education; (b) the opportunity to major in any subject; (c) completion of the undergraduate program in three to five years; and (d) a semester or year international study.

Students are expected to take Step 1 of the USMLE at the end of the second year of medical school, with a passing score required in order to begin clinical work. Passing both USMLE Steps 1 and 2 is a graduation requirement.

Expenses

In 2003–2004, residents of Wisconsin paid $5,140 per year to attend the University of Wisconsin–Madison and $22,450 per year at the University of Wisconsin Medical School.

Financial Aid

Scholarships and loans are available to students according to their need. More information can be obtained from the University of Wisconsin–Madison Financial Aid Office, 432 North Murray Street, Madison, Wisconsin 53706.

APPLICATION AND ACCEPTANCE POLICIES

Filing of application:
    Earliest date: September, 2004
    Latest date: January 15, 2005
Application fee: None
Acceptance notice:
    Earliest date: n/a
    Latest date: April 1, 2005
Applicant's response to acceptance offer:
    Latest date: 1 month (by May 1, 2005)
Deposit to hold place in class: None
Starting date: Mid-August 2005

INFORMATION ON 2003–2004 ENTERING CLASS

Number of	In-State	Out-of-State	Total
Applicants	n/a	n/a	243
Applicants Interviewed	n/a	n/a	n/a
New Entrants	n/a	n/a	44
Total number of students enrolled in program: 170			

CHAPTER

10

Information About U.S. Medical Schools
Accredited by the LCME

Information about individual medical schools is given in the following two-page entries for 122 schools in the United States and three schools in Puerto Rico that will be considering applications for fall 2005 entering classes. The schools presented here are fully accredited as of fall 2003 by the Liaison Committee on Medical Education (LCME), which is sponsored by the Association of American Medical Colleges (AAMC) and the American Medical Association (AMA).

Individual school entries provide the tuition and student fees for a 2003–2004 first-year student.

Each school entry provides statistics on the number of applicants, interviewed applicants, and new entrants (students entering medical school for the first time, excluding repeaters and re-entrants) to the 2003–2004 first-year class. These statistics are presented by residence status – in-state and out-of-state. Foreign nationals who do not have permanent resident status in the United States are included in the out-of-state figures.

Abbreviations

Listed below are the abbreviations used in the school entries in this chapter.

AMCAS–American Medical College Application Service
CLEP–College Level Examination Program
FAF–Financial Aid Form
FAFSA–Free Application for Federal Student Aid
FAP–Fee Assistance Program
GAPSFAS–Graduate and Professional School Financial Aid Service
GPA–Grade-point average
MCAT–Medical College Admission Test
VR–Verbal Reasoning
PS–Physical Sciences
WS–Writing Sample
BS–Biological Sciences
USMLE–United States Medical Licensing Examination
WICHE–Western Interstate Commission for Higher Education

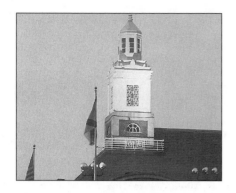

University of Alabama School of Medicine

Birmingham, Alabama

Dr. William B. Deal, *Dean*
Dr. Nathan B. Smith, *Assistant Dean for Admissions*
Mark H. Martin, *Associate Director of Medical Student Services for Financial Aid*
Dr. Johnny W. Scott, *Assistant Dean, for Minority Programs*

ADDRESS INQUIRIES TO:

Office of Medical Student Services/Admissions
University of Alabama
School of Medicine
Volker Hall 100
1530 3rd Ave. S.
Birmingham, Alabama 35294-0019
(205) 934-2433; 934-8724 (FAX)
E-mail: medschool@uab.edu
Web site: www.uab.edu/uasom/

MISSION STATEMENT

The School of Medicine is dedicated to the education of physicians and scientists in all of the disciplines of medicine and biomedical investigation for careers in practice, teaching, and research. Necessary to this educational mission are the provision of outstanding medical care and services and the enhancement of new knowledge through clinical and basic biomedical research.

GENERAL INFORMATION

The School of Medicine was founded in Mobile in 1859, moved to the campus of the University of Alabama in Tuscaloosa in 1920, and relocated to Birmingham in 1945. The University of Alabama School of Medicine, composed of the main campus in Birmingham and branch campuses in Huntsville and Tuscaloosa, was created in 1969. A six-story addition to the medical student education facility in Birmingham opened in the summer of 2003, and the Huntsville and Tuscaloosa campuses have new clinical education buildings.

CURRICULUM

The four-year academic program emphasizes the fundamentals that underlie clinical medical practice including attention to the emotional, cultural, and social characteristics of patients and to the importance of adapting care to meet their needs. First-year courses include anatomy, physiology, biochemistry, nutrition, behavioral science, neuroscience, medical ethics, and history of medicine. Second-year courses include microbiology, pharmacology, and pathology. In addition, both years include an Introduction to Clinical Medicine course providing training in medical professionalism, patient interviewing, and physical examination. All students are required to pass Step 1 of the USMLE at the end of the second year.

The third year and part of the fourth year consist of required rotations in internal medicine, surgery, pediatrics, obstetrics-gynecology, family medicine/rural medicine, psychiatry and neurology. This involves participation in the care of patients in both hospital and ambulatory settings. The remainder of the fourth year is elective and individualized experiences. All students are required to pass Step 2 of the USMLE and an Observed Structured Clinical Examination (OSCE) prior to graduation.

After completing the first two years in Birmingham, students are assigned to the Birmingham, Huntsville, or Tuscaloosa campus for their required clinical rotations. Other clinical rotations may be taken on any of the campuses during the fourth year.

There are three opportunities for combined degrees: MD/PhD (Medical Scientist Training Program), MD/MPH, and MD/MS. The University of Alabama, Birmingham and the University of Alabama School of Medicine offer an eight-year Early Medical School Acceptance Program (EMSAP) for exceptional high school students.

REQUIREMENTS FOR ENTRANCE

The MCAT and at least 90 semester hours from an accredited institution are required. With rare exceptions, completion of an undergraduate degree is expected. The MCAT should be taken during the spring before making application in early summer. Grades below C in required courses are not acceptable. Applicants should select a major that best suits their talents and interests since no specific major is preferred. Coursework in Spanish, social and behavioral sciences, and biochemistry is strongly encouraged. Applicants enrolled in a graduate-degree program must complete all requirements for that degree prior to matriculation to medical school. Specific requirements include:

Sem. hrs.

General Biology or Zoology 8
Inorganic (General) Chemistry (with labs). 8
Organic Chemistry (with lab). 8
General Physics (with lab). 8
College Mathematics 6
English (Composition and Literature) 6

SELECTION FACTORS

The UASOM Admissions Committee is committed to admitting those applicants who possess the intelligence, skills, attitudes, and other personal attributes to become excellent physicians and to meet the health care needs of the state of Alabama. While evidence of solid academic ability is essential for admission, other attributes are vital for becoming an excellent physician. Effective communication and interpersonal skills, evidence of service to others, empathy, emotional maturity, personal resilience, honesty, leadership ability, sense of purpose, and a growing understanding of what it means to be a physician are examples of these vital attributes. Other desirable attributes include a commitment and ability to meet healthcare needs of underserved populations, particularly urban and rural populations in Alabama, commitment to biomedical research careers, and commitment to primary care careers. While Alabama residents are given strong preference, the school is committed to a creative and a diverse student experience and encourages applications from nonresident applicants. Disadvantaged, rural, and minority residents of Alabama are encouraged to apply. Non-U.S. citizens must have a permanent U.S. resident visa. The school provides equal educational opportunities and is open to all qualified students without regard to race, religion, national origin, age, handicap or gender.

Secondary applications are requested of selected applicants after an initial review and must be completed online. All applications and supporting documents are read by members of the Admissions Committee. Selected applicants are interviewed individually on the Birmingham campus by members of the Admissions Committee. The average GPA for admitted applicants in recent years has been between 3.6 and 3.7. Successful applicants have undergraduate degrees in a broad range of subjects. There is a special acceptance program for state residents committed to rural practice in Alabama. Information is available at: http://bama.ua.edu/~ruralmed/.

Transfers from other LCME-accredited medical schools are considered for students in good academic standing, who have a compelling reason to transfer. Available positions are limited to attrition.

AP or CLEP coursework may be accepted to meet a premedical requirement on a case-by-case basis. Factors for acceptance include the overall strength the applicant's undergraduate academic record and MCAT scores. AP and CLEP coursework least likely to be accepted for biology and chemistry courses.

FINANCIAL AID

About 82 percent of our students receive financial aid. Available loan funds are disbursed primarily on the basis of demonstrated financial need. State scholarships/loans are available in limited numbers to Alabama residents who can demonstrate economic need. Other scholarships are awarded on a merit basis. Students are advised not to seek outside employment. Summer research opportunities, supported by stipends and fellowships, are available. Alabama residents who commit to practice in rural Alabama may receive aid from the state.

The School of Medicine will consider the waiver of application fees for disadvantaged students, and some interviewing costs may be defrayed.

INFORMATION ABOUT DIVERSITY PROGRAMS

Through the Office of Minority Programs, the Admission Committee attempts to identify and provide academic counseling and information to students from groups underrepresented in medicine early in their college careers to facilitate application processes.

Institution Type: *Public*
Application Process: *AMCAS, see chapter 4.*

APPLICATION AND ACCEPTANCE POLICIES FOR 2005–2006 FIRST-YEAR CLASS

Filing of AMCAS application
  Earliest date: June 1, 2004
  Latest date: Nov. 1, 2004
School application fee after screening: $65
Oldest MCAT scores considered: 2002
Does have Early Decision Program (EDP)
  For Alabama residents only
  EDP application period: June 1–Aug. 1, 2004
  EDP applicants notified by: Oct. 1, 2004
Acceptance notice to regular applicants
  Earliest date: Oct. 15, 2004
  Latest date: Until class is filled
Applicant's response to acceptance offer
  Maximum time: 2 weeks
Requests for deferred entrance considered: Yes
Deposit to hold place in class (applied to tuition):
  $50, due with response to acceptance offer
  ($500 out of state)
Deposit refundable prior to: May 16, 2005
Estimated number of new entrants: 160 (10 EDP)
Starting date: July 2005

TUITION AND STUDENT FEES PER YEAR FOR 2003–2004 FIRST-YEAR CLASS

Tuition   Student fees: $3,966
  Resident: $8,886
  Nonresident: $26,658

INFORMATION ON 2003-2004 FIRST-YEAR CLASS

Number of	*In-State*	*Out-of-State*	*Total*
Applicants	418	947	1,365
Applicants Interviewed	292	169	461
New Entrants*	144	16	160

*99% took the MCAT; 100% had baccalaureate degrees.

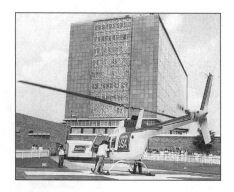

University of South Alabama
College of Medicine

Mobile, Alabama

Dr. Robert A. Kreisberg, *Dean*
Dr. M. Margaret O'Brien, *Vice Dean, Student Affairs and Medical Education*
Mark Scott, *Director for Admissions*
Dr. Hattie M. Myles, *Assistant Dean, Special Programs and Student Affairs*

ADDRESS INQUIRIES TO:

Office of Admissions, 2015 MSB
University of South Alabama
College of Medicine
Mobile, Alabama 36688-0002
(251) 460-7176; 460-6278 (FAX)
Web site: www.southalabama.edu/com/

MISSION STATEMENT

To prepare talented, highly qualified students to become physicians, providing them the opportunity to develop basic science and clinical skills that will carry them successfully through residency and their career in medicine.

GENERAL INFORMATION

The College of Medicine of the University of South Alabama was approved by the Board of Trustees of the university in 1967; the legislature of the state of Alabama passed a resolution authorizing the college on August 19, 1967. The college admitted a charter class of 25 students in January 1973 and a full class of 64 students in September 1973. No increase or decrease in the number of entering students is planned. The basic medical sciences are housed on the university campus in a building that was completed in March 1974. The largest site for the clinical education program is the University of South Alabama Medical Center. Operating continuously since 1831, this hospital has provided medical education for more than a century. It functions as the major physician-staffed emergency facility in South Alabama and has been named a Level I trauma center by the Alabama Committee on Trauma. Other clinical training facilities include the U.S.A. Springhill Campus, U.S.A. Cancer Center and Clinical Building, U.S.A. Health Services Building, and Searcy Hospital. U.S.A. Knollwood and U.S.A. Children's and Women's Hospitals, our most recent additions, provide our students with state-of-the-art clinical training facilities.

CURRICULUM

The first year is devoted to the basic sciences of anatomy, physiology, biochemistry, neuroanatomy, and embryology. However, opportunity for early introduction to clinical problems is afforded by courses such as Correlation Conferences and Medical Practice and Society. The second year includes pathology, physical diagnosis, microbiology-immunology, pharmacology, and behavioral science. Public health/epidemi-

ology and medical genetics round out the second-year curriculum. All students are required to take and pass Step 1 of the USMLE at the end of the second year. The third year is composed of clinical clerkships in medicine, surgery, pediatrics, psychiatry, obstetrics-gynecology, and family practice. The fourth year is composed of nine rotations of four weeks each. The student is required to select one rotation each in clinical neuroscience, surgical subspecialties, ambulatory care, primary care subspecialty in medicine, pediatrics, or obstetrics-gynecology, acting internship, and an in-house elective. Three of the rotations may be used for approved extramural experiences. Students are required to take and pass Step 2 of the USMLE in September of the fourth year. An A–F (A, B, C, D, F) grading system is used with the exception of the fourth year, during which an honors/pass/fail system is used.

The philosophy of the institution is to utilize all of the existing resources that provide opportunities for almost all of the experiences in clinical medicine. After acquiring a sound basis in scientific medicine, students then have the opportunity to select multiple tracks of study.

A combined M.D.-Ph.D. program in basic medical sciences is also offered.

REQUIREMENTS FOR ENTRANCE

The MCAT and three years of college are required; the baccalaureate degree is highly desirable. Each applicant must have at least 90 semester hours of acceptable credit from an accredited undergraduate institution. Required courses are:

Sem. hrs.

General Biology (with lab) 8
General Chemistry (with lab) 8
Organic Chemistry (with lab) 8
General Physics (with lab) 8
Humanities 6
English Composition and/or Literature 6
College Mathematics 8
Calculus is highly recommended.

The University of South Alabama College of Medicine does not accept pass/fail grades for required science courses, except in the rare instance in which an applicant's college assigns only pass/fail grades.

Applicants are strongly urged to take the MCAT in the spring of the year of application and to have their basic science requirements completed at the time of application. Required coursework in process or fall MCAT scores delay the processing of an application.

SELECTION FACTORS

The Committee on Admissions will consider seriously all candidates whose undergraduate academic work and scores on the MCAT indicate that they will be able to handle the rigorous curriculum of the College of Medicine. However, consideration will be given to more than scholastic achievement alone. Applicants will be considered from the standpoint of their potential to become conscientious and capable physicians. The University of South Alabama provides equal educational opportunities and is open to all qualified students without regard to race, creed, national origin, sex, or handicap with respect to all of its programs and activities. Because the college is state-supported, preference is shown to Alabama residents; however, residents of the Mississippi Gulf Coast and Florida Panhandle qualify for in-state tuition.

Disadvantaged, rural, and minority residents of Alabama are strongly encouraged to apply. The application process consists of two stages: the preliminary AMCAS application and the final application sent when requested by the Committee on Admissions. This latter application requires recommendations, a photograph, and a $50 fee. After review of the final application, the committee will select those applicants to be invited to the campus for interviews. Fee waivers, based solely on economic need, are granted when documented.

The 65 members of the 1998 entering class came from 31 different undergraduate schools. The *average undergraduate GPA* was 3.70; *average MCAT scores,* VR-10.0, PS-9.2, BS-9.9; 90 percent *residents* of Alabama.

FINANCIAL AID

The Office of Financial Aid coordinates the programs of assistance available to medical students demonstrating financial need. Scholarships are also available for entering freshmen and medical students who have demonstrated academic excellence and/or financial need.

A limited number of state scholarships/loans are available to Alabama residents who can demonstrate economic need. After graduation, repayment may be made by cash or by the practice of medicine in certain areas of the state for the number of years stipulated by law.

The Medical Student Summer Research Program is available to entering first-year students and rising second-year students. The participants are paid a stipend, and no previous research experience is necessary. Part-time employment is available; however, students are discouraged from accepting employment during academic periods.

INFORMATION ABOUT DIVERSITY PROGRAMS

The school is committed to the enrollment and education of individuals from all disadvantaged groups. For information, write Dr. Hattie M. Myles, assistant dean of special programs and student affairs.

Institution Type: *Public*
Application Process: *AMCAS, see chapter 4.*

APPLICATION AND ACCEPTANCE POLICIES FOR 2005–2006 FIRST-YEAR CLASS

Filing of AMCAS application
    Earliest date: June 1, 2004
    Latest date: Nov. 15, 2004
School application fee after screening: $50
Oldest MCAT scores considered: 2002
Does have Early Decision Program (EDP)
    For Alabama residents only and service area
    EDP application period: June 1–Aug. 1, 2004
    EDP application notified by: Oct. 1, 2004
Acceptance notice to regular applicants
    Earliest date: Nov. 15, 2004
    Latest date: Until class is filled
Applicant's response to acceptance offer
    Maximum time: 2 weeks
Requests for deferred entrance considered: Yes
Deposit to hold place in class (applied to tuition):
    $50, due with response to acceptance offer
Deposit refundable prior to: May 16, 2005, if requested in writing
Estimated number of new entrants: 64 (10 EDP)
Starting date: Aug. 2005

TUITION AND STUDENT FEES PER YEAR FOR 2003–2004 FIRST-YEAR CLASS

Tuition   Student fees: $2,951
    Resident: $9,770
    Nonresident: $19,540

INFORMATION ON 2003–2004 FIRST-YEAR CLASS

Number of	In-State	Out-of-State	Total
Applicants	371	395	766
Applicants Interviewed	170	21	191
New Entrants*	59	5	64

*All took the MCAT and had baccalaureate degrees.

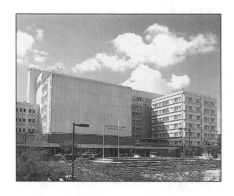

University of Arizona
College of Medicine

Tucson, Arizona

Dr. Kenneth J. Ryan, *Interim Dean*
Dr. Christopher A. Leadem, *Senior Associate Dean*
Maggie Gumble, *Program Coordinator Senior, Financial Aid*
Linda K. Don, *Director, Office of Minority Affairs*

ADDRESS INQUIRIES TO:

Admissions Office, Room 2209
University of Arizona
College of Medicine
P.O. Box 245075
Tucson, Arizona 85724-5075
(520) 626-6214; 626-3777 (FAX)
E-mail: admissions@medicine.arizona.edu
Web site: www.medicine.arizona.edu

MISSION STATEMENT

The mission of the College of Medicine, as it pertains to medical students, is to provide medical students with the knowledge and skills basic to the practice of medicine, and inculcate them with the fundamental attitudes of compassionate patient care and a spirit and desire for lifelong independent learning and scholarship.

GENERAL INFORMATION

The College of Medicine enrolled its first class of students in 1967. As a professional and graduate college of the University of Arizona located adjacent to the main campus, its programs provide education and training for both the M.D. and Ph.D. degrees.

The University of Arizona Health Sciences Center complex consists of several interconnected buildings and adjoining structures on a 30-acre site north of the main campus (Arthritis Center, Basic Sciences Building, Clinical Sciences Building, Life Sciences Building, Outpatient Clinic, Arizona Health Sciences Library, University Medical Center, Children's Research Center, Arizona Cancer Center, and Sarver Heart Center). The Colleges of Nursing and Pharmacy are located south of the Basic Sciences Building, and the College of Public Health is located within the Basic Sciences Building. A student wing of the Basic Sciences Building houses the multidisciplinary laboratories, anatomy laboratories, the learning resource center, lecture rooms, conference rooms, student lounge, and support facilities.

CURRICULUM

The overall purpose of the educational program is to give students the desire for lifelong learning in medicine by creating study habits that call for the continuous pursuit of knowledge and the capacity to modify previously acquired information. The program also aims to give students the skills to conduct patient care activities as well as the professional attitudes consonant with the charge to provide patients with preventive and curative advice and treatment.

Biologic, cultural, psychosocial, economic, and sociologic concepts and data are provided in the core curriculum. Increasing emphasis is placed on problem-solving ability, beginning with initial instruction and carried through to graduation. Excellence in performance is encouraged and facilitated. Awareness of the milieu in which medicine is practiced is also encouraged. The core curriculum comprises three years of required studies and one year of elective rotations. The learning environment encompasses lectures, small-group discussion and problem-solving sessions, independent study, clinical clerkships, practice in physical diagnosis, computer-based instruction, and a variety of other modes for the learner. Students learn in the classroom, conference room, laboratory, clinic and physician's office, bed units of hospitals, special sites for diagnostic and therapeutic maneuvers, University Medical Center, and a variety of inpatient and outpatient settings in Tucson, Phoenix, and throughout Arizona. All medical students will participate in an educational experience with an underserved population sometime during medical school. Upon graduation the physician is equipped to continue postgraduate education in general or specialty practice, teaching, or research. Combined M.D.-Ph.D. and M.D.-M.P.H. programs of study are also offered.

REQUIREMENTS FOR ENTRANCE

All applicants must be residents of Arizona or WICHE-certified and funded residents of Montana, or Wyoming. The MCAT and a minimum of three years of college are required. Each applicant must successfully complete at least 90 semester hours (135 quarter hours) at an accredited college or university, including 30 semester hours of upper division courses. A baccalaureate degree is preferred. Applicants educated outside the United States or Canada must have completed the same required courses as students in the U.S. or Canada, including 30 hours of upper-division courses, prior to submitting an application. Postbaccalaureate students should have recent courses in the required science areas. The following specific courses are required:

	Sem./Qtr.
General Biology or Zoology	2/3
General Chemistry	2/3
Organic Chemistry	2/3
Physics	2/3
English (Composition and Literature)	2/3

CLEP or AP credits are acceptable for the required courses. Applicants are strongly urged to take the MCAT in the spring of the year of application and to have their basic requirements completed at the time of application. All required courses must be completed by the spring semester prior to matriculation. Applicants are encouraged to take the required science courses that include laboratory experiences. No preference is given to any particular kind of undergraduate academic major, although applicants are encouraged to have a broad social science and/or humanities background.

Many Arizona residents and patients who receive care at the Arizona Health Sciences Center and its affiliated clinics and hospitals speak Spanish as their primary language, and it would be useful for our medical students to be conversant in Spanish.

SELECTION FACTORS

The University of Arizona College of Medicine accepts only Arizona residents; highly qualified applicants who are WICHE-certified and funded residents of Montana and Wyoming, and Native Americans who reside on reservations contiguous with the state of Arizona. In evaluating applicants the Admissions Committee considers many factors including the entire academic record, performance on the MCAT, the applicant's personal statement, interviews and letters of recommendation. Applicants are chosen on the basis of their career goal, motivation, academic ability, integrity, maturity, altruism, communication skills and leadership skills. Clinical, research or community service experience is viewed favorably. The Admissions Committee strives to accept a student body with diverse backgrounds in order to best meet the medical needs of the people of Arizona. Priority consideration is given to applicants who demonstrate a willingness to practice in medically underserved areas of Arizona.

Accepted students for the 2003 entering class had the following characteristics: *mean GPA,* 3.63; *sex,* 53 percent women; *residence,* 98 percent from Arizona; *overall acceptance rate,* 35 percent of those seriously considered received acceptances; and 151 acceptances were offered out of 429 applicants considered. Disadvantaged, rural, and minority residents of Arizona are strongly encouraged to apply. The College of Medicine does not discriminate on the basis of sex, age, race, creed, national origin, or handicap in its admission policies.

FINANCIAL AID

Federal and local scholarships and loans are available to students with financial need. Ninety-one percent of the students are receiving financial assistance. All determinations of need are made after an applicant is accepted for enrollment.

INFORMATION ABOUT DIVERSITY PROGRAMS AND FOR NONTRADITIONAL STUDENTS

The College of Medicine and the Office of Minority Affairs have an active program dedicated to the recruitment, admission, education, and graduation of an increased number of individuals from groups underrepresented in medicine. The program offers the Summer Medical Education Program for premed students and a summer Preprofessional Program for entering medical students. Learning specialists work closely with students during all phases of their medical education. The Commitment to Underserved People (CUP) project provides numerous opportunities to participate in neighborhood clinic settings. Tutoring, counseling, and a variety of student support services are also available. Faculty members participate in all aspects of the program.

Institution Type: *Public*
Application Process: *AMCAS, see chapter 4.*

APPLICATION AND ACCEPTANCE POLICIES FOR 2005–2006 FIRST-YEAR CLASS

Filing of AMCAS application
   Earliest date: June 1, 2004
   Latest date: Nov. 1, 2004
School application fee: $75.00
   Oldest MCAT scores considered: 2002
Does not have Early Decision Program
Acceptance notice to regular applicants
Earliest date: Jan. 31, 2005
   Latest date: Until class is filled
Applicant's response to acceptance offer
   Maximum time: 2 weeks
Requests for deferred entrance considered: Yes
Deposit to hold place in class: None
Estimated number of new entrants: 110
Starting date: July 2005

TUITION AND STUDENT FEES PER YEAR FOR 2003-2004 FIRST-YEAR CLASS

Tuition   Student fees: $95
   Resident: $11,483
   Nonresident: Not applicable

INFORMATION ON 2003-2004 FIRST-YEAR CLASS

Number of	In-State	Out-of-State	Total
Applicants	450	155	605
Applicants Interviewed	421	14	435
New Entrants†	108	2*	110

*Certified WICHE applicants from Montana, and Wyoming.
†All took the MCAT and had baccalaureate degrees or higher.

CHAPTER
11

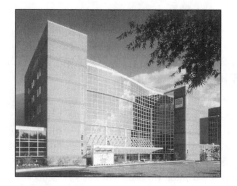

University of Arkansas for Medical Sciences College of Medicine

Little Rock, Arkansas

Dr. E. Albert Reece, *Vice Chancellor, UAMS, Dean, College of Medicine*
Tom G. South, *Director, Admissions and Financial Aid*
Dr. Richard Wheeler, *Executive Associate Dean, Academic Affairs*
Dr. Billy R. Thomas, *Assistant Dean, Office of Minority Affairs*

ADDRESS INQUIRIES TO:

Tom G. South
Office of the Dean
University of Arkansas for Medical Sciences
College of Medicine
4301 West Markham Street, Slot 551
Little Rock, Arkansas 72205-7199
(501) 686-5354; 686-5873 (FAX)
E-mail: SouthTomG@uams.edu
Web site: www.uams.edu

MISSION STATEMENT

The University of Arkansas for Medical Sciences was established in 1879 as the "Medical Department of the Arkansas Industrial University." Today it is a comprehensive health center with six colleges – Medicine, Nursing, Pharmacy, Health Related Professions, Graduate School, and our newest, the College of Public Health. It also encompasses clinical care facilities consisting of an Ambulatory Care Center, the 400-bed University Hospital, the Jones Eye Institute, the Donald W. Reynolds Center on Aging, and the Arkansas Cancer Research Center, seven Area Health Education Centers (AHECs) located in Fort Smith, Pine Bluff, El Dorado, Fayetteville, Jonesboro, Texarkana, and Helena, and research laboratories and programs located in the T. H. Barton Research Building, the Biomedical Research Building, and in virtually every other facility on campus. The education, service and research programs are closely integrated with the Arkansas Children's Hospital, the McClellan Veterans Administration Hospital adjacent to UAMS, and the North Little Rock Veterans Administration Hospital. Affiliated programs are conducted with the Arkansas State Hospital, the community hospitals in Little Rock, and the community hospitals in each AHEC region.

The mission of UAMS is to provide exemplary and comprehensive education in training programs for the health professions, to offer health and medical services in order to meet the needs of our patients in the state and region, and to conduct programs of research in human health and disease. Financial support for our mission is derived from state appropriations, tuition income, patient care fees, research grants from foundations and the federal government, and gifts from private donors. During the past decade a number of new facilities have been constructed and the University Hospital has been renovated.

The University of Arkansas for Medical Sciences has taken its place as the single major medical center in the state. We are the "sole source" for many of the educational programs in the health professions including medicine and pharmacy. We serve the state as a referral center for patients with special problems that demand the highest standards of complex medical care and we serve as the only biomedical research facility in the state. We have embarked into the 21st century with enthusiasm and confidence. Our strong base will allow us to alter existing programs and add new programs as we meet the challenges of the future.

CURRICULUM

Along with the standard courses in anatomy, biochemistry, and physiology, the first year includes a program to introduce the student to clinical contacts and concepts. This is accomplished with formal lectures in medico-socioeconomic topics, small-group discussions, faculty-supervised interviews with patients, and the extensive use of standardized patients.

The third year is a full 48 weeks with rotation through the major clinical services. This expanded clinical year provides substantial preparation for the predominantly elective fourth year, which consists of a minimum of 36 weeks to a maximum of 48 weeks of courses selected with the assistance of a faculty advisor. On- and off-campus electives are available to round out preparation for each student's career goals. The traditional grading system (A, B, C, D, F) is used throughout the first three years. Elective courses and a few selected ones in the first three years are graded as pass/fail. Opportunities are provided for students to engage in research activities and to pursue graduate courses leading to the M.D./Ph.D. and M.D./M.P.H. degrees. The number of M.D./Ph.D. scholarships has increased significantly in recent years. Plans are underway to provide students with expanded opportunities through the M.D./M.B.A. and M.D./J.D. degree programs.

REQUIREMENTS FOR ENTRANCE

The MCAT and at least 90 semester hours of college work are required; a baccalaureate degree is strongly recommended. The following courses must be completed prior to matriculation:

Semesters

Biology 2
General Chemistry 2
Organic Chemistry 2
Physics 2

Mathematics (or through Calculus I) 2
English 2

AP credit may be used to satisfy prematriculation course requirements provided the AP credit is accepted by and posted on the applicant's undergraduate college transcript.

No particular undergraduate field is given preference in the selection process; students from a variety of backgrounds are actively sought. While applicants are encouraged to follow their own interests in selecting college majors, courses such as embryology, genetics, quantitative analysis, psychology, history, statistics and logic are also recommended.

Applicants must have taken the MCAT no earlier than April 2002 and prior to the November 1 application deadline. Students enrolled in graduate/professional programs must have an advisor submit a letter assuring the completion of all graduate degree requirements prior to matriculation.

SELECTION FACTORS

Selection is based on scholastic attainment, performance on the MCAT, personal interviews with members of the faculty, and recommendations, particularly evaluations by college pre-professional advisory committees. Applicants should also demonstrate time and effort devoted to volunteerism and community service. Selection is made without regard to race, sex, creed, national origin, age, or handicap. Unsuccessful applicants may reapply without prejudice.

Matriculants for the 2003 entering class had the following profile: *mean GPA,* 3.66 (97 percent above 3.0); *sex,* 44 percent women; *undergraduate major,* 80 percent in science disciplines; *average MCAT score,* 9.0.

Although applications are accepted from students who are not residents of the state of Arkansas, preference must be given to qualified resident applicants. Nonresidents who do not have a GPA of at least 3.5 (based on a 4.0 scale) and above average scores on each section of the MCAT should not apply.

Qualified nonresidents will be considered. Preference is given to those who demonstrate strong ties to Arkansas.

FINANCIAL AID

Approximately 90 percent of our medical students receive financial aid. The average educational indebtedness for graduates in 2003 was $88,854. The financial status of applicants is not a factor in selection for admission.

The Community Match Program allows students who commit to practice primary care medicine in rural communities in Arkansas to receive up to $66,000 ($16,500 per academic year). The rural community provides one-half of the funds, and the remaining half is provided by the College of Medicine's Community Match Program. The student is obligated to return to the rural community following residency training and practice full time for the same number of years the student was assisted during medical school. For each year of service, one year of loans is forgiven until the debt is retired. A unique feature of the program allows alternates, who sign

rural practice contracts, the opportunity to advance to the top of the alternate list. For additional details, contact the Financial Aid Office.

INFORMATION ABOUT DIVERSITY PROGRAMS

Students from groups underrepresented in medicine are encouraged to apply for admission. The Office of Minority Student Affairs has developed an active recruitment and retention program. The Summer Science Program for students from groups underrepresented in the health care profession is available for five weeks during the summer and offers an introduction to the medical school curriculum, along with reading and study skill enrichment sessions designed to strengthen students in these areas. A prematriculation program is available to all students accepted for admission and has as its primary focus students who may have some problems mastering the medical college curriculum. Every effort is made by the faculty to assist students academically as these needs are identified.

Institution Type: *Public*
Application Process: *AMCAS, see chapter 4.*

APPLICATION AND ACCEPTANCE POLICIES FOR 2005–2006 FIRST-YEAR CLASS

Filing of AMCAS application
    Earliest date: June 1, 2004
    Latest date: Nov. 1, 2004
School application fee to all applicants: $60
Oldest MCAT scores considered: 2002
Does not have Early Decision Program
Acceptance notice to regular applicants
    Earliest date: Dec. 15, 2004
    Latest date: Until class is filled
Applicant's response to acceptance offer
    Maximum time: 2 weeks
Requests for deferred entrance considered: Yes
Deposit to hold place in class: None
Estimated number of new entrants: 150
Starting date: Aug. 2005

TUITION AND STUDENT FEES PER YEAR FOR 2003-2004 FIRST-YEAR CLASS

Tuition   Student fees: $563
    Resident: $11,642
    Nonresident: $23,284

INFORMATION ON 2003-2004 FIRST-YEAR CLASS

Number of	In-State	Out-of-State	Total
Applicants	313	346	659
Applicants Interviewed	309	28	337
New Entrants*	145	2	147

*All took the MCAT; 99% had baccalaureate degrees.

CHAPTER
11

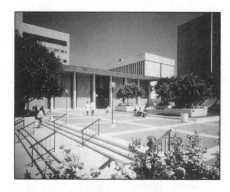

Keck School of Medicine of the University of Southern California

Los Angeles, California

Dr. Stephen J. Ryan, *Dean*
Dr. Erin A. Quinn, *Associate Dean for Admissions*
Robert J. McCann, *Director of Student Services*
Althea Alexander, *Assistant Dean for Minority Student Affairs*

ADDRESS INQUIRIES TO:

Office of Admissions
Keck School of Medicine of the
University of Southern California
1975 Zonal Avenue (KAM 100-C)
Los Angeles, California 90089-9021
(323) 442-2552; 442-2433 (FAX)
E-mail: medadmit@usc.edu
Web site: www.usc.edu/schools/medicine

MISSION STATEMENT

The mission of the Keck School of Medicine is to improve the quality of life for individuals and society by promoting health, preventing and curing disease, advancing biomedical research, and educating tomorrow's physicians and scientists.

GENERAL INFORMATION

USC, a privately supported, nondenominational, coeducational university, established its School of Medicine in 1885. The 31-acre campus is located directly across the street from its chief teaching hospital, the Los Angeles County+USC Medical Center. In addition to the Medical Center, which is one of the largest teaching centers in the United States, patient-care facilities include the 284-bed USC University Hospital, USC/Norris Cancer Center and Hospital, Doheny Eye Institute, Children's Hospital Los Angeles, Rancho Los Amigos Medical Center, Hospital of the Good Samaritan, Barlow Respiratory Hospital, California Medical Center, Huntington Memorial Hospital, Presbyterian Intercommunity Hospital, House Ear Institute, Veterans Administration Outpatient Clinic, and White Memorial Medical Center.

CURRICULUM

Students are progressively involved with regular patient contact beginning the first week of medical school. An important feature is Introduction to Clinical Medicine, a course that begins in the first year of medical school and runs through the second year. Doctor-patient relationships and interviewing are presented during the first year, and physical diagnosis and history-taking are taught in the second. Groups of six to seven students are led by a faculty member who serves as a clinical tutor to these students for their first two years.

The newly revised curriculum is designed to enhance the students' understanding of the basic sciences and their relevance to clinical medicine. This methodology improves students' problem-solving and independent-study skills. Curriculum themes are delivered in a case-centered format with the integration of small-group learning sessions, directed-independent study and newer instructional technologies emphasized.

The first year of the Year I–II continuum begins with 18 weeks of Core Principles of Health and Disease, followed by 49 weeks of organ system review, ending with a 10-week Integrated Case Study section. There is an eight-week summer break between the first and second years.

Each week of the academic year is composed of approximately 20 hours of lecture and small group sessions with an additional 20 hours of independent directed study or Introduction to Clinical Medicine. Examinations in all systems throughout the first two years are graded pass/fail. Dean's recognition is awarded on the basis of year-end comprehensive examinations and special projects.

The final two years are designed as a continuum of two academic calendar years. Each student's program is individually designed to include 55 weeks of required clerkships (i.e. medicine, general surgery, obstetrics-gynecology, pediatrics, psychiatry, neurology, family medicine, and surgical specialties), 12 weeks of selective clerkships at Keck School of Medicine, 16 weeks of free electives, and a one-week clinical orientation program. Grading for the final two years is on an honors, satisfactory, and unsatisfactory basis.

SPECIAL PROGRAMS

Students have an opportunity to engage in clinical or basic research through voluntary participation in a summer fellowship program between the first and second years.

The school sponsors an M.D.-Ph.D. program for those interested in obtaining these degrees jointly. A special fifth-year option is available for students who wish to pursue a research project and may be considering a career in academic medicine. A baccalaureate-M.D. program is offered and described in Chapter 10.

REQUIREMENTS FOR ENTRANCE

The MCAT and a minimum of four full years or 120 semester hours of academic work at an accredited college or university at the time of matriculation are required. Coursework must include the following subjects:

	Sem./Qtr.
General Biology (with lab)	2/3
Organic Chemistry (with lab)	1/2
General Physics (with lab)	2/3
Biochemistry	1/1

Additionally, a course in basic molecular biology and 30 semester hours (or quarter equivalent) of coursework in the social sciences, humanities, and English composition are required. Facility in the principles of college mathematics or calculus and in the use of computers as a tool for independent learning is recommended.

Applicants are strongly urged to take the MCAT in the spring of the year of application and to have their basic science requirements completed at the time of application.

Foreign students must have completed at least one year of study in an accredited university or college in the United States prior to application.

Individuals who have discontinued studies in medical school for academic reasons are not eligible to apply.

Applications for admission with advanced standing into the third year are accepted only from full-time medical students currently enrolled, or on approved leave-of-absence, and in good standing at an LCME-accredited medical school.

SELECTION FACTORS

The Admissions Committee seriously considers candidates whose academic achievement and MCAT performance indicate their ability to satisfactorily complete the rigorous curriculum of the medical school. Favorable consideration also reflects additional factors including motivation and evidence of qualities deemed desirable for the study and practice of medicine, significant achievements in nonacademic pursuits, and demonstrated commitment to service and community. The School of Medicine does not discriminate on the basis of race, creed, gender, nationality, residency, age, or handicap.

Receipt of the application from AMCAS is acknowledged. All candidates are requested to complete the supplemental application and arrange for submission of letters of recommendation. Interview selection is based upon careful evaluation of the application and all supporting documentation. Interviews are required of all applicants under serious consideration and are granted only by invitation of the Admissions Committee.

The 2003 entering class had a *mean GPA* of 3.62 and *mean MCAT* scores of 10.1 in Verbal Reasoning, 11 in Physical Sciences, and 11.3 in Biological Sciences. Women comprised 47 percent of the class, which came from 50 colleges and universities and 18 states. The mean age was 24 (range 20-34 years).

FINANCIAL AID

A variety of university scholarships and loans are available to supplement federal and state programs. Awards are based on need as demonstrated through a financial statement. Approximately 75 percent of students receive some type of financial assistance. For additional information, contact Linda Lewis, director of financial aid, (323) 442-1016.

INFORMATION ABOUT DIVERSITY PROGRAMS

The goal of the Office of Diversity is to recruit, retain and increase the number of students, from a variety of backgrounds, enrolled in the Keck School of Medicine. For more information, please call (323) 442-1050.

Institution Type: *Private*
Application Process: *AMCAS, see chapter 4.*

APPLICATION AND ACCEPTANCE POLICIES FOR 2005–2006 FIRST-YEAR CLASS

Filing of AMCAS application
    Earliest date: June 1, 2004
    Latest date: November 1, 2004
School application fee to all applicants: $90
Oldest MCAT scores considered: 2002
Does have Early Decision Program (EDP)
    EDP application period: June 1-Aug 1, 2004
    EDP applicants notified by: Sep. 1, 2004
Acceptance notice to regular applicants
    Earliest date: Oct. 15, 2004
    Latest date: Until class is filled
Applicant's response to acceptance offer
    Maximum time: 10 days
Requests for deferred entrance considered: Yes
Deposit to hold place in class (applied to tuition):
    $100, due with response to acceptance offer
Deposit refundable prior to: May 16, 2005
Estimated number of new entrants: 160 (10 EDP)
Starting date: Aug. 2005

TUITION AND STUDENT FEES PER YEAR FOR 2003–2004 FIRST-YEAR CLASS

Tuition: $35,928   Student fees: $1,148

INFORMATION ON 2003-2004 FIRST-YEAR CLASS

Number of	In-State	Out-of-State	Total
Applicants	2,924	1,732	4,656
Applicants Interviewed	388	138	526
New Entrants†	131	29	160

†All took the MCAT and had baccalaureate degrees.

CHAPTER

11

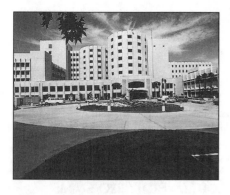

Loma Linda University School of Medicine

Loma Linda, California

Dr. H. Roger Hadley, *Dean*
Dr. John S. Thorn, *Associate Dean for Admissions*
Verdell Schaefer, *Financial Aid Director*
Dr. Daisy Deleon, *Associate Professor of Physiology and Pharmacology,
Assistant to the Dean for Diversity*

ADDRESS INQUIRIES TO:

Associate Dean for Admissions
Loma Linda University
School of Medicine
Loma Linda, California 92350
(909) 558-4467; 558-0359 (FAX)
Web site: www.llu.edu
E-mail: ledwards@som.llu.edu

MISSION STATEMENT

Our overriding purpose is the formation of Christian physicians, educated to serve as generalists or specialists providing whole-person care to individuals, families, and communities.

GENERAL INFORMATION

The School of Medicine was organized in 1909 at Loma Linda. The campus is composed of basic science facilities and Loma Linda University Medical Center, which includes the Children's Hospital and the Loma Linda University Community Medical Center. Also used for clinical instruction are Loma Linda Behavioral Medicine Center, Jerry L. Pettis Memorial Veterans Hospital, Riverside County Regional Medical Center, and the White Memorial Medical Center in Los Angeles. San Bernardino County General Hospital, Kaiser Foundation Hospital, and Glendale Adventist Medical Center are also affiliated with the School of Medicine and are utilized for undergraduate and postgraduate clinical training.

Objectives of the School of Medicine include providing the student with a solid foundation of medical knowledge, assisting the student in the attainment of professional skills, and motivating investigative curiosity and a desire to participate in the advancement of knowledge. The school endeavors to reinforce interest in the practical application of Christian principles through service to humanity.

CURRICULUM

The major objective of the School of Medicine is to prepare students who will be well grounded in the science and art of medicine and who also will be prepared after further training for the practice of general medicine or any specialty.

The first two years are primarily devoted to the study of the basic medical sciences, including the relationship to pathology and clinical application, and the introduction to physical diagnosis and human behavior. The last two years provide clinical rotations in the major areas of medical practice: surgery, internal medicine, pediatrics, obstetrics-gynecology, family medicine, emergency medicine, ambulatory care, and psychiatry, as well as didactic and practical experience in preventive medicine. Elective time is available for various types of additional educational experience in the clinical or research areas to prepare students in their selection of postgraduate medical education.

Qualified students interested in a career in academic medicine may earn an M.S. or Ph.D. degree along with the M.D. degree. Six to seven years are required to complete this program.

Performance of students is evaluated by means of standard or scaled scores. The grading system is on a pass/fail basis.

REQUIREMENTS FOR ENTRANCE

The MCAT and a minimum of three years (90 semester hours or 135 quarter hours) of collegiate preparation in an accredited college or university in the United States or Canada are required. Preference is given to applicants who will have completed the baccalaureate degree prior to matriculation. No major is preferred, but a broad educational background is encouraged. Demonstrated ability in the sciences is important. Rejected applicants may reapply and usually will receive the same consideration as first-time applicants.

Required courses are:

Sem./Qtr. hrs.
General Biology or Zoology (with lab) 8/12
General or Inorganic Chemistry (with lab) 8/12
Organic Chemistry (with lab) 8/12
Physics (with lab) 8/12
English equivalent to satisfy baccalaureate degree requirement.

Biochemistry and an introductory course in basic statistics are strongly recommended.

Additionally, keyboard and computer skills are considered essential.

CLEP and pass/fail performances are not acceptable for the required courses.

Applicants are urged to take the MCAT in the spring of the year of application and to have the basic requirements completed at the time of application.

SELECTION FACTORS

The Admissions Committee seeks candidates who have demonstrated the greatest potential for becoming capable physicians. A strong academic background is needed in preparation for medical studies. While special attention is given to the performance in science courses, candidates should also have a solid foundation in the humanities, social sciences, and human behavior.

The Admissions Committee looks for applicants who demonstrate problem-solving skills, critical judgment, and the ability to pursue independent study and thinking. In evaluating academic achievements, the Admissions Committee considers such factors as the difficulty of the program, the need to work, social and cultural hardship, and participation in meaningful extracurricular activities. For nonacademic qualifications, the committee looks for a commitment to medicine, judgment, a positive attitude, ability to make decisions, emotional stability, and integrity.

The School of Medicine is owned and operated by the Seventh-day Adventist church; therefore, preference for admission is given to members of this church. However, it is a firm policy of the Admissions Committee to admit each year a number of nonchurch-related applicants who have demonstrated a strong commitment to Christian principles. No candidate is accepted on the basis of religious affiliation alone. The school does not discriminate on the basis of race, sex, age, or handicap.

After receipt of the AMCAS application, each applicant is requested to submit the supplementary form and supply preprofessional faculty evaluations and/or personal letters of recommendation. Invitations for an interview are extended to selected applicants on the medical school campus and on a regional basis at selected locations throughout the country.

Applicants with an outstanding academic record and with a particular interest in Loma Linda University School of Medicine are encouraged to apply through the Early Decision Program (EDP). Contact the associate dean for admissions prior to submitting AMCAS application.

Final selection is made by the Admissions Committee on the basis of overall scholastic record, personal character qualifications, and promise of success as a physician. Matriculated students for the class of 2002 had a *mean overall GPA* of 3.69.

FINANCIAL AID

The School of Medicine has limited loan funds available through the Student Finance Office. All aid is awarded on the basis of a uniform needs analysis. Financial aid information is provided to all accepted students. In view of the costs of a medical education, students are urged to plan their financial program carefully.

Institution Type: *Private*
Application Process: *AMCAS, see chapter 4.*

APPLICATION AND ACCEPTANCE POLICIES FOR 2005–2006 FIRST-YEAR CLASS

Filing of AMCAS application
  Earliest date: June 1, 2004
  Latest date: Nov. 1, 2004
School application fee to all applicants: $75
Oldest MCAT scores considered: 2002
Does have Early Decision Program (EDP)
  EDP application period: June 1–Aug. 1, 2004
  EDP applicants notified by: Oct. 1, 2004
Acceptance notice to regular applicants
  Earliest date: Dec. 16, 2004
  Latest date: Until class is filled
Applicant's response to acceptance offer
  Maximum time: 30 days
Requests for deferred entrance considered: Yes
Deposit to hold place in class (applied to tuition):
  $100, due with response to acceptance offer
Deposit refundable prior to: May 16, 2005
Estimated number of new entrants: 159 (10 EDP)
Starting date: Aug. 2005

TUITION AND STUDENT FEES PER YEAR FOR 2003–2004 FIRST-YEAR CLASS

Tuition: $30,012   Student fees: $1,588

INFORMATION ON 2003–2004 FIRST-YEAR CLASS

Number of	In-State	Out-of-State	Total
Applicants	1,528	1,489	3,017
Applicants Interviewed	180	172	352
New Entrants*	80	85	165

*All took the MCAT; 99.4% had baccalaureate degrees.

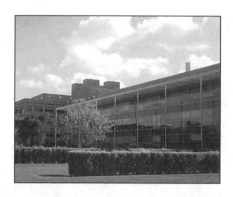

Stanford University School of Medicine

Stanford, California

Dr. Philip A. Pizzo, *Dean*
Dr. Gabriel Garcia, *Associate Dean of Medical School Admissions*
Charlene Hamada, *Assistant Dean of Student Affairs*
Dr. Ronald D. Garcia, *Assistant Dean of Minority Affairs*

ADDRESS INQUIRIES TO:

Office of Admissions
Stanford University School of Medicine
251 Campus Drive, MSOB XC301
Stanford, California 94305-5404
(650) 723-6861; 725-7855 (FAX)
E-mail: admissions@med.stanford.edu
Web site: www.med.stanford.edu

MISSION STATEMENT

The mission of the Stanford School of Medicine is to be a premier research intensive medical school that improves health through leadership and collaborative discoveries and innovation in patient care, education, and research.

GENERAL INFORMATION

The school is part of the Stanford University Medical Center and consists of 26 departments. The major clinical teaching facilities are: Stanford University Hospital (663 beds), Lucile Packard Children's Hospital (152 beds), Santa Clara County Valley Medical Center (791 beds), and the Palo Alto Veterans Administration Hospital (1,000 beds). This association of hospitals provides facilities for comprehensive clinical training, and the school offers opportunities in many areas of fundamental and clinical research. Lane Medical Library has one of the largest collections of medical books in the West. SUMMIT (Stanford University Medical Media and Information Technologies) produces faculty- and student-authored programs.

CURRICULUM

The goals of the curriculum are to develop outstanding clinical skills in all students as well as the capacity for leadership in the practice of scientific medicine, and to prepare as many students as possible for careers in research and teaching. Stanford's flexible curriculum is its major innovative approach to medical education. This curriculum was designed to create an environment that encourages intellectual diversity and to provide opportunities for students to develop as individuals. While traditional courses and clerkships are required for graduation, the duration of study leading to the M.D. degree may vary from four to six years. Students have flexibility in sequencing some courses and clerkships, and they may be exempt from certain basic science courses by demonstrating competency through examination. This curriculum stimulates self-directed learning, and it provides students time to pursue an investigative project, obtain teaching experience, perform community service, explore special interests, or obtain advanced degrees.

The required curriculum includes work in the basic medical sciences and clinical experiences in medicine, surgery, pediatrics, gynecology-obstetrics, and psychiatry. All M.D. candidates must satisfactorily complete at least 13 quarters of academic work. Fees for additional quarters are nominal. Students are encouraged to plan for a five-year course of study in order to include research activities, teaching assistantships, and a variety of elective courses both in the medical school and in other schools of the university in their educational enrichment plans. Thus, the time spent in medical school may vary with the individual student's background and study plans. Courses are graded pass/fail.

Stanford offers many opportunities for study in depth in the preclinical and clinical disciplines. Students with strong interests in careers in medical research should inquire of the Office of Admissions about the Medical Scientist Training Program (MSTP) or the training programs in cancer biology, immunology, medical information sciences, neurosciences, or pharmacology. These federally funded programs enable selected students to pursue research and coursework leading to both the M.D. and Ph.D. degrees. Students request MSTP application forms on the supplementary application to the School of Medicine. Applications for other programs are also supplied on request to the specific department.

REQUIREMENTS FOR ENTRANCE

The MCAT is required, preferably taken in the spring but no later than late summer of the year of application. Applicants from colleges and universities of recognized standing who hold a U.S. bachelor's degree or its equivalent are eligible to be considered for admission for graduate study. The minimal entry requirements are:

	Years
Biological Science (with lab)	1
Chemistry, including Organic Chemistry (with labs)	2
Physics (with lab)	1

Courses in calculus, physical chemistry, behavioral sciences, and particularly in biochemistry are strongly recommended.

An undergraduate major in any field is acceptable, provided the candidate presents a record of outstanding achievement. Breadth of education and/or experience in the humanities and social sciences and knowledge of a foreign language are desirable.

Medical School Admission Requirements, 2005-2006

SELECTION FACTORS

Stanford's educational milieu fosters rigorous scholarship and encourages students to develop investigative and innovative approaches to problems in medicine. The school seeks applicants who have a strong humanitarian commitment and whose originality, creativity, and independent critical thinking best equip them for this environment.

Stanford does not discriminate against applicants on the basis of race, religion, national origin, sex, marital status, age, or disability. The applicant's state of residence is irrelevant in the selection process. No preference is given to California residents. Foreign applicants must have completed a minimum of one year of study in a U.S., Canadian, or United Kingdom accredited college or university.

Acceptances are based upon standards of merit, and no quotas of any kind play a role in the evaluation or selection process.

In recent years, applicants granted admission have had a *mean GPA* of about 3.7 and *mean MCAT* scores as follows: *VR*-10, *PS*-12, *BS*-12. Applicants whose MCAT scores are below the national mean are highly unlikely to be admitted to the medical school.

The application fee applies to students who return the supplemental application and will be waived for applicants who have obtained a fee waiver from AMCAS.

Application during the summer or very early fall is strongly encouraged.

Transfer Students: For information on the transfer policy, you may visit our Web site at ✆www.med.stanford.edu.

FINANCIAL AID

Acceptance is independent of the applicant's financial status, and Stanford makes every effort to ensure that students are not excluded from admission to the school for financial reasons. Approximately 70 percent of students receive some form of financial assistance. Available grant and loan funds are awarded to students on the basis of demonstrated need, as determined by a needs analysis. For federal aid, students are considered independent. For university-based aid, students are considered dependent up until the age of 30, and the school will consider the student's parents' ability to contribute to the cost of financing the student's education in determining eligibility for university loans and grants. This applies regardless of your marital status, other graduate degrees, or the fact that you have been self-supporting for a number of years. Eligibility for aid is assessed according to the cost of attendance, and the student budget is standardized. Other approved expenses (outside the standard budget) will be met with a loan. The average debt of our 2002 graduates was $64,877; six of the graduates had debts over $100,000.

Foreign students who are not U.S. citizens or permanent residents are not eligible for federal or university-based aid. Foreign students must complete a certification of finances reflecting an escrow account of funds to cover their cost of education for the M.D. degree.

Teaching and research assistantships, for which students receive salary and tuition credit, can be used to offset loans, and may reduce the indebtedness of students on financial aid. However, these positions are not guaranteed, and should not be viewed as a way to meet expenses.

Applicants should complete the FAFSA at ✆www.fafsa.ed.gov and the needs analysis at ✆www.accessgrp.org as soon as possible after January 1 so that, if requested, a preliminary estimate of the financial aid award can be provided by the Office of Student Financial Services. The Supplemental Financial Aid application forms will be made available to all applicants that have been accepted. For additional information about financial aid, contact the Office of Student Financial Services at (650) 724-3181.

INFORMATION ABOUT DIVERSITY PROGRAMS

Stanford takes pride in its highly diverse and exceptionally qualified student body. Stanford is committed to increasing the representation in its student body of members of groups underrepresented in medicine and particularly encourages applications from such candidates and others that will contribute to the diversity of our school. An early matriculation program emphasizing leadership skills, professional development and scholarly activities is in place.

Institution Type: *Private*
Application Process: *AMCAS, see chapter 4.*

APPLICATION AND ACCEPTANCE POLICIES FOR 2005–2006 FIRST-YEAR CLASS

Filing of AMCAS application
  Earliest date: June 1, 2004
  Latest date: Oct. 15, 2004
School application fee after screening: $75
  Oldest MCAT scores considered: 2002
Deadline for complete application: Dec. 1, 2004
Does have Early Decision Program (EDP)
  EDP application period: June 1–Aug. 1, 2004
  EDP applicants notified by: Oct. 1, 2004
Acceptance notice to regular applicants
  Earliest date: Oct. 15, 2004
  Latest date: Varies
Applicant's response to acceptance offer
  Maximum time: 2 weeks
Requests for deferred entrance considered: Yes
Deposit to hold place in class: None
Estimated number of new entrants: 86 (2 EDP)
Starting date: Sept. 2005

TUITION AND STUDENT FEES PER YEAR FOR 2003–2004 FIRST-YEAR CLASS

Tuition: $34,716   Student fees: $1,457

INFORMATION ON 2003–2004 FIRST-YEAR CLASS

Number of	In-State	Out-of-State	Total
Applicants	2,024	3,421	5,445
Applicants Interviewed	216	340	556
New Entrants*	34	53	87

*All took the MCAT and had baccalaureate degrees.

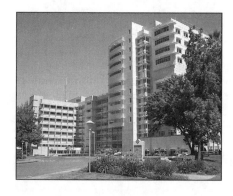

University of California, Davis
School of Medicine

Davis, California

Dr. Joseph Silva, Jr., *Dean*
Dr. Michael S. Wilkes, *Vice Dean*
Dr. Faith T. Fitzgerald, *Assistant Dean*
Edward D. Dagang, *Director of Admissions and Outreach*

ADDRESS INQUIRIES TO:

Office of Admissions and Outreach
School of Medicine
University of California
One Shields Avenue
Davis, California 95616-8661
(530) 752-2717
Web site: http://som.ucdavis.edu
E-mail: medadmisinfo@ucdavis.edu

MISSION STATEMENT

The University of California, Davis, School of Medicine's educational mission is to create a collegial, supportive learning environment that enables students to develop the skills, knowledge, and attitudes to excel and become tomorrow's leaders in areas related to patient care, public service, research, and education.

CURRICULUM

The relatively small class size (93 students) allows a personalized approach to medical education. Small group learning is important in all stages of the curriculum. Clinical and community exposure is provided beginning in the first year. Integrated and clinically oriented basic science courses are emphasized through active participation early in the first and second year. A strong emphasis is placed within the curriculum on problem-solving and active learning rather than passive learning. The third and fourth years of medical school provide intensive, interactive, clinical training in both required clerkships and flexible electives. Pass-fail grading in years one and two and class time limited to 27 hours per week increase the emphasis on collaboration and self-directed, life-long learning.

Overall governance of the curriculum is by the Committee on Educational Policy of the Academic Senate. The curriculum undergoes constant reexamination for excellence and topical coverage by students, faculty and administration. From the onset of the curriculum, students have the opportunity to take a broad range of elective courses, many of which involve clinical and community learning.

The Davis campus affords opportunities for interaction with other schools, colleges, departments, and laboratories of the University. Close educational relationships are enjoyed with the School of Veterinary Medicine, the California Primate Center, the Center for Developmental Nutrition, the Center for Health Services Research, the Clinical Cancer Center, the Center for Neurosciences, and the MIND Institute.

First and second year students have curriculum delivered at both the Davis campus and the medical center complex in Sacramento. The nationally renowned University of California, Davis, Medical Center consists of a 568-bed main hospital, the Shriners Hospital for Children, the extensive ambulatory clinic facilities including five student-run community-based clinics, the VA Medical Center, and the David Grant Medical Center located at Travis Air Force Base. The Health System offers a full range of state-of-the-art inpatient services, diagnostic services, and ambulatory care programs, with 150 subspecialty clinics, and 24-hour level-1 trauma emergency medical services. The university also has affiliation agreements with rural and urban hospitals located throughout Northern California.

In addition to the Doctor of Medicine degree, UC Davis offers a variety of dual-degree programs through coordination with other graduate schools and divisions. These advanced degrees can couple the M.D. degree with the M.P.H., Master of Informatics, Ph.D., and M.B.A. The requirements for entrance remain the same.

The School of Medicine seeks to attract students who are curious, motivated, and intelligent with a view toward meeting the needs of society. Ideal student's will have a demonstrated track record of achievement and leadership in an area of interest, demonstrable humanistic attitudes, and a realistic vision of the role they hope to play in health care delivery. In their pursuit of excellence, they will have demonstrated strong interpersonal skills, ethical judgment, and explored methods of inquiry.

The school embraces diversity in its student body. This is reflected in the school's commitment to expand opportunities in medical education for individuals from groups underrepresented in medicine as the result of social discrimination and to increase the number of physicians practicing in underserved areas. Therefore, the Admissions Committee, which is composed of individuals from a variety of cultural and professional backgrounds, evaluates each applicant in terms of the total person, carefully considering all relevant factors. These include academic credentials, with due regard to how they may have been affected by disadvantage experienced by the applicant; such personal traits as character and motivation; experience in the health sciences and/or the community; career objectives; and the ability of the individual to make a positive contribution to society, the profession, and the school.

Factors considered for admission include the applicant's scholastic record, GPA, MCAT performance, community service, leadership, and reports of teachers and advisors regarding intellectual capability, motivation, and emotional stability.

126

Characteristics that make applicants particularly attractive to the Admissions Committee are outstanding non-academic achievements, capability for independent study, maturity, and other factors that suggest good academic and leadership potential.

A personal interview will normally be required of each applicant who is accepted. Regional interviews are not usually available. We now expect that ten percent of our entering class will come from outside of the state of California. UC Davis School of Medicine participates in the WICHE Professional Student Exchange Program for applicants from certain western states that do not have medical schools.

REQUIREMENTS FOR ENTRANCE

The new MCAT and three years (90 semester hours or 135 quarter hours) in an accredited college or university in the United States or Canada are required. Applicants are urged to take the MCAT in April but no later than August when the application is made. A course of study leading to a bachelor's degree is recommended.

The school believes a medical student should have a sound background in the humanities and behavioral and social sciences as well as in the physical and biological sciences. Premedical requirements must be completed by June of the year of desired entry. The following college level courses are required:

	Years
English	1
Biological Sciences (with labs)	1.5*
General Chemistry (with lab)	1
Organic Chemistry	1
Physics	1
Mathematics (College level Mathematics)	1

*Upper Division Science Requirements for Admission: one (1) semester or two (2) quarters of upper division biology. This can be satisfied by courses in: biochemistry, molecular biology, cell biology or genetics.

Admission to medical school requires that the applicant will have an understanding of fundamental concepts of biomedical science. Although a biochemistry course is not absolutely required for admission, it is strongly recommended.

AP or CLEP credit is not acceptable for prerequisite courses.

FINANCIAL AID

A complete range of financial aid is available to medical students at the University of California, Davis: scholarships, fellowships, grants, and a variety of loans. The majority of financial aid is awarded based on demonstrated financial need. However, all accepted students are considered for university-awarded, merit- and need-based scholarships.

Historically, students at the School of Medicine have been able to receive full financial aid funding of their calculated financial need. Financial aid applications are available in December or early January. Students granted an interview can request an application by mail or pick up an application when they come to UC Davis for their interview. Early application

for aid is strongly recommended. Questions should be directed to the Financial Aid Office at (530) 752-6618, or by e-mail at medfinancialaid@ucdavis.edu.

INFORMATION FOR DISADVANTAGED APPLICANTS

The Office of Medical Education offers a variety of supplemental assistance programs and services for medical students, premed undergraduates, and high school students. The mission is to ensure diversity among students and faculty through outreach, development, and support activities for individuals from educationally and socioeconomically disadvantaged backgrounds, as well as to ensure that all medical students are prepared to give the best care to the wide variety of people in California and beyond.

Institution Type: *Public*
Application Process: *AMCAS, see chapter 4.*

APPLICATION AND ACCEPTANCE POLICIES FOR 2005–2006 FIRST-YEAR CLASS

Filing of AMCAS application & UC application
Earliest date: June 1, 2004
Latest date: Nov. 1, 2004
School application fee after screening: $60
Oldest MCAT scores considered: August 2001
Does not have Early Decision Program
Acceptance notice to regular applicants
   Earliest date: Oct. 15, 2004
   Latest date: Until class is filled
Applicant's response to acceptance offer
   Maximum time: 2 weeks
Requests for deferred entrance considered: Yes
Deposit to hold place in class: None
Estimated number of new entrants: 93
Starting date: Sept. 2005

TUITION AND STUDENT FEES PER YEAR FOR 2003–2004 FIRST-YEAR CLASS

Tuition   Student fees: $15,882
  Resident: None
  Nonresident: $12,245

INFORMATION ON 2003–2004 FIRST-YEAR CLASS

Number of	In-State	Out-of-State	Total
Applicants	3,014	621	3,635
Applicants Interviewed	364	2	366
New Entrants†	96	0	96

*Data not available.
†All took the MCAT and had baccalaureate degrees.

CHAPTER

11

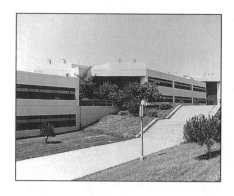

University of California, Irvine
College of Medicine

Irvine, California

Dr. Thomas C. Cesario, *Dean*

Dr. Ellena M. Peterson, *Associate Dean for Admissions and Outreach*

Gayle J. Pierce, *Director of Admissions*

ADDRESS INQUIRIES TO:

University of California, Irvine – College of Medicine
Office of Admissions and Outreach
Medical Education Building 802
Irvine, CA 92697-4089
(949)824-5388; (800)824-5388
(949)824-2485 (FAX)
E-mail: medadmit@uci.edu
Web site: www.ucihs.uci.edu/admissions/

MISSION STATEMENT

The University of California, Irvine, College of Medicine, is dedicated to advancing the knowledge and practice of medicine for the benefit of society. This mission will be achieved through programs of excellence in education, research, clinical care and service to the public.

GENERAL INFORMATION

Since its establishment at UCI, the College of Medicine has grown extensively, attaining national recognition. Approximately 380 medical students are enrolled at the college, and over 100 students are pursuing graduate degrees in the biomedical sciences. The faculty includes more than 650 full-time and 1,500 voluntary members in 25 academic departments. The faculty have expertise in a wide range of biomedical subjects. Research emphasized at the college includes the following multispeciality areas: the neurosciences, oncology, cardiovascular and pulmonary diseases, medical imaging, geriatric medicine, infectious diseases, molecular biology and human genetics.

The UCI Clinical Services System consists of the UCI Medical Center, off-site outpatient facilities, and numerous affiliated hospitals and clinics that participate in the educational and research programs of the college.

CURRICULUM

The medical curriculum at the UCI College of Medicine encourages medical students to become participants in their educational process, to be active rather than passive learners, to become life long learners and to use cooperative and team learning principles. The College of Medicine faculty views curriculum development as a continual process and feels that medical education and teaching innovations must be encouraged and supported.

The UCI College of Medicine is dedicated to the nurturing of humanistic, caring physicians with state-of-the-art clinical expertise and skills. This is achieved through a curriculum that is not only anchored in the science of medicine but also in the humanistic dimensions of medicine. The College of Medicine faculty feels that the curriculum should strive to integrate basic and clinical sciences, by bringing substantial clinical material into the early phases of medical education. To achieve this, in addition to the basic sciences, which are concentrated in the first two years, the College of Medicine has implemented vertical integration of the curriculum with the development of a series of "Patient-Doctor" courses. These courses are longitudinal multidisciplinary experiences broadly designed to prepare students for their future careers in medicine through the application of experiential and self-directed learning. In the first year students work with standardized patients to develop interview and physical examination skills. These clinical skills are further strengthened in the second year by working in the community with patients. Clinically oriented courses are designed to complement the material covered in the basic science courses.

Basic Science Advisors are assigned to all students during the first and second years and Clinical Advisors for the third and fourth years. A Learning Resource Program is available to provide tutorial assistance and study skills training. USMLE reviews are also provided.

SPECIAL PROGRAMS

M.D./Ph.D.

A combined M.D./Ph.D. degree is available to interested students through the Medical Scientist Training Program. Application forms to the M.D./Ph.D. program are included in the secondary application materials. Applicants not chosen for the M.D./Ph.D. program will be considered for acceptance into the M.D. class.

M.D./Masters

The College of Medicine offers a track to prepare students for medical careers in the Latino community. This unique five-year curriculum, Program in Medical Education for the Latino Community (PRIME-LC), prepares students to provide culturally and linguistically competent medical care as well as for academic or leadership careers. It is anticipated that in addition to the M.D. degree students will obtain a joint masters degree in a related field. Successful applicants must meet all the general admissions criteria for the UCI College of Medicine. They must also be able to demonstrate a history of significant commitment to the underserved or the Latino community and advanced conversational Spanish skills. Substantial financial support will be provided to those who participate in the program. Application forms for this program are included in the secondary application materials.

M.D./M.B.A.

A five- to six-year joint program with the Graduate School of Management affords medical students the opportunity to receive a M.B.A. while at the UCI-College of Medicine. Students interested in the M.D./M.B.A. program generally apply during the second year of medical school.

REQUIREMENTS FOR ENTRANCE

The MCAT is required. The latest MCAT that will be accepted is that given in August of the year before anticipated admission. A minimum of three years (90 semester units) of undergraduate coursework is required, including a minimum of one full-time year at an accredited U.S. college or university. The baccalaureate degree is strongly recommended but not required.

Minimum requirements include the successful completion of the following courses with a grade of C or better:

Sem. hrs.

Biology 12
   Courses must include a minimum of one semester or two quarters of upper-division biology, excluding botany
General Chemistry 8
Organic Chemistry 8
Physics 8
Biochemistry 4
   On the quarter system, a quarter of biochemistry must be taken in combination with either an additional quarter of biochemistry, molecular biology, or genetics
Calculus 4

Applicants who do not meet these requirements or who do not indicate that these subjects will be completed by the date of entrance will not be considered for admission.

No specific major is required; however, demonstrated ability in the sciences is of great importance. In addition, applicants are advised to take advantage of the intellectual maturation afforded by a well-rounded liberal arts education. English, the humanities, and the social and behavioral sciences are considered particularly important. The following courses are also recommended but not required: cell biology, genetics, molecular biology, psychology, statistics, vertebrate embryology, and Spanish.

SELECTION FACTORS

The UCI College of Medicine seeks to admit students who are highly qualified to be trained in the practice of medicine and whose backgrounds, talents, and experiences contribute to a diverse student body. The Admissions Committee carefully reviews all applicants whose undergraduate record and scores on the MCAT indicate that they will be able to handle the rigorous curriculum of medical school. In addition to scholastic achievement, attributes deemed desirable in prospective students include leadership ability and participation in extracurricular activities, such as exposure to clinical medicine and/or medically related research, as well as community service. Careful consideration is given to applicants from disadvantage backgrounds (i.e., disadvantaged due to social, cultural, and/or economic conditions). Preference is given to California residents and applicants who are

either U.S. citizens or permanent residents. The College of Medicine does not accept transfer students.

Information provided by the AMCAS application is used for the preliminary screening of applicants. Based on decisions reached by the Admissions Committee, applicants may be sent a secondary application. A limited number of applicants (approximately 500) are invited to be interviewed. Regional interviews are not available. The Admissions Committee in reviewing a candidate for acceptance takes a holistic approach, taking into consideration academics, activities, letters of recommendation, and results of interviews conducted at UCI-COM.

The UCI-College of Medicine participates in the WICHE Professional Student Exchange Program for applicants from certain western states without medical schools.

Statistics for the 2003 entering class were: *mean GPA*, 3.7; *mean MCAT scores*, VR-10, PS-11, and BS-11.

INFORMATION FOR DISADVANTAGED APPLICANTS

Qualified applicants from disadvantaged backgrounds are encouraged to apply. Programs for the recruitment and retention of disadvantaged students have been developed through the Office of Admissions and Outreach. The application fee will be waived to individuals granted a fee waiver by AMCAS.

Institution Type: *Public*
Application Process: *AMCAS, see chapter 4.*
All applicants must check our Web site for additional information regarding our current application requirements.

APPLICATION AND ACCEPTANCE POLICIES FOR 2005–2006 FIRST-YEAR CLASS

Filing of AMCAS application
   Earliest date: June 1, 2004
   Latest date: Nov. 1, 2004
School application fee after screening: $60
   Oldest MCAT scores considered: 2002
Does not have Early Decision Program
Acceptance notice to regular applicants
   Earliest date: Dec. 1, 2004
   Latest date: Until class is filled
Applicant's response to acceptance offer
   Maximum time: 2 weeks
Requests for deferred entrance considered: Yes
Deposit to hold place in class: None
Estimated number of new entrants: 104
Starting date: Sept. 2005

TUITION AND STUDENT FEES PER YEAR FOR 2003–2004 FIRST-YEAR CLASS

Tuition	Academic fees: $16,332
Resident: None	
Nonresident: $12,246	

INFORMATION ON 2003–2004 FIRST-YEAR CLASS

Number of	In-State	Out-of-State	Total
Applicants	3,037	423	3,460
Applicants Interviewed	417	1	418
New Entrants*	91	1	92

*All took the MCAT and had baccalaureate degrees.

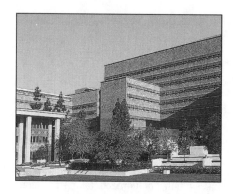

University of California, Los Angeles
David Geffen School of Medicine at UCLA

Los Angeles, California

Dr. Gerald Levey, *Dean*
Dr. Neil Parker, *Dean for Admissions and Students*
Lili Fobert, *Director of Admissions*
Patricia Pratt, *Director, Academic Enrichment and Outreach*

ADDRESS INQUIRIES TO:

David Geffen School of Medicine at UCLA
Office of Admissions, Box 957035
Los Angeles, California 90095-7035
(310) 825-6081
E-mail: somadmiss@mednet.ucla.edu
Web site: www.medstudent.ucla.edu/admissions

MISSION STATEMENT

The David Geffen School of Mission seeks to admit students who will be future leaders in their communities having distinguished careers in clinical practice, teaching, research, and public service. The school strives to create an environment in which students prepare for a future in which scientific knowledge, societal values and human needs are ever-changing.

GENERAL INFORMATION

The UCLA School of Medicine graduated its first class in 1955. The medical school is situated on the UCLA campus. The University Medical Center, UCLA Ambulatory Medical Plaza, UCLA Childrens Hospital, and Stein Eye Institute are adjacent to the school. These institutions, together with the Santa Monica Hospital and the Schools of Dentistry, Nursing, and Public Health, are integral parts of the School of Medicine and the Center for the Health Sciences. Close affiliation exists between the UCLA School of Medicine and the Los Angeles County Harbor/UCLA Medical Center, the Veterans Administration Medical Centers at West Los Angeles and Sepulveda, Cedars-Sinai Medical Center, and Olive View Medical Center.

CURRICULUM

The first two years of a four-year curriculum present a thorough knowledge of the sciences basic to medicine. An integrated approach to basic and clinical sciences is enhanced through problem-based learning in small-discussion groups in most courses of the first- and second-year curricula. Students are introduced to a holistic approach to patient care from the beginning of medical school and throughout the curriculum, through the innovative and nationally recognized doctoring courses. The first two years center on the processes of disease, with emphasis on organ-system oriented instruction. The third year has a core curriculum of clinical clerkships encompassing the areas of internal medicine, surgery, obstetrics and gynecology, pediatrics, psychiatry, family practice, radiology,

neurology, head and neck, orthopedics, urology, and ophthalmology. The school has a special focus in the fourth year through a set of "colleges" to provide a meaningful clinical and educational experience. Electives in the clinical continuum are designed to give students a foundation on which to develop and fulfill their personal interests, broaden their clinical knowledge, and give them an educational advantage in securing the clinical training calculated to best prepare them for postgraduate medical training. In 1993, UCLA initiated a pass-fail grading system with Letters of Distinction possible for outstanding performance.

Students are encouraged to participate in school and student organized activities. During the school year, students run clinics at the Salvation Army Homeless Center, Health Fairs, and DOC/STATS, which teach high school students about preventive health. Summers are filled with research projects and clinic and community work, as well as educational endeavors and opportunities such as international electives.

A Medical Scientist Training Program, leading to both M.D. and Ph.D. degrees, is available for a limited number of students who desire careers in medical research. This program requires six to seven years to complete and provides rigorous research training in addition to the medical curriculum. Stipends are available for some of the students in this program.

New programs leading to the M.D./M.B.A. and M.D./M.P.H. over a five-year period are available.

DREW/UCLA MEDICAL PROGRAM

Approximately 24 of the 169 students admitted each year have been admitted to the Drew/UCLA Medical Program. This program is designed to attract students who have an interest in addressing the concerns of underserved populations. Students will spend their first two years at the UCLA campus and their second two years at the Drew campus. Interested applicants should contact: Charles R. Drew University of Medicine and Science, 1621 East 120th Street, Los Angeles, California 90059; or call (323) 563-4960.

UCR/UCLA BIOMEDICAL SCIENCES PROGRAM

Additionally, 24 students are admitted to the UCLA School of Medicine through participation in the UCR/UCLA Biomedical Sciences Program, a cooperative venture with the University of California, Riverside (UCR). Students follow an integrated course of study through five to six years on the UCR campus and the final two years of clinical studies at the UCLA School of Medicine. Interested high school students should write to: Division of Biomedical Sciences; University of California, Riverside; Riverside, California 92521-0121.

REQUIREMENTS FOR ENTRANCE

The MCAT and three years of college are required. Ordinarily a baccalaureate degree is required, but in exceptional instances those who have completed three full academic years at an approved college or university will be considered. The required courses are:

	Years
English and Composition	1
College Physics (with lab)	1
Chemistry (with lab)	2
(Must include study of inorganic chemistry and organic chemistry)	
Biology	1
(One year of general biology with lab)	
College Mathematics	1
Study of introductory calculus and statistics is required.	

Courses in Spanish, computer skills, and the humanities are strongly recommended.

Candidates are urged to take the MCAT in the spring rather than in the summer of the year of application.

SELECTION FACTORS

The Admissions Committee gives preference to those applicants who present evidence of broad training and high achievement in their college education and possess, in the greatest degree, those traits of personality and character essential to success in medicine. Applicants whose records are judged by the Admissions Committee to qualify them for further consideration will receive a supplemental application. The completed applications are reviewed on the basis of letters of recommendation, supplemental applications, personal comments, GPA, and MCAT scores. Qualified applicants will receive an interview with members of the Admissions Committee.

For the 2003 entering class, accepted students had the following profile: *mean science GPA,* 3.64; *mean nonscience GPA,* 3.73. Applicants to the 2003 class had the following profile: *mean overall science GPA,* 3.31; *mean nonscience GPA,* 3.47.

Selections are made on the basis of individual qualifications and not on the basis of race, sex, creed, age, sexual orientation, national origin, or handicap. A third application is discouraged.

FINANCIAL AID

Scholarships and loan funds from private, state, and federal sources are available to all U.S. citizens and are awarded on the basis of need and/or scholarship. The school makes every effort to provide as much aid as possible. Outside employment is strongly discouraged.

DISADVANTAGED APPLICANTS

The UCLA School of Medicine Admissions Committee is composed of subcommittees, one of which is devoted exclusively to the consideration of applicants who have had a disadvantaged educational or financial background. This admissions subcommittee, which is composed of faculty and medical students, makes recommendations for action to be taken on disadvantaged applicants, although final decisions are made by the full Admissions Committee.

ADDITIONAL INFORMATION

The decision of which medical school to attend is extremely important. In addition to the school of medicine brochure, which is located on our Web site, we hope to provide the applicant with critical information through our School of Medicine and Student Affairs Web sites. Additionally, students may check their application status on the Admission Web page. Students invited for interviews will have the opportunity to have student-led tours and meet with faculty, staff, and members of the Admissions Committee.

Institution Type: *Public*
Application Process: *AMCAS, see chapter 4.*

APPLICATION AND ACCEPTANCE POLICIES FOR 2005–2006 FIRST-YEAR CLASS

Filing of AMCAS application
   Earliest date: June 1, 2004
   Latest date: Nov. 1, 2004
School application fee after screening: $60
Oldest MCAT scores considered: 2002
Does not have Early Decision Program
Acceptance notice to regular applicants
   Earliest date: Dec. 15, 2005
   Latest date: Aug. 6, 2005
Applicant's response to acceptance offer
   Maximum time: 2 weeks
Requests for deferred entrance considered: Yes
Deposit to hold place in class: None
Estimated number of new entrants: 169 (121 UCLA, 24 Drew/UCLA, 24 UCR/UCLA)
Starting date: Aug. 2005

TUITION AND STUDENT FEES PER YEAR FOR 2003–2004 FIRST-YEAR CLASS

Tuition   Academic fees: $15,173
   Resident: None
   Nonresident: 12,245

INFORMATION ON 2003–2004 FIRST-YEAR CLASS

Number of	In-State	Out-of-State	Total
Applicants	3,070	2,133	5,203
Applicants Interviewed	534	194	728
New Entrants*	106	15	121

*All took the MCAT and had baccalaureate degrees except in the UCR program.

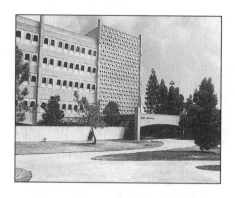

University of California, San Diego School of Medicine

La Jolla, California

Dr. Edward W. Holmes, *Vice Chancellor and Dean*
Dr. David H. Rapaport, *Acting Associate Dean for Admissions and Financial Aid*
Linda Whitson, *Director of Admissions*
Dr. Sandra Daley, *Assistant Dean of Diversity & Community Partnership*

ADDRESS INQUIRIES TO:

Office of Admissions, 0621
Medical Teaching Facility
University of California, San Diego
School of Medicine
9500 Gilman Drive
La Jolla, California 92093-0621
(858) 534-3880; 534-5282 (FAX)
E-mail: somadmissions@ucsd.edu
Web site: http://medschool.ucsd.edu/admissions

MISSION STATEMENT

The overall objective of the medical school curriculum is to instill graduates with the knowledge, skills, behaviors, and attributes that will lead to their becoming capable and compassionate physicians.

GENERAL INFORMATION

The simultaneous development of the School of Medicine and the general campus at the University of California, San Diego (UCSD), has fostered implementation of innovative programs enabling the medical students to benefit from the diversity of university faculty, from a wide variety of laboratory teaching facilities, and from a broad spectrum of clinical opportunities. Located on the main campus of the university at La Jolla, the School of Medicine is surrounded by learning resources and research institutions representing all disciplines. Unusual opportunities exist for integrating instruction in medical and related sciences with the natural sciences and disciplines centering on man in his social milieu. Clinical instruction is carried on at University of California Medical Center, Veterans Administration Hospital, Naval Regional Medical Center, San Diego Children's hospital, and seven other affiliated hospitals and clinics.

CURRICULUM

The goal of the medical curriculum and faculty-student interactions is to develop critical, objective, conscientious physicians prepared for changing conditions of medical practice and continuing self-education.

The curriculum is divided into two major components: the core curriculum and the elective programs. These are pursued concurrently, with the core curriculum predominating in the early years. The core curriculum includes those aspects of medical education deemed essential for every medical student regardless of background or ultimate career direction. The integrated core curriculum of the first two years is designed to provide each entering student with an essential understanding of the fundamental disciplines underlying modern medicine. The core curriculum of the last two years is composed of the major clinical specialties taught in hospital settings, out-patient situations, and relevant extended-care facilities.

Each student is required to plan and complete an Independent Study Project in consultation with a member of the faculty. A written document is required in all projects. Other components are devised by the student and faculty member.

Two combined M.D.-Master's programs are available, one in Public Health and the other in Leadership of Healthcare Organizations. Both programs require one additional year.

The Medical Scientist Training Program has been designed to provide the opportunity to earn both the M.D. and Ph.D. degrees over a seven- to eight-year period of study for a limited number of students.

A Medical Scholars Program (B.S.-M.D.) is available for outstanding California high school seniors planning careers in medicine. A maximum of 12 students accepted to UCSD undergraduate school will also be provisionally accepted into the School of Medicine to begin their medical studies following receipt of their undergraduate degree. This is not an accelerated program.

REQUIREMENTS FOR ENTRANCE

The MCAT is required, and must be taken within three years of application but no later than August of the year prior to matriculation. A minimum of three years of college is required, including one full-time year at an accredited U.S. four-year university; the baccalaureate degree is preferred. It is recommended that students take their course of study in the most demanding curricular environment possible. Minimum requirements include the successful completion of the following courses with a grade of C or better:

Biology: One year of college-level biology; (excluding Botany and Biochemistry (8 sem. hrs.).
Chemistry: Two years of college-level chemistry; must include one year of organic chemistry (16 sem. hrs.).
Physics: One year of college-level general physics (8 sem. hrs.).
Mathematics: One year of coursework; only calculus, statistics, or computer science will be considered (8 sem. hrs.).

English: Competence in speaking and writing English is required.

A broad base of knowledge is advantageous in preparing for the many roles of a physician and may include courses in: behavioral sciences, the biology of cells and development, genetics, biochemistry, English, or social sciences. Proficiency in a foreign language, such as Spanish, is considered highly desirable.

The Admissions Committee will only consider applicants who have taken the MCAT and completed the academic prerequisites.

SELECTION FACTORS

The Admissions Committee selects applicants who have demonstrated intelligence, maturity, integrity, and dedication to the ideal of service to society and who are best suited for an educational curriculum designed to prepare students for care of the total patient either in preparation for primary care specialization or as a groundwork for other fields of medicine. The school is seeking a student body with a broad diversity of backgrounds and interests reflecting our diverse population. The Admissions Committee has no preference as to undergraduate major but does prefer students with evidence of broad training and in-depth achievement in a particular area of knowledge, whether in the humanities, social sciences, or natural sciences.

Preference is necessarily afforded to California residents, and consideration is given only to applicants who are either U.S. citizens or permanent residents. Candidates are evaluated on the nature and depth of scholarly and extracurricular activities undertaken, academic record, performance on the MCAT, letters of recommendation, and personal interviews. The Admissions Committee interview evaluates the applicant's abilities and skills necessary to satisfy the nonacademic or technical standards established by the faculty and the personal and emotional characteristics that are necessary to become an effective physician. The UCSD School of Medicine participates in the WICHE Professional Student Exchange Program for applicants from certain western states without medical schools. The School of Medicine does not accept transfer students.

Accepted students for the 2003 entering class had the following credentials: *mean science GPA,* 3.8; *sex,* 54 percent women; *residence,* 92 percent from California; *undergraduate major,* 54 percent in biology or chemistry, with the remainder in the physical sciences, humanities, and social sciences. Approximately 50 percent of those interviewed receive acceptances.

FINANCIAL AID

Financial aid in the form of scholarships, grants, loans, and work opportunities is offered to help students in need of financial assistance. Approximately 90 percent of the students receive financial assistance during their four years of study. Medical Scientist Training Program participants may receive full tuition and a stipend for up to six years. An application form for financial aid is sent to every accepted student upon request.

DISADVANTAGED APPLICANTS

The UCSD School of Medicine is committed to expanding the educational opportunities for applicants coming from disadvantaged educational or economic backgrounds. This institutional commitment is expressed through a prematriculation summer program, tutorial support programs, and financial aid assistance.

Since its inception, the School of Medicine has been a national leader in maintaining a diverse student body and providing outreach programs for socioeconomically disadvantaged students at grade school through high school levels. The School of Medicine recognizes that disadvantaged students are underrepresented in the medical profession and regards a diverse student body as among its highest priorities.

Institution Type: *Public*
Application Process: *AMCAS, see chapter 4.*
All applicants must check our Web site for additional information regarding our current application requirements.

APPLICATION AND ACCEPTANCE POLICIES FOR 2005–2006 FIRST-YEAR CLASS

Filing of AMCAS application
  Earliest date: June 1, 2004
  Latest date: Nov. 1, 2004
School application fee after screening: $60
Oldest MCAT scores considered: 2002
Does not have Early Decision Program
Acceptance notice to regular applicants
  Earliest date: Oct. 15, 2004
  Latest date: Until class is filled
Applicant's response to acceptance offer
  Maximum time: 2 weeks
Requests for deferred entrance considered: Yes
Deposit to hold place in class: None
Estimated number of new entrants: 122
Starting date: Sep. 2005

TUITION AND STUDENT FEES PER YEAR FOR 2003-2004 FIRST-YEAR CLASS

Tuition   Academic fees: $15,570
  Resident: None
  Nonresident: $12,245

INFORMATION ON 2003-2004 FIRST-YEAR CLASS

Number of	In-State	Out-of-State	Total
Applicants	3,000	1,297	4,297
Applicants Interviewed	442	79	521
New Entrants†	111	10	121

*Data not available.
†All took the MCAT; All had baccalaureate degrees.

CHAPTER
11

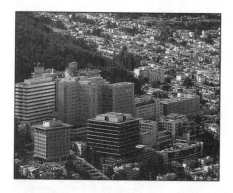

University of California, San Francisco School of Medicine

San Francisco, California

Dr. David A. Kessler, *Dean*
Dr. H.J. Ralston, *Associate Dean for Admissions*
Kathleen Ryan, *Admissions Officer*

ADDRESS INQUIRIES TO:

School of Medicine, Admissions
C-200, Box 0408
University of California, San Francisco
San Francisco, California 94143
(415) 476-4044
Web site: http://medschool.ucsf.edu

MISSION STATEMENT

The educational mission of the University of California, San Francisco (UCSF) School of Medicine is to provide a supportive and challenging educational environment in which students of diverse backgrounds prepare themselves for careers characterized by commitment to excellence, lifelong learning, and service to others through patient care, research, and teaching.

CURRICULUM

During the first two years, the primary focus is integrated core instruction in the basic, behavioral, social, and clinical sciences, and clinical experience is introduced within the first weeks of classes. Emphasis is placed on small-group teaching. Students begin longitudinal patient experiences during the foundations of patient care course. In the last two years the various clinical departments provide 46 weeks of core clerkships, which teach students the basic skills of clinical medicine. The third-year core includes additional weeks of advanced integration of basic and behavioral science experiences, including clinical intersessions. An additional 34 weeks of clinical and basic science courses must be elected from a wide range of offerings at UCSF medical center and other hospitals.

The grading system is pass/not pass. Honors recognition is assigned on an individual basis in third- and fourth-year courses of three units or more.

There are numerous opportunities for students to engage in research. They include the joint-degree programs, Student Research Fellowship Program, research electives, and various opportunities offered at UCSF and other institutions. Students who wish to do research should consult with the director of student research.

Special programs are available for students who wish to earn the M.D. degree jointly with the M.S., M.P.H., or Ph.D. degree. In addition, through the Medical Scientist Training Program,

approximately 12 students in each class may obtain the M.D. and Ph.D. degrees in six or more years of study.

The Joint Medical Program, sponsored by the University of California at Berkeley and San Francisco, is a five-year graduate and professional program leading to M.S. and M.D. degrees. The goal of the graduate segment (three years at Berkeley) is to develop students' abilities to approach problems of health and disease that require in-depth training in a variety of disciplines. Basic science and introductory clinical courses are enriched by individually structured Master's degree programs in selected areas of the medical sciences or in the social sciences pertinent to health care. Upon the student's completion of the Berkeley phase of the program, including a Master's thesis, an M.S. degree in health and medical sciences is awarded. Students then transfer to UCSF for the remainder of their training for the M.D. degree. The size of each class is limited to 12 students. Details are available from: Graduate Office, Health and Medical Sciences Program, 570 University Hall, #1190, University of California, Berkeley, California 94720; telephone (510) 642-5671; Web site: http://jmp.berkeley.edu/

REQUIREMENTS FOR ENTRANCE

The MCAT and a minimum of three years of college are required. A baccalaureate degree is strongly recommended but not required. The MCAT must be taken within three years of application but no later than August of the year prior to matriculation. However, applicants are strongly urged to take the test the preceding spring rather than the summer.

Applicants must complete 135 quarter units (90 semester units) of acceptable transfer college credit by June of the year of desired entry. These courses must be completed at an accredited institution; moreover, only 105 acceptable quarter units may be transferred from a community college. Courses must include:

	Qtr. hrs.
Biology or Zoology (with lab)	12

Must include the study of vertebrate zoology.

General Chemistry (with lab)	12
Organic Chemistry	8
Physics (with lab)	12

Survey courses in the sciences are not acceptable as fulfilling the requirements in science.

It is to the applicant's advantage to complete the above prerequisites before taking the MCAT and filing an application.

SECONDARY APPLICATION INFORMATION

Upon receipt of the verified AMCAS information a preliminary acknowledgment email is sent and checked on our applicant status Web site. All files are reviewed on a rolling basis; therefore supporting documents should not be sent unless specifically requested. Any letters of recommendation received prior to UCSF requesting them will be destroyed.

Applicant files pass through two screening processes within 10 to 12 weeks, and applicants are notified by emailed approval of a secondary application, or a letter of denial. Applicants approved for a secondary application are asked to submit a minimum of three letters of recommendation, including two letters from the applicant's instructors. A maximum of five letters is preferred. If the applicant's undergraduate school has a premedical committee or its equivalent (an office that gathers all letters), letters **must** be sent from that committee or office.

Applications to the Medical Scientist Training Program and the UC Berkeley/UC San Francisco Joint Medical Program are included in the secondary application materials. Applicants may apply to the regular medical program and one or both of these programs at that time.

MEDICAL SCHOOL ADMISSIONS INFORMATION

Selection is based on an appraisal of both intellectual and personal characteristics, which the Admissions Committee regards as desirable for prospective medical students and physicians. Based on these considerations, a limited number of applicants (500) are selected for interview. Personal interviews are required of applicants who pass the second screening. Regional interviews are not available.

Successful applicants tend to have strong academic records; firm and clear motivation for medicine, which is manifested in their work experience, activities, or interests; and outstanding personal qualities. Academic performance is evaluated in relation to background, with the aim of determining the influence of external factors on this parameter. Since preference is given to California residents, only nonresidents with superior qualifications are encouraged to apply. International applicants who are not permanent residents of the United States should not apply unless they have superior qualifications and adequate funding for their medical education and living expenses. The School of Medicine does not accept transfer students at any level, except for those students in the D.D.S.-M.D. program.

The School of Medicine has a long-standing commitment to increasing the number of physicians who are members of groups underrepresented in medicine. As a result, over the past 30 years UCSF has had one of the highest enrollment and graduation rates for these students of continental U.S. medical schools. In addition, the medical school welcomes applications from socioeconomically disadvantaged persons.

The UCSF School of Medicine does not discriminate on the basis of race, color, national origin, physical or mental disability, religion, sex, sexual orientation, or age in any of its policies, procedures, or practices. To obtain further information, please visit the following Web site: www.aaeo.ucsf.edu/nondispol.htm

Some statistics of the 2003 entering class were: *mean cumulative GPA,* 3.76; *mean science GPA,* 3.76; *mean MCAT scores,* VR-10, PS-11, BS-12; 58 percent women; *nonwhite ethnic groups,* 52 percent; *underrepresented in medicine,* 23 percent.

FINANCIAL AID

Scholarships are awarded to entering students on the basis of scholarship and/or need. General financial support is awarded through the Student Financial Services Office. Aid packages consist of a combination of loans, grants-in-aid, and scholarships. Financial aid is only available to U.S. citizens or permanent residents of the United States.

Institution Type: *Public*
Application Process: *AMCAS, see chapter 4.*
All applicants must check our Web site for additional information regarding our current application requirements.

APPLICATION AND ACCEPTANCE POLICIES FOR 2005–2006 FIRST-YEAR CLASS

Filing of AMCAS and any additional required primary material
    Earliest date: June 1, 2004
    Latest date: Nov. 1, 2004
School application fee after screening: $60
Oldest MCAT scores considered: 2002
Does not have Early Decision Program
Acceptance notice to regular applicants
    Earliest date: Dec. 15, 2004
    Latest date: Until class is filled
Applicant's response to acceptance offer
    Maximum time: 2 weeks
Requests for deferred entrance considered: Yes
Deposit to hold place in class: None
Estimated number of new entrants: 141
Starting date: Sept. 2005 (June 2005 for UCB-UCSF
    Joint Medical Program, 12 places)

TUITION AND STUDENT FEES PER YEAR FOR 2003–2004 FIRST-YEAR CLASS

Tuition   Academic Fees: $15,977
    Resident: None
    Nonresident: $12,245

INFORMATION ON 2003–2004 FIRST-YEAR CLASS

Number of	In-State	Out-of-State	Total
Applicants	2,352	1,693	4,045
Applicants Interviewed	*	*	553
New Entrants†	115	26	141

*Data not available.
†All took the MCAT and had baccalaureate degrees.

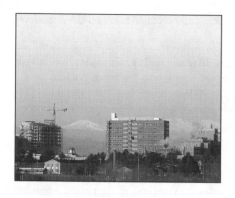

University of Colorado School of Medicine

Denver and Aurora, Colorado

Dr. Richard D. Krugman, *Dean*
Dr. Henry M. Sondheimer, *Associate Dean for Admissions*
Dominic Martinez, *Coordinator of Student Outreach and Support*

ADDRESS INQUIRIES TO:

Medical School Admissions
University of Colorado
School of Medicine
4200 East 9th Avenue, C-297
Denver, Colorado 80262
(303) 315-7361; 315-1614 (FAX)
E-mail: somadmin@uchsc.edu
Web site: www.uchsc.edu/sm/sm/mddgree.htm

MISSION STATEMENT

The mission of the University of Colorado School of Medicine is to provide Colorado, the nation, and the world with programs of excellence in:

• Education—through the provision of educational programs to medical students, allied health students, graduate students and house staff, practicing health professionals, and the public at large;

• Research—through the development of new knowledge in the basic and clinical sciences, as well as in health policy and health care education;

• Clinical Care—through state-of-the-art clinical programs, which reflect the unique educational environment of the university, as well as the needs of the patients it serves; and,

• Community Service—through sharing the school's expertise and knowledge to enhance the broader community, including our affiliated institutions, other health care professionals, alumni and other colleagues, and citizens of the state.

GENERAL INFORMATION

The University of Colorado School of Medicine admitted its first students in 1883. The School of Medicine is a part of the University of Colorado Health Sciences Center, located in Denver. The Health Sciences Center also includes the schools of dentistry, nursing, pharmacy, and the graduate school. Basic science and clinical opportunities for medical students are located throughout the Denver area in a number of hospitals and clinics, and rural health experiences are found throughout the state of Colorado. Although no official student housing is provided, the school is located in a neighborhood with a wide range of housing choices.

The medical school is home for approximately 1,200 full-time and 2,000 volunteer faculty members. In addition to educating students and participating in research, the faculty assumes considerable responsibility for patient care.

Opportunities for student research and a variety of extracurricular activities are available. The entire University of Colorado Health Sciences Center, including the School of Medicine will be moving to our new 270-acre campus in August 2006.

CURRICULUM

The curriculum is designed to provide the scientific and clinical background to prepare graduates for the practice of medicine. Most of the basic science courses are taught during the first two years. Foundations of Doctoring curricula are longitudinal courses, taught over the first three years, and are designed to introduce students to clinical problems early in their medical education. Students spend two to three days each month with a physician/preceptor who is practicing in one of the primary care areas. The third and fourth years consist of clinical clerkships with required clerkships primarily in the third year and electives primarily in the fourth year.

REQUIREMENTS FOR ENTRANCE

The MCAT and a baccalaureate degree or at least 120 semester hours of college credit with a major leading to a degree are required. The MCAT must be taken before the November 1 application deadline. The following courses are required:

	Sem. hrs.
General Biology (with lab)	8
General Chemistry (with lab)	8
Organic Chemistry (with lab)	8
General Physics (with lab)	8
College Mathematics	6

Should include at least college-level algebra and trigonometry or the equivalent by means of Advanced Placement.

English Literature, Composition, or equivalent 9

In addition to these required courses, the following information may be helpful as applicants plan their pre-medical coursework. In choosing from among the available courses, our experience indicates that a good basis in molecular biology and genetics will be helpful. Although biochemistry is not a specific requirement, many of our students have reported that this course was useful as a preparation.

Although a strong background in science is important, a broad-based education and experiences in other areas such as humanities and social sciences are also important assets for the future physician.

In order to receive credit for any Advanced Placement, the subject matter credited must be listed on the official college transcript.

SELECTION FACTORS

Places are offered to the applicants who appear to the Committee on Admissions to be the most highly qualified in terms of intelligence, achievement, character, motivation, maturity, and emotional stability. For this assessment, college grades, MCAT scores, recommendations, and personal interviews are used. Interviews are offered to selected applicants, and no applicant will be accepted without a personal interview.

Of the 132 places in each class, approximately 80 percent will be awarded to Colorado residents. Colorado residents from rural areas and from groups underrepresented in medicine are especially encouraged to apply. Thereafter, preference will be given to applicants from certain western states participating in the WICHE program and to applicants from other states who have high GPAs and MCAT scores.

A wide variety of undergraduate majors are considered acceptable in the selection of applicants, and no special preferences are given to science majors over non-science majors. However, demonstration of good performance in the required science courses is essential. Accepted students for the 2003 entering class had the following statistics: *mean GPA,* 3.7; *mean MCAT,* 31; *mean age,* 24 years; 45 percent women; 14 percent underrepresented students.

The medical school has an active M.D.-Ph.D. program for qualified applicants who wish to combine medical school with intensive scientific training. Information about this program may be obtained by calling (303) 315-8986. Graduate study and research for the doctoral degree are pursued after the student has completed the basic science curriculum in the first two years. Medical students not in the combined-degree program may also be provided with research opportunities in the basic science or clinical departments.

Colorado residents and nonresidents from U.S. medical schools are considered for transfer into the sophomore year if they are in good standing at their current school and if the curriculum is similar to the University of Colorado School of Medicine curriculum. Applicants from osteopathic or foreign medical schools are considered only if they are Colorado residents. These applicants are considered for transfer into the sophomore class after successful completion of two years in their school and receipt of a passing score on the USMLE Step 1. Applications are available after March 1 for entrance that fall.

The University of Colorado School of Medicine does not discriminate on the basis of race, sex, creed, national origin, age, or disability. Financial status is not a factor in the selection of applicants.

FINANCIAL AID

The medical school participates in the federal aid programs and has a number of other scholarship and loan funds that are distributed on the basis of financial need. Colorado student grant funds are available for Colorado residents. Financial aid questions should be directed to (303) 315-8364.

INFORMATION ABOUT DIVERSITY PROGRAMS

The University of Colorado encourages applications from qualified students from groups underrepresented in medicine. Acceptance is determined by the Committee on Admissions based on the same criteria applied to all applicants. Some disadvantaged students may have interview costs defrayed. Detailed information may be obtained from the Campus Office of Diversity at (303) 315-8558.

Institution Type: *Public*
Application Process: *AMCAS, see chapter 4.*

APPLICATION AND ACCEPTANCE POLICIES FOR 2005–2006 FIRST-YEAR CLASS

Filing of AMCAS application
    Earliest date: June 1, 2004
    Latest date: Nov. 1, 2004
School application fee to all applicants: $80
Oldest MCAT scores considered: 2002
Does not have Early Decision Program
Acceptance notice to regular applicants
    Earliest date: Oct. 16, 2004
    Latest date: Until class is filled
Applicant's response to acceptance offer
    Maximum time: 2 weeks
Requests for deferred entrance considered: Yes
Deposit to hold place in class (applied to tuition, fees, or other student obligations during last term): $200, due with response to acceptance offer
Deposit refundable prior to: July 1, 2005
Estimated number of new entrants: 132
Starting date: Aug. 2005

TUITION AND STUDENT FEES PER YEAR FOR 2003–2004 FIRST-YEAR CLASS

Tuition   Student fees: $2,174
   Resident: $15,333
   Nonresident: $67,000

INFORMATION ON 2003–2004 FIRST-YEAR CLASS

Number of	In-State	Out-of-State	Total
Applicants	630	1,752	2,382
Applicants Interviewed	341	237	578
New Entrants*	104	26	130

*All took the MCAT; 99% had baccalaureate degrees.

CHAPTER

11

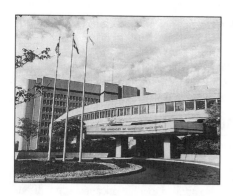

University of Connecticut School of Medicine

Farmington, Connecticut

Dr. Peter J. Deckers, *Dean*
Dr. Keat Sanford, *Assistant Dean for Admissions and Director of Student Services Center*
Patricia Lawson, *Director of Financial Assistance*
Dr. Marja Hurley, *Associate Dean of Minority Affairs*

ADDRESS INQUIRIES TO:

Admissions Center
University of Connecticut
School of Medicine
263 Farmington Avenue, Rm. AG-062
Farmington, Connecticut 06030-1905
(860) 679-4306; 679-1282 (FAX)
E-mail: sanford@nso1.uchc.edu
Web site:medicine.uchc.edu

MISSION STATEMENT

The School of Medicine's curriculum is designed to prepare professional men and women to practice medicine in a health care system that is evolving at an accelerated rate. In addition, it will equip them to formulate creative and courageous solutions to health care problems and issues. The primary goal of the curriculum is to develop in all students a fund of knowledge, skills, and attitudes that will enable them to pursue the postgraduate training necessary for their chosen career.

GENERAL INFORMATION

Established in 1968 as a unit of the University of Connecticut, the School of Medicine occupies the University of Connecticut Health Center complex in Farmington. The Health Center includes under one roof the School of Medicine and School of Dental Medicine, the 204-bed University Hospital and Ambulatory Unit, and the 160,000-volume Stowe Library. Clinical training programs exist in eight affiliated hospitals in the greater Hartford area and 11 allied community hospitals.

CURRICULUM

The curriculum plan for medical students is based on a multidepartmental approach. Basic medical sciences are taught from an organ-system approach. Normal structure/function is presented first, followed by pathophysiology and therapeutic approaches. Patient contact begins in Year 1 as part of the clinical medicine course. Students learn medical history taking, physical diagnosis, and various other aspects of the physician-patient relationship. In addition, students participate in a longitudinal ambulatory clinical experience throughout all four years. In the third year, the students rotate through ambulatory

and in-patient activities in each of the major clinical disciplines. In the fourth year, students complete clinical rotations in emergent and urgent care and have five months of electives. To aid individual development, students are assigned significant amounts of free time during the first two years and a wide choice of elective subjects in the clinical years. The USMLE examinations are required of all students. The grading system is strictly pass/fail; there are no class-rank scales or class standing. The third-year grading system is honors and pass/fail.

REQUIREMENTS FOR ENTRANCE

The MCAT and three years of college are required; four years of college and the baccalaureate degree are recommended. Prerequisite courses are:

	Sem. hrs.
General Biology or Zoology (with lab)	8
General Chemistry (with lab)	8
Organic Chemistry (with lab)	8
General Physics (with lab)	8

The level of these required courses should be equal to courses for those majoring in these respective fields. Courses in biochemistry, genetics and physiology are also recommended.

The School of Medicine supports the view that a broad liberal arts education provides the best background for those entering the medical profession. It will be difficult for students to master the programs in medicine unless they are adept in the use of the English language and in the handling of quantitative concepts. It is strongly recommended, therefore, that students include courses in their undergraduate curriculum that will provide them with a broad liberal arts background and aid them in the future development of their communicative and quantitative skills.

SELECTION FACTORS

The aim of the University of Connecticut School of Medicine is to accept qualified Connecticut residents, with special effort to include those who are disadvantaged. This assumes that places will be offered only to those whose achievements and/or capabilities are consistent with the rigor and high standards of the school's educational programs. A few exceptionally qualified out-of-state residents will be considered. An Early Assurance Program is available.

Occasionally, a couple of transfer positions are available in the third year.

The factors considered by the Admissions Committee are the applicant's career and clinical specialty interests, achievements, ability, motivation, and character. The applicant's GPA and MCAT scores are considered along with difficulty of the academic program, evidence of academic achievement beyond the regular coursework, and evidence of intellectual growth and development. Additional consideration is given for nonacademic activities and involvements and for letters of recommendation.

Requests to consider MCAT scores older than three years are handled individually. Personal interviews are arranged only at the request of the Admissions Committee. The 2003 entering class had a *mean GPA* of 3.66 and a *mean MCAT* of 30.5.

The University of Connecticut policy prohibits discrimination in education, in employment, and in the provision of services on account of race, religion, sex, age, marital status, national origin, ancestry, sexual orientation, disabled veteran status, physical or mental disability, mental retardation, other specifically covered mental disabilities, and criminal records that are not job related, in accordance with provisions of the Civil Rights Act of 1964, Title IX Education Amendments of 1972, the Rehabilitation Act of 1973, the Americans with Disabilities Act, and other existing federal and state laws and executive orders pertaining to equal rights.

FINANCIAL AID

Financial aid is available in three forms: scholarships; long-term, low-interest loans; and short-term, no-interest emergency loans. Eligibility for all programs is primarily based on demonstrated need. Approximately 90 percent of the students receive financial aid during the four-year educational period. Financial need is not considered relevant to the admissions process. A student's financial need is assessed after admission, and every effort is made to meet the student's minimum financial requirements. Further information is available from Patricia Lawson, director of financial aid.

INFORMATION ABOUT DIVERSITY PROGRAMS

The School of Medicine recruits disadvantaged applicants and applicants from groups underrepresented in medicine nationally through the Department of Health Careers Opportunity Programs (HCOP). Their applications are reviewed by the same general procedure for all applications and by the full Admissions Committee. Candidates for admission receive a full and sensitive review and are selected on a competitive basis. Candidates invited for an interview meet with the staff of the HCOP Department who answer questions in an informal setting. The School of Medicine has developed summer enrichment programs for high school and college students from groups traditionally underrepresented in American medicine in order to expand the pool of applicants to medical

school. Information about enrichment programs may be obtained by writing to the HCOP Department or by calling at (860) 679-3483.

Tutorial and counseling assistance is available to all students. The financial aid package is constructed on the basis of individual need, and every effort is made to meet this need. Application fees may be waived for disadvantaged students.

Institution Type: *Public*
Application Process: *AMCAS, see chapter 4.*

APPLICATION AND ACCEPTANCE POLICIES FOR 2005–2006 FIRST-YEAR CLASS

Filing of AMCAS application
  Earliest date: June 1, 2004
  Latest date: Dec. 15, 2004
School application fee to all applicants: $75
Oldest MCAT scores considered: 2001
Does have Early Decision Program (EDP)
  EDP application period: June 1–Aug. 1, 2004
  EDP applicants notified by: Oct. 1, 2004
Acceptance notice to regular applicants
  Earliest date: Oct. 15, 2004
  Latest date: Until class is filled
Applicant's response to acceptance offer
  Maximum time: 2 weeks
Requests for deferred entrance considered: Yes
Deposit to hold place in class (applied to tuition):
  $100, due with response to acceptance offer
Deposit refundable prior to: May 16, 2005
Estimated number of new entrants: 80 (8 EDP)
Starting date: Aug. 2005

TUITION AND STUDENT FEES PER YEAR FOR 2003–2004 FIRST-YEAR CLASS

Tuition   Student fees: $5,140
  Resident: $12,000
  Nonresident: $27,300

INFORMATION ON 2003–2004 FIRST-YEAR CLASS

Number of	In-State	Out-of-State	Total
Applicants	340	1,868	2,208
Applicants Interviewed	200	200	400
New Entrants*	53	21	74

*All took the MCAT and had baccalaureate degrees.

11

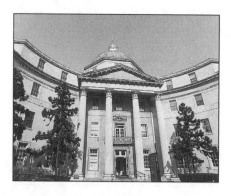

Yale University School of Medicine

New Haven, Connecticut

Dr. Dennis D. Spencer, *Interim Dean*
Dr. Thomas L. Lentz, *Associate Dean for Admissions and Financial Aid*
Pamela J. Nyiri, *Director of Financial Aid*
Dr. Forrester A. Lee, *Assistant Dean for Multicultural Affairs*

ADDRESS INQUIRIES TO:

Richard A. Silverman
Director of Admissions
Yale University
School of Medicine
367 Cedar Street
New Haven, Connecticut 06510
(203) 785-3046; 785-3234 (FAX)
E-mail: medical.admissions@yale.edu
Web site: http://info.med.yale.edu/medadmit

MISSION STATEMENT

The aim of the Yale University School of Medicine is to produce physicians who will be among the leaders in their chosen field, whether it be in the basic medical sciences, academic clinical medicine, or medical practice in the community. Belief in the maturity and responsibility of the students is emphasized by creating a flexible educational program, through anonymous examinations, by eliminating grades, and by encouraging independent study and research. The ideal Yale physician is a highly competent and compassionate practitioner of the medical arts, schooled in the current state of knowledge of both medical biology and patient care.

GENERAL INFORMATION

The Yale University School of Medicine was established by passage of a bill in the Connecticut General Assembly in 1810 granting a charter for the Medical Institution of Yale College. The Yale-New Haven Medical Center is composed of the School of Medicine, the School of Nursing, and the Yale-New Haven Hospital. The West Haven Veterans Hospital, Connecticut Mental Health Center, Hospital of St. Raphael, and Waterbury Hospital are also used for instruction. The Yale Medical Library has an extensive collection of current and historical medical literature.

CURRICULUM

The educational objective of the School of Medicine is to develop physicians who are highly competent and compassionate practitioners of the medical arts, schooled in the current state of knowledge of both medical biology and patient

care. It is hoped that Yale-trained physicians will establish a lifelong process of learning the medical, behavioral, and social sciences by independent study. The aim is to produce physicians who will be among the leaders in their chosen field, whether it be in the basic medical sciences, academic clinical medicine, or medical practice in the community. The program allows considerable freedom for planning according to the ability and interests of the student.

The first two years of the Yale School of Medicine are spent building a foundation in the basic sciences. The first year emphasizes normal biological form and function. The second-year curriculum emphasizes the study of disease. Throughout both years, a pre-clinical clerkship course meets weekly to teach physical diagnosis and the art of talking with patients. The third year is almost entirely devoted to clinical clerkships with 45 weeks of study in clerkships required for graduation. The fourth year is devoted to electives, a required primary care clerkship, and completion of the thesis work.

The thesis, a requirement since 1839, is an essential part of the curriculum and is designed to develop critical judgment, habits of self-education, and application of the scientific method to medicine. The thesis, based on original research in an area of the student's choosing, gives students the opportunity to work closely with faculty who are distinguished scientists, clinicians, and scholars.

A combined M.D.-Ph.D. program is available for qualified applicants with a strong motivation toward a career in academic medicine and the biomedical sciences. Support is made available through the Medical Scientist Training Program. The M.D.-Ph.D. program is flexible and normally takes seven to eight years to complete. Joint M.D.-J.D., M.D.-M.P.H., M.D.-M.Div. and M.D.-M.BA. programs are also available.

REQUIREMENTS FOR ENTRANCE

It is recommended that students enter medical school after four years of study in a college of arts and sciences or institute of technology. Students holding advanced degrees in science or other fields are also considered. Foreign students must complete one year of study and the pre-medical requirements in an American college or university prior to application. Students who have been refused admission on three prior occasions are ineligible to apply for admission to the first-year class. The MCAT and satisfactory completion of the following courses are required.

Sem. hrs.

General Biology or Zoology (with lab) 6–8
General or Inorganic Chemistry (with lab). 6–8
Organic Chemistry (with lab). 6–8
General Physics (with lab) 6–8

Acceptable courses in these subjects usually extend over one year and are given credit for six to eight semester hours. The medical faculty has no preference as to a major field for undergraduate study but recommends that students advance beyond the elementary level in their field of study. Students entering college with a strong background in the sciences, as demonstrated by Advanced Placement, are encouraged to substitute advanced science courses for the traditional requirements listed above.

The secondary application for Yale must be completed at the listed Web address and forwarded to the Office of Admissions electronically.

SELECTION FACTORS

The Committee on Admissions in general seeks to admit students who best suit the philosophies and goals of the school, which include providing an education in the scholarly and humane aspects of medicine and fostering the development of leaders who will advance medical practice and knowledge. It also seeks to ensure an adequate representation of women and groups underrepresented in medicine and a diversity of interests and backgrounds. The class entering in 2003 has 54 percent women, 23 percent underrepresented minority, and 28 percent Asian American and other students from groups underrepresented in medicine. Yale University School of Medicine does not discriminate on the basis of race, sex, religion, national origin, age, handicap, or sexual orientation.

All secondary applications are read and screened by members of the Admissions Committee. In considering applicants, the committee views the individual as a whole, taking into consideration each student's academic record, MCAT scores, pre-medical committee evaluations, letters of recommendation, outside accomplishments, personal qualities, and suitability for Yale.

Interviews are arranged only by invitation of the Admissions Committee. A large number of applicants have attained a high level of academic achievement as indicated by grades and test scores. Activities and accomplishments are of considerable importance in distinguishing candidates as individuals and demonstrating the ability to make significant independent contributions. The admissions committee also considers personal attributes thought to be important in a physician and suitability for the Yale program of medical education.

FINANCIAL AID

The school discourages excessive outside work and provides scholarship awards and loans for those who have serious financial needs. Financial aid applications will be mailed on or around January 1. All applicants for financial aid will be required to participate in FAFSA. A supplemental needs analysis will be required for students applying for institutional funds. This application will require student, spouse, and family financial statements.

INFORMATION ABOUT DIVERSITY PROGRAMS

Yale University School of Medicine seeks to obtain an adequate representation of all groups that are underrepresented in medicine and encourages qualified students from these groups to apply. Applicants invited for interviews will have the opportunity to meet with students from groups underrepresented in medicine and faculty to learn about the school. The membership of the Committee on Admissions is quite diverse.

Further information may be obtained from Dr. Forrester Lee, assistant dean for multicultural affairs.

Institution Type: *Private*
Application Process: *AMCAS, see chapter 4.*

APPLICATION AND ACCEPTANCE POLICIES FOR 2005–2006 FIRST-YEAR CLASS

Filing of AMCAS application
  Earliest date: June 1, 2004
  Latest date: Oct. 15, 2004
School application fee to all applicants: $75
Oldest MCAT scores considered: 2002
Does have Early Decision Program (EDP)
  EDP application period: June 1–Aug. 1, 2004
  EDP applicants notified by: Oct. 1, 2004
Acceptance notice to regular applicants
  Earliest date: March 15, 2005
  Latest date: Until class is filled
Applicant's response to acceptance offer
  Maximum time: 3 weeks
Requests for deferred entrance considered: Yes
Deposit to hold place in class (applied to tuition):
  $100, due with response to acceptance offer
Deposit refundable prior to: May 16, 2005
Estimated number of new entrants: 100 (1–3 EDP)
Starting date: Aug. 2005

TUITION AND STUDENT FEES PER YEAR FOR 2003–2004 FIRST-YEAR CLASS

Tuition: $33,800   Student fees: $375

INFORMATION ON 2003–2004 FIRST-YEAR CLASS

Number of	In-State	Out-of-State	Total
Applicants	197	3,128	3,325
Applicants Interviewed	67	742	809
New Entrants*	22	78	100

*All took the MCAT and had baccalaureate degrees.

CHAPTER

11

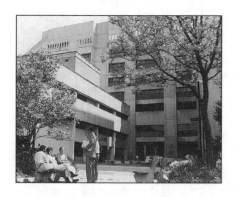

The George Washington University
School of Medicine and Health Sciences

Washington, D.C.

Dr. John F. Williams, *Provost and Vice President for Health Affairs,*
 School of Medicine and Health Sciences
Dr. James L. Scott, *Interim Dean, School of Medicine and Health Sciences*
Dr. Brian J. McGrath, *Associate Dean of Admissions and Financial Aid*
Diane P. McQuail, *Assistant Dean of Admissions*

ADDRESS INQUIRIES TO:

Office of Admissions
The George Washington University
School of Medicine and Health Sciences
2300 I Street, N.W., Ross Hall 716
Washington, D.C. 20037
(202) 994-3506
E-mail: medadmit@gwu.edu
Web site: www.gwumc.edu/edu/admis/

MISSION STATEMENT

With a vision to be the pre-eminent health institution in the Washington area, the George Washington University School of Medicine is dedicated to improving the health and well-being of our local community and beyond. We are committed to providing the highest quality of care and health services to the public; excellence and innovation in education; and research that expands the frontiers of science and knowledge. We strive to set standards of excellence by providing exemplary and innovative teaching programs that produce health professionals trained and prepared for the future; by generating and expanding health knowledge through superior programs in basic science, health policy, and applied research; and by delivering compassionate, high quality, and patient-focused clinical care. We are committed to the principles of altruism, collaboration, communication, compassion, innovation, integrity, respect, and service excellence.

GENERAL INFORMATION

Founded in 1825, the School of Medicine and Health Sciences (SMHS) is the 11th oldest medical school in the country. The School is housed in Ross Hall, a research, educational and administrative facility located in the nation's capital. Located adjacent to Ross Hall, the new, state-of-the-art GW Hospital opened in August 2002. This new facility boasts an Educational Center consisting of a clinical simulation facility, a standardized patient examination facility, a computer resource center and lounge/conference areas. In addition to the GW Hospital, the teaching services of the Children's Hospital National Medical Center, Fairfax Hospital, Holy Cross Hospital, National Naval Medical Center, St. Elizabeth's Hospital, Veterans Administration Hospital, and Washington Hospital Center are also available to students. A variety of ambulatory sites throughout the DC area are also utilized including neighborhood clinics that serve the indigent.

CURRICULUM

The curriculum is designed to provide students a medical education comprehensive enough to prepare them for careers in all areas of medicine and offer them a broad exposure on which to base residency selection. The faculty's objectives include imparting to students a substantial body of information, while stressing the attitude of compassion, the skill of problem-solving, the habit of self-education, and a high regard for the acquisition of new knowledge, both basic and applied. Emphasis is placed on education through cooperative effort, not through competition.

The Practice of Medicine (POM) portion of the curriculum integrates the building blocks of a traditional medical education—a strong foundation of basic and clinical sciences—by interweaving them throughout the four-year curriculum. The first phase of this course places every student with a practicing clinician on a regular basis throughout Years I and II. On alternate weeks, clinical assessment skills will be taught and evaluated in a small group format. A small group problem-based learning (PBL) model designed to integrate both basic and clinical sciences is incorporated in POM.

Clinical clerkships begin in the third year. In an effort to keep up with the changing practice of medicine, an optional pilot curriculum was recently introduced for the third year that provides ambulatory exposure over an extended period of time designed to be consistent with actual clinical practice. Choice of courses is largely elective during the fourth year. Opportunities for international clinical experiences are available for fourth year medical students. The honors/pass/conditional/fail system is used for grading.

A seven-year Bachelor of Arts/Medical Doctor program and an eight-year Integrated Engineering/MD program are available at The George Washington University. These programs are designed for high school honor students of high ability and maturity who demonstrate significant motivation for a medical career. Please visit ✍ http://gwired.gwu.edu/adm/ for more information on these programs for high school seniors. Early Selection Programs are available to sophomores in the spring semester at GW, University of Maryland-College Park, Franklin & Marshall, Claremont, McKenna, Scripps, George Mason, Colgate, and Hampden Sydney College. In addition, linkage agreements exist with postbaccalaureate programs at Goucher College, University of Pennsylvania, Brandeis University, Scripps College, Johns Hopkins University and Bryn Mawr College.

Both M.D./M.P.H. and M.D./Ph.D. programs are available to medical students. The M.D./M.P.H. can be obtained in four years. Coursework for the M.P.H. can begin the summer preceding medical school matriculation.

Transfer applications for the second- and third-year classes are accepted beginning in February.

REQUIREMENTS FOR ENTRANCE

Applicants must have completed 90 semester hours including the pre-medical coursework at an accredited U.S. or Canadian institution prior to matriculation. (Most students have completed four years of college.) Applicants must take the MCAT. Applicants must be a U.S. or Canadian citizen or must hold a U.S. permanent resident visa.

The International Medicine program is available to International applicants sponsored by their home governments or medical institution. This program prepares international students for medical practice and leadership roles in their own countries.

Sem. hrs.

Biology and/or Zoology (with lab) 8
Inorganic Chemistry (with lab) 8
Organic Chemistry (with lab) 8
Physics (with lab) 8
English Composition and/or Literature 6

With the exception of these specific requirements, applicants are urged to follow their personal interests in developing a pre-medical course of study. Applicants with an undergraduate emphasis in the arts, humanities, and social sciences are welcomed. Required courses must be completed by July 2005.

SELECTION FACTORS

The initial overall evaluation is based on data contained in the AMCAS and supplemental applications. This evaluation screens applicants on the basis of academic performance; MCAT scores; extracurricular, health-related, research, and work experiences; and evidence of non-scholastic accomplishments. Evidence of strong performance in recent, relevant coursework is to an applicant's advantage. Some additional consideration is given to applicants from the District of Columbia and its metropolitan area as well as to applicants from the University's undergraduate schools. The next phase of the selection procedure depends on careful examination of personal comments and letters of recommendation. The most promising applicants are then invited for a personal interview either at the school or with a regional interviewer. The last phase includes the review by the Committee on Admissions of the entire dossier. This phase is designed to select academically prepared students with motivational and personal characteristics the committee considers important in future physicians. There is no discrimination in the selection process because of race, gender, religion, age, marital status, sexual orientation, disability, or national or regional origin.

The 167 members of the 2003 entering class came from 92 different undergraduate schools. The *mean undergraduate GPA* was 3.55, although there was great variability. Some other characteristics of the 2003 entering class were: *undergraduate major,*

40 percent in non-science fields; *graduate degrees,* 23 students; *gender,* 94 women.

FINANCIAL AID

Information regarding financial aid is available at ✎ www.gwumc.edu/smhs/fin-aid/index.html. Detailed financial aid information is provided at the time of interview. Merit-based admissions scholarships are available. Financial aid is not readily available for non-U.S. citizens.

INFORMATION ABOUT DIVERSITY PROGRAMS

The School of Medicine is committed to providing an education to students from groups underrepresented in medicine. Twelve percent (12) of the class entering in 2003 self-identified as members of an underrepresented group. Visiting applicants are encouraged to meet with students from groups underrepresented in medicine and faculty.

Institution Type: *Private*
Application Process: *AMCAS, see chapter 4.*

APPLICATION AND ACCEPTANCE POLICIES FOR 2005–2006 FIRST-YEAR CLASS

Filing of AMCAS application
  Earliest date: June 1, 2004
  Latest date: Dec. 1, 2004
School application fee to all applicants: $90
Oldest MCAT scores considered: 2002
Does have Early Decision Program (EDP)
  EDP application period: June 1–Aug. 1, 2004
  (AMCAS applications are due in the Admissions
  Office by August 1, 2004.)
  EDP applicants notified by: Oct. 1, 2004
Acceptance notice to regular applicants
  Earliest date: Oct. 15, 2004
  Latest date: Until class is filled
Applicant's response to acceptance offer
  Maximum time: 2 weeks
Requests for deferred entrance considered: Yes
Deposit to hold place in class: $100, deposit is due
  between May 1–May 16, 2005
Deposit is refundable prior to: May 16, 2005
Estimated number of new entrants: 167 (2 EDP)
Starting date: Aug. 2005

TUITION AND STUDENT FEES PER YEAR FOR 2003–2004 FIRST-YEAR CLASS

Tuition: $39,005   Student fees: $280

INFORMATION ON 2003–2004 FIRST-YEAR CLASS

Number of	D.C.	Out-of-State	Total
Applicants	49	9,179	9,228
Applicants Interviewed	10	1,118	1,128
New Entrants*	1	166	167

*All had baccalaureate degrees and 88% took the MCAT.

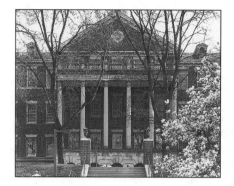

Georgetown University School of Medicine

Washington, D.C.

Dr. S. Ray Mitchell, *Dean for Medical Education*
Dr. Russell T. Wall III, *Associate Dean for Admissions and Student Services*
Eugene T. Ford, *Director of Admissions*
Joy P. Williams, *Assistant Dean for Students and Special Programs**

ADDRESS INQUIRIES TO:

Office of Admissions
Georgetown University School of Medicine
Box 571421
Washington, D.C. 20057-1421
(202) 687-1154; 687-3079 (FAX)
Web site: www.georgetown.edu/schmed

MISSION STATEMENT

Guided by the University's Jesuit tradition of *cura personalis*, of caring for the whole person, Georgetown University School of Medicine will educate, in an integrated way, knowledgeable, skillful, ethical, and compassionate physicians and biomedical scientists, dedicated to the care of others and the health needs of our society.

The Georgetown School of Medicine was established in 1851 and is a part of the oldest Catholic and Jesuit-sponsored university in the United States. Georgetown seeks to educate and produce future physicians who possess a strong general foundation of basic and clinical science knowledge well-developed clinical skills and the ability to make decisions based on scientific evidence; can address care for the community, as well as individuals; and can engage in continuous self-directed learning. The School of Medicine encourages attitudes and values that reflect the importance of ethical, spiritual, psychological, social, and cultural aspects of compassionate care and healing of the whole patient—a foundation that will equip Georgetown medical graduates for the pursuit of any one of the many possible avenues for medical practice in the 21st century, including primary care, specialization, and subspecialization.

Our educational approach involves excellent basic science and clinical faculty who are committed to providing first-rate scientific information in an environment conducive to learning and application. All of our students participate in small group and independent learning, including PBL and other forms of clinical decision-making/problem-solving, and utilize computer-based educational program supplements. Students also contribute heavily to our educational planning and evaluation activities and are valued members of all medical education committees.

GENERAL INFORMATION

The School of Medicine works in association with the 535-bed Georgetown University Hospital, which is part of a major regional not-for-profit health care system comprising of seven other hospitals. In addition, the school has affiliations with eight federal and community hospitals in the Washington metropolitan area. The medical center includes a Concentrated Care Center and Outpatient Surgical Center with state-of-the-art emergency, x-ray, and transplant facilities. The campus also contains a modern health science library and classroom and laboratory facilities dedicated to basic and preclinical science and research. Adjacent to the hospital is the Vincent T. Lombardi Cancer Research Center providing both research and clinical care. The school is near the National Institutes of Health and other internationally prominent health care and research facilities.

Georgetown also offers opportunities for the overall development of its student body. The Reverend Gerard F. Yates, S.J., Memorial Field House offers swimming facilities, jogging tracks, many athletic programs, and the availability of multi- and single-purpose courts. In the nearby Thomas and Dorothy Leavey Center, a variety of dining establishments and guest quarters complement space for conferences and the performing arts.

CURRICULUM

Georgetown's curriculum combines diverse teaching modalities. Courses in the first two years focus on the development of fundamental knowledge concerning the body's normal and altered structure and functions. Small-group teaching and exposure to patient assessment and care begin early. In the third year, clinical clerkships in hospitals and ambulatory care settings stress the skills required to acquire and interpret patient-based data, while the fourth year further develops skills in patient management. Sixteen weeks of electives are available during this final year.

At Georgetown, the grading system consists of honors, high pass, pass, and fail.

A research track for medical students and a combined M.D.-Ph.D. program are also available; the Ph.D. may be taken in a basic medical science department or in philosophy-bioethics. Applicants may also apply for a five-year combined M.D.-M.B.A. program.

REQUIREMENTS FOR ENTRANCE

In general, Georgetown requires the MCAT and a minimum of three years of college (90 semester hours) for consideration of admission to the School of Medicine. The baccalaureate degree is highly desirable. The minimum specific course requirements are:

	Sem./Qtr.
Biology (with lab)	2/3
Inorganic Chemistry (with lab)	2/3

Organic Chemistry (with lab) 2/3
General Physics (with lab) 2/3
English 2/3
Mathematics/Statistics . . . . (3 credits)

While a solid preparation in the basic sciences is essential, a broad background in the humanities and computer science is also important. Biochemistry is strongly recommended and can be substituted for second-semester organic chemistry.

Applicants should take the MCAT in the spring of the year they intend to apply and make sure that required courses will be completed. Georgetown allows six to eight hours of prerequisites to be taken during the application year. Applicants are cautioned that files are not reviewed until MCAT scores are received; a delay in the receipt of such credentials may delay consideration of an application.

SELECTION FACTORS

The Committee on Admissions selects students on the basis of academic achievement, character, maturity, and motivation. There are no geographical quotas. In rendering its decisions, the Committee on Admissions evaluates the applicant's entire academic record, performance on the MCAT, college premedical advisory committee evaluations, letters of recommendation, and personal interviews.

For the 2003 entering class, 7,547 candidates applied from over 624 undergraduate colleges. The applicants who enrolled had the following characteristics: *mean science GPA,* 3.61; *undergraduate major,* 55 percent in the biological sciences, 10 percent in the physical sciences, 18 percent in social sciences, 17 percent in various humanities and other majors; 52 percent *women.*

Georgetown requires personal interviews. These interviews are conducted on the medical center campus, and applicants are not invited to interview until all their credentials have been received and reviewed by the Committee on Admissions. A secondary application and essay are required for all applicants. Applicants are urged to submit their applications and supporting credentials as early as possible. The School of Medicine does not discriminate on the basis of race, sex, creed, age, handicap, or national or ethnic origin.

The School of Medicine has an Early Assurance Program with its undergraduate institution. Generally, applicants for transfer are considered only from LCME-accredited medical schools.

FINANCIAL AID

Georgetown's medical school participates in federal financial aid programs and awards school-administered grants, scholarships, and low-interest loans to students on the basis of financial need. Parents' financial information is required for students seeking school-administered aid.

Medical students at Georgetown are expected to take responsibility for their financial affairs in meeting deadlines for both tuition payment as well as in applying for financial aid. Loan indebtedness counseling is an important function of the Office of Student Financial Planning as a majority of students at the School of Medicine incur substantial educational debt. Candidates for admission are strongly encouraged to contact that office with questions about financial aid.

INFORMATION ABOUT DIVERSITY PROGRAMS

In 2003 the School of Medicine has a diverse student body, with students from groups underrepresented in medicine. Questions about programs and opportunities for applicants from the groups should be addressed to the director, Office of Programs for Minority Student Development. The Georgetown Experimental Medical Studies (GEMS) Program is a one-year postbaccalaureate program for qualified disadvantaged students and those from groups underrepresented in medicine. Priority consideration is given to residents of the District of Columbia. For more information, please telephone the GEMS program coordinator, at (202) 687-1406.

Institution Type: *Private*
Application Process: *AMCAS, see chapter 4.*

APPLICATION AND ACCEPTANCE POLICIES FOR 2005–2006 FIRST-YEAR CLASS

Filing of AMCAS application
  Earliest date: June 1, 2004
  Latest date: Nov. 1, 2004
School application fee to all applicants: $100
Oldest MCAT scores considered: 2002
Does not have Early Decision Program
Acceptance notice to regular applicants
  Earliest date: Oct. 15, 2004
  Latest date: Until class is filled
Applicant's response to acceptance offer
  Maximum time: 3 weeks
Requests for deferred entrance considered: Yes
Deposit to hold place in class (applied to tuition):
  $100, due March 15, 2005
Deposit refundable prior to: May 1, 2005
Partial tuition prepayment due: June 1, 2005
Estimated number of new entrants: 170
Starting date: Aug. 2005

TUITION AND STUDENT FEES PER YEAR FOR 2003–2004 FIRST-YEAR CLASS

Tuition: $33,670   Student Fees: $43

INFORMATION ON 2003–2004 FIRST-YEAR CLASS

Number of	D.C.	Out-of-State	Total
Applicants	41	7,506	7,547
Applicants Interviewed	9	1,127	1,136
New Entrants*	0	170	170

*All had baccalaureate degrees; 95% took the MCAT.

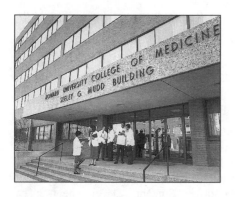

Howard University
College of Medicine

Washington, D.C.

Dr. Floyd J. Malveaux, *Dean*
Dr. Dawn L. Cannon, *Associate Dean for Student Affairs and Admissions*
Ann Finney, *Admissions Officer*

ADDRESS INQUIRIES TO:

Office of Admissions, Office of the Dean
Howard University
College of Medicine
520 W Street, N.W.
Washington, D.C. 20059
(202) 806-6270; 806-7934 (FAX)
Web site: www.med.howard.edu

GENERAL INFORMATION

The Howard University College of Medicine is the oldest and largest historically black medical school in the United States and the 36th oldest of all 125 medical schools in this country. Initially established as a medical department, the college opened in 1868 with eight students and seven faculty members. The medical department's primary goal then remains the college's today: to train students to become competent, compassionate physicians who will provide care in medically underserved communities.

In 1871, Howard University graduated its first medical class, consisting of two black men and three white men. One woman was graduated the following year. Subsequent classes throughout the College of Medicine's history have been similarly cosmopolitan in accordance with the spirit and intention of Howard University's founders. The college proudly cites its long history of training men and women of all races and ethnic origins, religions, creeds, nationalities, and economic backgrounds.

The college has more than 4,000 living alumni, including approximately 25 percent of all black practicing physicians in this country. During the first half of this century, the college contributed nearly half of the black physicians in the United States.

The 321-bed Howard University Hospital was completed in 1975. It is the college's primary teaching hospital for medical students and is used for postgraduate training in the various specialties of medicine. Medical students also serve clerkships at the Children's National Medical Center, Inova Fairfax Hospital, St. Elizabeths Hospital, the Washington Veterans Affairs Medical Center, Providence Hospital, the Washington Hospital Center, and Prince George's Hospital Center.

CURRICULUM

The curriculum is designed to provide a firm basis for the science and art of medicine and to provide effective integration of basic science concepts, clinical application, and research. Students are presented the essential knowledge and skills necessary for the practice of medicine in courses that are required of all medical students. In addition, time is provided in the schedule for students to pursue areas of their interest through elective courses.

An integrated curriculum was implemented in August 2001. Students in the first year complete curriculum blocks in Molecules and Cells, Structure and Function, and Medicine and Society. In year 2, pathophysiology, pathology and pharmacology are integrated according to organ systems. The Medicine and Society block continues throughout the second year, and a block in Physical Diagnosis is also included.

The third and fourth years consist of blocks of instruction in a continuum of clerkships and examinations in various clinical subjects. During the fourth year, opportunity is available for additional clinical or research experience through 20 or 24 weeks of required electives.

Satisfactory performance is required in all courses for promotion and graduation. Students are required to pass Step 1 of the USMLE for promotion to the third year. Passing Step 2 of the USMLE is required for graduation. Grades in the College of Medicine are reported as H (honors), S (satisfactory), or U (unsatisfactory).

A combined B.S./M.D. program was initiated in 1974 for students enrolling in the Howard University College of Arts and Sciences from high school. Both degrees may be obtained in a six-year period.

An M.D./Ph.D. degree program is available in anatomy, human genetics, microbiology, biochemistry, pharmacology, physiology, biology, and chemistry.

REQUIREMENTS FOR ENTRANCE

The MCAT is required. It is recommended that all applicants take the MCAT in the spring rather than in the fall of the year in which they apply. A minimum of 62 semester hours at an accredited U.S. or Canadian university or college is required. Course work should include:

	Sem. hrs.
Biology or Zoology	8
General Chemistry	8
Organic Chemistry	8
General Physics	8
College Mathematics	6
English	6

SELECTION FACTORS

There are four major criteria used in the selection of applicants for admission to the College of Medicine: (1) character and discernible motivation for a career in medicine, (2) scholastic record, (3) results of the MCAT, and (4) letters of recommendation from preprofessional advisors and faculty. Candidates for admission and alternates are selected from those applicants who satisfy the criteria and who are most likely to serve in communities needing physician services. MCAT scores and GPAs are used for initial screening.

An invitation for an interview may be extended to an applicant after the Committee on Admissions has made a preliminary examination of the applicant's credentials and has decided that an interview is desirable. Although the total student is evaluated, the Committee on Admissions gives strongest consideration to those who have GPAs of 3.0 and above.

There are no residence restrictions. All applicants will be evaluated regardless of their sex, race, religion, national or ethnic origin, age, marital status, or handicap.

A nonrefundable $150 enrollment fee (due with response to acceptance) is required of accepted students who have never previously enrolled at Howard University. This is in addition to the $100 refundable good faith deposit.

FINANCIAL AID

Approximately 85 percent of the students enrolled in the College of Medicine receive some sort of financial assistance. Financial aid applicants must submit the FAFSA. Students with demonstrated need may receive school-based scholarships and loans, and those who qualify are recommended for federally guaranteed and private educational loans. Some merit awards are offered to outstanding entering freshmen and for exceptional academic performance in the medical curriculum. Some students receive scholarships funded by the National Health Service Corps or by the military.

Institution Type: *Private*
Application Process: *AMCAS, see chapter 4.*

APPLICATION AND ACCEPTANCE POLICIES FOR 2005–2006 FIRST-YEAR CLASS

Filing of AMCAS application
    Earliest date: June 1, 2004
    Latest date: Dec. 15, 2004
School application fee to all applicants: $45
Oldest MCAT scores considered: 2002
Does not have Early Decision Program
Acceptance notice to regular applicants
    Earliest date: Oct. 15, 2004
    Latest date: Until class is filled
Applicant's response to acceptance offer
    Maximum time: 30 days
Requests for deferred entrance considered: Yes
Deposit to hold place in class (applied to tuition):
    $100, due with response to acceptance offer
Deposit refundable prior to: May 16, 2005
Estimated number of new entrants: 110
Starting date: August 2005

TUITION AND STUDENT FEES PER YEAR FOR 2003–2004 FIRST-YEAR CLASS

Tuition: $20,010   Student fees: $3,771

INFORMATION ON 2003–2004 FIRST-YEAR CLASS

Number of	D.C.	Out-of-State	Total
Applicants	44	4,222	4,268
Applicants Interviewed	19	411	430
New Entrants*	3	108	111

*All took the MCAT; 96% had baccalaureate degrees.

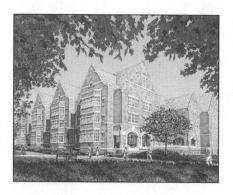

Florida State University College of Medicine

Tallahassee, Florida

Dr. J. Ocie Harris, *Dean*
Dr. Helen Livingston, *Assistant Dean for Student Affairs and Admissions*
Dr. Myra Hurt, *Associate Dean of Student Affairs, Admissions and Outreach*
April Qualls, *Enrollment Services Coordinator*

ADDRESS INQUIRIES TO:

Office of Student Affairs and Admissions
Florida State University College of Medicine
Administration Building, Room 117
Tallahassee, Fl 32306-4300
(850) 644-7904; 645-1420 (FAX)
E-mail: medadmissions@med.fsu.edu
Web site: www.med.fsu.edu

MISSION STATEMENT

The mission of the Florida State University College of Medicine is to educate and develop exemplary physicians who practice patient-centered health care, discover and advance knowledge, and respond to community needs, especially through service to elder, rural, and other medically underserved populations.

GENERAL INFORMATION

The Florida State University (FSU) College of Medicine was created in July 2000 by a legislative act, to train physicians with a focus on serving medically underserved populations in rural and inner-city areas, and the growing geriatric population in the state. The College of Medicine was built on the foundation of the successful Program in Medical Sciences, which was founded in 1971 as an expansion program of the University of Florida College of Medicine.

The FSU College of Medicine is composed of the main campus in Tallahassee and Regional Medical Campuses, where students will complete their 3rd- and 4th-year clerkships, in Pensacola, Orlando, and Tallahassee.

CURRICULUM

The academic program consists of a four-year sequence of instruction in the biopsychosocial sciences and community-based clinical training. An integrated approach in the first and second year is enhanced through case-based and problem-based learning in small group discussions and through simulated standardized-patient interviews. The first two years include biopsychosocial courses which include anatomy, embryology, and radiologic anatomy; microanatomy; clinical neuroscience; physiology; medical biochemistry and genetics; pathology; pharmacology and immunology; pharmacology

and laboratory medicine; psychosocial aspects of medicine; health issues; and microbiology. A two-year doctoring course composed of lecture, small group discussion and patient encounters, clinical skills instruction, and preceptorships provides application models to complete the integrated program of study for years one and two. In the preceptorship component, each student is paired with a primary care physician for 60 hours in the first year and 135 hours in the second year.

The third year and part of the fourth year consist of required rotations through the clinical science disciplines (medicine, surgery, pediatrics, obstetrics-gynecology, family medicine/rural medicine, geriatrics, emergency medicine, advanced medicine (critical care unit), advanced family practice, and psychiatry. After the required clerkships are completed students will spend up to 24 weeks in electives in the clinical continuum which are designed to give students a foundation on which to develop and fulfill their personal interests, broaden their clinical knowledge, and prepare for postgraduate medical training. A faculty advisor is selected in the third year when students relocate to the regional medical campuses and assumes an important role in assisting students in achieving their own special educational goals.

REQUIREMENTS FOR ENTRANCE

The MCAT, all pre-medical pre-requisites, and all requirements for a bachelor's degree must be completed by the time of matriculation. The MCAT should be taken during the spring or summer before submitting an application. The required prerequisites are:

Sem. hrs.

English and Composition 6
Mathematics 6
General Biology I & II (with lab) .8
General Chemistry I & II (with lab) 8
Organic Chemistry I & II (with lab) 8
General Physics I & II (with lab) .8
*Biochemistry I & II 6

*Some universities have a one-semester biochemistry with lab rather than a two-course, two-semester sequence. If that course is recommended by your institution for pre-medical students it will meet the biochemistry pre-requisite.

Genetics and psychology are strongly recommended.

SELECTION FACTORS

Although scholastic aptitude is necessary in order to complete studies in medical school, neither high GPAs nor high MCAT scores alone or in combination are adequate to obtain admission. Only Florida residents will be considered for admission to the FSU College of Medicine. International applicants must have a permanent resident visa. Applicants who have grades and test scores predictive of success in medical school, who have demonstrated through their experiences a high degree of motivation for medicine and a strong commitment to the service of others, and who have a likelihood of practicing medicine with medically underserved populations will receive an interview with two members of the Admissions Committee. The committee evaluates all aspects of the applicant's academic record, including trends in scholastic performance. Those invited to interview will have lunch with the medical students serving as hosts for that day.

Acceptances were issued to 64 applicants to obtain a class of 46 entering students. In the 2003 class, accepted students had the following profile: *mean science* GPA, 3.53; *mean total* GPA, 3.62. The *mean MCAT*, VR-7.9, PS-9.1, BS-9.7; *mean age*, 23; 33 percent *multi-cultural*; 41 percent *women* and 59 percent *men*. *Biology* majors made up 26 percent of the class, 13 percent were *Microbiology majors* and 13 percent were Exercise Science and Physiology majors, with the remainder from a variety of fields.

FINANCIAL AID

About 90 percent of our students receive financial aid. Scholarships and loan funds from private, state, and federal sources are available to qualified students and are awarded on the basis of need and/or scholarship. For additional details and assistance in financial planning, please contact the Coordinator of Enrollment Services at (850) 644-5323.

INFORMATION ABOUT DIVERSITY PROGRAMS

Because of the mission of the College of Medicine and because the medical school seeks to admit a diverse cohort of students each year, the need to provide all students with the opportunity to study medicine is recognized as an important guiding tenet. The Postbaccalaureate Bridge Program is designed to provide opportunities for applicants from groups underrepresented in medicine and rural and inner-city populations to attend medical school. Five students from these groups who embody the characteristics valued by the College of Medicine are selected each year from the applicant pool. The Bridge year is used to develop and enhance study, time management, and test-taking skills; the psychosocial and basic science backgrounds; and the clinical experiences of these students. If the Bridge students meet all requirements established for the year, they are then admitted to the next year's medical school class. Students may contact the Director of Outreach at (850) 644-4607.

Institution Type: *Public*
Application Process: *AMCAS, see chapter 4.*

APPLICATION AND ACCEPTANCE POLICIES FOR 2005–2006 FIRST-YEAR CLASS

Filing of AMCAS application
  Earliest date: June 1, 2004
  Latest date: December. 15, 2004
School application fee: None
Oldest MCAT scores considered: 2001
Does have Early Decision Program (EDP)
  Florida residents only
  EDP application period: June 1–Aug. 1, 2004
  EDP applicants notified by: Oct. 1, 2004
Acceptance notice to regular applicants
  Earliest date: Oct. 15, 2004
  Latest date: May 28, 2004
Applicant's response to acceptance offer
  Maximum time: 2 weeks
Requests for deferred entrance considered: Yes
Deposit to hold place in class: None
Estimated number of new entrants: 60 (5 EDP)
Starting date: June 2005

TUITION AND STUDENT FEES PER YEAR FOR 2003–2004 FIRST-YEAR CLASS

Tuition   Student fees: $670
  Resident: $14,208
  Non-Resident: $43,530

INFORMATION ON 2003-2004 FIRST-YEAR CLASS

Number of	In-State	Out-of-State	Total
Applicants	473	39	512
Applicants Interviewed	105	1	106
New Entrants*	46	0	46

*All took the MCAT and had baccalaureate degrees.

CHAPTER

11

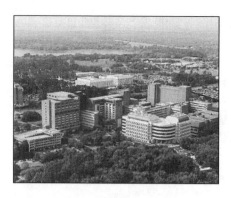

University of Florida College of Medicine

Gainesville, Florida

Dr. Craig C. Tisher, *Dean*
Robyn Sheppard, *Coordinator of Admissions*
Eileen M. Parris, *Coordinator of Financial Aid*
Dr. Donna M. Parker, *Assistant Dean for Minority Affairs*

ADDRESS INQUIRIES TO:

Chair, Medical Selection Committee
Box 100216
UF Health Sciences Center
University of Florida
College of Medicine
Gainesville, Florida 32610–0216
(352) 392-4569; 392-1307 (FAX)
Web site: www.med.ufl.edu/

MISSION STATEMENT

To educate medical students in humanistic, scientific and practical principles of medicine to become, and remain, exemplary practitioners, academicians and leaders. To educate scientistists for research, teaching or industry careers. To provide compassionate, skilled and innovative healthcare. To foster discovery. To promote health, prevent disease, and so educate the public. To promote the professional and personal growth of faculty and staff.

GENERAL INFORMATION

The College of Medicine, a component college of the University of Florida Health Science Center, admitted the first class in September 1956. Situated at the southeast corner of the 2,000-acre campus of the University of Florida, the College of Medicine enjoys the benefit of strong ties with other programs within the university as well as a close relationship to the other Health Science Center colleges (dentistry, health professions, nursing, pharmacy, and veterinary medicine). The University of Florida Health Science Center complex also includes the Chandler A. Stetson Medical Science Building, the Communicore Building (library, teaching laboratories, and classrooms), the Academic Research Building, the Cancer Research Building, Shands Hospital, the Brain Institute, and the Veterans Administration Medical Center, located across the street from the Health Science Center. The University of Florida Health Science Center—Jacksonville is our urban campus. Formal educational affiliations have also been established in Ft. Lauderdale, Miami, Orlando, and Pensacola.

CURRICULUM

The four years of medical education are divided into three blocks of time—Preclinical Coursework (two years), Clinical Clerkships (one year), and Postclerkship Electives and Required courses (one year).

Preclinical coursework provides students with essential basic science and general clinical information necessary for clinical training. Faculty from both basic and clinical science departments participate. Students may elect the option of taking the preclinical basic science courses over an extended track. This option allows the M.D./Ph.D candidates (joint degree), and other students, to begin research activities earlier and in more depth. It also lets these students pursue additional coursework as necessary. An extended time track may assist students with less intensive science backgrounds who would benefit from more moderately paced coursework. A student's request to participate in an extended track must receive prior review and approval by that Associate Dean for Education and the Chair of the Academic Status Committee. A student who either fails any coursework or meets the standards for dismissal, and is given the option of repeating an entire academic year, is not eligible to elect an extended track option.

The third year is devoted to clinical clerkships, in which student groups experience the major clinical services. The required clerkships include family medicine/geriatrics, medicine, neurology, pediatrics, psychiatry, obstetrics/gynecology, and surgery. Students spend 10 to 12 weeks participating in clerkships at UF Health Science Center—Jacksonville. Housing will be provided during Jacksonville clerkships. During these clinical clerkships, the student becomes an integral member of the medical team and has direct responsibility for assigned patients during rotation.

The fourth year includes seven elective periods and three required courses: anesthesiology, emergency medicine and either senior medicine, community medicine or pediatrics. An eleventh period is available for accomplishing residency interviews. For students who have already chosen a specialty, fourth-year programs may be designed to provide experiences related to their career choice. Elective courses in the basic sciences also are available. Independent study programs may be designed to allow study of areas in medicine not represented by formal course offerings. Students ranked in the upper 2/3 of their class may take up to three electives at other institutions.

JOINT PROGRAMS:

M.D./Ph.D.

This program offers an opportunity for students who are motivated toward an academic career in the medical sciences. The M.D.-Ph.D. program is designed to be intensive, yet flexible, and to provide a smooth interface between clinical and research training. Candidates for this program must satisfy admission requirements for the college of medicine and the graduate school and have significant research experience.

M.D./J.D.

The faculties of the College of Law and the College of Medicine have approved a joint degree program culminating in both M.D. and J.D. degrees conferred from each college. Under the joint degree program, a student can obtain both degrees in approximately one year less than it would take to obtain both degrees if pursued consecutively.

M.D./M.B.A.-M.S.W.

The College of Business Administration have approved joint degree programs with the College of Medicine which culminates in obtaining both degrees in approximately one year less than it would take to obtain both degrees if pursued consecutively. The purpose of the joint degree program is to produce physicians with an understanding of business management principles to be used in their medical practices or to prepare them for careers as health care systems administrators.

B.S./M.D.: Junior Honors Medical Program

Students accepted into the Junior Honors Medical Program at the end of their second year of college enroll in basic medical science seminars and undergraduate courses during their third year. They become full-time first year medical students in their fourth year and receive a B.S. degree at the end of that year from the College of Liberal Arts and Sciences. Although primarily intended for students in their second year at the University of Florida, applications from students enrolled at other colleges and universities will be considered. Further information may be obtained by writing to the admissions office.

REQUIREMENTS FOR ENTRANCE

Only U.S. citizens and permanent resident aliens will be considered. The MCAT is required and must be taken within three years before matriculation, and before the December 1 application deadline. The student should complete the requirements for a bachelor's degree at an accredited American college or university prior to matriculation. In exceptional instances students upon whom the degree has not been conferred may be admitted. College work must include:

Sem. hrs.

Biochemistry (with lab) 4
Biology (with lab) 8
General Chemistry (with lab) 8
Organic Chemistry (with lab) 4
Physics (with lab) 8

SELECTION FACTORS

Applicants will be appraised on the basis of personal attributes, academic record, evaluation of past activities, the MCAT,

and letters of recommendation. A personal interview is required to complete the application process and is granted at the discretion of the Medical Selection Committee. The school does not discriminate on the basis of race, sex, age, disability, creed, or national origin. Although Florida residents are given preference in admission, a limited number of nonresidents are considered each year. Nonresident applicants must demonstrate superior qualifications. The College of Medicine welcomes applications from members of groups underrepresented in medicine and from persons who demonstrate a clear, long-standing commitment to underserved populations.

Students matriculating into the 2002 entering class had the following characteristics: *mean GPA,* 3.71; *MCAT,* 30.75; *female,* 53 percent; 11 percent *minorities.*

FINANCIAL AID

Financial assistance is available to all enrolled students who show need. The College has scholarships and low interest loans available. Applications are mailed to all accepted applicants. Summer and school-year research fellowships are also available.

Institution Type: *Public*
Application Process: *AMCAS, see chapter 4.*

APPLICATION AND ACCEPTANCE POLICIES FOR 2005–2006 FIRST-YEAR CLASS

Filing of AMCAS application
    Earliest date: June 1, 2004
    Latest date: Dec. 1, 2004
School application fee: $30
Oldest MCAT scores considered: August 2002
Does not have Early Decision Program
Acceptance notice to regular applicants
    Earliest date: Oct. 15, 2004
    Latest date: August 15, 2005
Applicant's response to acceptance offer
    Maximum time: 2 weeks
Requests for deferred entrance considered: Yes
Deposit to hold place in class: $200
Estimated number of new entrants: 120
Starting date: Aug. 2005

TUITION AND STUDENT FEES PER YEAR FOR 2003–2004 FIRST-YEAR CLASS

Tuition	Student fees
Resident: $13,925	Resident: $1,815
Nonresident: $40,082	Nonresident: $3,123

INFORMATION ON 2002-2003 FIRST-YEAR CLASS

Number of	In-State	Out-of-State	Total
Applicants	1,026	977	2,003
Applicants Interviewed	229	73	302
New Entrants*	113	3	116

*All took the MCAT and had baccalaureate degrees.

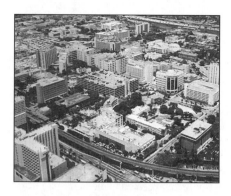

University of Miami
School of Medicine

Miami, Florida

Dr. John G. Clarkson, *Senior Vice President for Medical Affairs and Dean, School of Medicine*
Dr. R.E. Hinkley, *Assoc. Dean for Admissions and Enrollment Management*
Laura L. Horsley, *Assistant Dean for Student Financial Assistance*
Dr. Astrid Mack, *Associate Dean for Minority Affairs*

ADDRESS INQUIRIES TO:

Office of Admissions
University of Miami
School of Medicine
P.O. Box 016159
Miami, Florida 33101
(305) 243-6791; 243-6548 (FAX)
E-mail: med.admissions@miami.edu
Web site: www.miami.edu/medical-admissions

MISSION STATEMENT

The University of Miami has four interrelated missions: patient care, teaching, research, and community service.

GENERAL INFORMATION

The University of Miami School of Medicine is the largest and oldest medical school in the state of Florida. Since its founding in 1952, the School of Medicine has experienced a remarkable growth rate and has been the catalyst in the development of one of the largest and most comprehensive health care centers in the nation. In 2003 the school had a full-time faculty of 1,077, an annual budget of $650 million, and research expenditures of $188 million.

The School of Medicine is located on the medical campus next to Jackson Memorial Hospital in the Civic Center area of Miami. Classrooms used by students during the first two years, as well as administrative offices and research laboratories, are located in the Rosenstiel Medical Sciences Building and the Glaser Medical Research Building. Jackson Memorial Hospital and the Veterans Affairs Medical Center provide the primary settings in which third- and fourth-year students acquire their clinical skills. Six hospitals containing nearly 3,000 beds are located on the medical campus and provide a complete spectrum of clinical experiences.

Also located on the medical campus and affiliated with the University of Miami School of Medicine are the Mailman Center for Child Development, the Bascom Palmer Eye Institute and Anne Bates Leach Eye Hospital, the Applebaum Magnetic Resonance Imaging Center, the Ambulatory Care Center, the UM Hospitals and Clinics, the Diabetes Research Institute, and the Ryder Trauma Center. The Sylvester Comprehensive Cancer Center was the first facility in the state of Florida to be designated as a comprehensive center by the National Cancer Institute. The new Lois Pope LIFE Center houses research and clinical facilities for the Miami Project to cure spinal cord paralysis. The Bachelor Children's Research Institute opened in 2001 and houses many research initiatives in children's health.

CURRICULUM

The curriculum is a modern, integrated program that employs a variety of educational methodologies that require students to be active and responsible learners. It emphasizes faculty and student-led small group experiences wherein basic science concepts are introduced and assimilated in light of common disease states and clinical relevancy. It also includes material not traditionally emphasized: professionalism, humanism and ethics, population medicine, prevention and screening, quality and outcome assessment, medical informatics, geriatrics, alternative medicine, nutrition, medical economics, and end-of-life care. An over-arching theme throughout all four years is the acquisition and refinement of clinical skills through expert teaching and patient encounters. This starts in the first weeks of the first year when students begin the Clinical Skills program and start developing their clinical skills under the personal tutelage of a faculty physician, either in a private office setting, ambulatory clinic, or hospital ward.

Each medical student belongs to one of twelve Academic Societies which play unique roles in the curriculum by emphasizing cooperation in the learning process, fostering active learning styles, and providing a collegial environment in which faculty and more advanced students mentor and tutor newer students in the basic sciences, the art of medicine, medical decision-making, and the acquisition of diagnostic skills.

The School of Medicine has two B.S.-M.D. programs. Information about these special programs may be obtained from the Office of Undergraduate Admissions at (305) 284-4323. The school sponsors an M.D.-Ph.D. program, which is not limited to residents of Florida.

REQUIREMENTS FOR ENTRANCE

The School of Medicine only accepts U.S. citizens and permanent residents of the United States who have completed a minimum of 90 semester hours of college work. Credits earned at foreign institutions are not accepted. Courses specifically required are:

	Sem. hrs.
English	6
Chemistry (with lab)	8
Organic Chemistry (with lab)	8
Physics (with lab)	8
General Biology or Zoology	6
Other science courses*	6

*A course in biochemistry is strongly recommended and can be substituted for one semester of organic chemistry.

AP credit may be used as part of the 90-semester-hour total, but the credits listed above should be graded credits. CLEP credits are not accepted.

All applicants must take the MCAT exam no later than the fall preceding the year in which they hope to enroll in the School of Medicine.

SELECTION FACTORS

The University of Miami School of Medicine participates in AMCAS and accepts applications **only** from US citizens and permanent residents of the United States. Although Florida residents are given preference in all admissions decisions, the School of Medicine has made a commitment to enroll up to 35 exceptionally qualified non-Floridians in each first year class. To receive a secondary application, Florida residents must have a 3.2 or higher undergraduate cumulative GPA, or a post-bacc or graduate GPA of at least 3.5 (minimum of 15 credits). Non-Floridians must have a cumulative undergraduate GPA of at least 3.6 to receive a secondary application. Factors used by the Committee to rate all completed paper applications include: quality of undergraduate education and preparedness to study medicine, MCAT scores, diversity of life experiences, meaningfulness of direct patient contact experiences, writing ability, and quality of letters of recommendation. Applicants with the highest ratings are invited for an interview which is an integral part of the selection process. Interviews are arranged only at the initiative of the Office of Admissions and are held on the medical campus. Some of the factors evaluated at the time of interview are: maturity, knowledge about the profession of medicine, interpersonal skill level, depth and source of motivation to study medicine, and desire to serve others. Applicants' files are reviewed without regard to race, creed, sex, national origin, age, or handicap.

The 2003 entering class (141 new entrants) had the following profile: *mean cumulative* GPA, 3.66; *mean science* GPA, 3.64; *mean MCAT scores*: VR 9.5, PS 9.3, BS, 10.3, writing sample, P; *46% women, 6% underrepresented minorities*, 70 percent *biology or chemistry majors*; 49 undergraduate colleges represented.

FINANCIAL AID

Eighty percent of all medical students receive some type of financial aid. In 2003-2004 the amount awarded totaled about $20 million. The school participates in all major federal and state programs. Several scholarships are awarded each year for academic promise and for proven financial need. Information concerning financial assistance and student budgets may be obtained by calling the Office of Student Financial Assistance at (305) 243-6211.

INFORMATION ABOUT DIVERSITY PROGRAMS

The Health Careers Motivation Program is a special seven-week summer program that provides pre-medical undergraduates with the opportunity to gain first-hand knowledge of the requirements of a medical education. The program gives participants a "mini" medical school experience and consists of courses in human anatomy, biochemistry, and microbiology, along with a specialized course in reading and study skills, and an MCAT prep course. Books, supplies, meals, and housing are provided by the program and all accepted students receive a stipend. Applications and information may be obtained by calling (305) 243-5998.

Institution Type: *Private*
Application Process: *AMCAS, see chapter 4.*

APPLICATION AND ACCEPTANCE POLICIES FOR 2005–2006 FIRST-YEAR CLASS

Filing of AMCAS application
  Earliest date: June 1, 2004
  Latest date: Dec. 15, 2004
School application fee after screening: $65
Oldest MCAT scores considered: 2002
Does not have Early Decision Program (EDP)
Acceptance notice to regular applicants
  Earliest date: Oct. 15, 2004
  Latest date: Until class is filled
Applicant's response to acceptance offer
  Maximum time: 3 weeks
Requests for deferred entrance considered: No
Deposit to hold place in class (applied to tuition):
  $100, due by May 15, 2005
Deposit refundable prior to: May 16, 2005
Estimated number of new entrants: 150
Starting date: Aug. 2005

TUITION AND STUDENT FEES PER YEAR FOR 2003–2004 FIRST-YEAR CLASS

Tuition   Student fees: $140
  Resident: $28,050
  Nonresident: $36,740

INFORMATION ON 2002-2003 FIRST-YEAR CLASS

Number of	In-State	Out-of-State	Total
Applicants	1,183	1,440	2,623
Applicants Interviewed	225	100	325
New Entrants*	106	35	141

*All took the MCAT; 81% had baccalaureate degrees.

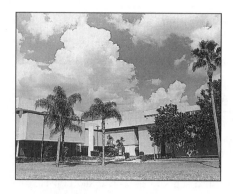

University of South Florida College of Medicine

Tampa, Florida

Dr. Robert S. Belsole, Interim *Dean*
Dr. Steven Specter, *Associate Dean for Admissions and Student Affairs*
Robert E. Larkin, *Director of Admissions and Records*
Dr. Marvin T. Williams, *Associate Dean for Diversity Initiatives*

ADDRESS INQUIRIES TO:

Office of Admissions
Box 3
University of South Florida
College of Medicine
12901 Bruce B. Downs Boulevard
Tampa, Florida 33612-4799
(813) 974-2229; 974-4990 (FAX)
Web site: www.med.usf.edu/medicine

GENERAL INFORMATION

The College of Medicine, one of the three Colleges of the University of South Florida (USF) Health Sciences Center, admitted the first class of medical students in 1971. At present, the freshman class consists of 115 new students each year. In addition to the three colleges, the Health Sciences Center includes a medical science area, auditorium, cafeteria, medical library, and medical clinics. Clinical instruction for College of Medicine students is in large part based in Tampa at the USF Medical Clinics, Tampa General Hospital, James A. Haley Veterans Hospital, Tampa Unit Shriners Hospital for Crippled Children, H. Lee Moffitt Cancer Center and Research Institute, University Psychiatry Center, University Diagnostic Institute, Genesis Clinic, USF Eye Institute, USF Dialysis Center, and the 17 Davis Pediatric Ambulatory Care Centers. Clinical instruction is also provided at All Children's Hospital, Bayfront Medical Center, Bay Pines Veterans Hospital in St. Petersburg, and the Orlando Regional Medical Center.

CURRICULUM

The four-year curriculum is designed to permit the student to learn the fundamental principles of medicine, to acquire skills of critical judgment based on evidence and experience, and to develop an ability to use principles and skills wisely in solving problems of health and disease. It includes the sciences basic to medicine, the major clinical disciplines, and other significant elements such as behavioral science, medical ethics, and human values.

The intent is to foster in students the ability to learn through self-directed, independent study throughout their professional lives. Using both ambulatory and hospital settings, students are given increasing responsibility for patient care in preparation to enter graduate medical education residencies.

Some students begin medical school with future plans such as primary care practice, clinical research, or preventive medicine and public health. For these students, special opportunities are available in medical school. For students seriously considering primary care, there are special opportunities to test and to reinforce this interest through a variety of existing and newly developed programs. Special programs are available for a select few students interested in an intense research career or to acquire both the M.D. and Ph.D. degrees in less time than would ordinarily be required for each separately. Likewise, it is possible for a student interested in public health, preventive medicine, epidemiology, health care systems, and related areas to achieve both an M.D. and master's in public health (M.P.H.) degree with minimal additional time. The M.P.H. degree is awarded through the College of Public Health.

PREMEDICAL HONORS PROGRAM

This is an integrated program in which the USF College of Medicine has an agreement with the USF Honors College and the University of Central Florida (UCF) Burnett Honors College. Superior students who satisfy requirements for the honors college and the college of medicine will be admitted into the M.D. program. All questions concerning the premedical options in the university honors programs should contact the specific university honors program directly.

USF: by post: USF Honors College, Director of Honors/FAO 274, 4202 E. Fowler Ave., Tampa, FL, 33620; or via telephone at (813) 974-3087.

UCF: by post: UCF Burnett Honors College, Dr. Madi Dogariu/BHC 110A, PO Box 161800, Orlando, FL, 32816-1800; or by telephone at (407) 823-2076.

REQUIREMENTS FOR ENTRANCE

The MCAT is required. Students applying should plan to complete the requirements for a bachelor's degree at an accredited university or college by the time of matriculation. Required courses are as follows:

	Semesters
General Biology (with lab)	2
General Chemistry (with lab)	2
Organic Chemistry (with lab)	2
General Physics (with lab)	2
Mathematics	2
English	2

Applicants are strongly urged to take the MCAT in the spring of the year of application and to have their basic science requirements completed at the time of application. No applicant will be considered for admission until the application materials are complete and received in the Admissions Office. Applications from individuals who wait to take the MCAT in the spring of the year in which they anticipate matriculating will not be considered.

SELECTION FACTORS

The selection of students of medicine is based on character, integrity, motivation, academic achievement, emotional maturity, stability, and the applicant interview. In addition, course load and types of courses taken will be evaluated and will constitute a factor in the overall evaluation.

Although the selection process is essentially competitive, with evaluation of students by their college faculty being a significant factor, there are some general guidelines on suitability of an applicant to the college. Because the University of South Florida is a state institution, preference is given to Florida residents. In those instances where residency is in question, for tuition purposes, an applicant is requested to submit a Declaration of Domicile.

Applicants requesting an application should clearly indicate their state of residency. This program is state-supported and the vast majority of our matriculating class will be residents of the state of Florida. Beginning with the entering class of August 2004, a limited number of exceptionally qualified non-Florida residents may be considered for entry into our M.D. Program.

To be considered, Florida residents should have an overall GPA and science GPA of 3.0 or better on a 4.0 scale and a minimum MCAT total score of 24 or better.

The 2003 entering class profile was: science *GPA,* 3.6; overall *GPA* 3.7; *MCAT scores, VR*-9.5 PS-9.9, *BS*-10.1; *minorities 44* (38%) women 53 (46%), men 62 (54%).

The Admissions Office may at its discretion invite the applicant to come for a personal interview. An invitation for an interview means only that the initial evaluation is sufficiently high to warrant further consideration by the Medical Student Selection Committee. Eligibility for admission will be determined without regard to race, creed, sex, age, religion, national origin, or handicap.

Applicants are encouraged to apply early and complete their applications as soon as possible. We will begin to interview applicants as early as September. The committee may vote to admit highly qualified applicants in such a way that the class could be filled earlier than the final application deadline. Once the class is filled, interviewed applicants will be able to enter the class via a wait list process.

FINANCIAL AID

The financial status of applicants does not affect their acceptance. Limited funds are available for loans and scholarships.

First-year students are not permitted to engage in outside employment. There are employment opportunities in Tampa and the surrounding area for spouses.

Questions may be addressed to Michelle Williamson, director of financial aid, by telephoning (813) 974-2068.

INFORMATION ABOUT DIVERSITY PROGRAMS

Events, activities, programs, and facilities of the University of South Florida are available to all without regard to race, sex, religion, national origin, Vietnam or disabled veteran status, handicap, or age, as provided by law and in accordance with its respect for personal dignity. Qualified applicants from groups underrepresented in medicine who are Florida residents are strongly encouraged to apply; the telephone number is (813) 974-3609.

Institution Type: *Public*
Application Process: *AMCAS, see chapter 4.*

APPLICATION AND ACCEPTANCE POLICIES FOR 2005–2006 FIRST-YEAR CLASS

Filing of AMCAS application
  Earliest date: June 1, 2004
  Latest date: Dec. 1, 2004
School application fee to all applicants: $30
Oldest MCAT scores considered: 2002
Does have Early Decision Program (EDP)
  For Florida residents only
  EDP application period: June 1–Aug. 1, 2004
  EDP applicants notified by: Oct. 1, 2004
Acceptance notice to regular applicants
  Earliest date: Oct. 15, 2004
  Latest date: Until class is filled
Applicant's response to acceptance offer
  Maximum time: 2 weeks
Requests for deferred entrance considered: Yes
Deposit to hold place in class: None
Estimated number of new entrants: 115 (20 EDP)
Starting date: Aug. 2005

TUITION AND STUDENT FEES PER YEAR FOR 2003–2004 FIRST-YEAR CLASS

Tuition	Student fees
Resident: $13,925	Resident: $1,780
Nonresident: $41,782	Nonresident: $3,173

INFORMATION ON 2003–2004 FIRST-YEAR CLASS

Number of	In-State	Out-of-State	Total
Applicants	1,239	346	1,585
Applicants Interviewed	360	0	360
New Entrants*	115	0	115

*All took the MCAT and had baccalaureate degrees.

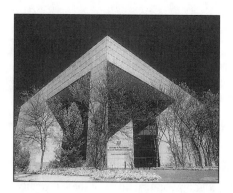

Emory University School of Medicine

Atlanta, Georgia

Dr. Thomas J. Lawley, *Dean*

Dr. J. William Eley, *Associate Dean for Medical Education, Student Affairs and Director of Admissions*

Dr. Jonas A. Shulman, *Executive Associate Dean for Medical Education/Student Affairs*

Dr. Robert Lee, *Assoc. Dean and Director, Office of Multicultural Affairs*

ADDRESS INQUIRIES TO:

Emory University School of Medicine
Office of Admissions
Woodruff Health Sciences Center Administration Building
1440 Clifton Rd., NE Suite 115
Atlanta, Georgia 30322-4510
(404) 727-5660; 727-5456 (FAX)
E-mail: medadmiss@emory.edu
Web site: www.med.emory.edu

MISSION STATEMENT

Emory University School of Medicine is committed to providing leadership in medicine and science through the development of recognized programs of excellence and innovation in medical education, biomedical research, and patient care.

GENERAL INFORMATION

The Emory University School of Medicine, a private school, was founded in 1915, resulting from several reorganizations dating from 1854 when the Atlanta Medical College was founded. Students spend the first two years primarily on the university campus. The last two years are spent in the school's teaching hospitals, in which there are more than 3,000 beds and large outpatient clinics.

Emory University is accredited by the Commission on Colleges of the Southern Association of Colleges and Schools.

CURRICULUM

The curriculum is intended to lay a comprehensive foundation for a career in practice, teaching, research, or other medical areas. The first two years consist primarily of basic health sciences and incorporate multimedia teaching aids. Recent curricular changes include a reduction in lecture hours, a parallel increase in small-group/problem-based learning, and introduction to patients in the first year of medical school. Courses are often interdisciplinary (for example, neurobiology, molecular and human genetics, medical problem solving, patient-doctor, and human values in medicine). In the second year, students complete their basic science background and spend a major portion of their time in integrated courses in pathology, pathophysiology, and clinical methods, which extend broadly into the various clinical fields. The third and fourth years are devoted exclusively to instruction in all major clinical subjects, including primary care. The 19-month period of actual coursework includes time for elective clerkships that encompass a large variety of studies at both local and distant sites.

A combined M.D.-Ph.D. degree program is available for highly qualified students interested in careers in academic medicine. This six- to eight-year program provides the in-depth clinical experience and biomedical research training necessary for future medical scientists. A five-year dual-degree M.D.-M.P.H. program is also available to prepare medical students for leadership roles in public health.

REQUIREMENTS FOR ENTRANCE

The MCAT and a minimum of three years of college are required. Ninety semester or 135 quarter hours in arts and sciences at an institution accredited by its regional association must be completed to be eligible for enrollment.

The premedical program should be aimed toward a balanced liberal education and should ensure thorough grounding in the stated requirements. Majors in the sciences or non-sciences are equally acceptable. The latter must show competence in the natural sciences and mathematics. Majors in the natural sciences or mathematics should always include subjects of broad educational value in their premedical curricula.

Specific minimum requirements are:

	Sem. hrs
Biology (with lab)	8
Inorganic Chemistry (with lab)	8
Organic Chemistry (with lab)	8
Physics (with lab)	8
English	6
Humanities, social and/or behavioral sciences	18

Biochemistry is highly recommended.

Undergraduate degree credit that has been granted to the student on the basis of CLEP will be accepted provided (1) the credit appears on the official transcript and (2) CLEP credits are not the sole fulfillment of any specific course requirement listed above. CLEP credit in excess of 25 percent of a student's total undergraduate credit will not be accepted.

SELECTION FACTORS

Students are selected on the basis of scholastic achievement, fitness and aptitude for the study of medicine, and personal qualifications, without regard to race, sex, sexual orientation, age, disability, creed, veteran status, or national origin. All applicants must (a) present a very high level of scholarship; (b) take the MCAT within four years of the matriculating year (e.g. 2001 for 2005 enrollment); (c) apply through AMCAS and submit the required Emory supplemental application form and fee (this form is available on-line upon Emory's receipt of the AMCAS application); (d) have the required evaluation(s) submitted; and (e) appear for a personal interview before the Admission Committee, if invited. Applications are screened for possible interview only after all required items have been received. Interview is by invitation and is conducted only at Emory University. Students from foreign schools must have completed at least one year of academic work in an accredited U.S. or Canadian institution. It is anticipated anyone enrolled in a graduate degree program will have completed all required work for the degree by the date of matriculation. Only students enrolled in U.S. LCME-accredited medical schools are eligible to apply for transfer to Emory's third-year class. Advanced standing is not given for work completed in other professional or graduate schools.

The 2003 class had the following credentials at the time of application: *mean GPA*, 3.75; *mean MCAT scores, VR*-10.7, *PS*-11.1, *BS*-11.1; *undergraduate major*, 37% biological sciences, 21% physical sciences, 27% non-sciences, 3% other health professions (nursing, pharmacy, etc.), 12% all others, including double majors and mixed disciplines. Of the entering class of 113, 52% were women.

FINANCIAL AID

A limited number of scholarships and loans are available through the Financial Aid Office of Emory University. Approximately 83 percent of all the enrolled medical students receive scholarships and loans through Emory University. Most scholarships and loans are awarded on the basis of documented financial need. Application information may be requested prior to acceptance from the university Financial Aid Office. Approximately two percent of the students receive U.S. Armed Forces scholarships. A limited number of highly qualified students in the first-year class are awarded merit scholarships. Foreign citizens who are not permanent residents of the United States must provide and document their own funding for tuition, fees, and living expenses. Although foreign citizens are not eligible for any federally based aid, they may be considered for merit scholarships and loans from sources outside of Emory. The university's Financial Aid Office may be reached at 1-800-727-6039.

Seven Robert Woodruff Fellowships, not based on need, are awarded yearly to entering students. Additional information on this competitive, merit-based program is available from the Medical School Admissions Office.

INFORMATION ABOUT DIVERSITY PROGRAMS

Emory University School of Medicine is strongly committed to increasing opportunities for students from groups underrepresented in medicine. The Office of Multicultural Affairs works in conjunction with the Admission Committee and the Office of Student Affairs in the recruitment, selection, and retention of qualified students from groups underrepresented in medicine. Further inquiries may be addressed to Dr. Robert Lee, director of multicultural affairs.

Institution Type: *Private*
Application Process: *AMCAS, see chapter 4.*

APPLICATION AND ACCEPTANCE POLICIES FOR 2005–2006 FIRST-YEAR CLASS

Filing of AMCAS application
    Earliest date: June 1, 2004
    Latest date: Oct. 15, 2004
School application fee to all applicants: $80
Oldest MCAT scores considered: 2001
Does not have Early Decision Program
Acceptance notice to regular applicants
    Earliest date: Oct. 25, 2004
    Latest date: Until class is filled
Applicant's response to acceptance offer
    Maximum time: 2 weeks
Requests for deferred entrance considered: Yes
Deposit to hold place in class: None
Estimated number of new entrants: 112
Starting date: July 2005

TUITION AND STUDENT FEES PER YEAR FOR 2003–2004 FIRST-YEAR CLASS

Tuition: $32,576   Student fees: $492

INFORMATION ON 2003–2004 FIRST-YEAR CLASS

Number of	In-State	Out-of-State	Total
Applicants	499	4,665	5,164
Applicants Interviewed	125	607	734
New Entrants*	36	77	113

*All took the MCAT and had baccalaureate degrees.

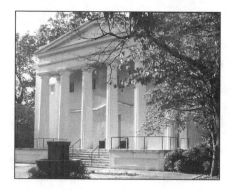

Medical College of Georgia
School of Medicine

Augusta, Georgia

Dr. David M. Stern, *Dean*
Dr. Mason P. Thompson, *Associate Dean for Admissions*
Cynthia A. Parks, *Interim Director of Student Financial Aid*
Dr. Rosie Allen-Noble, *Associate Dean for Special Academic Programs*

ADDRESS INQUIRIES TO:

Dr. Mason P. Thompson
Associate Dean for Admissions
School of Medicine
Medical College of Georgia
Augusta, Georgia 30912-4760
(706) 721-3186; 721-0959 (FAX)
E-mail: stdadmin@mail.mcg.edu
Web site: www.mcg.edu

MISSION STATEMENT

The Medical College of Georgia is a unit of the University System of Georgia and as such is committed to the following:

• a supportive campus climate, necessary services, and leadership and development opportunities, all to educate the whole person and meet the needs of students, faculty, and staff

• cultural, ethnic, racial, and gender diversity in the faculty, staff, and student body, supported by practices and programs that embody the ideals of an open democratic and global society

• technology to advance educational purposes, including instructional technology, student support services, and distance learning

• collaborative relationships with other System institutions, state agencies, local schools and technical institutes, and business and industry, sharing physical, human, information, and other resources to expand and enhance programs and services available to the citizens of Georgia

GENERAL INFORMATION

The School of Medicine of the Medical College of Georgia was founded in 1828 and is the nation's 11th oldest medical school. The institution is a separate university under the Georgia Higher Education System and consists of five schools: medicine, allied health, dentistry, graduate studies, and nursing.

The Medical College of Georgia Hospital and Clinics is the primary clinical teaching facility. Other hospitals in Augusta and in cities throughout the state have affiliate agreements with the Medical College of Georgia to provide clinical teaching facilities.

CURRICULUM

During the first year (Phase I), students study the structure and functions of the human body through courses in anatomy, histology and development, biochemistry and genetics, neuroscience, physiology, and psychiatry. A new course named Essentials of Clinical Medicine containing topic areas of ethics, community medicine, health promotion, behavioral science/psychiatry, and the patient-doctor clinical experience introduce students to ethical and interpersonal aspects of the practice of medicine. Contact with patients begins with physical diagnosis I and patient-doctor courses during the first year.

The second year (Phase II) emphasizes the pathophysiologic basis of clinical medicine with courses in pathology, pharmacology, clinical microbiology, reproductive endocrinology, and introduction to clinical medicine. The second year course in Essentials of Clinical Medicine brings together ethics, disease prevention, problem-based learning, and a continuation of physical diagnosis. A student-led, faculty-facilitated, problem-based learning course emphasizes skills of case-based and self-directed learning, development of information retrieval and analysis skills, group dynamics, and evaluation.

Interdepartmental cooperation and clinical relevance are stressed throughout the first two years. During part of the first year, two afternoons a week are available for electives.

During Phase III, students are required to take 19 months of academic work, which must include 12 months of basic clerkships in the departments of medicine, surgery, obstetrics and gynecology, family medicine, pediatrics, psychiatry and neuroscience. The remaining 7 months consist of an acting internship, emergency medicine, critical care medicine, and electives. Students are required to pass Step 1 of the USMLE at the end of their second year and Step 2 of the USMLE prior to graduation.

REQUIREMENTS FOR ENTRANCE

The MCAT and three years of undergraduate college work leading to a baccalaureate degree in an institution accredited by its regional association are required. However, preference is given to students who will have completed the baccalaureate degree prior to enrollment at the School of Medicine.

College work must include:

	Years
Biology or Zoology (with lab)	1
Inorganic Chemistry (with lab)	1
Advanced Chemistry (with lab)	1
Must include one semester or two quarters of Organic Chemistry.	
Physics (with lab)	1
English (sufficient to satisfy baccalaureate degree requirements.)	
Biochemistry is highly recommended.	

These required courses must be taken on a letter or number grading system (not pass/fail) if at all possible.

SELECTION FACTORS

Applicants for admission to the School of Medicine are evaluated on a competitive basis utilizing our admission guidelines. Information used for assessing an individual's academic accomplishments, personal attributes, and interests includes, but is not limited to, the applicant's responsibilities prior to application to medical school; involvement in extracurricular and community activities; ethnic, socioeconomic, and cultural background; region of residence with respect to its health professional needs; commitment to practice in an underserved area of Georgia; letters of recommendation by the premedical advisor and two personal references; motivation and potential for serving as a physician; personal interviews; performance on the Medical College Admission Test; and college grades including undergraduate, graduate, and postbaccalaureate. In addition, the medical school faculty has specified nonacademic (technical) standards, which all students must meet in order to participate effectively in the medical education program and in the practice of medicine.

Preference is given to residents of Georgia. A maximum of five percent of the entering class may be nonresidents of Georgia.

Application through the Early Decision Program is encouraged for Georgia residents interested in attending the Medical College of Georgia. Early Decision applicants must take the MCAT prior to making application. All other applicants must take the MCAT no later than the fall of the year application is made.

Interviews are by invitation and are with members of the Admissions Committee, faculty, students, and/or individuals from the community. About 420 applicants are interviewed each year. Regional interviews are not available.

Applicants must have received at least the last two years of their education at an accredited U.S. or Canadian college or university in order to be considered. Transfer admission with advanced standing is on a space-available basis, and only students who are currently in good academic standing in an LCME-accredited medical school may be considered for transfer admission. Anyone enrolled in a graduate-degree program is expected to complete all requirements for that degree prior to the date of matriculation.

The Medical College of Georgia does not discriminate on the basis of age, race, sex, creed, or national origin in its admissions process.

FINANCIAL AID

The Office of Financial Aid coordinates the programs of assistance that are available to medical students.

An applicant's financial status does not affect acceptance for admission. Information and applications may be obtained at www.mcg.edu/students/finaid.

INFORMATION ABOUT DIVERSITY PROGRAMS

The School of Medicine at the Medical College of Georgia seeks to encourage qualified students from groups underrepresented in medicine to apply to our school. A summer program is designed for undergraduate, disadvantaged college students who show academic promise and who desire to practice medicine. Students may apply for this program by writing to Dr. R. Allen-

Noble, Associate Dean for Special Academic Programs. For further information, please contact Special Academic Programs, School of Medicine (AA-153), Medical College of Georgia, Augusta, GA 30912-1900; (706) 721-2522.

GENERALIST PHYSICIAN INITIATIVE

The Medical College of Georgia in an effort to graduate more physicians who choose to practice family medicine, general internal medicine, or general pediatrics has participated in the generalist physician initiative program funded in part by the Robert Wood Johnson Foundation. The initiative involves all aspects of medical education, from pre-entry through undergraduate and residency education, to practice entry and support of generalist physicians. It is anticipated that ultimately 50 percent of MCG graduates will select generalist residency and generalist practice.

Institution Type: *Public*
Application Process: *AMCAS, see chapter 4.*

APPLICATION AND ACCEPTANCE POLICIES FOR 2005–2006 FIRST-YEAR CLASS

Filing of AMCAS application
   Earliest date: June 1, 2004
   Latest date: Nov. 1, 2004
School application fee after screening: none
Oldest MCAT scores considered: 2002
Does have Early Decision Program (EDP)
   For Georgia residents only
   EDP application period: June 1–Aug. 1, 2004
   EDP applicants notified by: Oct. 1, 2004
Acceptance notice to regular applicants
   Earliest date: Oct. 15, 2004
   Latest date: Until class is filled
Applicant's response to acceptance offer
   Maximum time: 2 weeks
Requests for deferred entrance considered: Yes
Deposit to hold place in class (applied to tuition):
   $100, due with response to acceptance offer
Deposit refundable prior to: May 16, 2005
Estimated number of new entrants: 180 (55 EDP)
Starting date: Aug. 2005

TUITION AND STUDENT FEES PER YEAR FOR 2003–2004 FIRST-YEAR CLASS

Tuition   Student fees: $783
   Resident: $9,772
   Nonresident: $29,976

INFORMATION ON 2003–2004 FIRST-YEAR CLASS

Number of	In-State	Out-of-State	Total
Applicants	825	623	1,448
Applicants Interviewed	453	20	473
New Entrants*	177	3	180

*All took the MCAT; 100% had baccalaureate degrees.

CHAPTER

11

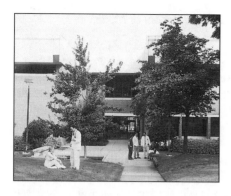

Mercer University School of Medicine

Macon, Georgia

Dr. Ann C. Jobe, *Dean*
Dr. A. Peter Eveland, *Associate Dean for Admissions and Student Affairs; Minority Affairs*
Youvette D. Hudson, *Director for Financial Aid; Registrar*

ADDRESS INQUIRIES TO:

Office of Admissions and Student Affairs
Mercer University School of Medicine
1550 College Street
Macon, Georgia 31207
(478) 301-2524; 301-2547 (FAX)
E-mail: faust_ek@mercer.edu
Web site: http://medicine.mercer.edu

MISSION STATEMENT

Mercer University School of Medicine (MUSM) admitted its charter class in August 1982. The school's mission is to educate physicians to meet the health care needs of rural and other underserved areas of Georgia. The program's educational format is that of problem-based, student-centered learning.

GENERAL INFORMATION

The medical education building located on the campus of Mercer University serves as the primary center for learning during the first two years. Mercer Health Systems, a 40-room ambulatory care facility, the Medical Center of Central Georgia, in Macon, and the Memorial Health University Medical Center, in Savannah, serve as the primary affiliate clerkship sites. Clinical teaching is also provided at the Floyd Medical Center in Rome, Phoebe Putney Memorial Hospital in Albany, the Medical Center in Columbus, and several rural hospitals throughout Georgia.

CURRICULUM

While the major emphasis during the first two years is placed on the acquisition and practical application of basic science knowledge, there are also programs in bioethics and those that are designed to prepare the students for contact with patients in various inpatient, outpatient, community, and rural settings.

The Biomedical Problems Program is the educational vehicle for motivating students to obtain and apply the basic scientific knowledge germane to the practice of medicine. The onus of gathering this knowledge is on the individual student through a program of self-directed learning. The application occurs in small-group tutorials in which theme-based cases are discussed.

In the Clinical Skills Program students learn the basic skills necessary for interaction with patients. These skills include interview/medical history and physical examination techniques. Students interview and examine actual and "standardized" patients. The latter group is composed of persons who have been trained to portray specific medical problems and behavioral roles, and to give constructive feedback to students.

The Community Office Practice Program (COPP) provides students with the opportunity to learn and experience current administrative practices while observing and participating in the clinical aspects of a community-oriented, primary care medical practice. In the Community Science Program students become familiar with the nature of a primary care practice in rural Georgia, while being educated on the health needs of individuals, families, and communities. It extends throughout the four years and culminates in a 4-week senior rural clerkship.

The third year consists of required clinical rotations in internal medicine, surgery, pediatrics, obstetrics-gynecology, ambulatory family medicine, and psychiatry. In addition, there are weekly programs in radiology. The fourth year is devoted to advanced clinical work, which includes 20 weeks of electives and required clerkships in acute or critical care, surgery subspecialties, rural and community medicine, and substance abuse.

REQUIREMENTS FOR ENTRANCE

The MCAT and the equivalent of three academic years or a minimum of 90 semester hours in an approved college or university are required for admission. Students are advised to balance their work in the biological sciences with courses in the social sciences and humanities. In addition, they are urged to follow their own inclinations in choosing a subject to pursue as a major. Required courses are:

	Years
General Biology (with lab)	1
General or Inorganic Chemistry (with lab)	1
Organic Chemistry or Organic/Biochemistry sequence (with lab)*	1
General Physics (with lab)	1

*Must include one semester or two quarters of organic chemistry. Biochemistry is highly recommended.

SELECTION FACTORS

The Admissions Committee has accepted only applicants who are legal residents of Georgia. Each applicant must also show promise of learning effectively in Mercer's curriculum and show strong potential of practicing a medical specialty commensurate with the health care needs of rural and other underserved areas of Georgia.

In addition to the AMCAS application, a supplementary application is required of applicants who meet preliminary selection criteria. This application has a $50 fee and requests the following: two letters of recommendation or one premedical committee evaluation, a personal history (a chronological list of residences and activities since the beginning of high school), certification of Georgia residency, practice vision statement, and a list of the required premedical courses.

Interviews are by invitation only and are held at the medical school. In making the final decisions for acceptance or rejection, the Admissions Committee considers all criteria but emphasizes strongly an applicant's potential for complying with the mission of the institution. The committee does not discriminate on the basis of race, sex, creed, national origin, age, or handicap.

The 60 students that matriculated in 2003 consisted of 32 men and 28 women, and 2 students from groups underrepresented in medicine; and the average age was 25.

FINANCIAL AID

Financial aid in the form of loans and scholarships is available. Awards are made on the basis of need and merit, with 93 percent of the students receiving aid. Although acceptance to MUSM is not based on an applicant's ability to pay, the responsibility for adequate funding rests with the student. The financial aid officer conducts financial management conferences and assists students in obtaining needed support.

INFORMATION ABOUT DIVERSITY PROGRAMS

The school is committed to the recruitment of qualified individuals from groups underrepresented in medicine and disadvantaged backgrounds.

Institution Type: *Private*
Application Process: *AMCAS, see chapter 4.*

APPLICATION AND ACCEPTANCE POLICIES FOR 2005–2006 FIRST-YEAR CLASS

Filing of AMCAS application
  Earliest date: June 1, 2004
  Latest date: Nov. 1, 2004
School application fee after screening: $50
Oldest MCAT scores considered: 2002
Does have Early Decision Program (EDP)
  For Georgia residents only
  EDP application period: June 1–Aug. 1, 2004
  EDP applicants notified by: Oct. 1, 2004
Acceptance notice to regular applicants
  Earliest date: Oct. 15, 2004
  Latest date: Until class is filled
Applicant's response to acceptance offer
  Maximum time: 2 weeks
Requests for deferred entrance considered: Yes
Deposit to hold place in class (applied to tuition):
  $100, due with response to acceptance offer
Deposit refundable prior to: May 16, 2005
Estimated number of new entrants: 60 (15 EDP)
Starting date: Aug. 2005

TUITION AND STUDENT FEES PER YEAR FOR 2003–2004 FIRST-YEAR CLASS

Tuition and student fees: $26,372

INFORMATION ON 2003–2004 FIRST-YEAR CLASS

Number of	In-State	Out-of-State	Total
Applicants	547	180	738
Applicants Interviewed	228	0	228
New Entrants*	60	0	60

*All took the MCAT and had baccalaureate degrees.

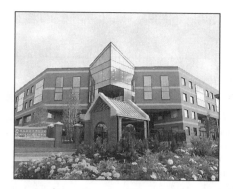

Morehouse School of Medicine

Atlanta, Georgia

Dr. Angela Walker Franklin, *Associate Dean for Student Affairs*
Marvell Nesmith, *Director of Admissions*
Cynthia Handy, *Director of Student Fiscal Affairs*

ADDRESS INQUIRIES TO:

Admissions and Student Affairs
Morehouse School of Medicine
720 Westview Drive, S.W.
Atlanta, Georgia 30310-1495
(404) 752-1650; 752-1512 (FAX)
Web site: www.msm.edu

MISSION STATEMENT

Morehouse School of Medicine's main mission is to recruit and train minority and other students as physicians, biomedical scientists, and public health practitioners committed to meeting the primary health care needs of the underserved.

GENERAL INFORMATION

Morehouse School of Medicine is one of three medical schools in the nation founded by historically black institutions and was the first such medical school begun in the 20th century. The School of Medicine admitted its first students to a two-year basic medical science curriculum in September 1978. The inaugural M.D. degree class graduated in May 1985.

Basic science teaching facilities are located in the lecture halls and multidisciplinary laboratories of the Hugh Gloster Sciences Building, which also houses research laboratories, preclinical departments, and administrative offices. The Hugh Gloster building, dedicated in May 1987, also houses clinical departments, study areas, and the library. In May 1996, the new Multidisciplinary Research Center was dedicated.

Facilities expansion continued through 2000 and 2001 with the opening of the new parking deck and research wing of the medical education building. In 2002 the new National Center for Primary Care opened. This facility features a 570 seat auditorium, cafeteria services, as well as additional office and teaching space.

Clinical instruction takes place in affiliated hospitals and clinics, including Grady Memorial Hospital and Southwest Community Hospital. The school also administers the Area Health Education Center Program.

CURRICULUM

An educational experience focusing both on scientific medicine and on meeting more effectively the primary health care needs of underserved inner-city and rural patients is offered. The concept of the patient as a whole person is fostered through a variety of teaching experiences that relate social, environmental, emotional, and cultural factors to medical disorders.

The first two years of the curriculum emphasize an understanding of the principles, concepts, and major factual background of the basic medical sciences. Exposure to clinical medicine begins in the first year through assignment to a preceptor and increases in the second year with introduction to clinical medicine. Clinical education is continued through core clerkships during the third and fourth years with 20 weeks of electives in the senior year. The major strengths of the curriculum include small class size, a highly diversified faculty, and courses that are taught by departmental and/or interdisciplinary faculty.

All students are required to pass Step 1 and Step 2 of the USMLE for promotion and graduation, respectively. Student performance is evaluated primarily by letter grades. Promotion into the next year's class is recommended by the Student Academic Progress and Promotions Committee.

First-year classes begin in early July with a required summer program. Learning resources and other support services are available to all students throughout their four years. Morehouse School of Medicine also offers the Ph.D. in Biomedical Sciences and Master of Public Health degrees.

REQUIREMENTS FOR ENTRANCE

The MCAT and completion of a baccalaureate degree are required. It is highly recommended that the MCAT be taken in the spring of the year in which the application is made.

The faculty has no preference as to the major field of undergraduate study; students should determine their fields of major study according to their personal interest. Applicants are expected to present a sound, well-balanced academic background with evidence of competency in the stated requirements. Specific minimum requirements are:

	Year
Biology (with lab)	1
Inorganic or General Chemistry (with lab)	1
Organic Chemistry (with lab)	1
Physics (with lab)	1
College Mathematics	1
English (including composition)	1

Coursework in behavioral sciences is strongly recommended.

SELECTION FACTORS

Selection of students for admission is made by the Committee on Admissions after careful consideration of many factors. These include MCAT scores, the undergraduate academic record, the extent of academic improvement, balance and depth of academic program, difficulty of courses taken, and other indicators of maturation of learning ability. Additional factors considered by the committee include the nature of extracurricular activities, hobbies, the need to work, research projects and experiences, evidence of activities that indicate concurrence with the school's mission, and evidence of pursuing interests and talents in depth. Finally, the committee looks for evidence of those traits of personality and character essential to success in medicine: compassion, integrity, motivation, and perseverance.

All information available about each applicant is considered without assigning priority to any single factor. Students are admitted on the basis of individual qualifications regardless of sex, age, race, creed, national origin, or handicap. Preferential consideration is given to qualified applicants who are residents of the state of Georgia. However, all well-qualified applicants are encouraged to apply. Foreign applicants must have a permanent resident visa.

After receipt and preliminary screening of the AMCAS application, qualified applicants will be invited via email to submit the online supplementary application and letters of evaluation. After review of all submitted materials, applicants who are competitive in this stage of the admissions process are invited to Atlanta for a personal interview. Interviews are arranged only by invitation of the Committee on Admissions.

Medical education requires that the accumulation of scientific knowledge be accompanied by the simultaneous acquisition of skills and professional attitudes and behavior. Technical standards have been established as a prerequisite for admission and graduation from the Morehouse School of Medicine. All courses in the curriculum are required in order to develop essential skills required to become a competent physician.

A candidate for the M.D. degree must have aptitude, abilities, and skills in five areas: observation, communication, motor, conceptual integrative and quantitative, and behavioral and social.

Morehouse School of Medicine's Technical Standards for Medical School Admission and Graduation are provided at interview.

Applicants are not considered for admission who have been dismissed from another medical school for academic or disciplinary reasons. Transfer applications are considered only from students in good standing at an LCME-accredited U.S. or Canadian medical school (foreign medical schools, osteopathic, veterinary, or dental schools are not acceptable). Transfers are allowed into the second year only on a space-available basis. Transfer application deadline is May 1.

FINANCIAL AID

A broad financial aid program is available. In addition to federally insured loan programs, a number of scholarships and loans are available. Scholarships and loans are awarded on the basis of documented financial need as determined by the College Scholarship Service needs analysis system (see Part 1). Applicants with an AMCAS fee waiver can waive the $50 school application fee. Accepted applicants are eligible to apply for financial aid to the Office of Student Fiscal Affairs. Approximately 94 percent of the students receive some form of financial aid during a part or all of their four years of study. Students are discouraged from accepting outside employment because of the lack of available time during a heavy academic schedule.

Institution Type: *Private*
Application Process: *AMCAS, see chapter 4.*

APPLICATION AND ACCEPTANCE POLICIES FOR 2005–2006 FIRST-YEAR CLASS

Filing of AMCAS application
    Earliest date: June 1, 2004
    Latest date: Dec. 1, 2004
School application fee to all applicants: $50
Oldest MCAT scores considered: 2002
Does have Early Decision Program (EDP)
    For URM residents of Georgia only
    EDP application period: June 1–Aug. 1, 2004
    EDP applicants notified by: Oct. 1, 2004
Acceptance notice to regular applicants
    Earliest date: November 2004
    Latest date: Until class is filled
Applicant's response to acceptance offer
    Maximum time: 14 days
Requests for deferred entrance considered: Yes
Deposit to hold place in class (applied to tuition):
    $100, due with response to acceptance offer
Deposit refundable prior to: May 16, 2005
Estimated number of new entrants: 52 (1 EDP)
Starting date: July 2005

TUITION AND STUDENT FEES PER YEAR FOR 2003–2004 FIRST-YEAR CLASS

Tuition: $20,966   Student fees: $4,405

INFORMATION ON 2003–2004 FIRST-YEAR CLASS

Number of	In-State	Out-of-State	Total
Applicants	311	1,736	2,047
Applicants Interviewed	85	162	247
New Entrants*	27	25	52

*All took the MCAT and had baccalaureate degrees.

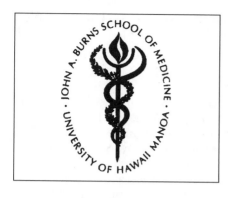

University of Hawai'i at Mānoa
John A. Burns School of Medicine

Honolulu, Hawaii

Dr. Edwin C. Cadman, *Dean*
Dr. Satoru Izutsu, *Senior Associate Dean/Chair, Admissions Committee*
Marilyn M. Nishiki, *Admissions Officer/Registrar*

ADDRESS INQUIRIES TO:

Office of Admissions
Marilyn Nishiki, Admissions Officer
University of Hawai'i at Mānoa
John A. Burns School of Medicine
1960 East-West Road
Honolulu, Hawaii 96822
(808) 956-8300; 956-9547 (FAX)
E-mail: mnishiki@hawaii.edu
Web site: http://hawaiimed.hawaii.edu

MISSION STATEMENT

The school's mission is to educate students to become outstanding physicians, scientists and other healthcare professionals and to conduct research and community service in areas of specific interest to our region and community.

GENERAL INFORMATION

The University of Hawai'i at Manoa John A. Burns School of Medicine is in the College of Health Sciences and Social Welfare, which also includes schools of public health, nursing, and social work. The School of Medicine is located on the Manoa campus of the university in Honolulu and has some elements at nearby Leahi Hospital. It also has teaching facilities in affiliated community hospitals and primary care clinics throughout the state.

CURRICULUM

The school utilizes a problem-based learning curriculum, in which basic sciences are learned in the context of the study of clinical problems. These activities are supplemented by selected lecture and laboratory sessions. Clinical skills and community health activities are prominent, and begin in the first year of the curriculum.

Special features of the program include an emphasis on problem-based learning as the primary instructional method in the pre-clinical years; early introduction of clinical training, community service and research experiences; rural health training opportunities; a longitudinal, interdisciplinary clerkship opportunity in the third-year; and opportunities for training experiences in various communities throughout Hawaii, the Pacific and Asia.

REQUIREMENTS FOR ENTRANCE

The MCAT (taken within three years of the expected date of matriculation and no later than August of the year of application) and at least 90 college credits are required. Course work must include:

	Sem. hrs.
Biology (with lab)	8
Chemistry (with lab)	4
Molecular and Cell Biology (with lab)	4
Biochemistry	3
Physics (with lab)	8

Applicants are strongly urged to complete their requirements at the time of application. All required coursework must be completed prior to matriculation. These courses should be rigorous and the type acceptable for students majoring in these areas and where indicated should include laboratory experience. Additional enrichment in the biological social sciences is encouraged (e.g., immunology, genetics, microbiology, human anatomy, physiology, embryology, psychology, and sociology). Applicants also must be fully competent in reading, speaking, and writing the English language.

SELECTION FACTORS

All applicants are considered without discrimination as to age, sex, race, creed, national origin, or handicap. The school admits 62 students to its regular freshman class. The University of Hawai'i at Manoa John A. Burns School of Medicine's first priority is to admit applicants with strong ties to the state of Hawaii. Applications go through two screens. The first admissions screen determines an applicant's ties to the State of Hawaii. This screen reviews an applicant's a) state or country of legal residence, b) birthplace, c) high school graduated, d) college attended, and e) parents' legal residence. An applicant who meets three of the five categories demonstrates ties to the state of Hawaii. The second admissions screen is the academic screen which a resident or nonresident candidate must pass in order to be invited for interviews. Selection depends upon the prospective medical student's character, scholarship, ideals, motivation, and aptitude. An evaluation of what the potential student might contribute to the health profession in the Pacific is an integral part of the selection process. For the limited number of applicants who reach a secondary screening level, interviews are conducted in Hawaii.

All interviewed applicants are reviewed and rated by the Admissions Committee. Acceptance, alternate, and rejection letters are mailed in May. Offers of acceptance are sent out to the top-ranked applicants to fill the entering first-year class. Nonresident candidates must be highly ranked, preferably with some ties to Hawaii or the American Pacific Basin, to be accepted. No additional supplemental materials are requested of applicants on the alternate list.

The 2003 regular entering class had the following profile: *median cumulative GPA,* 3.63; *median MCAT scores, VR*-9, *PS*-9, *BS*-10, *WS*-O.

Some candidates for the M.D. degree may also work toward master's or Ph.D. degrees within the university. Such joint programs require the explicit permission of the associate dean for student affairs, the university's Graduate Division, and the appropriate graduate faculty. Separate applications must be made to the Graduate Division and to the medical school. Applicants are accepted independently by the respective degree programs.

FINANCIAL AID

Financial status is not a factor in considering applicants for acceptance. Although financial aid is limited, efforts are made to assist medical students in obtaining loans and scholarships wherever possible. Loan funds from federal sources are only available to U.S. citizens. In general, students are discouraged from seeking outside employment. Approximately 80 percent of the student body currently receive financial assistance.

INFORMATION ABOUT DIVERSITY PROGRAMS

The student body and faculty are culturally diverse.

The John A. Burns School of Medicine is actively involved in the recruitment, admission, and retention of students from disadvantaged backgrounds, who are interested in pursuing an M.D. degree. The school provides a range of student services and faculty development programs through its Native Hawaiian Center of Excellence. In addition the school offers the Imi Hó ola Postbaccalaureate Program for students from disadvantaged backgrounds, but who are deemed capable of succeeding in medical school. The curriculum emphasizes the integration of concepts and principles in the sciences and humanities, and further develops communication and learning skills. Interested persons are encouraged to contact Dr. Nanette L.K. Judd, Project Director, Imi Hó ola Postbaccalaureate Program, 1960 East-West Road, Honolulu, Hawaii 96822; or call (808) 956-3466.

Institution Type: *Public*
Application Process: *AMCAS, see chapter 4.*

APPLICATION AND ACCEPTANCE POLICIES FOR 2005–2006 FIRST-YEAR CLASS

Filing of AMCAS application
   Earliest date: June 1, 2004
   Latest date: Dec. 1, 2004
School application fee after screening: $50
Oldest MCAT scores considered: 2002
Does have Early Decision Program (EDP)
   For residents of Hawaii only
   EDP application period: June 1–Aug. 1, 2004
   EDP applicants notified by: Oct. 1, 2004
Acceptance notice to regular applicants
   Earliest date: Oct. 15, 2004
   Latest date: Until class is filled
Applicant's response to acceptance offer
   Maximum time: 2 weeks
Requests for deferred entrance considered: Yes
Deposit to hold place in class: None
Estimated number of new entrants: 62 (1 EDP)
Starting date: July 2005

TUITION AND STUDENT FEES PER YEAR FOR 2003–2004 FIRST-YEAR CLASS

Tuition   Student fees: $142.40
   Resident: $14,808
   Nonresident: $28,512

INFORMATION ON 2003–2004 FIRST-YEAR CLASS

Number of	In-State	Out-of-State	Total
Applicants	205	1,079	1,284
Applicants Interviewed	156	100	256
New Entrants*	56	6	62

*All took the MCAT and 98% had baccalaureate degrees.

CHAPTER

11

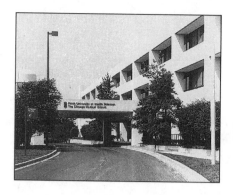

Rosalind Franklin University of Medicine and Science
Chicago Medical School

North Chicago, Illinois

Dr. K. Michael Welch, *Interim Dean*
Kristine A. Jones, *Director of Admissions and Registrar*
Maryann DeCaire, *Director of Financial Aid*
Dr. Timothy R. Hansen, *Associate Dean of Educational Affairs*
Dr. Monica Miles, *Director of Multicultural Affairs*

ADDRESS INQUIRIES TO:

Office of Admissions
Chicago Medical School
3333 Green Bay Road
North Chicago, Illinois 60064
(847) 578-3204/3205
E-mail: jonesk@finchcms.edu
Web site: www.finchcms.edu/

MISSION STATEMENT

The mission of the Chicago Medical School is to acquire, preserve, enhance, and communicate knowledge of the health sciences for the welfare of humanity and improvement of the environment. The school is dedicated to the education and training of professionals in the health sciences at all levels of training and experience. These goals are continually evaluated in terms of the school nurturing education, research, and health care delivery.

GENERAL INFORMATION

The Chicago Medical School, founded in 1912, is part of the Rosalind Franklin University of Medicine and Science, which is located in North Chicago, Illinois. It is a private, nonsectarian, coeducational institution chartered by the state of Illinois and administered by a Board of Trustees. The Chicago Medical School is the core component of four allied units. One unit is the School of Graduate and Postdoctoral Studies, which grants degrees at the master and doctoral levels in the major basic science areas, as well as the doctorate in clinical psychology. The College of Health Professions currently offers programs in physical therapy, medical technology, clinical laboratory sciences, nutrition, physician assistant practice and pathologist's assistant, leading to DPT, baccalaureate, and master's degrees. The fourth component is the Dr. William M. Scholl College of Podiatric Medicine. Upon successful completion of all requirements, students receive the Doctor of Podiatric Medicine degree. In addition, the university has a B.S.–M.D. honors program in engineering/medicine, in conjunction with the Illinois Institute of Technology. Clinical training at various levels is provided at Cook County Hospital, Edward Hines Veterans Affairs Medical Center, Christ Hospital, Mt. Sinai Hospital,

North Chicago Veterans Affairs Medical Center, Elgin Mental Health Center, Illinois Masonic Medical Center, Swedish Covenant Hospital, Norwalk (CT) Hospital, Lutheran General Hospital, Highland Park Hospital, and Great Lakes Naval Hospital.

CURRICULUM

To meet the changing needs of the future physician, the content of the curriculum is under continual evaluation and revision. The curriculum offers students a strong foundation in both the science and practice of medicine by providing an interface between basic science and clinical science.

Currently, the four-year curriculum consists of 13 terms. Of the 6 terms of basic science, the first 3 are devoted primarily to the study of the structure and function of the human body. Many courses, including medical ethics, genetics, and epidemiology, are offered in didactic and small-group sessions. The following 3 terms are devoted to the study of disease etiology, processes, therapy, and prevention. Concomitantly, there is extensive training in physical diagnosis, medical interviewing, and history-writing. Of the last 7 terms, 50 weeks are devoted to junior clinical rotations and 36 weeks are spent in senior clinical selectives, electives, and/or basic science courses. The required junior clinical clerkships include medicine, surgery, obstetrics-gynecology, psychiatry, family medicine, pediatrics, neurology, emergency medicine, and ambulatory care medicine. The senior requirements include a medical subinternship plus 32 weeks of approved electives (14 of which must be done on campus). The elective period gives students an opportunity, through both intramural and extramural experiences, to explore and strengthen their personal career interests.

Along with passing all courses and clerkships, students are required to pass Step 1 and Step 2 of the USMLE as a requisite for graduation.

All students are required to complete the first two years within three academic years; clinical clerkships and electives are to be completed within 2½ years. Thus, students must complete their education at the Chicago Medical School in no more than 5½ years, unless enrolled in a combined-degree program, or on an approved extended program, or on an approved leave of absence.

Combined M.D.-Ph.D. degree programs are available for students interested in biomedical or clinical research. These programs provide an opportunity for a limited number of students to pursue a program of individualized coursework and research leading to the M.D. and Ph.D. degrees. Candidates who complete their Ph.D. degrees may receive full tuition scholarships for all four years of medical school and their graduate studies. Applications and additional information are available from the director, combined M.D.-Ph.D. degree program.

REQUIREMENTS FOR ENTRANCE

The MCAT and three years of college (minimum of 135 quarter hours) are required; the baccalaureate degree is preferred. The college work must include the following:

	Years
Biology or Zoology (with lab)	1
Inorganic Chemistry (with lab)	1
Organic Chemistry (with lab)	1
General Physics (with lab)	1

Science courses beyond those required will be helpful in preparing for study in medical school; however, the applicant is expected to have a broad foundation in general education, and any major field of interest is acceptable.

SELECTION FACTORS

Students are selected on the basis of various criteria, including scholarship, character, motivation, and educational background without regard to race, creed, religion, sex, sexual orientation, disability, age, or national origin. One's potential for the study and practice of medicine will be evaluated on the basis of academic achievement, MCAT results, personal appraisals by a preprofessional advisory committee or individual instructors, and a personal interview, if requested by the Student Admissions Committee.

Successful applicants for the 2003 entering class had the following credentials: *mean GPA,* 3.42; *residence,* 25 percent from Illinois, with the remainder from 29 other states; *undergraduate major,* 46 percent in biology or chemistry, with the remainder from a variety of fields.

Applicants working on advanced degrees will be considered on the same basis as all other applicants. Applicants who have not been accepted previously and who make reapplication will be treated on the same basis as first-time applicants.

The University offers other programs that produce applicants who are considered for admission by the Chicago Medical School. Acceptance of graduates from the MS Applied Physiology program and others may effectively reduce the number of places available for general AMCAS applicants.

FINANCIAL AID

Limited university-administered financial aid is available to students who are unable to meet school costs through family resources and major financial aid programs. Awards are made to eligible students based on the availability of funds and demonstrated financial need (expenses minus resources). The university utilizes FAFSA to uniformly measure student resources. Approximately 89 percent of the medical students receive financial assistance. An average award through university-administered funds is $3,000 for full-need medical students.

INFORMATION ABOUT DIVERSITY PROGRAMS

The school maintains an extensive recruitment and retention program for students from groups underrepresented in medicine. Application fees may be waived for financially disadvantaged students. Deceleration of basic science curriculum is an option available to all students with demonstrated need.

Institution Type: *Private*
Application Process: *AMCAS, see chapter 4.*

APPLICATION AND ACCEPTANCE POLICIES FOR 2005–2006 FIRST-YEAR CLASS

Filing of AMCAS application
  Earliest date: June 1, 2004
  Latest date: Nov. 15, 2004
School application fee to all applicants: $95
Oldest MCAT scores considered: 2002
Does have Early Decision Program (EDP)
  EDP application period: June 1–Aug. 1, 2004
  EDP applicants notified by: Oct. 1, 2004
Acceptance notice to regular applicants
  Earliest date: December 1, 2004
  Latest date: Until class is filled
Applicant's response to acceptance offer
  Maximum time: 2 weeks
Requests for deferred entrance considered: Yes
Deposit to hold place in class (applied to tuition):
  $100, due with response to acceptance offer
Deposit refundable prior to: May 16, 2005
Estimated number of new entrants: 185 (3EDP)
Starting date: July 2005

TUITION AND STUDENT FEES PER YEAR FOR 2003–2004 FIRST-YEAR CLASS

Tuition: $36,740   Student fees: $120

INFORMATION ON 2003–2004 FIRST-YEAR CLASS

Number of	In-State	Out-of-State	Total
Applicants	919	6,857	7,776
Applicants Interviewed	143	444	587
New Entrants*	46	138	184

*All took the MCAT and had baccalaureate degrees.

CHAPTER

11

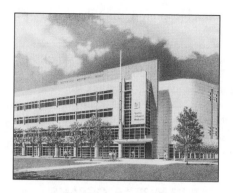

Loyola University Chicago
Stritch School of Medicine

Maywood, Illinois

Dr. Stephen Slogoff, *Dean*
LaDonna E. Norstrom, *Assistant Dean for Admissions*
Donna J. Sobie, Director, *Financial Aid*
Leibert Morris, *Assistant Dean for Student Affairs*

ADDRESS INQUIRIES TO:

Loyola University Chicago
Stritch School of Medicine
Office of Admissions
2160 South First Avenue
Maywood, Illinois 60153
(708) 216-3229
Web site: www.meddean.luc.edu

GENERAL INFORMATION

Loyola University Chicago is a private university founded in 1870 by the Jesuits. It is one of the largest Catholic universities in the United States. By 1920 the university had organized several small medical colleges into a new medical school. In 1948 the school was named in honor of Samuel Cardinal Stritch, Archbishop of Chicago. In 1969 the university opened the Loyola University Medical Center, built on land given by the Veterans Administration, in Maywood, a suburban community located 12 miles west of the Chicago Loop. The medical center is home to the Stritch School of Medicine, Loyola Hospital, Cardinal Bernardin Cancer Center, and Loyola Outpatient Center. Students receive their clinical training at the 523-bed Loyola Hospital, 625-bed Hines Veterans Administration Hospital, and other affiliated hospitals in the Chicago area.

CURRICULUM

The primary purpose of the Stritch School of Medicine is to train physicians who will care for their patients with skill, respect, and compassion. The personal and intellectual development of each student is promoted through close contact with members of the faculty and administration. Students are exposed to the operation of a large academic medical center, as well as to VA and community offices and hospitals, where they learn in an atmosphere of cooperation and mutual assistance. The first year of the curriculum concentrates on the basic principles and processes related to the normal structure, function, and regulation of the human body. In addition, the first year includes instruction in health promotion/disease prevention, health care finance and access, medical ethics, medical/legal issues, and the doctor/patient relationship. Students also have the opportunity to visit ambulatory care sites to experience the delivery of medical care in the ambulatory setting. The second year of the curriculum focuses on basic science principles related to the mechanisms of human disease, neuroscience, and the therapeutic approach to disease. Additionally, students have

the opportunity to continue to develop their knowledge about human behavioral science, physical examination skills, basic clinical skills, evidence-based clinical decision making, and medical ethics and humanities. The third and fourth years are organized into clinical clerkships. The core curriculum includes medicine (12 weeks), a critical care subinternship (4 weeks), an inpatient medicine subinternship (4 weeks), surgery (12 weeks), pediatrics (6 weeks), psychiatry (6 weeks), family medicine (6 weeks), neurology (4 weeks), and obstetrics and gynecology (6 weeks). The curriculum also includes up to 34 weeks of elective time during the fourth year. There is an option for a third year elective for which the student may apply. Through these electives, students are able to broaden their general educational foundation and anticipate their residency training and preparation for careers in medicine suited to their particular talents and interest.

Special curricular features include an emphasis on Bioethics and Professionalism and intensive training in history taking, physical examination, and communication skills using our extensive Clinical Skills Center, which combines the latest in educational technology and patient simulation activities. A Dual Degree Program is offered that allows medical students to earn M.D. and Ph.D. degrees in order to prepare for careers as medical scientists and teachers.

Passage of USMLE Step 1 and Part A of Step 2-CK is a requirement for graduation. Students also must take Step 2-CS.

REQUIREMENTS FOR ENTRANCE

A bachelor's degree and the MCAT, preferably taken by the spring but no later than the fall of the year of application, are required. The following courses are required:

	Years
Biology or Zoology (with lab)	1
Inorganic Chemistry (with lab)	1
Organic Chemistry (with lab)	1
Physics (with lab)	1

A semester or quarter of biochemistry can be substituted for part of the organic chemistry requirement.

Any undergraduate major is acceptable. Applicants are expected to take challenging coursework in the humanities and social sciences, and they should be able to speak and write the English language correctly. Coursework in molecular biology and genetics is strongly recommended. An introduction to statistics is helpful, but not required.

Applicants must be U.S. citizens or hold a permanent resident visa. As a rule, applicants are limited to applying no more than twice. Applicants enrolled in advanced-degree programs must expect to complete their degrees prior to matriculation.

SELECTION FACTORS

The academic record will be evaluated for both depth and breadth of study. Circumstances, such as need to work, which affect a student's academic performance will be taken into account when the record is evaluated. The 2003 entering class had a mean GPA of 3.62. Applicants who present academic credentials that indicate they are capable of succeeding in the rigors of a medical education will be evaluated for evidence of the personal qualifications they can bring to the medical profession. Essential characteristics include an interest in learning, integrity, compassion, and the ability to assume responsibility. Of particular concern will be an applicant's exploration of the field of medicine and the nature of the motivation to enter this career. Each year approximately 600 applicants are invited to interviews with members of the Committee on Admissions. These interviews are conducted only at the medical center campus.

A typical entering class is about 50 percent Illinois residents and 50 percent women. The age range of accepted applicants is quite broad. Early submission of the AMCAS application and prompt return of all supporting material will enhance an applicant's chance of being offered a place in the class.

Loyola University does not discriminate on the basis of race, religion, national origin, sex, age, or handicap. The Committee on Admissions attempts to select students with diversified backgrounds for the contributions they can make to the educational process and the medical profession. Members of groups underrepresented in medicine are encouraged to apply.

FINANCIAL AID

Over 90 percent of Stritch students receive some form of financial aid during the four years of medical school. Student aid is primarily in the form of loans, but limited scholarship and grant money is also available. Some students have found it possible to work during their first two years, often in jobs at the medical center. The school's financial aid office attempts to keep student debt at a manageable level through workshops on budgeting and financial planning. Applicants should receive a preliminary financial aid award approximately two months after submitting financial aid forms.

TRANSFER/ADVANCED STANDING

Medical students who wish to transfer to Stritch for their third year must be enrolled in an allopathic medical school located in the United States that is accredited by the Liaison Committee on Medical Education. Space for transfer students depends on attrition; consequently few, if any, spaces are available each year.

Students who wish to transfer to Stritch may contact our Admissions Office beginning March 1 to request a special application; submission deadline for all materials is May 1.

Applicants must take Step 1 of the United States Medical Licensing Examination (USMLE) under the sponsorship of their present medical school.

INFORMATION ABOUT DIVERSITY PROGRAMS

The Loyola University Chicago Stritch School of Medicine sponsors a summer enrichment program for pre-medical students from groups underrepresented in medicine. The six-week program includes an integrated science oriented curriculum, community based clinical experiences, community health care service projects, and presentations by Loyola clinical faculty on a variety of health care topics. This program provides experiences uniquely directed towards the needs and preparatory background of participants who have completed the first three years of their undergraduate education. Applications and program information are available annually each Fall on the Stritch School of Medicine Student Affairs Web site.

Institution Type: *Private*
Application Process: *AMCAS, see chapter 4.*

APPLICATION AND ACCEPTANCE POLICIES FOR 2005–2006 FIRST-YEAR CLASS

Filing of AMCAS application
  Earliest date: June 1, 2004
  Latest date: Nov. 15, 2004
School application fee after screening: $60
Oldest MCAT scores considered: 2001
Does not have Early Decision Program
Acceptance notice to regular applicants
  Earliest date: Oct. 15, 2004
  Latest date: Until class is filled
Applicant's response to acceptance offer
  Maximum time: 2 weeks
Requests for deferred entrance considered: Yes
Deposit to hold place in class: None
Estimated number of new entrants: 140
Starting date: July 2005

TUITION AND STUDENT FEES PER YEAR FOR 2003–2004 FIRST-YEAR CLASS

Tuition: $32,800   Student fees: $700

INFORMATION ON 2003–2004 FIRST-YEAR CLASS

Number of	In-State	Out-of-State	Total
Applicants	1,125	5,372	6,497
Applicants Interviewed	204	415	619
New Entrants*	59	81	140

*All took the MCAT and had baccalaureate degrees.

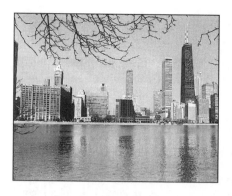

Northwestern University
Feinberg School of Medicine

Chicago, Illinois

Dr. Lewis Landsberg, *Dean*
Delores G. Brown, *Associate Dean for Admissions*
Effie N. Barnett, *Director of Financial Aid*
Dr. John E. Franklin, *Associate Dean for Minority and Cultural Affairs*

ADDRESS INQUIRIES TO:

Northwestern University
Feinberg School of Medicine
Office of Admissions
303 East Chicago Avenue, Morton I-606
Chicago, Illinois 60611-3008
(312) 503-8206
E-mail: med-admissions@northwestern.edu
Web site: www.med-admissions.northwestern.edu

MISSION STATEMENT

Students graduated from Northwestern University's Feinberg School of Medicine are well grounded scientifically and clinically. Committed to the ethical and humane practice of medicine, they learn how to approach patients, perform physical examinations, and formulate a plan of investigation for optimal health management. Beyond diagnosis and treatment, they appreciate the importance of disease prevention, utilizing the skills of allied health professionals, and ascertaining the role of the patient's relationships with family, friends, and the community in producing and alleviating symptoms. Students become lifelong learners, understanding that knowledge at any time is only a prologue to new facts and concepts. They are well prepared for their choice of careers in either the practice of medicine or a research-oriented career in academic medicine.

GENERAL INFORMATION

Founded in 1859, the Feinberg School is located on the university's lakefront Chicago campus. Medical students may live on campus at Lake Shore Center or, in one of the several subsidized apartment buildings. More than 3,000 full-time, part-time, and contributed services faculty members offer instruction in the basic sciences and clinical medicine. The school also offers opportunities in basic science research and clinical research. Students gain clinical experience at the McGaw affiliated group of hospitals, a network of urban, suburban, specialized, and general care facilities. They include Northwestern Memorial, Children's Memorial, Evanston, Northwestern Health Care; Rehabilitation Institute of Chicago; and VA Chicago Health Care System.

CURRICULUM

Northwestern medical students are trained through an integrated, organ system-based curriculum that contains the essential basic science and the biopsychosocial foundations of medicine during the first year. There are two hours of lecture and two hours of directed, independent, active learning (problem-based learning, laboratories, small-group discussions, student presentations, and group projects) each weekday morning.

The first year integrates biochemistry, cell and molecular biology, genetics, cell physiology, gross and microscopic anatomy, physiology, and neuroscience. The second year combines immunology, microbiology, infectious diseases, pharmacology, pathology, and pathophysiology. Three short blocks of time are devoted to Medical Decision Making, which develops a student's abilities in analyzing and managing information, dealing with uncertainty and clinical decision-making.

In the first two years, students also take Patient, Physician, and Society (PPS), which meets two afternoons a week. Each student participates as a member of one of four colleges, led by a faculty mentor. Designed to facilitate student collaboration, faculty-student interaction, and active patient contact, the course involves learning skills physicians should possess to practice medicine (e.g., interviewing and physical examination skills, communication skills, and an understanding of human behavior.) PPS also prepares students to confront and learn to deal with attitudes and knowledge reflecting the interface of medicine with society. These include such topics as ethics and human values, epidemiology, preventive medicine, health care economics, and organized medicine. Periodic PPS sessions also make up part of the third and fourth year curricula.

In the third and fourth years, students learn from attending physicians and residents during clinical clerkships in medicine, surgery, and several of its subspecialties, neurology, psychiatry, pediatrics, obstetrics and gynecology, primary care, urology, emergency medicine, and physical medicine and rehabilitation. A subinternship in medicine or pediatrics and electives round out the curriculum.

Feinberg offers three combined-degree programs: M.D.-Ph.D., M.D.-M.B.A., and M.D.-M.P.H. The M.D.-Ph.D. (Medical Scientist Training Program), offered by the medical school in cooperation with the graduate school, prepares students for careers in academic medicine. Inquiries about the M.D.-Ph.D. program should be directed to the MSTP Program Office, Ward 12-363, 303 East Chicago Avenue, Chicago, IL 60611.

The M.D.-M.B.A. program with the Kellogg Graduate School of Management enables students to obtain both medical and business degrees in five calendar years. Students apply to the M.D.-M.B.A. program during their second year of medical school. The M.D.-M.P.H. program provides students with a broader and deeper experience in public health. Students obtain both degrees in four years. Inquiries should be directed to the

170

M.D.-M.P.H. Office at 680 North Lake Shore Drive, Suite 1102, Chicago, IL 60611. Special research, clinical, and other programs can be arranged to meet individual student interests.

REQUIREMENTS FOR ENTRANCE

The Committee on Admissions seeks applicants who have demonstrated academic excellence, leadership qualities, intellectual curiosity and personal maturity. Applicants should be liberally educated men and women who have studied in some depth subjects beyond the conventional required premedical courses. The medical school has a particular interest in students with promise as physician scholars. Experience in research and evidence of a commitment to medicine as a service profession are positive factors for selection.

Northwestern requires the MCAT and 135 quarter hours (90 semester hours) of undergraduate coursework from an accredited college or university in the United States or Canada. Applicants may have chosen any field for their major; however, year-long courses in biology, general and organic chemistry, and physics are recommended as preparation for the MCAT and for medical school.

Candidates are expected to take the Spring MCAT and to have completed at least their baccalaureate degree requirements prior to medical school matriculation.

SELECTION FACTORS

Reviewers look for evidence of emotional maturity, motivation, past achievement, and character as well as academic excellence. A premium is placed on breadth and depth of the academic program, life experiences of the individual, and clinical and research exposure. Applicants should be liberally educated men and women who have studied in some depth subjects beyond the conventional premedical sciences. Panel interviews are required of all students considered seriously for acceptance. Interview invitations are issued solely upon the request of the Committee on Admissions and are conducted at the medical school.

Some characteristics of the 2003 entering class were: mean *GPA*, 3.69; *MCAT scores* averaged 10.4-Verbal Reasoning, 10.8-Physical Sciences, and 11-Biological Sciences; *average age*, 23 (range 20-33); *gender*, 50.5 percent women.

The Medical School faculty has established technical performance standards. Candidates for admission should demonstrate the mental capability, moral integrity, and physical skills required to function effectively in a broad variety of clinical situations. Northwestern University does not discriminate on the basis of race, religion, national origin, gender, sexual orientation, age, or handicap in its educational programs or activities.

FINANCIAL AID

Financial considerations do not influence admissions decisions. About 75 percent of the student body receives financial aid. Support is provided primarily through national and local loan programs. Northwestern University offers a loan program to international students who have a co-signer on the loan.

Accepted applicants wishing to receive further information may write the assistant director for financial aid, 710 North Lake Shore Drive, Room 629, Chicago, Illinois 60611.

INFORMATION ABOUT DIVERSITY PROGRAMS

The Feinberg School is committed to diversity in the student body, and makes a concerted effort to recruit, admit, and graduate students from groups underrepresented in medicine. The admissions committee, interview committee, minority affairs committee, and faculty are comprised of diverse members.

HONORS PROGRAM

One of the oldest combined baccalaureate-M.D. programs in the country, the Honors Program in Medical Education (HPME) each year selects approximately 40 highly motivated, talented high school graduates for a course of study leading to baccalaureate and M.D. degrees in seven years. Inquiries should be directed to the Office of Undergraduate Admission, P.O. Box 3060, Evanston, Illinois 60204.

Institution Type: *Private*
Application Process: *AMCAS, see chapter 4.*

APPLICATION AND ACCEPTANCE POLICIES FOR 2005–2006 FIRST-YEAR CLASS

Filing of AMCAS application
  Earliest date: June 1, 2004
  Latest date: October 15, 2004
School application fee after screening: $70
Oldest MCAT scores considered: 2002
Does not have Early Decision Program
Acceptance notice to regular applicants
  Earliest date: late November 2004
  Latest date: late February 2005
Applicant's response to acceptance offer
  Maximum time: 2 weeks
Requests for deferred entrance considered: Yes
Deposit to hold place in class: None
Estimated number of new entrants: 170
Starting date: Sept. 2005

TUITION AND STUDENT FEES PER YEAR FOR 2003–2004 FIRST-YEAR CLASS

Tuition: $34,998   Student fees: $2,048

INFORMATION ON 2003–2004 FIRST-YEAR CLASS

Number of	In-State	Out-of-State	Total
Applicants	860	5,097	5,957
Applicants Interviewed	117	514	631
New Entrants*	46	124	170

*All took the MCAT and had baccalaureate degrees (excluding the HPME entrants).

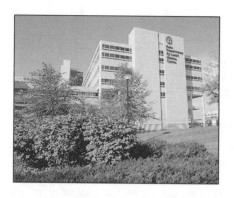

Rush Medical College of Rush University

Chicago, Illinois

Dr. Thomas A. Deutsch, *Dean*
Jan L. Schmidt, *Director of Admissions*
Robert Dame, *Director of Student Financial Aid*
Dr. Cynthia E. Boyd, *Assistant Dean for Minority Affairs*

ADDRESS INQUIRIES TO:

Office of Admissions
524 Armour Academic Center
Rush Medical College of Rush University
600 South Paulina Street
Chicago, Illinois 60612
(312) 942-6913; 942-2333 (FAX)
Web site: www.rushu.rush.edu
E-mail: rmc_admissions@rush.edu

MISSION STATEMENT

The purpose of Rush University is to educate students as practitioners, scientists, and teachers who will become leaders in advancing health care and to further the advancement of knowledge through research. As a major component of Rush University Medical Center, the university integrates patient care, education, and research through the practitioner-teacher model. Rush University encourages the growth of its students by committing itself to the pursuit of excellence, to the advancement of knowledge, to free inquiry, and to the highest intellectual and ethical standards.

GENERAL INFORMATION

Rush Medical College, founded in 1837, is the oldest component of Rush University. The original medical college graduated over 10,000 physicians before closing in 1942. Rush Medical College, a private school, reopened in 1971 and is part of Rush University.

Through the academic and health care network of more than a dozen affiliated hospitals and a neighborhood health center, Rush-Presbyterian-St. Luke's Medical Center serves 1.5 to 2 million people. Thus, the students of Rush University train in urban and suburban areas in a variety of socioeconomic and ethnic settings.

CURRICULUM

Rush Medical College provides a firm background in the science of medicine and a balanced introduction to the practice of clinical medicine in a four-year curriculum designed to provide educational flexibility. A major goal of the college and its faculty is to create an environment that fosters commitments to competent and compassionate patient care and to attitudes of inquiry and lifelong learning.

The four-year curriculum at Rush provides students with a solid foundation in the basic sciences and clinical medicine through a core of required courses and by offering a wide range of electives in our own medical center and affiliated hospitals.

Preclinical Curriculum — The primary objective of the first year is to provide students with exposure to the vocabulary and the fundamental concepts upon which clinical medicine is based. The courses are taught by discipline and utilize lecture, laboratory, small group and workshop formats. The second year curriculum centers on the causes and effects of disease and therapeutics. In addition to the learning formats listed above, the pathophysiology course utilizes a case-based approach during its workshops. Students in the preclinical years also participate in the Generalist Curriculum, which has three components: the Primary Care Preceptorship, Interviewing and Communication and Physical Diagnosis.

Clinical Curriculum — The third and fourth years provide students with training in clinical skills, diagnosis and patient management in a variety of clinical settings. Required clerkships include family medicine, internal medicine, neurology, obstetrics and gynecology, pediatrics, psychiatry, surgery, surgical selectives and a subinternship in either family medicine, internal medicine, pediatrics or surgery. In addition, students are required to complete 18 weeks of electives prior to graduation; at least 8 weeks must be done at Rush or a network hospital. Rush students will complete the majority of their required clinical rotations at either Rush University Medical Center or the John H. Stroger, Jr. Hospital of Cook County.

Rush University offers qualified students who aspire to careers in academic medicine and research the opportunity to enroll in a combined M.D.-Ph.D. program. Ph.D. programs are offered in the Graduate College in the following areas: anatomical sciences, biochemistry, immunology, microbiology, medical physics, neurosciences, pharmacology, and physiology. Students in concurrent programs must meet the full conditions and requirements of the Graduate College, Graduate Division, and the Medical College.

Upon entering Rush Medical College, each student is assigned an academic advisor to help define goals, aid in the selection of courses of study, provide other counseling, and serve as a role model. This advisor will continue with the student as the student progresses through school.

REQUIREMENTS FOR ENTRANCE

The MCAT and 90 semester hours of undergraduate work in an accredited college are required. College work must include the following science areas:

| | | *Sem. hrs.* |
Biology or Zoology 8
Inorganic Chemistry 8
Organic Chemistry. 8
General Physics 8

Four semester hours of biochemistry may be substituted for the second semester of organic chemistry.

Sound preparation in the basic sciences is essential, but a broad background in the humanities and wide exposure to people and their problems are equally necessary.

Applicants are strongly urged to take the MCAT in the spring of the year of application; however, those who take it in the fall will also be considered.

SELECTION FACTORS

Students who enter the Rush Medical College program are carefully selected for their intellectual and social maturity and represent a wide variety of educational and social backgrounds. Problem-solving skills, critical judgment, and the capability to pursue independent study are considered important. Majors in science and majors in other areas with demonstrated excellence in the required science courses are considered equally appropriate to a medical education at Rush Medical College. All applicants to Rush are invited to complete the supplemental application and submit letters of recommendation. The Committee on Admissions looks for objective evidence that the applicant will be able to handle the academic demands of the medical curriculum. In evaluating academic achievement, the committee does consider factors such as the degree of difficulty of the program, the need to work, social and cultural backgrounds, and other factors that may affect the record. In the nonacademic realm, maturity, a balanced education, personal integrity, and motivational factors are considered essential determinants.

Undergraduate academic achievement, recommendations of premedical committees and/or undergraduate faculty, performance on the MCAT, and personal interviews (which are requested of those applicants who are considered competitive candidates by the Committee on Admissions) are considered in the evaluation of applicants. Interviews are held only on the Rush campus and strong preference is given to residents of Illinois. Only applications from U.S. citizens or permanent residents are considered. The average GPA and MCAT scores approximate those of nationally accepted applicants. All applicants are considered without regard to sex, religion, race, age, handicap, or national origin. Applicants from groups underrepresented in medicine are encouraged to apply. Rush will waive its application fee for applicants who receive an AMCAS fee waiver.

FINANCIAL AID

Determination of a financial aid award is made after acceptance into medical school. The financial aid package will consist primarily of loans. Due to limited institutional scholarship assistance, scholarship eligibility is based on parents' resources regardless of the student's age or status. Students are awarded financial aid packages to meet 100 percent of the demonstrated financial need during each year of their medical education. Approximately 80 percent of the medical students receive financial assistance from state, federal, institutional, or other sources outside the family.

TRANSFER

Only those students who are currently enrolled and in good academic standing at LCME-accredited medical schools are considered eligible to apply for transfer. Students must also pass USMLE Step 1 at the conclusion of their second year of medical studies. The number of positions available for transfer is strictly limited by attrition.

Institution Type: *Private*
Application Process: *AMCAS, see chapter 4.*

APPLICATION AND ACCEPTANCE POLICIES FOR 2005–2006 FIRST-YEAR CLASS

Filing of AMCAS application
   Earliest date: June 1, 2004
   Latest date: Nov. 15, 2004
School application fee to all applicants: $65
Oldest MCAT scores considered: 2001
Does have Early Decision Program (EDP)
   EDP application period: June 1–Aug. 1, 2004
   EDP applicants notified by: Oct. 1, 2004
Acceptance notice to regular applicants
   Earliest date: Oct. 15, 2004
   Latest date: varies
Applicant's response to acceptance offer
   Maximum time: 2 weeks
Requests for deferred entrance considered: Yes
Deposit to hold place in class (applied to tuition):
   $100, due with response to acceptance offer
Deposit refundable prior to: May 16, 2005
Estimated number of new entrants: 120 (5 EDP)
Starting date: Sept. 2005

TUITION AND STUDENT FEES PER YEAR FOR 2003–2004 FIRST-YEAR CLASS

Tuition: $32,268   Student fees: $1,284

INFORMATION ON 2003–2004 FIRST-YEAR CLASS

Number of	In-State	Out-of-State	Total
Applicants	1,180	2,748	3,928
Applicants Interviewed	340	108	448
New Entrants*	95	25	120

*All took the MCAT and had baccalaureate degrees.

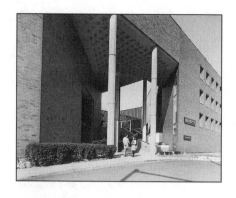

Southern Illinois University School of Medicine

Springfield, Illinois

Dr. Kevin Dorsey, *Dean and Provost*
Erin L. Graham, *Director of Admissions*
Nancy Calvert, *Director of Financial Aid*
Dr. Wesley Robinson-McNeese, *Assistant Dean for Minority Affairs*

ADDRESS INQUIRIES TO:

Office of Admissions
Southern Illinois University
School of Medicine
P.O. Box 19624
Springfield, Illinois 62794-9624
(217) 545-6013; 545-5538 (FAX)
E-mail: admissions@siumed.edu
Web site: www.siumed.edu

MISSION STATEMENT

SIU School of Medicine is guided by a clear mandate to assist the people of central and southern Illinois in meeting their present and future health care needs through education, research and service.

GENERAL INFORMATION

Southern Illinois University School of Medicine was established in 1969 and graduated its first class in 1975. Students spend the first 12 months of the program at the medical education facilities on the Carbondale campus and the remaining three years at the Medical Center in Springfield.

CURRICULUM

SIU School of Medicine conducts its four-year program on two campuses. The overall focus of the curriculum is on student-directed learning in a small group setting, with close integration of basic science and clinical information throughout the four-year course of study. Continuity clinic assignments will allow students to follow a patient group over time beginning in the first year.

The curriculum also provides students with the opportunity to participate in a Mentored Professional Enrichment Project, an optional experience between the first and second years that allows students to work on a project with a mentor over the course of 12 weeks. The objective of the project is to increase their knowledge in a wide variety of areas ranging from rural practice to population and/or community health to academic medicine to bench research.

The first two years of the curriculum engages students in case-based learning, with much student time spent in small group learning activities. Basic sciences are emphasized, and clinical activities center on building basic clinical skills and enhancing the learning of basic science concepts in a clinical context. Thirty to fifty percent of students' scheduled time is spent in clinical activities during these first two years. An increased emphasis on issues such as community health care and the psychosocial issues of medicine continues SIU School of Medicine's emphasis on caring while curing—treating patients as people, rather than medical conditions.

The third year consists of a series of multidisciplinary clinical rotations, with emphasis on both hospital-based and ambulatory practice. These activities take place at various locations throughout the state. Basic sciences are re-emphasized throughout the third year as students work with patients.

The fourth year comprises a series of electives designed to help students with final preparations for residency. Basic sciences will again be re-emphasized as a part of patient care.

Our curriculum is designed to prepare students for careers as professionals in the rapidly changing field of health care while providing a means for developing the knowledge and skills necessary for licensure, residency, and future certification examinations. Its recent development offers students and faculty an opportunity to be participants in an innovative medical school known for a medical education program that trains the best possible physicians and scientists.

The grading system is honors/pass/fail.

The school also offers a six-year M.D.-J.D. program.

REQUIREMENTS FOR ENTRANCE

Applications for the M.D. program are accepted from Illinois residents who are U.S. citizens and those foreign citizens possessing a permanent resident visa. A minimum of 90 semester hours of undergraduate work in an accredited degree-granting college or university is required. Foreign students are advised to have completed at least 60 semester hours of coursework in the United States. The M.D.-J.D. program is open to out-of-state applicants. All applicants are expected to have a good foundation in the natural sciences, social sciences, and humanities and to demonstrate facility in writing and speaking the English language.

To perform well on the MCAT, it is advisable to have had a minimum of two years of college chemistry (including organic), one year of physics, one year of biological or life sciences, mathematics (including statistics), and one year of English composition. Completion of one semester of biochemistry, one semester of cell/molecular biology and one semester of microbiology is also highly recommended.

SELECTION FACTORS

Preference is given to those with sufficient recent academic activity to demonstrate the potential for successful completion of the rigorous educational program and to those who demonstrate the necessary noncognitive characteristics of a successful medical student and physician. Although the Admissions Committee establishes no quotas, an effort is made to recruit qualified applicants from groups that have been underrepresented in the medical profession. Applicants are selected for interview according to their strengths in academics, extracurricular activities, employment, and volunteer experiences, in addition to area of residence with preference given to central and southern Illinois residents. Selected applicants are interviewed in either Springfield or Carbondale; an interview is a prerequisite to acceptance.

The School of Medicine does not discriminate on the basis of race, religion, age, sex, handicap, or national or ethnic origin in administration of its education policies, admissions policies, scholarship and loan programs, and other school-administered programs.

FINANCIAL AID

Southern Illinois University School of Medicine participates in all major federal student aid programs. Students receive financial aid on the basis of their need as calculated on the FAFSA. Scholarship and grant aid is generally limited to students who demonstrate exceptional need.

The financial aid office provides short-term emergency loans as well as loan indebtedness counseling and assistance with securing outside loans and scholarships. Accepted applicants may contact the Office of Student Affairs—Financial Aid at (217) 545-2224 for additional information.

INFORMATION FOR STUDENTS FROM GROUPS UNDERREPRESENTED IN MEDICINE

The School of Medicine sponsors the Medical/Dental Education Preparatory Program (MEDPREP) for disadvantaged undergraduate or postbaccalaureate students, as well as underrepresented, rural, or low-income students. MEDPREP is a non-degree-granting program located on the Carbondale campus. Students who are admitted to the program must begin their matriculation during the fall. The MEDPREP curriculum is designed to meet students' individual preparatory needs. It consists of developmental and enrichment tutorials in small class format, preparation for the MCAT, and medical school application assistance. Additionally, students enroll in preprofessional courses offered by other departments on the campus. Personal, academic, and career counseling is also provided. MEDPREP does not offer a guarantee of eventual acceptance to the School of Medicine or to any other medical school, but

MEDPREP students who meet the criteria established for the MEDPREP Alliance are offered acceptance to the S.I.U. School of Medicine. Careful consideration will be given to MEDPREP participant applicants by the School of Medicine and those selected medical schools working cooperatively with MEDPREP. Inquiries should be addressed to: Director, MEDPREP, Southern Illinois University School of Medicine, Carbondale, Illinois 62901-4323.

Institution Type: *Public*
Application Process: *AMCAS, see chapter 4.*

APPLICATION AND ACCEPTANCE POLICIES FOR 2005–2006 FIRST-YEAR CLASS

Filing of AMCAS application
   Earliest date: June 1, 2004
   Latest date: Nov. 15, 2004
School application fee after screening: $50
Oldest MCAT scores considered: 2002
Does not have Early Decision Program
Acceptance notice to regular applicants
   Earliest date: Oct. 15, 2004
   Latest date: Varies
Applicant's response to acceptance offer
   Maximum time: 2 weeks
Requests for deferred entrance considered: Yes
Deposit to hold place in class (applied to tuition):
   $100, due with response to acceptance offer
Deposit refundable prior to: May 16, 2005
Estimated number of new entrants: 72
Starting date: Aug. 2005

TUITION AND STUDENT FEES PER YEAR FOR 2003–2004 FIRST-YEAR CLASS

Tuition   Student fees: $1,428
   Resident: $16,149
   Nonresident: $48,447

INFORMATION ON 2003–2004 FIRST-YEAR CLASS

Number of	In-State	Out-of-State	Total
Applicants	827	312	1,139
Applicants Interviewed	277	5	282
New Entrants*	72	0	72

*All had baccalaureate degrees and took the MCAT.

CHAPTER
11

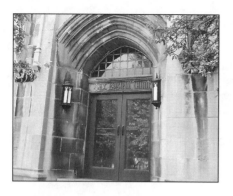

University of Chicago Pritzker School of Medicine

Chicago, Illinois

Dr. James L. Madara, *Dean, Division of Biological Sciences and Pritzker School of Medicine*

Dr. R. Eric Lombard, *Associate Dean for Admissions and Financial Aid*

Sylvia Robertson, *Assistant Dean of Admissions and Financial Aid*

Dr. William McDade, *Associate Dean for Multicultural Affairs*

ADDRESS INQUIRIES TO:

Office of Admissions
Pritzker School of Medicine
924 E. 57th Street, BSLC 104
Chicago, Illinois 60637-5416
(773) 702-1937; 834-5412 (FAX)
Web site: http://pritzker.bsd.uchicago.edu

MISSION STATEMENT

The University of Chicago Pritzker School of Medicine provides more than training in medicine. It provides a total experience: an immersion into the scholarship of a prestigious university, where the medical school, the hospital, and the University share the same campus; where interdisciplinary research and teaching is the norm not the exception; where recognized experts from all disciplines contribute to the development of young physicians in training.

Our mission is to educate students to become accomplished physicians who are capable of functioning as outstanding clinicians, physician-scientists, medical educators, and clinical scholars. Pritzker graduates are known to acquire superb skills in medical reasoning, problem solving, team building and life-long learning which help them assume leadership roles in their residency training programs and as faculty in academic medicine.

GENERAL INFORMATION

The University of Chicago is located on the south side of Chicago in the ethnically diverse community of Hyde Park, just 12 minutes from downtown Chicago. Organized into four major divisions—biological sciences, physical sciences, humanities, and social sciences—the university is made up predominantly of graduate and professional students. In addition to the four major divisions are six professional schools including the Pritzker School of Medicine, all on one campus. Nationally, Pritzker School of Medicine is unique in that it is a part of an academic Division of the Biological Sciences. As an integral part of a world-class university, it offers medical students diverse opportunities for interdisciplinary learning, clinical training, and research. In this environment, the school's mission is to train academic physicians. Over 90 percent of all students engage in some form of scholarly activity prior to completing the M.D. degree, and nearly 20 percent pursue combined M.D.-Ph.D. degrees. Of graduates from 1978–87, 19.1 percent became faculty members.

CURRICULUM

Ten basic competencies underlie the curriculum at Pritzker, and these are grouped into four general areas: the scientific basis of medicine; the scientific basis of diagnosis, prevention, and treatment of disease; interpersonal communication and teaching; and professional growth and development. Significant resources and programs are devoted to helping students excel in these educational objectives. The science library provides a comprehensive set of on-line medical and scientific materials with off-site access by students and faculty. This complements a Web-based curriculum that includes multimedia presentation and searchable text. Students are regularly exposed to evidence-based medicine and taught how to appraise the literature of science and medicine in a critical fashion. A Clinical Performance Center uses standardized patients and videotaped performance to educate students in taking a history, performing a physical examination, and clinical decision-making.

The scientific foundation of medicine is achieved through lectures, laboratories, case-based problem solving, and computer-based guided self-study and self-assessment; this foundation is revisited in senior year in courses designed to apply basic science principles to clinical medicine. The clinical biennium consists of eight clinical clerkships and electives taught entirely by full-time clinical faculty and by highly selected residents who are trained in the humanistic teaching of medical students. Over 90% of the clinical instruction takes place in the hospital and clinics on campus. The curriculum undergoes continued evaluation by faculty and student members of an active curriculum review process; programs identifying, enhancing, and rewarding teaching excellence facilitate curriculum renewal.

Selected students can pursue the M.D. and Ph.D. degrees in basic science through the Medical Scientist Training Program and the Pediatric Growth and Development Training Grant. Ph.D. and other programs of the University are open to medical students with appropriate credentials, and the Medicine in the Arts and Social Sciences Program facilitates combined degrees in the humanities and social sciences. Pritzker students may also pursue M.B.A. or J.D. degrees if accepted to those programs.

REQUIREMENTS FOR ENTRANCE

The MCAT is required of all applicants. Applicants are required to have completed at least 90 credit hours of college-level work, although a four-year baccalaureate degree is preferable. Pritzker's academic program is rigorous, and applicants are encouraged to obtain a strong course foundation in general education (English composition, mathematics, social sciences, and humanities), as well as the required science courses. The specific course requirements for admission are:

Years

Biology or Zoology (with lab) 1
General Chemistry (with lab) 1
Organic Chemistry (with lab) 1
Physics (with lab) 1

Pritzker has a rigorous graduate-level curriculum in biochemistry, and applicants are encouraged to have a working knowledge of biochemical principles prior to matriculation. Biochemistry with lab may be substituted for one half of the organic chemistry requirement. Visit our Web site for additional clarification of requirements.

SELECTION FACTORS

A supplementary application is made available to everyone who submits an application to the Pritzker School of Medicine through AMCAS. The Committee on Admissions reviews an application once the supplementary application is returned and the required letters of evaluation are received. About 500 applicants are invited to interview on the University campus from September through February. Offers of admission are extended on a rolling basis from October through March.

Offers of admission are made solely on the basis of ability, achievement, motivation, and humanistic qualities. Outstanding personal characteristics and a strong career commitment are as important as excellence in academics. Successful applicants passion for continual learning, a commitment to others and the goals of medicine, and have leadership among their peers. Students in the 2003 entering class had the following academic profile: average *GPA - science*, 3.58; *cumulative GPA*, 3.63; *average* MCAT, 9.8; 10.4; 10.6. The entering class is typically comprised of about 10-12 students in the MST Program, 2 in the MAS Program, 4-6 in the Early Acceptance Program (open to undergraduates from the University of Chicago), 1-2 in Early Decision, and 86 in regular admissions. Pritzker does not discriminate on the basis of race, gender, creed, sexual orientation, national origin, age or handicap, and has no residency restrictions.

One to two positions may be open each year for transfer into the second or third year classes. To apply for transfer, an individual must be a spouse or University registered partner of a current member of the University of Chicago faculty, administration, house staff, student body, or staff. Transfer applications are available after February 1, 2005.

FINANCIAL AID

The Pritzker School of Medicine believes no student should be denied admission or be unable to attend for financial reasons. Scholarships and low-interest loans are made available to all students who have demonstrated need. There are both federally subsidized loans and low or no interest loans from the University. Approximately 82 percent of students receive some form of financial assistance. Current levels of indebtedness for Pritzker students are below the national mean for   private institutions. Financial aid packets are mailed to all accepted applicants after January 1. Financial aid resources for international applicants are extremely limited.

INFORMATION ABOUT DIVERSITY PROGRAMS

Pritzker is particularly interested in providing a diverse educational experience for its students. Medical students from groups underrepresented in medicine who have attended Pritzker often assume strong leadership roles, both within their class and at the national level.

Institution Type: *Private*
Application Process: *AMCAS, see chapter 4.*

APPLICATION AND ACCEPTANCE POLICIES FOR 2005–2006 FIRST-YEAR CLASS

Filing of AMCAS application
    Earliest date: June 1, 2004
    Latest date: Oct. 15, 2004
School application fee to all applicants: $75
Oldest MCAT scores considered: 2002
    Does have Early Decision Program (EDP)
    EDP application period: June 1–Aug. 1, 2004
    EDP applicants notified by: Oct. 1, 2004
Acceptance notice to regular applicants
    Earliest date: Oct. 15, 2004
    Latest date: Until class is filled
Applicant's response to acceptance offer
    Maximum time: 30 days
Requests for deferred entrance considered: Yes
Deposit to hold place in class (applied to tuition): None
Estimated number of new entrants: 104 (2 EDP)
Starting date: Sept. 2005

TUITION AND STUDENT FEES PER YEAR FOR 2003–2004 FIRST-YEAR CLASS

Tuition: $29,046   Student fees: $1,949

INFORMATION ON 2003–2004 FIRST-YEAR CLASS

Number of	In-State	Out-of-State	Total
Applicants	747	4,872	5,619
Applicants Interviewed	132	449	581
New Entrants*	41	63	104

*All took the MCAT and had baccalaureate degrees.

CHAPTER

11

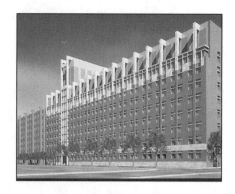

University of Illinois at Chicago College of Medicine

Chicago, Illinois

Dr. Gerald S. Moss, *Dean*
Dr. Jorge A. Girotti, *Associate Dean and Director*
Carmelita Gee, *Director of Financial Aid*

ADDRESS INQUIRIES TO:

Medical College Admissions
University of Illinois
College of Medicine
808 South Wood Street, Room 165 CME M/C 783
Chicago, Illinois 60612-7302
(312) 996-5635; 996-6693 (FAX)
E-mail: medadmit@uic.edu
Web site: www.uic.edu/depts/mcam

MISSION STATEMENT

The mission of the UIC College of Medicine is to enhance the health of the citizens of Illinois through the education of physicians and biomedical scientists, the advancement of our understanding and knowledge of health and disease, and the provision of health care in a setting of education and research. In pursuit of this mission, the College of Medicine is committed to the goal of achieving excellence in teaching, research, and service in the science, art, and practice of medicine. This goal is best attained by applying valid educational principles, demonstrating high-quality patient care, and establishing a spirit of inquiry leading to scholarly achievement in basic and clinical research.

GENERAL INFORMATION

Founded in 1881 as the College of Physicians and Surgeons of Chicago, the name was changed to the University of Illinois College of Medicine in 1900. Following a reorganization of college structure approved by the Board of Trustees in 1982, the College of Medicine programs are now conducted on two educational tracks at four geographic sites. The College of Medicine at Chicago is located at the Health Sciences Center of the university. The College of Medicine at Urbana-Champaign offers a four-year medical curriculum integrated with the programs of a comprehensive campus. The College of Medicine at Peoria includes facilities in each of the hospitals in that community and a modern downtown campus. The College of Medicine at Rockford has a centrally located campus and conducts programs in each of the Rockford hospitals and in several nearby smaller communities.

CURRICULUM

There are two separate curricular tracks within the College of Medicine. Students assigned to the Chicago campus will pursue

their full four-year program of undergraduate medical education under the supervision of the faculty at that site. Students assigned for their first year of instruction to the Urbana-Champaign campus either will remain assigned to that site for the last three years or will transfer to Peoria or Rockford for the three remaining years of the program. Once students begin in either Chicago or Urbana-Champaign, transfers between curricular tracks will be limited.

Each clinical curriculum presents techniques and information necessary for examination and care for the patient, and each provides supervised experiences in a wide variety of clinical settings under direction of the faculty. Through college-level faculty committees consisting of representation from all sites, the standards of quality are regularly evaluated for admissions, instruction, student appraisal, and student promotion.

The college also offers a number of special programs. The Medical Scholars Program on the Urbana-Champaign campus links the medical school with over 40 other academic units, including the natural and biological sciences, social sciences, humanities, business administration, and law, so that students can earn a combined graduate and medical degree. A combined-degree program on the Chicago campus enables medical students to carry out graduate work in the basic medical sciences, business administration, and public health. The Chicago, Rockford, and Peoria campuses offer independent study programs through which medical students can design their own curricula and carry out in-depth studies of health care topics in which they have a special interest.

REQUIREMENTS FOR ENTRANCE

All candidates must take the MCAT no later than the fall of the academic year in which application is made. The Committee on Admissions uses in its evaluation the highest MCAT scores reported of three previous years.

Applicants must be citizens of the United States or permanent legal residents in order to apply.

Applicants must receive the baccalaureate degree prior to matriculation in the College of Medicine. Students may elect any major field of interest. Biology, chemistry (through organic), physics or biophysics, and behavioral science will be particularly helpful in preparing for study in the college. However, the undergraduate major may be chosen from the humanities, fine arts or behavioral, biological, or physical sciences. Mathematics through calculus is useful for those anticipating advanced work in basic or clinical research.

The following courses are required:

	Semesters
Biology or equivalent (with lab)	2
Inorganic Chemistry or equivalent (with lab)	2
Organic Chemistry (with lab)	2
(Note: introductory biochemistry may substitute for a semester of organic chemistry)	
General Physics or equivalent	2
Social Science with an emphasis in the behavioral sciences	3

A minimum of two semesters must be taken in a sequence within the same department and an additional semester within the social sciences. Letters of recommendation are required of all applicants.

SELECTION FACTORS

All candidates apply to the Committee on Admissions, and admitted applicants are given their choices of study sites insofar as places permit. Prospective and admitted students are provided with detailed information to help in their selection of sites.

The College of Medicine endeavors to select applicants who in the judgment of the Committee on Admissions demonstrate best the academic achievement, emotional stability, maturity, integrity, and motivation adjudged necessary for successful study and practice of medicine. The committee is interested in evidence of the applicant's capacity for mature and independent scholarship, while discouraging rigid patterns of coursework. The committee will consider the quality of work of each applicant in all subject areas, the breadth of education, achievement in advanced projects, and work and extracurricular experiences that demonstrate the applicant's imagination, initiative, and creativity. The College of Medicine does not discriminate against applicants on the basis of race, creed, sex, religion, national origin, age, disability, or status as a disabled veteran or veteran of the Vietnam era.

Selection of students is based on a critical evaluation of all available data on each applicant and on the changing needs of society. The Committee on Admissions gives strong preference to candidates who are Illinois residents and who also: (1) possess a GPA of B or better, (2) have attained an MCAT score above the national mean, and (3) meet the safety and technical standards set by the college. Candidates whose formal education has been interrupted are reviewed with respect to their potential contribution to the practice of medicine and to their competitive status with other applicants. An interview of selected candidates will be required.

FINANCIAL AID

Entering students are encouraged to provide timely application through the College of Medicine's Office of Student Financial Aid for loan funds and grant-in-aid scholarship assistance based on need. Grants and scholarships to meet proven financial need are awarded each year to students from all classes.

Financial aid consultation and information can be obtained by calling (312) 413-0127.

INFORMATION FOR DIVERSITY PROGRAMS AND FOR RURAL CANDIDATES

The College of Medicine has developed programs to encourage applications from qualified individuals from medically underserved areas of Illinois. The college maintains a professional staff to provide guidance and counseling to motivated students from groups underrepresented in medicine and resident candidates whose backgrounds indicate potential for rural Illinois practice. The Committee on Admissions reviews all applications, and students are accepted on the basis of their potential for successfully meeting all college standards leading to the M.D. degree.

Institution Type: *Public*
Application Process: *AMCAS, see chapter 4.*

APPLICATION AND ACCEPTANCE POLICIES FOR 2005–2006 FIRST-YEAR CLASS

Filing of AMCAS application
 Earliest date: June 1, 2004
 Latest date: Dec. 15, 2004
School application fee after screening: $70
Oldest MCAT scores considered: 2002
Does have Early Decision Program (EDP)
 For Illinois residents only
 EDP application period: June 1–Aug. 1, 2004
 EDP applicants notified by: Oct. 1, 2004
Acceptance notice to regular applicants
 Earliest date: Oct. 15, 2004
 Latest date: Until class is filled
Applicant's response to acceptance offer
 Maximum time: 2 weeks
Requests for deferred entrance considered: Yes
Deposit to hold place in class (applied to tuition):
 $100, due with response to acceptance offer
Deposit refundable prior to: May 16, 2005
Estimated number of new entrants: 300 (10 EDP)
Starting date: Aug. 2005

TUITION AND STUDENT FEES PER YEAR FOR 2003–2004 FIRST-YEAR CLASS

Tuition   Student fees: $1,900
 Resident: $20,874
 Nonresident: $48,310

INFORMATION ON 2003–2004 FIRST-YEAR CLASS

Number of	In-State	Out-of-State	Total
Applicants	1,478	3,000	4,478
Applicants Interviewed	623	289	912
New Entrants*	254	59	313

*All took the MCAT and had baccalaureate degrees.

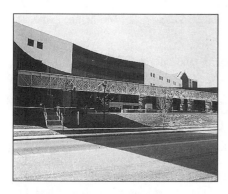

Indiana University School of Medicine

Indianapolis, Indiana

Dr. D. Craig Brater, *Dean*
Robert M. Stump, Jr., *Director of Admissions*
Karen Smartt, *Associate Director of Admissions*

ADDRESS INQUIRIES TO:

Medical School Admissions Office
Fesler Hall 213
Indiana University
School of Medicine
1120 South Drive
Indianapolis, Indiana 46202-5113
(317) 274-3772
E-mail: inmedadm@iupui.edu
Web site: www.medicine.iu.edu/home.html

MISSION STATEMENT

The goal of the Indiana University School of Medicine is the education of physicians, scientists, and other health professionals in an intellectually rich environment with research as its scientific base. In education, we are committed to imparting a fundamental understanding of both clinical practice and the basic scientific knowledge upon which it rests, to provide a firm foundation for lifelong learning. In research, we are committed to the advancement of knowledge. In patient care, we are committed to the highest standards of medical practice in an atmosphere of respect and empathy for our patients. Education, research, and delivery of health care are inseparable components of our mission. Excellence can only be achieved when all components are of highest quality, well integrated, and mutually supportive.

GENERAL INFORMATION

Indiana University School of Medicine, founded in 1903, is the sole institution responsible for providing medical education in the state of Indiana and operates the Indiana Statewide Medical Education System. The school has centers for medical education at Bloomington, Evansville, Fort Wayne, Gary, Lafayette, Muncie, South Bend, and Terre Haute, where students may spend their first two years of medical school. The medical center in Indianapolis has students enrolled in all four years of the medical curriculum.

In addition to its role and responsibilities in teaching, patient care, and service, Indiana University School of Medicine is a major academic research center.

Indiana University School of Medicine utilizes a number of integrated teaching hospitals on or near the medical center campus, as well as other affiliated hospitals in Indianapolis and throughout the state.

CURRICULUM

The School of Medicine's faculty have adopted a competency-based curriculum which equips students with excellent clinical skills balanced by development of interpersonal and professional skills. The basic medical sciences are presented in the first two years. In addition, a multidisciplinary course, Introduction to Clinical Medicine, spans the first two years. Students' skills, knowledge, and attitudes about patient care begin to take shape in this course as they encounter patients for the first time.

A 12-month clinical clerkship program at the medical center in Indianapolis occupies the third year and includes units in family medicine, internal medicine, surgery, obstetrics and gynecology, pediatrics, and psychiatry. In the fourth year, students complete clerkships in neurosensory science, radiology, and surgical specialties, and select seven one-month elective units from an approved list of hundreds of choices. With the permission of the faculty, students may arrange for elective experiences around the country and abroad.

Students interested in research or academic medicine may enroll in the combined-degree program and pursue a Ph.D. degree in addition to the M.D. degree.

In Indianapolis, the School of Medicine's basic science departments offer combined-degree programs in nine basic science disciplines. A special Indiana Medical Scientist Program offers financial support and research opportunities for outstanding students.

The Medical Sciences Program in Bloomington offers graduate studies in anatomy, biochemistry, pathology, pharmacology, and physiology. Also available to combined-degree students in Bloomington are studies in the humanities, law, and social and behavioral sciences as well as in the biological and physical sciences.

In cooperation with Purdue University, combined-degree programs are offered in engineering, medicinal chemistry, molecular biology, and neuroscience at the Lafayette Center for Medical Education.

There are also programs leading to the M.B.A. and M.P.H. degrees in addition to the M.D.

REQUIREMENTS FOR ENTRANCE

The School of Medicine recommends that students preparing for the study of medicine take a variety of courses commonly included in a traditional liberal arts and sciences curriculum.

The MCAT and a minimum of three college years (90 semester hours) are required. Physical education and ROTC courses will not be accepted as part of the 90 semester hours. The undergraduate coursework must include:

	Years
Biology (with labs)	1
General Chemistry (with labs)	1
Organic Chemistry (with labs)	1
Physics (with labs)	1

Applicants should take the MCAT in the spring prior to making application.

The Admissions Committee shows preference to applicants who will have at least a baccalaureate degree prior to matriculation in medical school.

SELECTION FACTORS

Students are offered places in the class on the basis of scholarship, character, personality, references, residence, interview, and performance on the MCAT. In addition, the medical school faculty has specified non-academic criteria (technical standards), which all applicants must meet in order to participate effectively in the medical education program and the practice of medicine.

Because the School of Medicine is state-supported, the Admissions Committee shows preference to Indiana residents in selecting the class. Nevertheless, a number of nonresidents are offered acceptances each year (88 for the 2001 entering class). The applications of nonresidents who have significant ties to the state of Indiana may be given greater consideration.

The average GPA of the 2001 entering class was 3.66/4.0. Average MCAT scores were: *VR*-9.5, *PS*-9.7, *WS*-O, *BS*-9.8.

The School of Medicine does not discriminate on the basis of age, color, disability, ethnicity, gender, marital status, national origin, race, religion, sexual orientation or veteran status.

FINANCIAL AID

Scholarships and long-term, low-interest loans are available to students with financial need. There are also scholarships for students who have demonstrated academic excellence.

There is a significant scholarship for Indiana residents who commit to practicing primary care medicine in a medically underserved location.

INFORMATION ABOUT DIVERSITY PROGRAMS

Applications from disadvantaged individuals and members of groups underrepresented in medicine are encouraged.

The school recruits college students from these groups and provides counseling for high school and college students interested in the health professions.

The School of Medicine has instituted a pre-matriculation program. Selected students are invited to participate in a two-week medical preparatory program prior to the medical school's orientation activities.

There is a graduate program in the medical sciences for disadvantaged students and students from groups underrepresented in medicine whose applications show promise, but are not quite competitive for admission to medical school.

All applications are reviewed by the full Admissions Committee, which accepts students on an individual basis according to their potential and promise for medical school and for service as physicians. For additional information, please contact Karen Smartt, Associate Director of Admissions.

Institution Type: *Public*
Application Process: *AMCAS, see chapter 4.*

APPLICATION AND ACCEPTANCE POLICIES FOR 2005–2006 FIRST-YEAR CLASS

Filing of AMCAS application
  Earliest date: June 1, 2004
  Latest date: Dec. 15, 2004
School application fee to all applicants: $45
Oldest MCAT considered: 2000
Does have Early Decision Program (EDP)
  EDP application period: June 1–Aug. 1, 2004
  EDP applicants notified by: Oct. 1, 2004
Acceptance notice to regular applicants
  Earliest date: Oct. 15, 2004
  Latest date: until class is filled
Applicant's response to acceptance offer
  Maximum time: 3 weeks
Requests for deferred entrance considered: Yes
Deposit to hold place in class: None
Estimated number of new entrants: 280 (20 EDP)
Starting date: Aug. 2005

TUITION AND STUDENT FEES PER YEAR FOR 2003–2004 FIRST-YEAR CLASS

Tuition   Student fees: $2,497
  Resident: $17,993
  Nonresident: $36,827

INFORMATION ON 2003–2004 FIRST-YEAR CLASS

Number of	In-State	Out-of-State	Total
Applicants	605	1,424	2,029
Applicants Interviewed	534	339	873
New Entrants*	267	13	280

*All took the MCAT and had baccalaureate degrees.

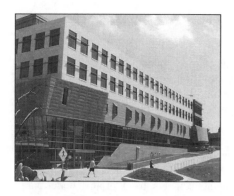

University of Iowa Roy J. and Lucille A. Carver College of Medicine

Iowa City, Iowa

Dr. Jean Robillard, *Dean*
Catherine M. Solow, *Assistant Dean of Student Affairs*
Linda G. Bissell, *Director of Financial Services*
Barbara E. Barlow, *Recruitment Coordinator and Minority Affairs Coordinator*

ADDRESS INQUIRIES TO:

Office of Admissions
University of Iowa
Roy J. and Lucille A. Carver, College of Medicine
100 Medicine Administration Building
Iowa City, Iowa 52242-1101
(319) 335-8052; 335-8049 (FAX)
E-mail: medical-admissions@uiowa.edu
Web site: www.medicine.uiowa.edu

MISSION STATEMENT

The UI Carver College of Medicine has three inextricably linked missions: education, research, and service. The college aspires to be responsive to the needs of society, and in particular the citizens of Iowa, through the excellence of its educational programs in the health professions and biomedical sciences, by the outstanding quality of its research, and through the provision of innovative and comprehensive health care and other services.

GENERAL INFORMATION

The College originated in 1868 and has evolved into a major health center serving the entire state and region. The health sciences campus includes the University of Iowa Hospitals and Clinics; Veterans Administration Hospital; Hardin Health Sciences Library; and medical college, basic sciences, dental, nursing, and pharmacy buildings. A new Medical Education and Biomedical Research Facility opened Fall 2001. The new facility (approximately 203,000 square feet) provides teaching, research, and student spaces. The medical school has a full-time teaching faculty.

CURRICULUM

The curriculum is intended to more efficiently incorporate advances in medical knowledge, to better prepare students to address developing health care issues, to enable students to utilize current health care delivery patterns, and to allow students and faculty to take advantage of improved instructional approaches. Case-based and self-directed learning, clinical correlation, computer-based learning, small-group activities, and vertical integration of material are emphasized.

Year 1 is devoted to the investigation of the normal structure and function of the human body. Core material from the traditional basic science disciplines is presented in the first semester. The second semester is devoted to an integrated, interdisciplinary core of material arranged on an organ system basis. Year 2 is devoted to the investigation of abnormal structure and function. Discipline-specific courses are utilized to present core material in the first half of the year. Early patient contact, an introduction to medical history taking and physical diagnosis, and coverage of emerging topic areas such as continuity of care and behavioral medicine are presented in the Foundations of Clinical Practice, a course that runs concurrently throughout the first two years of the curriculum. In the fourth semester, introduction to the clinical disciplines provides students with a foundation in clinical medicine that will prepare them to perform effectively in the clinical arena.

The two clinical years of the curriculum afford a broad base of clinical experiences and training to provide the student with the essential skills and knowledge required to enter residency training. A generalist core, which includes community-based primary care experiences as well as exposure to the generalist specialties and required selective segments in a variety of other specialty areas, is a feature of the clinical years. Ample time for electives is provided.

In order to prepare academicians in medicine, a Medical Scientist Training Program is offered, which leads to both the M.D. and Ph.D. degrees over a six- to seven-year period.

There are also combined degree programs with business, law and public health.

REQUIREMENTS FOR ENTRANCE

The MCAT is required and must be taken within five years of application, but no later than August of the application year. Applicants must receive a baccalaureate degree prior to matriculation. Candidates must have earned college credit in the following coursework, with appropriate laboratory experience:

Biological Sciences: A complete introductory course in the principles of biology, or zoology and botany, (i.e., 1 year) and one advanced course in biology (1 semester or quarter).

Chemistry: A complete introductory course in organic chemistry (1 year), which would ordinarily follow a complete introductory course in modern general chemical principles.

Physics: A complete introductory course (1 year).

Mathematics: College algebra and trigonometry or advanced college mathematics when college algebra and trigonometry were completed in high school.

The remaining hours are chosen by the student. It is assumed that rhetoric, literature, social and behavioral science, and historical culture are generally among the courses taken as requirements for a baccalaureate degree. A natural science major is not required as the college recognizes the value of a broadly educated student body.

Applicants for admission to the College must demonstrate the capability to complete the entire medical curriculum, which requires proficiency in a variety of cognitive, problem-solving, manipulative, communicative, and interpersonal skills.

Only U.S. citizens or those holding a U.S. permanent resident visa at the time of application may apply.

SELECTION FACTORS

The Admissions Committee selects those applicants best qualified for the study and practice of medicine. To be eligible for admission, the applicant must have attained at least a 2.5 GPA (based on a 4.0 scale) for all college work undertaken. Fulfillment of the basic requirements does not guarantee admission. The major factors considered are:

1. Overall undergraduate academic record as reflected in the GPA: 3.7 class average.

2. Science GPA: 3.7 class average.

3. MCAT: 9–10 class average on each section.

4. Residence: Preference is given to Iowa residents with high scholastic standing. Consideration is also given to outstanding nonresidents.

5. Personal characteristics: Evaluated through letters of recommendation completed by evaluators who are chosen by the applicant, from information on the AMCAS application, and from a supplemental information form.

6. On-site personal interviews (by invitation).

Applications for transfer or admission with advanced standing are generally not considered.

FINANCIAL AID

Applicants are selected without consideration of their ability to meet the expenses of attending medical school. Students receive financial aid solely on the basis of need as calculated using the FAFSA. Scholarship assistance is also available.

While students are responsible for their own financial support, the college provides information and advice on locating sources of funds. Loan and grant funds from private, state, collegiate, and federal sources are available through the college. Approximately 96% of students receive some form of financial aid.

INFORMATION FOR DISADVANTAGED APPLICANTS

The Carver College of Medicine is committed to the recruitment, selection and retention of a diverse student body. To this end, the college provides financial and academic assistance to educationally and economically disadvantaged students and those from groups underrepresented in American medicine. Financial aid packages are designed individually on the basis of need and grant assistance is available for financially disadvantaged students. The application fee and admission deposit also may be waived for financially disadvantaged students upon request.

Institution Type: *Public*
Application Process: *AMCAS, see chapter 4.*

APPLICATION AND ACCEPTANCE POLICIES FOR 2005–2006 FIRST-YEAR CLASS

Filing of AMCAS application
  Earliest date: June 1, 2004
  Latest date: Nov. 1, 2004
School application fee after screening: $50
Oldest MCAT scores considered: 1999
Does have Early Decision Program (EDP)
  EDP application period: June 1–Aug. 1, 2004
  EDP applicants notified by: Oct. 1, 2004
Acceptance notice to regular applicants
  Earliest date: Oct. 15, 2004
  Latest date: Aug. 2005
Applicant's response to acceptance offer
  Maximum time: 2 weeks
Requests for deferred entrance considered: Yes
Deposit to hold place in class (applied to tuition):
  $50, due March 1, 2005, or within 3 weeks after
  acceptance offer if accepted after March 1, 2005
Deposit refundable prior to: June 15, 2005
Estimated number of new entrants: 142
Starting date: Aug. 2005

TUITION AND STUDENT FEES PER YEAR FOR 2003–2004 FIRST-YEAR CLASS

Tuition   Student fees: $1,472
  Resident: $17,838
  Nonresident: $36,306

INFORMATION ON 2003–2004 FIRST-YEAR CLASS

Number of	In-State	Out-of-State	Total
Applicants	325	2,001	2,326
Applicants Interviewed	243	304	547
New Entrants*	97	45	142

*All took the MCAT and had baccalaureate degrees.

CHAPTER
11

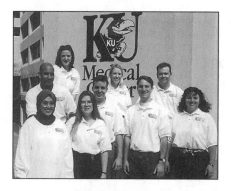

University of Kansas School of Medicine

Kansas City, Kansas

Dr. Barbara F. Atkinson, *Executive Dean*
Sandra J. McCurdy, *Assistant Dean for Admissions*
Lisa Erwin, *Director of Student Financial Aid*
Dr. Patricia A. Thomas, *Associate Dean for Cultural Enhancement and Diversity*

ADDRESS INQUIRIES TO:

Assistant Dean for Admissions
University of Kansas
School of Medicine
Mail Stop 1049
3901 Rainbow Boulevard
Kansas City, Kansas 66160
(913) 588-5245; 588-5259 (FAX)
Web site: www.kumc.edu/som/som.html

MISSION STATEMENT

The University of Kansas School of Medicine commits to enhance the quality of life and serve our community through the discovery of knowledge, the education of health professionals, and by improvement the health of the public.

GENERAL INFORMATION

The University of Kansas School of Medicine was established in 1899 with a two-year program, which expanded to four years in 1906. It is located on the Medical Center campus in Kansas City, Kansas, which also houses the schools of nursing, allied health, and graduate studies. There are 1,500 faculty members in the School of Medicine, including 450 full-time faculty members in general and specialty medicine and the basic sciences. Full-time members actively participate in the teaching, service, and research mission of the school. Facilities at the Medical Center include the Delbert D. Neis, M.D., Clinical Skills Laboratory; the Archie R. Dykes Library of the Health Sciences; the Orr-Major basic sciences facility, containing classrooms, laboratories, an auditorium, and a learning resources center; the Ernst F. Lied Biomedical Research Building; and the University Hospital. This 485-bed hospital offers complete primary and tertiary care for patients of all ages and care for a wide range of problems from traumatic injuries to specialized care for those with chronic conditions.

The School of Medicine-Wichita campus was accredited in 1974, and a portion of every class completes clinical training in a community-based program at three Wichita hospitals.

CURRICULUM

The School of Medicine's curriculum ensures a sequential and interdisciplinary medical education with an emphasis on a generalist approach to the diagnosis, treatment, and management of patients' illnesses. This curriculum is designed to assist students in their acquisition of the knowledge, skills, and attitudes needed to become highly competent and caring physicians.

The first two years of the curriculum provide the basic biomedical and social sciences foundation essential to the practice of medicine. Didactic and self-directed learning are balanced between small-group activities and lectures. In addition, first- and second-year medical students are paired with a mentoring physician in a longitudinal ambulatory clinical experience.

During years three and four, students participate in the delivery of health care in ambulatory and hospital settings, both in the community and at the KU Medical Center. The curriculum consists of required clerkships in the core clinical areas as well as a one-month preceptorship with a practicing Kansas physician. Students also choose from a large selection of basic science and clinical electives to complete a well-rounded educational program. Seminars facilitate continuing student discussion of issues raised during their first two years of study, and a comprehensive advising system assists medical students with academic, personal, and professional development.

A five-level grading system of superior, high satisfactory, satisfactory, low satisfactory, or unsatisfactory is utilized. Students must pass the USMLE Step 1 to continue their clinical training and Step 2 to graduate from the School of Medicine.

A combined M.D./Ph.D. program in basic medical sciences is offered. Further information may be obtained at ☞www3.kumc.edu/mdphd/ or from the Office of Graduate Studies at (913) 588-5241. Information about the M.D./M.P.H. program is available by calling (913)588-2974.

REQUIREMENTS FOR ENTRANCE

The MCAT is required. Applicants must complete a course of study leading to a baccalaureate degree, which will be conferred prior to the planned date of enrollment in medical school. The degree requirement may be modified under exceptional circumstances. Specific minimum coursework requirements are:

	Semesters
General Biology (with lab)	2
Inorganic Chemistry (with lab)	2
Organic Chemistry (with lab)	2
Physics (with lab)	2
English	2
(sufficient credit to meet the prerequisites for a liberal arts degree)	
Mathematics (college-level algebra, or above)	1

Undergraduate courses should be rigorous and, in general, equivalent to courses taken by students majoring in those subject areas. The Admissions Committee does not give preference to a major field of study, and students are strongly advised to balance their work in the natural sciences with courses in the social sciences and humanities. Although no other specific courses are required, statistics, biochemistry and upper-level biology courses provide additional preparation for the medical school curriculum.

SELECTION FACTORS

Applicants are strongly encouraged to submit their AMCAS applications no later than September 1, 2004. Early application allows sufficient time for preliminary screening, for mailing of secondary applications, and for the subsequent screening for invitation to interview. Qualified residents of Kansas are given strong first preference for receipt of secondary applications, for interview, and for selection to the entering class. Successful nonresident applicants are those who have significant ties to Kansas or who will add breadth to the class.

The selection of students is made after careful consideration of the entire application, letters of evaluation, and a personal interview. Each applicant's scholarship is evaluated, but it is recognized that individual capabilities and professional promise cannot always be completely measured by traditional systems of grading. Trends in academic performance, the AMCAS essay, impressions gained from interviews, and the record of extracurricular activities and involvement in community affairs will be assessed in considering the applicant's candidacy. The University of Kansas does not discriminate on the basis of race, sex, religion, sexual orientation, national origin, age, or handicap.

The 2003 entering class was made up of 87 percent *Kansans*, 42 percent *women*, and 16 percent *minorities*, and 38 percent of the class was 25 years of age or older. The *mean GPA* was 3.6 with *mean MCAT scores* above the 60th percentile.

Applications for transfer are taken only upon the rare occasion of an available position in the third-year class. Kansas residents with a compelling need to transfer are given highest priority.

FINANCIAL AID

Numerous loans and scholarships are available for students attending the University of Kansas School of Medicine. The majority are based on financial need, determined by filing a Free Application for Federal Student Aid. Over 95 percent of students receive some type of financial assistance.

A major source of assistance is the Kansas Medical Student Loan Program, which provides payment of tuition and a stipend of up to $1,500 per month. Recipients may receive loan forgiveness by practicing primary care medicine in a small town or rural area in Kansas. Application forms and additional information can be obtained by contacting the Office of Student Financial Aid at (913) 588-5170.

INFORMATION ABOUT DIVERSITY PROGRAMS

The School of Medicine has an active program dedicated to the recruitment, admission, retention, education, and graduation of increased numbers of individuals from groups underrepresented in medicine. Several scholarships are available for qualified students. For additional information contact the associate dean for cultural enhancement and diversity at (913) 588-5292.

Institution Type: *Public*
Application Process: *AMCAS, see chapter 4.*

APPLICATION AND ACCEPTANCE POLICIES FOR 2005–2006 FIRST-YEAR CLASS

Filing of AMCAS application
  Earliest date: June 1, 2004
  Latest date: Oct. 15, 2004
School application fee after screening: $40 for
  nonresidents who are invited to complete
  secondary application.
Oldest MCAT scores considered: 2001
Does have Early Decision Program (EDP)
  EDP application period: June 1–Aug. 1, 2004
  EDP applicants notified by: Oct. 1, 2004
Acceptance notice to regular applicants
  Earliest date: Nov. 1, 2004
  Latest date: Varies
Applicant's response to acceptance offer
  Maximum time: 2 weeks
Requests for deferred entrance considered: Yes
Deposit to hold place in class (applied to tuition):
  $50, due with response to acceptance offer
Deposit refundable prior to: May 16, 2005
Estimated number of new entrants: 175 (35 EDP)
Starting date: Aug. 2005

TUITION AND STUDENT FEES PER YEAR FOR 2003–2004 FIRST-YEAR CLASS

Tuition   Student fees: $396
  Resident: $14,584
  Nonresident: $29,115

INFORMATION ON 2003–2004 FIRST-YEAR CLASS

Number of	In-State	Out-of-State	Total
Applicants	413	880	1,293
Applicants Interviewed	297	101	398
New Entrants*	153	22	175

*All took the MCAT and had baccalaureate degrees.

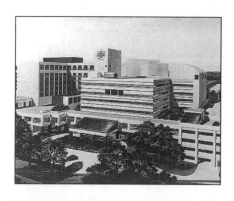

University of Kentucky College of Medicine

Lexington, Kentucky

Dr. Jay Perman, *Dean*
Dr. Carol L. Elam, *Assistant Dean for Admissions*
Linda A. Gilbert, *Financial Aid Coordinator*

ADDRESS INQUIRIES TO:

Admissions, Room MN-102
Office of Academic Affairs
University of Kentucky College of Medicine
Chandler Medical Center
800 Rose Street
Lexington, Kentucky 40536-0298
(859) 323-6161; 323-2076 (FAX)
Web site: www.mc.uky.edu/medicine

MISSION STATEMENT

The mission of the College of Medicine is to assume a leadership role in addressing the health care needs of the Commonwealth of Kentucky and to be preeminent among medical schools in selected areas of education, research, and service.

GENERAL INFORMATION

Established in 1956 by the Commonwealth of Kentucky and the University of Kentucky Board of Trustees, the University of Kentucky College of Medicine admitted its first class in 1960. The College of Medicine is part of the University of Kentucky Chandler Medical Center located on the university campus in Lexington.

The medical center comprises five colleges: medicine, nursing, pharmacy, dentistry, and health sciences and the new school of public health. The majority of on-site clinical teaching occurs at the 473-bed University of Kentucky Hospital, the 407-bed Veterans Affairs Medical Center, and the Kentucky Clinic. Hospitals throughout Lexington and across the Commonwealth hold affiliation agreements with the college for clinical teaching and patient service.

Basic science teaching areas for lecture, laboratory, and small-group instruction, as well as the Medical Center Library, are located in the Medical Sciences Building. Adjacent are the Health Science Learning Center, Critical Care Center, Sanders-Brown Center on Aging, Lucille Parker Markey Cancer Center, Mills-Davis Magnetic Resonance Imaging and Spectroscopy Center, and University of Kentucky Student Health Service.

CURRICULUM

In a curriculum designed to integrate basic and clinical sciences, medical students are taught the fundamental problems of human biology, how to recognize the causes of these problems, and how to prevent disease and treat patients. Year 1 of the Kentucky medical curriculum focuses on normal function of the human body (human structure, cellular structure and function, neurosciences, and human function). First-year students receive early exposure and experience in patient care through the study of interviewing, history taking, physical examination skills, and clinical decision making. In the first two years, medical students also explore principles of prevention and assess the impact of social, ethical, legal, economic, and psychological factors using case studies and small-group discussions. Year 2 exposes students to abnormal functions of the human body as related to disease processes. Coursework is designed to integrate studies of infectious disease, immunology, pathology, and pharmacology. Computer-based instruction reinforces basic science studies and provides linkages to clinical applications.

Clinical students work with patients in both inpatient hospital and outpatient clinic settings and are required to take medical histories, perform physical examinations on patients, and monitor laboratory tests. Year 3 of the Kentucky medical curriculum includes an integrated women's maternal and child health clerkship, along with clinical neurosciences, primary care, internal medicine, and surgery. Year 4 is highlighted by required rotations in emergency medicine, clinical pharmacology, rural medicine, two acting internships, and a three-month elective period.

Selected students may opt to pursue a combined M.D.-Ph.D. in anatomy and neurobiology, biochemistry, microbiology and immunology, pharmacology, or physiology and biophysics. Combined-degree programs are also available in preventive medicine, nutritional sciences, toxicology, and biomedical engineering. Students may also opt to pursue M.D./M.B.A. or M.D./M.P.H. degrees.

REQUIREMENTS FOR ENTRANCE

Applicants are expected to have a broad foundation in the natural sciences, social sciences, and humanities and should demonstrate facility in writing and speaking the English language.

186

Applicants are strongly urged to complete their baccalaureate degrees. The MCAT is required for admission. Applicants are strongly encouraged to take the spring exam. Specific course requirements are:

	Semesters
Biology (with labs)	2
General Chemistry (with labs)	2
Organic Chemistry (with labs)	2
Physics (with labs)	2
English	2

Emphasis is placed on written and spoken communication.

SELECTION FACTORS

The University of Kentucky College of Medicine gives preference to qualified applicants who are residents of Kentucky. Determination of state residence is made by the registrar's office. Applicants' files are reviewed without regard to race, sex, creed, national origin, age, or handicap. Secondary applications are sent to all Kentucky residents and to those nonresidents with undergraduate GPAs of 3.75 or higher and MCAT scores of 10 or higher on each section. Selected candidates are invited for interviews conducted at the University of Kentucky College of Medicine.

Necessary personal attributes of applicants include time management abilities, interpersonal skills, leadership, and demonstrated service to others. Admission decisions are made based upon review of academic and nonacademic factors including scholastic excellence, MCAT performance, personal attributes, breadth of experience, exposure to the profession, premedical recommendations, and admission interviews.

The students enrolled in the 2000 entering class had the following profile: *mean GPA,* 3.68; *women,* 48 percent; *residence,* 87 percent; *undergraduate major,* 68 percent in the natural sciences with the remainder from the social and behavioral sciences, engineering, and liberal arts. Transfers from LCME-accredited schools only are considered on a space-available basis. The University of Kentucky College of Medicine does not discriminate on the basis of race, sex, creed, national origin, age, or handicap.

FINANCIAL AID

A limited number of scholarship grants are awarded to selected students with exceptional achievement. Approximately 85 percent of the student body receives financial assistance through loans and scholarships. Institutional loan/scholarship assistance is available for eligible resident and nonresident students. Kentucky residents who plan to practice in rural Kentucky may receive aid from the Rural Kentucky Medical Scholarship Fund.

The Office of Academic Affairs provides financial aid counseling and assists students in applying for aid. Only in rare circumstances are students given permission to seek employment.

INFORMATION ABOUT DIVERSITY PROGRAMS

The University of Kentucky College of Medicine is committed to the recruitment and retention of disadvantaged students and students from groups underrepresented in medicine. Interested applicants are encouraged to contact the admissions office.

Institution Type: *Public*
Application Process: *AMCAS, see chapter 4.*

APPLICATION AND ACCEPTANCE POLICIES FOR 2005–2006 FIRST-YEAR CLASS

Filing of AMCAS application
    Earliest date: June 1, 2004
    Latest date: Nov. 1, 2004
School application fee after screening: $30
Oldest MCAT scores considered: Aug. 2002
Does have Early Decision Program (EDP)
    EDP application period: June 1–Aug. 1, 2004
    EDP applicants notified by: Oct. 1, 2004
Acceptance notice to regular applicants
    Earliest date: October 15, 2004
    Latest date: Until class is filled
Applicant's response to acceptance offer
    Maximum time: 2 weeks
Requests for deferred entrance considered: Yes
Deposit to hold place in class (applied to tuition):
    $100, due with response to acceptance offer
Deposit refundable prior to: May 16, 2005
Estimated number of new entrants: 103 (15 EDP)
Starting date: Aug. 2005

TUITION AND STUDENT FEES PER YEAR FOR 2003–2004 FIRST-YEAR CLASS

Tuition   Student fees: $666
    Resident: $13,604
    Nonresident: $31,996

INFORMATION ON 2003–2004 FIRST-YEAR CLASS

Number of	In-State	Out-of-State	Total
Applicants	400	541	941
Applicants Interviewed	242	66	308
New Entrants*	88	7	95

*All took the MCAT and had baccalaureate degrees.

CHAPTER

11

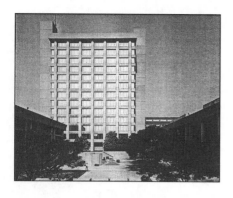

University of Louisville
School of Medicine

Louisville, Kentucky

Dr. Laura Schweitzer, *Acting Dean*
Pamela D. Osborne, *Director, Medical School Admissions*
Leslie Kaelin, *Director of Financial Aid*
Michael Byrne, *Director of Health Science Center, Special Programs*

ADDRESS INQUIRIES TO:

Office of Admissions
School of Medicine
Abell Administration Center
323 East Chestnut
University of Louisville
Louisville, Kentucky 40202-3866
(502) 852-5193; 852-0302 (FAX)
Web site: www.louisville.edu/medschool/admissions/

MISSION STATEMENT

The University of Louisville School of Medicine has a mandated statewide mission to meet the educational, research, and patient-care needs of the Commonwealth of Kentucky, within the resources available, and to cooperate with other health sciences center schools and colleges in educating health care teams. The educational program is designed to train physicians who are sensitive to medical ethics and who will meet the diverse health care needs of the Commonwealth of Kentucky.

GENERAL INFORMATION

The School of Medicine was established at the Louisville Medical Institute in 1833 and became affiliated with the University of Louisville in 1846. In 1970 the university became a member of the state system of higher education. The School of Medicine is part of the modern Health Sciences Center located near downtown Louisville that also includes the Schools of Dentistry and Nursing.

The major clinical teaching activities take place in the 404-bed acute and trauma care University Hospital. Within one or two blocks are three formally affiliated hospitals, which include the only full-service children's hospital in the state of Kentucky—Kosair-Children's Hospital, Jewish Hospital, and Norton Hospital. Other facilities include the world-renowned Kentucky Lions Eye Research Institute; James Brown Cancer Center; the Veterans Administration Medical Center; the Child Evaluation Center; Amelia Brown Fazier Rehabilitation Center; and the Trover Clinic, an off-campus teaching center located in Madisonville, Kentucky.

CURRICULUM

At the University of Louisville School of Medicine, an educational program has been developed that provides an efficiently organized, penetrating presentation of the general

information considered essential for all physicians, yet has sufficient flexibility to allow effective development of a student's individual abilities and interests. The major components of this program are the Core Curriculum, the Preclinical Elective Program, the Clinical Elective Program, and combined study.

The purpose of the Core Curriculum, which extends over the four-year course of study, is to provide each student with the general education and training considered essential to all physicians. It stresses understanding of concepts and general principles instead of a superficial knowledge of details. It provides opportunity for correlation among the sciences so that information received in one subject can reinforce ideas and build upon concepts developed in another. The incorporation of clinical correlations into the first two years demonstrates how knowledge of the basic sciences applies directly to the solution of problems of human disease. The Core Curriculum for the first two academic years is divided into four quarters (one-half-semester intervals) of nine weeks each. Within these smaller subdivisions it is possible to vary the balance of departmental activities to accommodate a better integrated presentation of subject matter.

The Core Curriculum for the last two years follows a track system of clerkships and electives, which exposes students to all of the major clinical fields of medicine. The curriculum includes an emphasis on primary care and ambulatory health care delivery sites. Students are also required to complete rotations at rural or urban AHEC sites in the third and fourth years. The schedule provides considerable flexibility and opportunities for selecting elective courses.

The Preclinical Elective Program allows each student to extend his/her education in specific areas of interest. The electives make it possible to construct a program of medical education that best meets the needs, abilities, and goals of the individual student. Students also are permitted to take courses as electives in divisions of the University of Louisville other than the School of Medicine, class schedule permitting. In addition to the courses listed, students with a research interest are permitted to participate in an approved research activity for credit. Elective courses constitute an integral part of the student's total program in medical school. Second-year students take two credit hours of elective courses.

In the Clinical Elective Program, the student selects a faculty member who works in a preceptorial relationship in the area of the student's interest. Virtually every member of the full-time clinical faculty participates in the program, as do many members of the basic science faculty. Students may select intensive exposure to any of the clinical areas or contribute to research advances in any of the basic science or clinical areas. During this time, a student also may select courses from the second-year elective program.

Especially capable students enrolled in the School of Medicine may work toward an M.S. or Ph.D. degree while pursuing the M.D. degree. A certain number of core and elective courses may be used to fulfill requirements for these degrees. A formal combined M.D./Ph.D. program is available.

REQUIREMENTS FOR ENTRANCE

The MCAT is required and may not be more than two years old. A bachelor's degree is recommended and most successful candidates have earned the bachelor's degree by the time they enroll in the medical school. Required courses are:

	Sem. hrs.
Biology (with lab)	8
General or Inorganic Chemistry (with labs)	8
Organic Chemistry (with labs)	8
Physics (with labs)	8
College Mathematics	8
Or one semester of Calculus	
English	8

Proficiency in written and oral English is required.

SELECTION FACTORS

Because the University of Louisville is a state institution, the School of Medicine gives preference to qualified residents of Kentucky. Applicants are selected on the basis of their individual merits without bias concerning sex, race, creed, national origin, age, or handicap.

Applicants are chosen on the basis of intellect, integrity, maturity, and the ability to interact with sensitivity towards others. In the selection of applicants, consideration is given to the past academic record, evaluations of college preprofessional committees or faculty letters of recommendations, extracurricular activities, and personal interviews. The interviews are given considerable weight and are held at the medical school.

Some characteristics of students in the 2003 entering class were: *mean MCAT* 9.2, *mean GPA,* 3.6; *sex,* 46 percent women; *minority,* 9 percent.

FINANCIAL AID

Financial needs of the applicant are not a consideration in the selection process. After acceptance, every effort is made to assist students in meeting their financial requirements. Approximately 85 percent of the student body receive some degree of financial aid during the academic year. Scholarships are available on a limited basis and are granted according to demonstrated financial need and scholastic and professional promise. Student Research Scholarships are available to qualified students during the summer months.

INFORMATION ABOUT DIVERSITY PROGRAMS

Applications from disadvantaged individuals and members of groups underrepresented in medicine are encouraged. The School of Medicine has a prematriculation program. Applicants are reviewed by the full Admissions Committee, which accepts students on an individual basis according to their potential and promise of medical school and service as physicians.

Institution Type: *Public*
Application Process: *AMCAS, see chapter 4.*

APPLICATION AND ACCEPTANCE POLICIES FOR 2005–2006 FIRST-YEAR CLASS

Filing of AMCAS application
  Earliest date: June 1, 2004
  Latest date: Nov. 1, 2004
School application fee after screening: $75
Oldest MCAT scores considered: 2002
Does have Early Decision Program (EDP)
  EDP application period: June 1–Aug. 1, 2004
  EDP applicants notified by: Oct. 1, 2004
Acceptance notice to regular applicants
  Earliest date: Oct. 15, 2004
  Latest date: April 30, 2005
Applicant's response to acceptance offer
  Maximum time: 2 weeks
Requests for deferred entrance considered: Yes
Deposit to hold place in class (applied to tuition):
  $100, due with response to acceptance offer
Deposit refundable prior to: May 16, 2005
Estimated number of new entrants: 149 (10 EDP)
Starting date: Aug. 2005

TUITION AND STUDENT FEES PER YEAR FOR 2003–2004 FIRST-YEAR CLASS

Tuition   Student fees: $660
  Resident: $14,544
  Nonresident: $36,262

INFORMATION ON 2003–2004 FIRST-YEAR CLASS

Number of	In-State	Out-of-State	Total
Applicants	397	914	1,311
Applicants Interviewed	211	79	290
New Entrants*	123	26	149

*All took the MCAT and had baccalaureate degrees.

CHAPTER
11

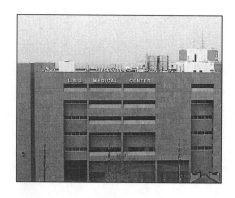

Louisiana State University School of Medicine in New Orleans

New Orleans, Louisiana

Dr. J. Patrick O'Leary, *Interim Dean*
Dr. Sam G. McClugage, *Associate Dean for Admissions*
Patrick Gorman, *Director of Student Financial Aid*
Dr. Edward Helm, *Associate Dean, Office of Community and Minority Health Education*

ADDRESS INQUIRIES TO:

Admissions Office
Louisiana State University
School of Medicine in New Orleans
1901 Perdido Street, Box P3-4
New Orleans, Louisiana 70112-1393
(504) 568-6262; 568-7701 (FAX)
E-mail: ms-admissions@lsuhsc.edu
Web site: www.medschool.lsuhsc.edu/admissions

MISSION STATEMENT

The Louisiana State University (LSU) School of Medicine in New Orleans is dedicated to providing the opportunity for an excellent medical education to all Louisiana applicants who are prepared to benefit from its curriculum and instruction. To this end, the Admissions Committee will strive to recruit and admit residents from Louisiana from every geographic, economic, social, and cultural dimension of the state of Louisiana.

GENERAL INFORMATION

The LSU School of Medicine in New Orleans was established in 1931 by authorization provided in the charter of Louisiana State University and Agricultural and Mechanical College adopted in 1877. The original building was constructed at 1542 Tulane Avenue, adjacent to the Medical Center of Louisiana at New Orleans (Charity Hospital). Over the years, additions were added to the original structure, and new buildings were erected as the school expanded, including a Residence Hall and Student Center, a Medical Education Building, the Lions-LSU Clinics Building, and a new Clinical Sciences Research Building. The School of Medicine is one component of the LSU Health Sciences Center in New Orleans, which includes Schools of Allied Health, Dentistry, Graduate Studies, and Nursing.

The major teaching hospitals are the Medical Center of Louisiana in New Orleans and University Hospital. Other hospitals in the city such as Children's Hospital are also used for clinical instruction and residency training. Also, some residency programs and clerkships are available at the University Medical Center in Lafayette, and the Earl K. Long Hospital in Baton Rouge.

Two student housing facilities are available. Furnished and unfurnished apartments are available for married and single students, and regular dormitory-type space is also available.

CURRICULUM

The first two years of the medical school curriculum emphasize several basic sciences and their relevancy to clinical medicine. Clinical experiences begin in the first year in courses such as Science and Practice of Medicine. The second year of medical school utilizes an integrated approach to the teaching of basic science and preclinical courses within an environment that fosters an early exposure to patient care. Clerkships begin in the third year where students rotate through the various clinical disciplines. In the fourth year, students are given several months for electives in addition to required rotations in Ambulatory Medicine, Acting Internships, etc. Some of these rotations can be completed at the institutions associated with the LSU School of Medicine throughout the state or at other approved institutions outside the state or country.

Computer-assisted instruction is an important component of the curriculum. Entering students are now required to purchase laptop computers.

Although major emphasis is placed on training primary care physicians, there are many opportunities for research and the pursuit of more specialized training. There are several Centers of Excellence that provide opportunities for research and training in such areas as cancer, neuroscience, genetics, alcohol and drug abuse, and asthma.

The Honors Programs at LSUHSC supplements the regular curriculum and is designed to challenge the exceptional student while stimulating the interests of the individual. It entails an independent research program that encompasses basic and clinical sciences in the pursuit of a problem of scientific interest.

The M.D.-Ph.D. program is available for highly motivated students interested in academic medicine. Only applicants who are first accepted to medical school can be considered for this program. Information can be obtained by calling the School of Graduate Studies, (504) 568-2211. Medical students can also apply for a Master of Public Health degree program.

Students are required to pass Step 1 of the USMLE before progressing to the third year. They must pass Step 2 prior to graduation.

The curriculum is under constant evaluation and review by both faculty and students.

REQUIREMENTS FOR ENTRANCE

The MCAT is required and must be taken at a time that enables scores to be received by the Admissions Office prior to the November application deadline to be considered for admission the following August. Applicants are strongly urged to complete the regular four-year undergraduate curriculum and take the appropriate recommended courses before entering the study of medicine. The school encourages a balance among the natural sciences, social sciences, and the humanities.

Specific course requirements are:

	Sem. hrs.
Biology or Zoology (with lab)	8
General or Inorganic Chemistry (with lab)	8
Organic Chemistry (with lab)	8
Physics (with lab)	8

Demonstrated proficiency in spoken and written English is required.

Current policy precludes acceptance of Advanced Placement courses for credit toward fulfilling specific requirements in the sciences (biology, chemistry, and physics). The School of Medicine does not accept pass/fail grades for required science courses.

SELECTION FACTORS

The Admissions Committee will evaluate all applicants who are residents of the state of Louisiana. Applicants who are children of alumni who no longer reside in the state or who are applying for the M.D.-Ph.D. program can also be considered for admission. Some of the criteria for admission are: academic factors such as grades and test scores, (average GPA was 3.6; average MCAT was 9.3), strength of the letters of recommendation, strength of the interviews, employment history and whether or not the applicant had to work to go to college, demonstrated history of leadership, demonstrated history of community service, an assessment of all extracurricular activities in which the applicant participated, special honors that have been awarded to the applicant, hobbies and interests, socioeconomic background, where in the state the applicant was raised, and whether there were any factors in the applicant's background that may have hindered him/her from achieving a higher level of academic achievement. There is no discrimination on the basis of race, religion, sex, age, handicap, national origin, or financial status. Transfer students from U.S. medical schools who are nonresidents may be considered for upper-level classes. Interviews are arranged by invitation and are conducted at the medical campus in New Orleans.

FINANCIAL AID

Financial assistance is available for students through several different methods. There are direct scholarship programs, scholarships for disadvantaged students, state and federal loan programs, work-study programs, and employment opportunities in the New Orleans area for students in their third and fourth years. Financial assistance information is available from the Student Financial Aid Office at (504) 568-4820.

INFORMATION ABOUT DIVERSITY PROGRAMS

Members of groups underrepresented in medicine are encouraged to apply. The School of Medicine's Office of Community and Minority Health Education actively recruits students from groups underrepresented in medicine and provides counseling for high school and college students.

Further information may be obtained by contacting Dr. Edward Helm, Associate Dean for Community and Minority Health Education, at (504) 568-8501 or at the address listed on the previous page.

Institution Type: *Public*
Application Process: *AMCAS, see chapter 4.*

APPLICATION AND ACCEPTANCE POLICIES FOR 2005–2006 FIRST-YEAR CLASS

Filing of AMCAS application
    Earliest date: June 1, 2004
    Latest date: Nov. 15, 2004
School application fee to all applicants: $50
Oldest MCAT scores considered: 2001
Does have Early Decision Program (EDP)
    For Louisiana residents only
    EDP application period: June 1, 2004
    EDP applicants notified by: Oct. 1, 2004
Acceptance notice to regular applicants
    Earliest date: Oct. 15, 2004
    Latest date: Varies
Applicant's response to acceptance offer
    Maximum time: 2 weeks
Requests for deferred entrance considered: Yes
Deposit to hold place in class (applied to tuition):
    $100, due with response to acceptance offer
Deposit refundable prior to: May 16, 2005
Estimated number of new entrants: 165 (10 EDP)
Starting date: Aug. 2005

TUITION AND STUDENT FEES PER YEAR FOR 2003–2004 FIRST-YEAR CLASS

Tuition*   Student fees: $2,632
    Resident: $10,426
    Nonresident: $24,574
*Includes one-time cost for laptop computer.

INFORMATION ON 2003–2004 FIRST-YEAR CLASS

Number of	In-State	Out-of-State	Total
Applicants	800	132	932
Applicants Interviewed	401	5	406
New Entrants*	166	1	167

*All took the MCAT and 100% had baccalaureate degrees.

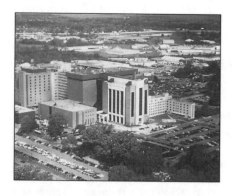

Louisiana State University Health Sciences Center School of Medicine in Shreveport

Shreveport, Louisiana

Dr. John C. McDonald, *Chancellor and Dean*
Dr. F. Scott Kennedy, *Assistant Dean for Student Admissions*
Sherry Gladney, *Associate Director of Student Financial Aid*
Shirley Roberson, *Director for Multicultural Affairs*

ADDRESS INQUIRIES TO:

Office of Student Admissions
Louisiana State University Health Sciences Center
School of Medicine in Shreveport
P.O. Box 33932
Shreveport, Louisiana 71130-3932
(318) 675-5190; 675-8690 (FAX)
E-mail: shvadm@lsuhsc.edu
Web site: www.sh.lsuhsc.edu

MISSION STATEMENT

The Louisiana State University Health Sciences Center (LSUHSC) provides education, research, patient care services, and community outreach. LSU Health Sciences Center encompasses six professional schools: the School of Medicine in New Orleans, the School of Medicine in Shreveport, the School of Graduate Studies in New Orleans and Shreveport, the School of Nursing, the School of Dentistry, and the School of Allied Health Professions in New Orleans and Shreveport.

LSU Health Sciences Center educates health professionals and scientists at all levels. Its major responsibility includes the advancement and dissemination of knowledge in medicine, dentistry, nursing, allied health, public health, and basic sciences. Statewide programs of clinical and basic health science research are developed and expanded by LSU Health Sciences Center. This research results in publications, technology transfer, and related economic enhancements to meet the changing needs of the state of Louisiana and the nation.

LSU Health Sciences Center provides vital public service through direct patient care, including care of indigent patients. Health care services are provided through the LSU Clinics in New Orleans, the LSU Hospital and Clinics in Shreveport, Dental Clinics and Nursing Clinics in New Orleans, the Allied Health Professions Clinics in New Orleans and Shreveport, and numerous affiliated hospitals and clinics throughout Louisiana. LSUHSC also provides coordination and referral services, continuing education, and public information.

LSU Health Sciences Center administers the Health Care Services Division of the LSU System. This division has a dual mission: 1) to assure the availability of acute and primary health care services to the uninsured, to the underinsured, and to others with problems of access to medical care, and 2) to serve as the principal sites for the clinical education of future doctors and other health care professionals.

LSUHSC created and oversees the operation of Area Health Education Centers (AHECs). These corporate entities, governed by boards of prominent citizens, act as liaison agencies between Louisiana's schools of health professions and Louisiana communities. AHEC programs seek to improve the number and distribution of health care providers in rural and urban underserved areas of Louisiana and support existing rural health care providers through continuing education programs.

GENERAL INFORMATION

The Louisiana State University (LSU) School of Medicine in Shreveport, a four-year school, admitted its first class in 1969; the first M.D. degrees were awarded in 1973. Teaching takes place at the school's principal teaching hospital, Louisiana State University Hospital (436 beds), and at the affiliated Shreveport Veterans Administration Hospital (450 beds). Permanent medical school facilities, consisting of a basic and clinical science building, library, and Comprehensive Care Teaching Facility, were occupied in the winter of 1975.

CURRICULUM

The curriculum is traditional in general features but not entirely classical in detail. It is flexible to permit experimentation without disruption. Contact with patients begins early, paralleling a thorough grounding in the basic medical sciences. In addition to short courses in radiology, psychiatry, biometry, and physical examination, live clinics throughout the first and second years serve to indicate application of the basic sciences in clinical medicine. A wide variety of elective instruction is available to first- and second-year students, and one-third of the senior year is elective time on campus or at other institutions. A program of comprehensive care is woven through all four years. The third and fourth years are essentially rotating clerkships in the clinical disciplines. A letter grading system is employed: A, B, C, and F.

REQUIREMENTS FOR ENTRANCE

The MCAT and a minimum of three years of college (at least 90 semester hours) are required. A baccalaureate degree is desirable. Required courses are:

	Sem. hrs.
Biology or Zoology (with lab)	8
Inorganic Chemistry (with lab)	8
Organic Chemistry (with lab)	8
General Physics (with lab)	8
English	6

Prospective applicants are strongly urged to take the MCAT by the spring prior to the year of application and to complete most of the required coursework by the time of application. They should pursue their own particular interests in selecting college courses not required for admission; a broad educational background is desirable.

SELECTION FACTORS

Admission is based upon character, motivation, intellectual ability, and achievement as judged by recommendations of premedical advisors, personal interviews with members of the faculty at the School of Medicine, college grades, and MCAT scores. In recent years, the number of applications filed by well-qualified residents of Louisiana has been in excess of the number of places available. For this reason, places have not been offered to nonresidents. Determination of state residence is provided by LSU system regulations.

Accepted students for the 2003 entering class had the following credentials: *mean science GPA,* 3.6; *mean overall GPA,* 3.7; *sex,* 40 percent *women* (acceptance rate the same for men and women per number of applicants); *residence,* 100 percent from Louisiana; *undergraduate major,* 83 percent in the sciences and chemistry; undergraduate college, 25 schools represented.

The School of Medicine in Shreveport does not discriminate in applicant selection on the basis of race, sex, creed, national origin, age, or handicap.

FINANCIAL AID

Scholarship and long-term, low-interest loan funds are available to students with financial need. In the past, no accepted students have been unable to meet their financial needs. Scholarships and loans are available to students all four years and are based on applicants showing verified need. Certain awards are given in recognition primarily of academic accomplishment and promise. The school offers summer employment to many students but does not advise employment during school sessions, which would interfere with academic performance. Financial need has no bearing on an applicant's acceptance. Applications for financial assistance are furnished by the Financial Aid Office after students have been accepted. Approximately 81 percent of the student body obtain financial aid in the form of loans.

INFORMATION ABOUT DIVERSITY PROGRAMS

Applications from students from groups underrepresented in medicine are encouraged and will be given every consideration.

Institution Type: *Public*
Application Process: *AMCAS, see chapter 4.*

APPLICATION AND ACCEPTANCE POLICIES FOR 2005–2006 FIRST-YEAR CLASS

Filing of AMCAS application
  Earliest date: June 1, 2004
  Latest date: Dec. 15, 2004
School application fee to all applicants: $50
Oldest MCAT scores considered: April 2001
Does have Early Decision Program (EDP)
  For Louisiana residents only
  EDP application period: June 1–August 1, 2004
  EDP applicants notified by: Oct. 1, 2004
Acceptance notice to regular applicants
  Earliest date: Oct. 15, 2004
  Latest date: Until class is filled
Applicant's response to acceptance offer
  Maximum time: 2 weeks
Requests for deferred entrance considered: Yes
Deposit to hold place in class (applied to tuition):
  $250, due by May 1, 2005
Estimated number of new entrants: 100 (8 EDP)
Starting date: August 2005

TUITION AND STUDENT FEES PER YEAR FOR 2003–2004 FIRST-YEAR CLASS

Tuition   Student fees: $487
  Resident: $8,846
  Nonresident: $22,994

INFORMATION ON 2003–2004 FIRST-YEAR CLASS

Number of	In-State	Out-of-State	Total
Applicants	681	214	895
Applicants Interviewed	212	0	212
New Entrants*	100	0	100

*All took the MCAT; 98% had baccalaureate degrees.

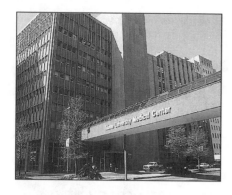

Tulane University School of Medicine

New Orleans, Louisiana

Dr. Ian L. Taylor, *Dean*
Dr. Joseph C. Pisano, *Associate Dean of Admissions*
Michael T. Goodman, *Director of Financial Aid*

ADDRESS INQUIRIES TO:

Office of Admissions
Tulane University School of Medicine
1430 Tulane Avenue, SL67
New Orleans, Louisiana 70112-2699
(504) 588-5187; 988-6735 (FAX)
E-mail: medsch@tulane.edu
Web site: www.mcl.tulane.edu

MISSION STATEMENT

Tulane has a rich tradition of education characterized by an environment that is both supportive and enriching in every sense. It strives to present the ideal environment for preparing students to be expert and compassionate clinicians.

GENERAL INFORMATION

Tulane University School of Medicine, a private, nonsectarian institution, was founded in 1834. Today it is one of the eleven colleges comprising Tulane University and is the 15th oldest medical school in the U.S. The School of Medicine is located in downtown New Orleans, a few blocks from the New Orleans Superdome and the Vieux Carré (French Quarter). While the School of Medicine has affiliation agreements with more than 10 hospitals and clinics in New Orleans and other communities, four of its principal clinical teaching facilities are in close proximity to the School of Medicine: the Medical Center of Louisiana in New Orleans (Charity Hospital), University Hospital (a Charity Hospital), Veterans Affairs Medical Center, and the Tulane University Hospital and Clinic. The School of Medicine and the Tulane University Hospital and Clinic are two components of the Tulane University Health Sciences Center. Other components of the center include: the School of Public Health and Tropical Medicine, the J. Bennett Johnston Center for Bioenvironmental Research, the Tulane National Primate Research Center, and the F. Edward Hébert Research Center. Within the Tulane University Health Science Center are 12 Centers of Excellence that serve as specialized health care education and research hubs for the region. These centers include the Depaul-Tulane Behavioral Health Center, Tulane Cancer Center, Tulane Center for Abdominal Transplant, Tulane Institute of Sports Medicine, Tulane-Xavier National Women's Center, The Tulane Center for Gene Therapy, and Tulane Cardio-Vascular Center of Excellence.

Through the full use of its varied resources, Tulane University School of Medicine is dedicated to conducting the highest-quality educational programs, which will result in academically and clinically prepared physicians (generalists and specialists) and biomedical scientists to satisfy regional, national, and international health needs.

CURRICULUM

The School of Medicine offers a four-year program leading to the M.D. degree. While the emphasis in the first two years is on the principles of the basic medical sciences, the goal of the first two years is helping students develop clinical problem-solving skills instead of emphasizing the transmission of facts devoid of clinical context. The program in Foundations in Medicine, which spans the first two years, is responsible for instructing students in the complex art and science of the patient-doctor interaction. This objective is accomplished through lectures, small-group discussions, clinical demonstrations, visits to community health facilities, and interactions with both real patients and individuals trained as patient instructors. The third and fourth years provide experience in clinical settings where the emphasis is on patient care and community health. Flexibility is attained throughout the four years by allowing approximately one-third of scheduled curriculum time for elective courses and selected advanced studies. Throughout all four years a number of interdisciplinary courses are offered by the combined faculties of the basic and clinical science departments. The course of study and grading methods are under review at all times by faculty and students.

Several combined-degree programs are available to medical students. Work towards a Ph.D. degree in combination with the doctorate in medicine requires concurrent enrollment in the Graduate School and the School of Medicine. Medical students may choose to concurrently enroll in the School of Public Health and Tropical Medicine to complement their doctorate in medicine with an M.P.H. or an M.P.H. and T.M. degree. Students wishing to obtain a public health degree are encouraged to begin their studies in the School of Public Health and Tropical Medicine during the summer before their matriculation into medical school.

Tulane offers a wide variety of support systems for medical students. Such support systems include an academic year tutorial program, study and test-taking skills workshops, and review programs for the USMLE. Academic, career, and personal counseling is available for students upon request.

REQUIREMENTS FOR ENTRANCE

The MCAT and a minimum of three years of college, or 90 semester hours, are required. Four years of college and the baccalaureate degree are strongly recommended.

Applicants are strongly urged to take the MCAT in the spring of the year of application and to have their basic science requirements completed at the time of application. The required courses are:

	Sem./hrs.
Biology or Zoology (with lab)	6
Inorganic Chemistry (with lab)	6
Organic Chemistry (with lab)	6
General Physics (with lab)	6
English	6

In premedical preparation, the major program need not be in one of the science fields. Students are urged to follow their own inclinations in choosing a course of study, recognizing that a physician should have a broad educational background. Approximately one-third of the entering class each year has come from a non-science background.

SELECTION FACTORS

In evaluating applicants, the Committee on Admissions relies on such criteria as grade point averages, MCAT scores, faculty appraisals from the applicant's college, special accomplishments and talents, and the substance and level of courses taken in a particular college. While most successful applicants have attained at least a GPA of 3.5 and a composite MCAT score of 31, Tulane has not established mandatory minimal scores, as all components of the application, cognitive and noncognitive, are taken into account. Because of national priorities, most students accepted must be U.S. citizens. Personal character of the highest order is required along with strong motivation, great potential, and evidence of high-level performance. Tulane University does not discriminate on the basis of race, sex, creed, age, national origin, or handicap.

All completed applications are read in full by members of the Committee on Admissions. Selected applicants are invited for personal interviews, which are held in New Orleans on the medical school campus. Following interview sessions, the committee reviews again an applicant's record during one of its regular weekly meetings. The committee holds the authority to decide whether a candidate should be accepted, rejected, or held for further evaluation at a later date.

FINANCIAL AID

Scholarships and loans (federal, private, and Tulane programs) are available to students based on an analysis of the individual's financial needs. Additionally, each year approximately 25 students are awarded scholarships which are based exclusively upon academic merit. More than 90 percent of the students receive some form of financial assistance during their four years of study.

First-year students ordinarily are encouraged not to undertake employment during the session; this is also true for students in the other years if their scholastic standing would be jeopardized.

INFORMATION ABOUT DIVERSITY PROGRAMS

Tulane encourages qualified disadvantaged students and students from groups underrepresented in medicine to apply. Special activities available for, but not limited to, students from groups underrepresented in medicine include tutorial and counseling services for students in medical school. The diversity in composition of the members of the Committee on Admissions is reflected in the composition of the medical student body.

Institution Type: *Private*
Application Process: *AMCAS, see chapter 4.*

APPLICATION AND ACCEPTANCE POLICIES FOR 2005–2006 FIRST-YEAR CLASS

Filing of AMCAS application
  Earliest date: June 1, 2004
  Latest date: Dec. 15, 2004
School application fee to all applicants: $95
Oldest MCAT scores considered: 2001
Does have Early Decision Program (EDP)
  EDP application period: June 1–Sept. 1, 2004
  EDP applicants notified by: Oct. 1, 2004
Acceptance notice to regular applicants
  Earliest date: Oct. 15, 2004
  Latest date: Until class is filled
Applicant's response to acceptance offer
  Maximum time: 2 weeks
Requests for deferred entrance considered: Yes
Deposit to hold place in class (applied to tuition): $500
Deposit is due on: May 16, 2005
Deposit is nonrefundable
Estimated number of new entrants: 155 (10)
Starting date: Aug. 2005

TUITION AND STUDENT FEES PER YEAR FOR 2003–2004 FIRST-YEAR CLASS

Tuition: $34,986   Student fees: $2,100

INFORMATION ON 2003–2004 FIRST-YEAR CLASS

Number of	In-State	Out-of-State	Total
Applicants	539	6,088	6,627
Applicants Interviewed	240	765	1,005
New Entrants*	39	116	155

*All had baccalaureate degrees and 100% took the MCAT.

CHAPTER
11

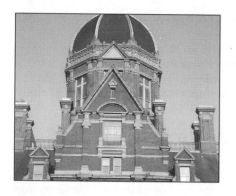

Johns Hopkins University School of Medicine

Baltimore, Maryland

Dr. Edward D. Miller, *The Baker Dean of the Medical Faculty and Chief Executive Officer, Johns Hopkins Medicine*
Paul T. White, *Assistant Dean for Admissions and Financial Aid*
Dr. James L. Weiss, *Associate Dean for Admissions*
Dr. Roland T. Smoot, *Assistant Dean for Student Affairs*

ADDRESS INQUIRIES TO:

Committee on Admission
Johns Hopkins University
School of Medicine
733 North Broadway, Suite G-49
Baltimore, Maryland 21205
(410) 955-3182; (410) 955-7494 FAX
Web site: www.hopkinsmedicine.org

MISSION STATEMENT

The Johns Hopkins University School of Medicine is dedicated to preparing students to practice compassionate medicine of the highest standards and to contributing to the advancement of medical knowledge.

GENERAL INFORMATION

Johns Hopkins University School of Medicine, founded in 1893, is a private, nondenominational institution, which fosters the training of medical practitioners, teachers, and biomedical scientists. The medical center provides: library facilities, the Reed Residence Hall, off-campus housing assistance, cafeterias, recreational sports in the Cooley Center, and performing arts programs.

Preclinical courses are given in the adjacent basic science complex. Medical care facilities such as the Johns Hopkins Hospital and the Outpatient Center provide an extensive and diverse patient base for the teaching of all clinical subjects. Students also attend educational programs conducted at community hospitals in Baltimore and pursue elective experiences at other medical schools in the United States and foreign countries.

The Ross building and other facilities house exceptional opportunities for students to engage in research. A new oncology center, dedicated to patient care and research, has recently opened. Within the Johns Hopkins Medical Institutions are the School of Hygiene and Public Health, School of Nursing, and affiliated centers such as the Kennedy Krieger Institute for children with disorders of the brain.

CURRICULUM

The Johns Hopkins curriculum provides sound foundations in basic sciences and clinical medicine while retaining the flexibility required for students to identify and to develop

diverse career interests. All students receive Honors, High Pass, Pass or Fail grades in lieu of letter grades.

The M.D. program includes the integration of basic sciences and clinical experiences and the expanded use of case-based small-group learning sessions. Students have contact with clinical medicine throughout the first year by working with community physicians. The Physician and Society course spans the four-year program and covers topics such as ethics, finances, legal and political issues, fine arts as they relate to medicine (literature, music, art), and history of medicine.

First Year: Includes integrated coverage of introductory basic sciences, neuroscience, epidemiology, and introduction to clinical medicine.

Second Year: Study of advanced basic sciences, behavioral sciences, clinical skills, and beginning clerkships.

Third and Fourth Years: With the assistance of faculty advisors, students develop individualized programs incorporating required clerkships in major clinical areas and electives. Students may use electives for specialized clerkships, research, and public health experience.

Students interested in academic medicine can obtain combined M.D.-Ph.D. degrees by pursuing coordinated graduate studies in biochemistry and molecular biology, biological chemistry, biomedical engineering, biophysics, cell biology and anatomy, cellular and molecular medicine, epidemiology, history of medicine, human genetics, microbiology and immunology, neurosciences, pathobiology, pharmacology, and physiology. Candidates accepted for M.D.-Ph.D. studies can apply for financial support through the Medical Scientist Training Program, which provides full tuition and stipend. Students may also enroll for special studies or seek advanced degrees in any component of the Johns Hopkins University, including the M.P.H. degree at the School of Hygiene and Public Health.

The deferral plan for admitted applicants provides opportunities for delayed matriculation into the School of Medicine. Deferred admission enables students to plan and pursue alternative education, research, work experience, international fellowships, or humanitarian service, which will enhance their future careers in medicine. For more information on the deferral plan, please contact the Admissions Office.

REQUIREMENTS FOR ENTRANCE

The MCAT is required for admission. The B.A. degree or equivalent is required of all students entering the School of

Medicine. Students are encouraged to complete coherent studies of sciences and liberal arts consistent with their undergraduate major. Required courses are:

Sem. hrs.

General Biology (with lab) 8
General Chemistry (with lab). 8
Organic Chemistry (with lab) 8
 or one term of organic/biochemistry
General Physics (with lab) 8
Humanities and Social and Behavioral Sciences 24
Calculus or Statistics 6

Advanced Placement credit is acceptable for meeting the calculus, general chemistry (plus one semester of advanced chemistry) and physics requirements. A semester of biochemistry may be substituted for one semester of organic chemistry. Students are expected to be proficient in the use of computers. Required courses must be evaluated by a traditional grading system other than pass/fail grades. CLEP credit may not be used to satisfy required courses.

Johns Hopkins participates in AMCAS. Prospective applicants are advised to consult the admissions Web site or contact the Admissions Office for the latest information on admissions requirements and policies. The Hopkins secondary application is available on-line at ☞ www.hopkinsmedicine.org/admissions.

SELECTION FACTORS

In addition to proven academic competence, previous achievements and activities help the Committee on Admission to evaluate applicants' suitability for medicine. Students who have unusual talents, strong humanistic qualities, demonstrated leadership, and creative abilities are sought. There are no residence requirements for U.S. citizens, and applications are invited from candidates in all sections of the country. Medical students in good academic standing may apply for transfer admission. Generally there are few, if any, positions available. The Johns Hopkins University complies with federal and state law prohibiting discrimination.

FINANCIAL AID

Financial aid in the form of federal and institutional grants and loans is awarded solely on the basis of need. Financial considerations do not influence admissions decisions. Approximately 85 percent of matriculating students receive financial assistance. Parents' financial information is required of all students requesting institutional aid. Students are awarded financial aid packages to fully meet their demonstrated financial need. The cost for living expenses is based on a twelve-month budget. Students are able to maintain a moderate lifestyle, because the cost of living in Baltimore is highly affordable. Student fellowship stipends are frequently available for projects carried out in summers.

Non-U.S. citizens without permanent resident or immigrant visa status are not eligible to receive financial aid because of

government restrictions on funds that support the aid program. Qualified foreign students receive final acceptance only after establishing an escrow account acceptable to the School of Medicine that is sufficient to meet all tuition, fees, and living expenses for the anticipated period of enrollment. This amount is currently $200,000 USD.

INFORMATION ABOUT DIVERSITY PROGRAMS

Johns Hopkins is committed to the enrollment and education of individuals from all disadvantaged groups. The school values having a diverse student population from all areas of the country. Hopkins has an excellent record of enrolling students from groups underrepresented in medicine. For information, write Dr. Roland Smoot, assistant dean for student affairs.

Institution Type: *Private*
Application Process: *AMCAS, see chapter 4.*

APPLICATION AND ACCEPTANCE POLICIES FOR 2005–2006 FIRST-YEAR CLASS

Filing of AMCAS application
 Earliest date: June 1, 2004
 Latest date: Oct. 15, 2004
School application fee to all applicants: $75
Oldest MCAT scores considered: 2001
Does have Early Decision Program (EDP)
 EDP application period: June 1–Aug. 15, 2004
 EDP applicants notified by: Oct. 1, 2004
Acceptance notice to regular applicants
 Earliest date: Oct. 15, 2004
 Latest date: April 30, 2005
Applicant's response to acceptance offer
 Maximum time: 3 weeks
Requests for deferred entrance considered: Yes
Deposit to hold place in class: None
Estimated number of new entrants: 120 (3 EDP)
Starting date: Sept. 2005

TUITION AND STUDENT FEES PER YEAR FOR 2003–2004 FIRST-YEAR CLASS

Tuition: $30,900   Student fees: $2,565

INFORMATION ON 2003–2004 FIRST-YEAR CLASS

Number of	In-State	Out-of-State	Total
Applicants	398	5,720	6,118
Applicants Interviewed	63	595	658
New Entrants*	18	101	119

*All students matriculating into four-year program had baccalaureate degrees; 100% took the MCAT.

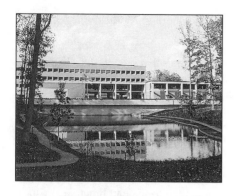

Uniformed Services University of the Health Sciences F. Edward Hébert School of Medicine

Bethesda, Maryland

Dr. Larry W. Laughlin, *Dean*
Peter J. Stavish, LTC, MS, USA (Ret), *Assistant Dean for Admissions and Academic Records*
Joan C. Stearman, *Director, Office of Admissions*

ADDRESS INQUIRIES TO:

Admissions Office, Room A-1041
Uniformed Services University
of the Health Sciences
F. Edward Hébert School of Medicine
4301 Jones Bridge Road
Bethesda, Maryland 20814-4799
(301) 295-3101; 295-3545 (FAX);
1 (800) 772-1743
Web site: www.usuhs.mil
E-mail: admissions@usuhs.mil

MISSION STATEMENT

The Uniformed Services University of the Health Sciences is the nation's federal health sciences university and is committed to excellence in military medicine and public health during peace and war. Our mission is to provide the nation with health professionals dedicated to career service in the Department of Defense and the United States Public Health Service and with scientists who serve the common good.

GENERAL INFORMATION

Created by public law in 1972, the Uniformed Services University of the Health Sciences (USUHS) was founded to prepare young men and women for careers as health care professionals in the uniformed services. The USUHS School of Medicine admitted its charter class in 1976. The school is located on the grounds of the Naval Hospital in Bethesda, Maryland. The school operates in close association with many federal health resources located in the greater Washington, D.C., area to provide students with a broad range of educational experiences in both the basic sciences and clinical medicine. The school's charter is to provide a comprehensive education in medicine to select individuals who demonstrate potential for, and commitment to, careers as medical officers in the uniformed services.

CURRICULUM

The school has a four-year program culminating in the doctor of medicine degree. Each of the first three academic years is 48 weeks, and the final year runs 40 weeks. Basic science instruction predominates in the initial two academic years, with the final two years being devoted to clinical education. Basic science instruction is correlated, as appropriate, both interdisciplinarily and clinically. The integration between the clinical and basic sciences is progressive and proceeds with involvement in patient care activities early in the curriculum, starting with the first semester of the first year. While the overall program is designed to educate students to serve as providers of primary health care, there is sufficient flexibility in the curriculum to accommodate differences in interests among students and also sufficient substances to enable graduates to pursue postgraduate activities such as research. Elective courses are offered in clinical and research facilities in this country and in areas of the world where diseases rarely seen in the United States are responsible for 80 percent of the morbidity and mortality. The curriculum also includes basic military orientation and concentration on unique aspects of military medicine. A conventional letter grading system is employed to record student progress.

REQUIREMENTS FOR ENTRANCE

Applicants must be U.S. citizens between the ages of 18 and 30 and must meet the physical and personal qualifications for a commission in the uniformed services. Applicants cannot be more than 30 years of age as of June 30 in the year of matriculation. Military applicants who have the appropriate creditable commissioned service will be given an age waiver through age 35. Individuals who exceed these age limits will be considered for an age waiver on a case-by-case basis. The MCAT and a baccalaureate degree are required.

The following courses are required:

	Sem. hrs.
General Biology (with lab)	8
General or Inorganic Chemistry (with lab)	8
Organic Chemistry (with lab)	8
Physics (with lab)	8
Calculus	3
English	6

CLEP and Advanced Placement credits are acceptable for required courses. However, individuals exempted from prerequisites through these programs are required to take formal coursework in the same areas at a more advanced level.

Both qualified civilians and military personnel are eligible to apply. However, individuals who are in military service or a program of study sponsored by the Armed Forces (including ROTC and the service academies) must obtain a "Letter of Approval to Apply" from their respective services before making application.

198

SELECTION FACTORS

The school employs a three-stage, progressive screening process for selecting entrants. The first stage consists of the submission of the standard AMCAS application form; the second, the submission of supplementary materials (a premedical committee recommendation and a personal statement describing the applicant's knowledge of and interest in a career in the service are required); and the third, personal interviews, which are conducted at the medical school campus. Advancement in the process is competitive, based on candidates' personal and intellectual characteristics. Applicants should not send transcripts, letters of recommendation, or other such materials unless specifically requested to do so by the Committee on Admissions. The Committee on Admissions does not discriminate on the basis of sex, race, religion, marital status, or national origin.

There were 1,686 applicants for the 2003 first-year class; of this total 465 were interviewed. The 167 entrants had the following credentials: *mean GPA,* 3.53; *mean MCAT,* 9.4; *mean age at time of application,* 24.1 years; *sex,* 40 percent women; *undergraduate major,* 35 percent in biology, with engineering, biochemistry, chemistry, english, and history among others represented; *residence,* 20 percent from northern states, 33 percent from southern states, 38 percent from western states, 9 percent from central states.

SERVICE BENEFITS AND MILITARY OBLIGATION

Upon entering the first-year class of the School of Medicine, the student will be commissioned and will serve on active duty in the grade of second lieutenant in either the Army or Air Force or ensign in the Navy or Public Health Service, receiving the appropriate pay and benefits of that grade. All incoming students will be affected by the new military retirement system if not in the military prior to August 1, 1986. The time spent in medical school is not creditable toward retirement until retirement eligibility has been established.

If current promotion policies continue, the student can expect a promotion in rank to captain in the Air Force or Army or lieutenant in the Navy and Public Health Service upon receipt of the M.D. degree. Graduates are obligated to serve on active duty as medical officers for not less than seven years as well as six years inactive ready reserve. The period of time spent in internship or residency training shall not be acceptable toward satisfying this seven-year obligation. A student who is dropped from the program for either academic deficiencies or other reasons may be required to perform active duty in an appropriate military capacity for a period equal to the time spent in the program. A disenrolled student may also be required to reimburse the government for tuition and fees. However, one year will be the minimum required active duty for persons separated from the school regardless of the time spent in the program.

INFORMATION ABOUT DIVERSITY PROGRAMS

The Office of Recruitment and Diversity at the Uniformed Services University School of Medicine is designed to provide a welcoming environment to all students by promoting and encouraging expression of their diverse ethnic, cultural, economic, and experiential backgrounds. Competitive applicants from groups underrepresented in medicine are actively encouraged to apply. The application and admissions processes are the same for all students.

The Vice President and staff seek to support all students throughout the four years of medical school, recognizing that each individual's unique circumstances may require various levels of support and encouragement. The learning environment is enhanced by participation in the Faculty-Student Mentor Program (administered by the Commandant's office) and the three major student sponsored groups: Women in Medicine and Science, the Asian Pacific American Medical Student Association, and the Student National Medical Association. Administrative and faculty support is provided by the Office of Recruitment and Diversity to advance the community outreach efforts of these student groups.

Institution Type: *Public*
Application Process: *AMCAS, see chapter 4.*

APPLICATION AND ACCEPTANCE POLICIES FOR 2005–2006 FIRST-YEAR CLASS

Filing of AMCAS application
    Earliest date: June 1, 2004
    Latest date: Nov. 1, 2004
School application fee: None
Oldest MCAT scores considered: 2002
Does not have Early Decision Program
Acceptance notice to regular applicants
    Earliest date: Oct. 15, 2004
    Latest date: Until class is filled
Applicant's response to acceptance offer
    Maximum time: 2 weeks
Requests for deferred entrance considered: Yes
Deposit to hold place in class: None
Estimated number of new entrants: 167
Starting date: June 2005

TUITION AND STUDENT FEES PER YEAR FOR 2003–2004 FIRST-YEAR CLASS

There are no tuition or fees for attending the USUHS. Required books, equipment, and instruments are furnished without charge. Students are required to pay for housing, food, and other expenses from their annual salary, which is equivalent to the salary of a second lieutenant in the Army or Air Force, or an ensign in the Navy or Public Health Service.

INFORMATION ON 2003–2004 FIRST-YEAR CLASS

Number of	Total
Applicants	1,686
Applicants Interviewed	465
New Entrants*	167

*All took the MCAT and had baccalaureate degrees.

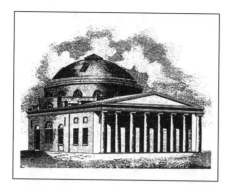

University of Maryland School of Medicine

Baltimore, Maryland

Dr. Donald E. Wilson, *Dean*
Dr. Milford M. Foxwell, Jr., *Associate Dean for Admissions*
Tara Jones, *Acting Director of Financial Aid*
Dr. Donna L. Parker, *Associate Dean for Student and Faculty Development*

ADDRESS INQUIRIES TO:

Committee on Admissions
Room 1-005
University of Maryland
School of Medicine
655 West Baltimore Street
Baltimore, Maryland 21201
(410) 706-7478; (410) 706-0467 (FAX)
Web site: www.medschool.umaryland.edu/admissions

MISSION STATEMENT

The University of Maryland School of Medicine is dedicated to providing excellence in biomedical education, basic and clinical research, quality patient care, and service to improve the health of the citizens of Maryland and beyond. The School is committed to the education and training of M.D., M.D.–Ph.D., graduate, physical therapy, and medical research technology students. The school will recruit and develop faculty to serve as exemplary role models for our students.

GENERAL INFORMATION

The University of Maryland School of Medicine is the fifth oldest medical college in the United States. It was organized in 1807 and chartered in 1808 under the name of the College of Medicine of Maryland; the first class was graduated in 1810. Among the first to erect its own hospital for clinical instruction in 1823, the University of Maryland established the first intramural residency for senior students.

Along with the other professional schools of the University of Maryland (dentistry, law, nursing, pharmacy, social work, and the graduate schools of basic sciences), the School of Medicine is located on the Baltimore City Campus, which is adjacent to the downtown Charles Center, Inner Harbor, Oriole Park at Camden Yards, and M&T Stadium.

CURRICULUM

The basic sciences during the first two years of medical school will be integrated and taught as systems, using interdisciplinary teaching with both basic and clinical science faculty. Problem-based learning has been implemented throughout the basic science years. Contact hours have been reduced, with an emphasis on independent study with the availability of mentors and learning resources. A half-day course in Introduction to Clinical Practice will begin at the inception of the first year and will continue throughout the first two years; the course is dedicated to the instruction of interviewing, physical examination, intimate human behavior, biomedical ethics, and the dynamics of ambulatory care. Much of this experience will be off-site in clinical settings. The clinical clerkships during the last two years of medical school will include a mandatory ambulatory month in family medicine, an emphasis on ambulatory teaching in all other disciplines, and a longitudinal half-day experience in a clinical setting in which the student will have continuity of care for patients and families.

A program offering a combined M.D.-Ph.D. is available for selected applicants. Application forms are included in the Stage II packet. After the preclinical years, M.D.-Ph.D. students perform as full-time graduate students for approximately two years, taking the required graduate courses and seminars and focusing on dissertation research. Following this period, students begin the two years of clinical clerkships, using elective time if necessary to complete Ph.D. research.

REQUIREMENTS FOR ENTRANCE

The MCAT and at least 90 semester hours of accredited arts and science college credit are required. Preference is given to applicants who will have earned a bachelor's degree. The following courses must be completed prior to matriculation:

	Sem. hrs.
Biological Sciences	8
Inorganic Chemistry	8
Organic Chemistry	8
General Physics	8
English	6

Applicants should major in the academic area of their interest. If a nonscience major is selected, sufficient science courses should be taken to acquaint the applicant with the demands of a science-oriented curriculum.

The MCAT must be taken no later than the fall test period of the year in which application is made. It is required that the MCAT be taken within four years preceding the anticipated date of matriculation.

SELECTION FACTORS

Applications are accepted from citizens and permanent residents of the United States and Canada only. All applicants are permitted to submit a direct application (Stage II) after the AMCAS application is received. The deadline for the Stage II application is December 1.

Interviews are arranged for those applicants who appear to have the academic and personal qualities required for successful completion of the requirements for the practice of medicine. All interviews are conducted on campus. Applications may be rejected from both residents and nonresidents without an interview.

Selections are based on a careful appraisal of the individual's character, motivation for medicine, academic achievement, performance on the MCAT, letters of recommendation, extracurricular activities, community service, and interviews by faculty members.

Accepted students for the 2003 entering class had the following characteristics: *average GPA,* 3.63 (range 3.0–4.0); *MCAT average,* 10 (range 6–14); *undergraduate major,* approximately 75 percent science majors; *sex,* 61 percent women; *minorities,* 19 percent.

The University of Maryland School of Medicine does not discriminate on the basis of race, sex, creed, national origin, age, or handicap.

FINANCIAL AID

The school makes available financial aid in the form of scholarships and loans to those students with demonstrable financial need. The amount of the award varies according to the student's needs and the level of funding available. About 70 percent of the students receive some degree of financial aid.

INFORMATION ABOUT DIVERSITY PROGRAMS

The University of Maryland School of Medicine is committed to the recruitment and retention of disadvantaged students and students from groups underrepresented in medicine. A major focus of our recruitment effort is to provide information on admissions requirements, the admissions process, undergraduate preparation for medicine, and education opportunities including the M.D.-Ph.D. program.

All students in the above categories are encouraged to apply. The admissions procedures for students from groups underrepresented in medicine are the same as those for all applicants. Among the selection factors emphasized by the Admissions Committee are undergraduate or graduate GPA, MCAT scores, application essay, and personal characteristics of the applicant, including work or research experience. The interview, letters of recommendation, and the applicant's life experiences help us to evaluate the subjective qualifications.

The school's recruitment coordinator, in conjunction with other support personnel, makes a special effort to provide information relevant to applicants from these groups. There is no fixed quota for any special group within the applicant pool. Information may be obtained from Hermione M. Hicks, director of recruitment, Room 1-005 in the Office of Admissions.

Institution Type: *Public*
Application Process: *AMCAS, see chapter 4.*

APPLICATION AND ACCEPTANCE POLICIES FOR 2005–2006 FIRST-YEAR CLASS

Filing of AMCAS application
  Earliest date: June 1, 2004
  Latest date: Nov. 1, 2004
School application fee to all applicants: $50
Oldest MCAT scores considered: 2001
Does have Early Decision Program (EDP)
  EDP application period: June 1–Aug. 1, 2004
  EDP applicants notified by: Oct. 1, 2004
Acceptance notice to regular applicants
  Earliest date: Oct. 15, 2004
  Latest date: Until class is filled
Applicant's response to acceptance offer
  Maximum time: 3 weeks
Requests for deferred entrance considered: Yes
Deposit to hold place in class: None
Estimated number of new entrants: 150 (10 EDP)
Starting date: Aug. 2005

TUITION AND STUDENT FEES PER YEAR FOR 2003–2004 FIRST-YEAR CLASS

Tuition   Student fees: $2,998
  Resident: $17,493
  Nonresident: $32,558

INFORMATION ON 2003–2004 FIRST-YEAR CLASS

Number of	In-State	Out-of-State	Total
Applicants	772	2,536	3,258
Applicants Interviewed	301	219	520
New Entrants*	112	38	150

*All took the MCAT and 100% had baccalaureate degrees.

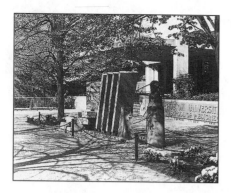

Boston University
School of Medicine

Boston, Massachusetts

Dr. Aram V. Chobanian, *Dean*
Dr. Robert A. Witzburg, *Associate Dean and Director of Admissions*
Dr. Kenneth Edelin, *Associate Dean for Student and Minority Affairs*
Dr. Phyllis L. Carr, *Associate Dean for Student Affairs*

ADDRESS INQUIRIES TO:

Admissions Office
Building L, Room 124
Boston University
School of Medicine
715 Albany Street
Boston, Massachusetts 02118
(617) 638-4630; (617) 638-4718 (FAX)
E-mail: medadms@bu.edu
Web site: www.bumc.bu.edu

MISSION STATEMENT

To educate and train students, physicians, and scientists who will bring superior qualities to the practice of medicine, biomedical research, and public health and who will be prepared for changes in the social, legal and economic climate that will affect the practice of medicine.

GENERAL INFORMATION

In 1848 the New England Female Medical College was founded as the first medical college for women in the world. In 1873 the original buildings and endowment were acquired by Boston University and the name was changed to Boston University School of Medicine. At present the School of Medicine, School of Dental Medicine, School of Public Health, Centers for Advancement in Health and Medicine, and Boston Medical Center constitute the Boston University Medical Campus. All clinical activities at Boston Medical Center are vested in the School of Medicine, and that hospital, together with 21 other health care facilities affiliated with the Medical Center, affords students varied and rich clinical experiences.

CURRICULUM

The curriculum provides the opportunity to study medicine in a flexible environment that stimulates a spirit of critical inquiry and provides sound knowledge in the biological, social, and behavioral sciences. In 1992, Integrated Problems, a course using problem-based learning, was added and Introduction to Clinical Medicine was reinforced. These courses link the discipline-specific work in basic sciences with applications in clinical medicine. They integrate longitudinally through the first two years.

During the first year, the basic medical sciences are emphasized in both departmental and interdisciplinary courses along with human development and community medicine.

The second-year program emphasizes changes in normal structure and function that lead to disease. Major systems pathophysiology is presented in an integrated, multidisciplinary format.

The third year represents the major clerkship year. In addition to the conventional clerkships in medicine, surgery, pediatrics, obstetrics, family medicine and psychiatry, a clerkship in out-patient primary care is included in either the third or fourth year.

The fourth year includes four mandatory clerkships: neurology, radiology, ambulatory primary care, and home medicine. The remainder of the fourth year is devoted to an individual program of electives developed by each student in concert with his/her advisor. Research opportunities are available in basic science and clinical settings in an independent study program. Students may also pursue electives in international health.

A dynamic generalist curriculum in the primary care disciplines of internal medicine, family practice, and pediatrics is presented throughout the four years. Faculty in on-campus practices, as well as in nearby urban and suburban practices serve as mentors and teachers. Primary care medicine is taught in these physicians' office practices, in community health centers, patients' homes, day care centers, and shelters. Experience in rural practice (in the United States and abroad) is also available during the fourth year.

With the approval of the promotions committee, students may complete the first-year requirements over two academic years by taking half the normal course load each year without paying any additional tuition.

In addition to the traditional M.D. degree, students may also pursue a pathway of study leading to the M.D./Ph.D. M.D./M.P.H., or M.D./M.B.A. degrees.

REQUIREMENTS FOR ENTRANCE

Applicants are required to have a baccalaureate degree from an accredited college of arts and sciences. The following courses are required:

	Years
Biology (with lab)	1
Inorganic Chemistry (with lab)	1

Organic Chemistry (with lab)........................ 1
Physics 1
Humanities 1
English Composition or Literature.................. 1

A knowledge of a quantitation in chemistry and calculus is recommended.

Applicants are urged to acquire a broad background in the humanities and behavioral and social sciences in their college years.

All required courses must be completed before medical school work begins. If an applicant has been excused from a required college-level course, another course at the same or higher level must be substituted.

The MCAT is required. Applicants are strongly urged to take the MCAT in the spring of the year of application and to have most of their basic science requirements completed at the time of application. Applicants who have not taken the MCAT by the fall of the application year will not be considered.

SELECTION FACTORS

The Committee on Admissions chooses applicants who seem best qualified not only by scholastic record, college recommendations, and involvement in college and community activities, but also by qualities of personality, character, and maturity. An on-campus interview is an integral part of the admissions process. Applicants who have not heard from the School of Medicine by December 15 and still wish to be considered for an interview should contact the Admissions Office. All interviews are granted at the discretion of the Committee on Admissions. The School of Medicine does not discriminate on the basis of race, sex, age, creed, or national origin. If places are available, applications for transfer may be requested in January.

FINANCIAL AID

The school is committed to equal financial access for all students demonstrating need. Financial assistance is available to students in all years of the medical school curriculum; 78 percent of the student body receive institutional and/or outside support. The school's Office of Student Financial Management administers its portfolio of revolving loans, assists students in securing aid from outside sources, conducts debt management seminars and activities, conducts all required entrance and exit counseling, and provides daily student financial management information. A new series of funds, the Primary Care Pool, has been introduced to promote primary care; students are eligible if they demonstrate need and express interest. Grant aid is minimal, equaling 8 percent of student aid in full-need cases. Most assistance is based upon need. Upon acceptance, students are automatically sent a student assistance response card which generates all necessary forms and information. Financial aid applications and information are available on our Web site at www.bumc.bu.edu/osfs. Financial need is not considered in the admissions process.

There are no special institutional financial funds disbursed for international students. Unless a student has an I-551 or I-151 resident alien card, federally insured loans are not available. Students may secure private educational loans with a co-applicant who is a creditworthy, US citizen or resident alien.

INFORMATION ABOUT DIVERSITY PROGRAMS

Programs for the recruitment and support of students from groups underrepresented in medicine have been developed through the Office of Minority Affairs. Applications are processed through the Committee on Admissions. It is possible to have application fees waived.

Institution Type: *Private*
Application Process: *AMCAS, see chapter 4.*

APPLICATION AND ACCEPTANCE POLICIES FOR 2005–2006 FIRST-YEAR CLASS

Filing of AMCAS application
　Earliest date: June 1, 2004
　Latest date: Nov. 1, 2004
School application fee to all applicants: $100
Oldest MCAT scores considered: 2002
Does have Early Decision Program (EDP)
　EDP application period: June 1–Aug. 1, 2004
　EDP applicants notified by: Oct. 1, 2004
Acceptance notice to regular applicants
　Earliest date: December 2004
　Latest date: Until class is filled
Applicant's response to acceptance offer
　Maximum time: 2 weeks
Requests for deferred entrance considered: No
Deposit to hold place in class (applied to tuition):
　$500, due May 16, 2005; nonrefundable
Estimated number of new entrants: 155 (3 EDP)
Starting date: August 2005

TUITION AND STUDENT FEES PER YEAR FOR 2003–2004 FIRST-YEAR CLASS

Tuition: $36,530　　　　Student fees: $450

INFORMATION ON 2003–2004 FIRST-YEAR CLASS

Number of	In-State	Out-of-State	Total
Applicants	556	8,142	8,698
Applicants Interviewed	135	810	945
New Entrants*	23	132	155

*All took the MCAT; 88% had baccalaureate degrees.

Harvard Medical School

Boston, Massachusetts

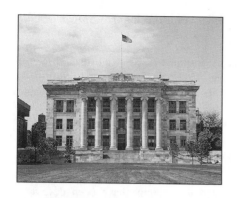

Dr. Joseph B. Martin, *Dean*
Dr. Jules L. Dienstag, *Faculty Associate Dean for Admissions;
    Chair, Committee on Admissions*
Theresa J. Orr, *Associate Dean for Admissions and Student Services*
Dr. Alvin F. Poussaint, *Associate Dean for Student Affairs*

ADDRESS INQUIRIES TO:

Admissions Office
Harvard Medical School
25 Shattuck Street
Boston, Massachusetts 02115-6092
(617) 432-1550; 432-3307 (FAX)
E-mail: admissions_office@hms.harvard.edu
Web site: www.hms.harvard.edu

MISSION STATEMENT

The mission of Harvard Medical School is to create and nurture a community of the best people committed to leadership in ending human suffering caused by disease.

GENERAL INFORMATION

Harvard Medical School was established in 1782. It has occupied its present site in the Longwood Avenue Quadrangle since 1906. Adjacent are the Harvard School of Public Health, the Harvard School of Dental Medicine, and the Francis A. Countway Library. Clinical teaching is carried out in several general and specialized hospitals. These include Massachusetts General, Brigham and Women's, Children's, Beth Israel Deaconess Medical Center, Massachusetts Eye and Ear, Mount Auburn, and Cambridge hospitals. The Massachusetts Mental Health Center and the McLean Hospital are psychiatric facilities. Harvard Vanguard Medical Associates and other community-based health centers provide additional opportunities for patient care, teaching, and research. Other affiliated institutions include the West Roxbury and Brockton VA Medical Centers, the Shriners Burns Institute, and the Spaulding Rehabilitation Hospital. Vanderbilt Hall provides living facilities for single students. Apartments for married students may be found nearby.

PROGRAMS

The New Pathway Program is designed to accommodate the variety of interests, educational backgrounds, and career goals that characterize the student body. Basic science and clinical content are interwoven throughout the four years. In the first and second years, a problem-based approach that emphasizes small-group tutorials and self-directed learning is complemented by laboratories, conferences, and lectures. Students are expected to analyze problems, locate relevant material in library and computer-based resources, and develop habits of lifelong learning and independent study. Clinical clerkships and a wide variety of elective courses and research opportunities are available at Harvard Medical School, its affiliated hospitals, Harvard University, and the Massachusetts Institute of Technology (M.I.T.). One hundred thirty-five students are admitted to this program each year.

A second M.D. pathway is the Harvard–M.I.T. Division of Health Sciences and Technology Program (HST). This program was established jointly by the faculties of these two institutions. The curriculum of this program is designed for the student with a strong interest and background in quantitative science. Courses in the first two years are taught both at Harvard Medical School and M.I.T. with faculty drawn from both institutions. The curriculum is in a semester format. HST students join students of the New Pathway Program for their clinical rotations. A thesis is required for graduation. Thirty students are admitted to this program each year.

The M.D.-Ph.D. Program exists for qualified applicants who wish to integrate medical school and intensive scientific training. Graduate study and research for the Ph.D. are pursued through one of the basic science departments or committees of the Division of Medical Sciences, other departments of the Harvard Graduate School of Arts and Sciences, or the Graduate Schools of Science and Engineering at M.I.T.

Other joint programs are offered in collaboration with the Harvard School of Public Health and the John Fitzgerald Kennedy School of Government.

An internet portal Web site, MyCourses, provides a fully mobile and wireless e-learning educational tool that supports our medical curriculum. Announcements, calendars, course materials (syllabi, images, videos, web links, etc.) are among the materials accessible to students and faculty on their computers and hand-held computing devices.

ACADEMIC SOCIETIES

All students are assigned to one of five academic societies. The societies offer the perspective of smaller groupings of students and faculty who will work together during their time at Harvard Medical School. Each society has a home base in the Tosteson Medical Education Center—a state-of-the-art teaching facility.

REQUIREMENTS FOR ENTRANCE

The MCAT, at least three years of college (preferably four), and a baccalaureate degree are required.

Biology—One year with laboratory experience. Courses taken should focus upon the cellular and molecular aspects as well as the structure and function of living organisms.

Chemistry—Two years with laboratory experience. Full-year courses in general (inorganic) and organic chemistry meet this requirement. Other options that adequately prepare students for the study of biochemistry and molecular biology in medical school will be acceptable.

Physics—One year.

Mathematics—One year of calculus.

Expository writing—One year. May be met with writing, English, or nonscience courses that involve expository writing.

HST Program—Requirements are the same as above except that calculus through differential equations and calculus-based physics are required. A course in biochemistry and preparation in molecular biology are encouraged.

A variety of course formats and combinations that provide equivalent preparation will be accepted. Advanced Placement credits may be used to satisfy the calculus requirement and one semester of the chemistry and physics requirements for the New Pathway program. In addition to the writing requirement, at least 16 credit hours should be completed in nonscience courses. No preference is shown toward students majoring in the sciences over students majoring in nonscience areas.

Applicants educated abroad must have completed at least one year of study in an approved college or university in the United States or Canada before applying. Foreign students who do not have a baccalaureate or advanced degree from an institution in the United States or Canada are rarely accepted for admission.

Students who have been enrolled in medical school or who have applied to us on two prior occasions are ineligible to apply.

SELECTION FACTORS

Academic excellence is expected. For the 2003 entering class, the *average GPA* was 3.8, with a range that was broader, and the *average MCAT scores* were VR-10.6, PS-11.8, and BS-11.6, with a range that was in keeping with the national average. Other factors considered include the essay, out-of-classroom activities, and life experiences. Research and community work and comments contained in letters of recommendation are considered. We look for evidence of integrity, maturity, humanitarian concerns, leadership potential, and an aptitude for working with people. Interviews are scheduled selectively and are conducted on campus. Please note that secondary applications are automatically sent to all applicants, and early application is strongly encouraged.

The Committee on Admissions welcomes applications from qualified students representing groups that historically have been underrepresented in medicine. Harvard Medical School is committed to the enrollment of a diverse body of talented students who will reflect the character of the American people whose health needs the medical profession must serve.

Harvard Medical School does not discriminate on the basis of race, color, religion, sex, sexual preference, age, or disability unrelated to course of study requirements.

The 2003 entering class came from 66 different colleges. Fifty-one percent were women, and 23 percent were from groups underrepresented in medicine.

Harvard Medical School does not invite applications for advanced standing because opportunities for transfer are not available.

FINANCIAL AID

All financial aid is awarded on the basis of need. A vigorous effort is made to assist accepted applicants in meeting their medical education costs through loans, medically related employment, and scholarships.

Foreign students who are not U.S. permanent residents are eligible to be considered for need-based institutional scholarships and loans. Approximately 70 percent of the student body receives financial aid.

For further information, contact the Financial Aid Office at (617) 432-1575.

Institution Type: *Private*
Application Process: *AMCAS, see chapter 4.*

APPLICATION AND ACCEPTANCE POLICIES FOR 2005–2006 FIRST-YEAR CLASS

Filing of AMCAS application
  Earliest date: June 1, 2004
  Latest date: Oct. 15, 2004
School application fee to all applicants: $75
Oldest MCAT scores considered: 2001
Does not have Early Decision Program
Acceptance notice to regular applicants
  Earliest date: Feb. 28, 2004
  Latest date: March 10, 2004
Applicant's response to acceptance offer
  Maximum time: 3 weeks
Requests for deferred entrance considered: Yes
Deposit to hold place in class: None
Estimated number of new entrants: 165
Starting date: Sept. 2005

TUITION AND STUDENT FEES PER YEAR FOR 2003–2004 FIRST-YEAR CLASS

Tuition: $32,000   Student fees: $2,776

INFORMATION ON 2003–2004 FIRST-YEAR CLASS

Number of	In-State	Out-of-State	Total
Applicants	342	4,979	5,321
Applicants Interviewed	65	655	720
New Entrants*	14	151	165

*All took the MCAT and had baccalaureate degrees.

CHAPTER

11

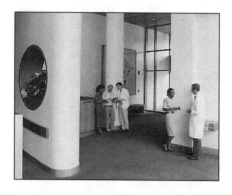

Tufts University School of Medicine

Boston, Massachusetts

Dr. Michael Rosenblatt, *Dean*
Dr. Robert C. Sarno, *Dean for Admissions*
Thomas M. Slavin, *Director of Admissions*
Colleen Romain, *Director of Minority Affairs*

ADDRESS INQUIRIES TO:

Office of Admissions
Tufts University
School of Medicine
136 Harrison Avenue
Boston, Massachusetts 02111
(617) 636-6571
E-mail: med-admissions@tufts.edu
Web site: www.tufts.edu/med

MISSION STATEMENT

To produce a competent, compassionate physician who is skilled and well-educated in a core of general knowledge; one who is capable of building on this core to achieve educational and career goals and to maintain the task of lifelong learning.

GENERAL INFORMATION

Tufts University was founded in 1852 as a liberal arts college in Medford, Massachusetts, and has since grown into a modern university whose School of Medicine was established in Boston in 1893. The medical school is located within a health sciences complex, which includes the dental school, veterinary school, Sackler School of Graduate Biomedical Sciences, Sackler Center for Health Communications, Nutrition Center, and the New England Medical Center. The medical school buildings, located in the center of Boston, house the preclinical departments, research laboratories, administrative offices, seminar rooms, lecture rooms, and the library. Close association of the School of Medicine with 30-plus hospitals affords ample facilities for clinical experience.

CURRICULUM

The initial phase of the curriculum focuses on the biology of cells and their constituent molecules followed by a segment dealing with the structure and development of tissues and organs. This is followed by the functions of the organs and the organism and its environment. The biology of normal cells, tissues, and organs is presented before the students are exposed to the pathological manifestations of these components. The curriculum also includes those aspects of the nonbiological sciences that are relevant to health care delivery and patient care, such as nutrition, health care economics, family medi-

cine, ethics, and history of medicine. The program also emphasizes problem solving and critical, analytical discussion in small groups instead of rote learning based on a large number of lectures. A strong emphasis on the use of problem-based learning, teaching based on case studies, is an aspect of the curriculum. The cases chosen have been closely coordinated with the material from the ongoing segments of the curriculum but provide opportunities for student learning in a wide range of areas, including ethics, socioeconomics, history, culture, and the physician-patient relationship. The Preclinical Elective Program is designed to encourage students to pursue outside interests and talents as well as to foster meaningful faculty-student relationships. Students can explore opportunities in basic science, clinical medicine, or community aspects of medicine. In addition, faculty are able to work more closely with students and to serve as role models, mentors, and informal advisors.

The third year consists of rotations through the major clinical specialties and an elective period.

The fourth year consists of a minimum of eight four-week rotations. Five of these eight must be taken at Tufts-affiliated hospitals; of these, two must be ward service rotations and one must be the clinical specialties rotation. Beyond these requirements, students are free to schedule approved learning experiences as part of their elective rotations at the Tufts-associated hospitals or elsewhere in the United States or abroad.

Tufts offers a combined M.D.-M.P.H. program, leading to the awarding of both degrees in four years. The program is fully accredited by the Council on Education for Public Health and provides basic grounding in epidemiology and biostatistics, health planning and management, environmental health, and the behavioral sciences. A public health field experience and advanced coursework are essential parts of the program, which is fully integrated into the medical curriculum.

Tufts, in collaboration with Northeastern and Brandeis Universities, now offers a combined M.D.-M.B.A. degree in health management. The changing nature of the nation's health care system has created a demand for physicians who are trained to plan and manage these changes in the best interests of patients, health care organizations, and the community. The curriculum is designed to provide students with a foundation in business problem-solving skills and knowledge in health care management. M.D.-M.B.A. candidates will begin their studies the summer before the start of medical school and devote the summer between the first and second years of medical school to M.B.A. courses. Tufts also offers an M.D.-Ph.D. program.

REQUIREMENTS FOR ENTRANCE

The MCAT and a minimum of three years of college are required. College credits must include:

	Years
Biology (with lab)	1
Inorganic Chemistry (with lab)	1
Organic Chemistry (with lab)	1
Physics (with lab)	1

SELECTION FACTORS

The selection of candidates for admission to the first year is based not only on performance in the required premedical courses, but also on the applicant's entire academic record and extracurricular experiences. Letters of recommendation and additional information supplied by the applicant are reviewed for indications of promise and fitness for a medical career. Personal interviews are a prerequisite for admission and are granted only by invitation of the Admissions Committee. Preference is given to American citizens and permanent residents who will receive a bachelor's degree from an American college or university prior to matriculation.

Tufts has a strong commitment to affirmative action and seeks to provide an atmosphere of nondiscrimination for members of groups underrepresented in medicine as well as an accessible campus and support services for persons with disabilities.

Tufts accepts transfers from other American, LCME-accredited medical schools into the second- and third-year classes in years when vacancies have been created by attrition. The number of seats available has traditionally been extremely limited. In some years, no transfer openings are available.

FINANCIAL AID

Up to 75 percent of students participate in the federal government's student loan programs at some time during their four years of study. Additionally, limited scholarship and loan assistance is available directly from Tufts for students who qualify on the basis of need. Approximately 33 percent of the students receive financial aid directly from Tufts at some time during their four years of study.

There are no rules prohibiting outside employment; however, first- and second-year students are urged not to seek outside work. Some opportunities for part-time employment are available in the various hospitals and in the medical school.

In situations of extreme financial need, the $95 application fee may be waived if AMCAS has first granted a similar waiver.

Institution Type: *Private*
Application Process: *AMCAS, see chapter 4.*

APPLICATION AND ACCEPTANCE POLICIES FOR 2005–2006 FIRST-YEAR CLASS

Filing of AMCAS application
    Earliest date: June 1, 2004
    Latest date: Nov. 1, 2004
School application fee to all applicants: $95
Oldest MCAT scores considered: 2002
Does have Early Decision Program (EDP)
    EDP application period: June 1–Aug. 1, 2004
    EDP applicants notified by: Oct. 1, 2004
Acceptance notice to regular applicants
    Earliest date: Dec. 1, 2004
    Latest date: Until class is filled
Applicant's response to acceptance offer
    Maximum time: 2 weeks
Requests for deferred entrance considered: Yes
Deposit to hold place in class (applied to tuition):
    $100, due with response to acceptance offer
Deposit refundable prior to: May 16, 2005
Estimated number of new entrants: 168 (2 EDP)
Starting date: Aug. 2005

TUITION AND STUDENT FEES PER YEAR FOR 2003–2004 FIRST-YEAR CLASS

Tuition: $39,579   Student fees: $555

INFORMATION ON 2003–2004 FIRST-YEAR CLASS

Number of	In-State	Out-of-State	Total
Applicants	583	7,624	8,207
Applicants Interviewed	225	692	917
New Entrants*	57	113	170

*All took the MCAT and had baccalaureate degrees.

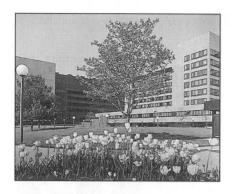

University of Massachusetts Medical School

Worcester, Massachusetts

Dr. Aaron Lazare, *Chancellor/Dean*
Dr. John Paraskos, *Associate Dean for Admissions*
Judith L. Case, *Director of Financial Aid*
Dr. Danna B. Peterson, *Assistant Dean of Student Affairs*

ADDRESS INQUIRIES TO:

Associate Dean for Admissions
University of Massachusetts Medical School
55 Lake Avenue, North
Worcester, Massachusetts 01655
(508) 856-2323
E-mail: admissions@umassmed.edu
Web site: www.umassmed.edu/education/admit.cfm

MISSION STATEMENT/GENERAL INFORMATION

Established in 1962, the University of Massachusetts Medical School accepted its first class in 1970. The school's founding mission was to provide high-quality and accessible medical education for the residents of Massachusetts. The University of Massachusetts Medical School is committed to training physicians in a wide range of medical disciplines and also emphasizes training for practice in general medicine and the primary care specialties, in the public sector and in underserved areas of Massachusetts. This mission has since been expanded to include graduate education in the biomedical sciences and nursing, graduate medical education, and continuing medical education for health professionals. The school's clinical partner is UMass Memorial Medical Center, which comprises two acute care hospitals with a total of 761 beds. Clinical education is also conducted at a number of affiliated community hospitals and health centers in the region. UMass Worcester is adjacent to the Massachusetts Biotechnology Research Park, which houses a number of UMass research programs including the Program in Molecular Medicine, the Cancer Center, and the Worcester Foundation for Biomedical Research.

CURRICULUM

The educational program stresses interdisciplinary learning and integration of the basic and clinical sciences, with special attention to clinical correlation of subject matter in the preclinical years. Emphasis in the first year is on normal structure and function, with a balance of small-group learning and large-group teaching. Through a longitudinal preceptorship program, students are provided with patient involvement beginning immediately in year one and continuing throughout the first two years. Emphasis in the second year is on the etiology of disease, pathophysiology, pharmacology, and clinical diagnosis. The two-year course on the Patient, Physician, and Society (PPS) runs throughout the preclinical program and integrates the basic sciences into

medical interviewing, clinical problem solving, biomedical ethics, preventive medicine, epidemiology, and medical informatics. Led by a diversity of senior faculty, students in the PPS course learn through an interdisciplinary model and work in small groups to experience a collaborative team approach to patient care and case-based clinical problem solving.

The third and fourth years are a continuum of required clerkships and both clinical and research electives. Elements of the PPS course are revisited in the clinical years through one-week interclerkship courses, which address a broad range of important issues using an interdisciplinary approach, which combines the clinical and basic sciences. Interclerkships have addressed diverse subjects including domestic violence, environmental medicine, managed care, nutrition, and substance abuse. An International Health Program is also available for students interested in clinical and/or research experience abroad and in underserved areas of the United States. Over one-third of UMass students benefit from an international health experience. The program coordinates and oversees the placement of students in electives worldwide, and provides a learning opportunity in which students experience and understand different cultures while serving those populations most in need.

The faculty of the medical school also encourages medical students to participate in research programs in basic and clinical science departments. A combined Ph.D./M.D. program in basic medical sciences is also offered.

REQUIREMENTS FOR ENTRANCE

The MCAT is required and must be taken within the last three years. A baccalaureate degree is required. Required courses that must be taken within the last six years are:

Years

Biology (with lab) 1
Inorganic Chemistry (with lab) 1
Organic Chemistry (with lab). 1
Physics (with lab) 1
English 1

Credit for any secondary school course may be given only if such credit appears on the college transcript. Applicants may major in the areas of either sciences or humanities, and in either case independent study is encouraged. Students able to do so are encouraged to take such courses as biochemistry, calculus, statistics, sociology, or psychology. Applicants are encouraged to complete the basic science requirements by the time of application since consideration will be delayed if required courses are in progress.

SELECTION FACTORS

Current policy limits admission to the M.D. program to students who are Massachusetts residents. Residents and non-residents of Massachusetts are eligible for admission to the joint PhD/MD Program through the Graduate School of Biomedical Sciences and the School of Medicine. All applicants must be United States citizens or have permanent resident status. The Committee on Admissions bases its evaluation of applicants on academic ability and achievement, scores on the MCAT, and such factors as extracurricular achievement, maturity, motivation, and character as these are reflected in letters of recommendation from preprofessional advisory committees and other persons. Interviews are arranged by invitation only. Applicants are selected on the basis of their individual merits without regard to race, sex, creed, national origin, age, or disability. UMass has a set of technical standards for admission and promotion, which are available upon request. All supplementary materials must be received by December 15.

Accepted students for the class entering August 2000 had the following credentials: *science GPA,* approximately 3.6; *sex,* 55 percent women; *undergraduate major,* 60 percent in science and 40 percent in nonscience.

FINANCIAL AID

Students otherwise unable to finance their medical education should consider applying for financial aid. The Financial Aid Office sends appropriate materials and establishes individual financial aid application deadlines when applicants are accepted or placed on the alternate list. Applicants for only Federal Stafford Loans need not supply parental information on the FAFSA. Applicants for campus-based funds are required to provide complete parental financial information and signatures on both the FAFSA and the CSS Profile Form.

The financial aid application comprises the UMass Medical School Financial Aid Application, the FAFSA, the Profile Form of the College Scholarship Service, and parental and student federal income tax returns and W-2 forms.

Financial aid funds are disbursed according to institutional packaging policy established by the Student Affairs Committee. Approximately 99 percent of the student body receive some combination of scholarships, loans, and/or employment. UMass Medical School offers all students, regardless of financial need, the option of entering into a learning contract that gives students the choice of paying full tuition or deferring a portion (currently two-thirds) of tuition until after residency training. Graduates must begin payment with either money or service no later than six months after completing residency or fellowship training. Service to the Commonwealth may be provided by practicing primary care medicine anywhere in the state, practicing medical specialties in under-

served areas in the state, or completing an approved activity of particular benefit to the Commonwealth. Students not able to provide service will be charged eight percent interest; interest begins accruing after completion of the medical internship. Payment may not exceed eight years.

INFORMATION FOR DISADVANTAGED STUDENTS

Please contact the associate vice chancellor for school services for additional information on programs for disadvantaged students.

Institution Type: *Public*
Application Process: *AMCAS, see chapter 4.*

APPLICATION AND ACCEPTANCE POLICIES FOR 2005–2006 FIRST-YEAR CLASS

Filing of AMCAS application
   Earliest date: June 1, 2004
   Latest date: Nov. 1, 2004
School application fee to all applicants: $75
Oldest MCAT scores considered: 2002
Does have Early Decision Program (EDP)
   EDP application period: June 1–Aug. 1, 2004
   EDP applicants notified by: Oct. 1, 2004
Acceptance notice to regular applicants
   Earliest date: Oct. 15, 2004
   Latest date: Varies
Applicant's response to acceptance offer
   Maximum time: 2 weeks
Requests for deferred entrance considered: Yes
Deposit to hold place in class (applied to tuition):
   $100, due with response to acceptance offer
Deposit refundable prior to: May 16, 2004
Estimated number of new entrants: 100 (10 EDP)
Starting date: Aug. 2005

TUITION AND STUDENT FEES PER YEAR FOR 2003–2004 FIRST-YEAR CLASS

Tuition   Student fees: $4,750
   Resident: $8,352
   Nonresident: N/A

INFORMATION ON 2003–2004 FIRST-YEAR CLASS

Number of	In-State	Out-of-State	Total
Applicants	621	0	621
Applicants Interviewed	349	0	349
New Entrants*	100	0	100

*All took the MCAT and had baccalaureate degrees.

CHAPTER

11

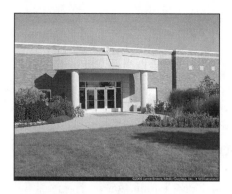

Michigan State University College of Human Medicine

East Lansing, Michigan

Dr. Glenn C. Davis, *Dean*
Dr. Christine L. Shafer, *Assistant Dean for Admissions*
Dr. Wanda D. Lipscomb, *Assistant Dean for Student Affairs and Services*

ADDRESS INQUIRIES TO:

College of Human Medicine
Office of Admissions
A-239 Life Sciences
Michigan State University
East Lansing, Michigan 48824-1317
(517) 353-9620; 432-0021 (FAX)
E-mail: MDAdmissions@msu.edu
Web site: www.chm.msu.edu

MISSION STATEMENT

The mission of the College of Human Medicine is to educate physicians who are exemplary in the art and science of medicine, responsive to the needs of medically underserved communities in Michigan, and considerate of the dignity, diversity, and values of patients and their families.

GENERAL INFORMATION

The College of Human Medicine (CHM) was founded in 1964 in response to Michigan's need for primary care physicians. CHM, a four-year medical school located on an active Big 10 campus, provides a small college atmosphere with an entering class of 106. The average student age is 25 (range 21–45) with men and women equally represented. Students spend the first two years at the East Lansing campus where they are taught in the classroom, laboratory, and clinical settings before moving on to one of the six community campuses for clinical training in realistic health care settings. Approximately 2,500 clinical and adjunct faculty join the more than 200 clinical and basic science faculty members in providing this unique learning environment.

CURRICULUM

The curriculum is divided into three blocks organized around a commitment to the integration of the basic biological, behavioral, and social sciences; a developmental approach to learning; early teaching of clinical skills; and clinical training utilizing a community-integrated approach.

Grading is on a modified pass/no pass system. Honors-level performance is recognized with a letter of recognition during the first two years and by a grade of "pass with honors" during the clerkship years.

Block I is a three-semester experience comprising the first year in which fundamental basic science concepts and principles are presented in a structured, discipline-based format. Basic clinical skills teaching begins, along with a mentor group experience, a longitudinal patient care experience, and opportunity to participate in independent as well as supplementary learning experiences. A clinical correlations course integrates basic science information, connects these sciences to medicine, and models a team approach to the practice of medicine.

Block II is a two-semester experience comprising the second year in which advanced basic science concepts are organized in an integrated, problem-based format. Emphasis is on small-group instruction and problem solving. A clinical context for learning basic science concepts is also provided. Clinical skills training continues along with special topics seminars, which deal with contemporary issues in society and medicine.

Block III includes 60 weeks of required and 20 weeks of elective clerkships. Students live in Flint, Grand Rapids, Kalamazoo, Lansing, Saginaw, or the Upper Peninsula during their required clerkships. Their experiences are in a variety of hospital and ambulatory care settings. The required clerkships include a family practice/primary care clerkship with exposure to the comprehensive and continuous care of patients and families. Students have the option to complete elective clerkships in other locations including third world countries.

REQUIREMENTS FOR ENTRANCE

The MCAT and a baccalaureate degree from an accredited college or university are required. Fifteen percent of the 2003 entering class hold graduate or professional degrees.

Applicants should select the academic major that best links their interests and talents since no specific major is preferred over another. A solid background in the arts, humanities, and social sciences is recommended.

Specific course requirements with no grade less than a 2.0 are:

Sem./Qtr. hrs.

General Biology sequence (one lab) 8/12
General Chemistry sequence (one lab) 8/12
Organic Chemistry sequence (one lab) 8/12
General Physics sequence (one lab) 8/12
English Writing (writing in the major) 8/12
Humanities/Social Science 8/12

Mathematics through college algebra or statistics and probability (waived with AP credit for Calculus 1, or first-year mathematics placement above college algebra) is required.

Completion of one upper-level (third- or fourth-year) biological science course from the following: biochemistry, cell biology, embryology, genetics, microbiology, molecular biology, neuroscience, or physiology, is also required.

SELECTION FACTORS

All application materials are reviewed prior to an initial decision. Approximately 800 applicants will be invited to complete the secondary application. Because MSU/CHM is a state school, approximately 80 percent of the entering class will be Michigan residents.

The college seeks to admit a class that is academically competent, reflective of both the rural and urban character of Michigan, and representative of a wide spectrum of personalities, backgrounds, and talents. Students who have the desire and aptitude to become physicians but who may be disadvantaged due to economic, cultural or educational background, or to family circumstances are encouraged to apply.

From approximately 3,000 applicants reviewed by the Committee on Admissions, approximately 400 applicants will be invited to Interview Day at the East Lansing campus for interviews with faculty and medical students. Selection is based on many factors, including the GPA, both year to year and cumulative; MCAT scores; fit with the school's mission; relevant community service experience; interviewers' assessments of motivation, ability to communicate, problem-solving ability, maturity, and suitability for the MSU program; state of residence; and potential to contribute to the overall quality of the entering class.

Special Programs include the Rural Physicians Program (RPP), which incorporates the successful Upper Peninsula Program that was established to meet special health care needs of patients in remote, medically underserved rural areas of Michigan through training physicians to provide on-site health care in these areas. Applicants to this program will need to complete additional essays and interviews. The Medical Scholars Program, available to high school seniors, awards combined B.A./B.S.-M.D. degrees. Opportunity exists for M.D.-Ph.D. programs as well as master's degrees in epidemiology, and ethics and humanities in the life sciences.

FINANCIAL AID

Information about specific scholarships and about financial aid can be obtained from the Office of Financial Aid, 252 Student Services Building or their Web site at www.finaid.msu.edu. Ability to pay is not considered in the selection process.

INFORMATION ABOUT DIVERSITY PROGRAMS

The College of Human Medicine enjoys a diverse student body. Approximately 17% of each entering class is from groups underrepresented in medicine with overall enrollment from these groups greater than 20% of the 2003 entering class. The college also offers a postbaccalaureate program, ABLE, for a few selected students. ABLE is designed for disadvantaged medical school applicants who have been invited to participate in a 13-month enriched academic experience that will result in regular admissions if successfully completed. Questions about the pre-matriculation programs and services afforded to students from groups underrepresented in medicine should be addressed to the Assistant Dean for Admissions.

Institution Type: *Public*
Application Process: *AMCAS, see chapter 4.*

APPLICATION AND ACCEPTANCE POLICIES FOR 2005–2006 FIRST-YEAR CLASS

Filing of AMCAS application
  Earliest date: June 1, 2004
  Latest date: Nov. 15, 2004
School application fee to all applicants: $60
Oldest MCAT scores considered: 2002
Does have Early Decision Program (EDP)
  EDP application period: June 1–Aug. 1, 2004
  EDP applicants notified by: Oct. 1, 2004
Acceptance notice to regular applicants
  Earliest date: Oct. 15, 2004
  Latest date: Varies
Applicant's response to acceptance offer
  Maximum time: 2 weeks
Requests for deferred entrance considered: Yes
Deposit to hold place in class: $100, due with response to acceptance offer
Deposit refundable prior to: May 16, 2005
Estimated number of new entrants: 106 (10 EDP)
Starting date: Aug. 2005

TUITION AND STUDENT FEES PER YEAR FOR 2003–2004 FIRST-YEAR CLASS

Tuition (3 semesters)   Student fees: $2,303
  Resident: $19,726
  Nonresident: $43,526

INFORMATION ON 2003–2004 FIRST-YEAR CLASS

Number of	In-State	Out-of-State	Total
Applicants	1,025	1,825	2,850
Applicants Interviewed	251	111	362
New Entrants*	85	21	106

*100% had baccalaureate degrees; 88% took the MCAT.

CHAPTER 11

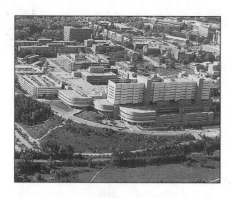

University of Michigan Medical School

Ann Arbor, Michigan

Dr. Allen S. Lichter, *Dean*
Dr. Daniel G. Remick, *Assistant Dean of Admissions*
Dr. David Gordon, *Assistant Dean for Diversity and Career Development*

ADDRESS INQUIRIES TO:

Admissions Office
4303 Medical Science I Building
University of Michigan Medical School
Ann Arbor, Michigan 48109-0624
(734) 764-6317; 763-0453 (FAX)
Web site: www.med.umich.edu/medschool/

MISSION STATEMENT

The University of Michigan Medical School seeks to graduate a diverse cohort of physicians who are dedicated to life-long learning. Our goals include educating individuals committed to achieving the highest standards of competency required to provide exemplary patient care. We seek to graduate culturally competent physicians who will assume leadership roles in the areas of clinical medicine, research, and teaching. Physicians who graduate from the University of Michigan will demonstrate a strong foundation in biomedical sciences; empathetic interpersonal skills; an ability to identify and reduce health risk factors; an ability to obtain and interpret relevant patient information and to make effective clinical decisions; a commitment to achieving personal and professional excellence; and the critical attributes of compassion, honesty, and integrity.

GENERAL INFORMATION

The University of Michigan Medical School was founded in 1850. This school was the first to establish a university-owned hospital. Today, the medical center occupies more than 30 buildings, the world's largest one-site complex devoted to health care, education, and research. The Health System consistently ranks as one of the top ten in the nation. Instructional sites also include nearby tertiary care hospitals and ambulatory care facilities.

CURRICULUM

The medical school instituted a revised curriculum in August 2003. In planning curriculum improvements, the faculty designed a robust and multi-faceted program that provides structured learning opportunities to help students achieve very high-level skills. In the first year, the introductory Patients and Populations course acquaints medical students with genetics, principles of disease, epidemiology, and evidence-based medicine. After that, most of the material is structured within Normal Organ Systems sequences and a Microbiology and Infectious Disease course.

Clinical skills are taught in focused one- and two-week modules throughout the first and second years, beginning with the medical interview and history-taking skills and moving to physical examination practice. In the two-year Family Centered Experience, pairs of first-year students are assigned to a family in the community. These families will serve as resources to help medical students understand how health changes, chronic conditions, and serious illnesses affect patients and those close to them.

The second year curriculum features Abnormal Organ Systems sequences. It includes additional patient cases and continuing reinforcement of information gathering and critical appraisal skills. Clinical skills modules will continue with expectations for mastery of more advanced physical examination, history-taking, and communication skills.

Clinical training in the third year includes required rotations, but also includes opportunities for career exploratory electives. Fourth-year requirements include a subinternship and an ICU experience, as well as a course in Advanced Medical Therapeutics. In the subinternship, students are assigned their own patient caseload and they perform with almost the same level of responsibility as a resident. The fourth year includes eight weeks of vacation and interviewing time, as well as twelve weeks of electives, with opportunities for off-campus and international rotations.

All courses in the first year are graded pass/fail. In the subsequent years, faculty assign students grades of honors, high pass, pass, or fail. Students are required to pass the USMLE, Step 1, before promotion to the clinical phase in the third year, and are required to pass USMLE, Step 2, before graduation.

Opportunities exist for individual research summer programs or for special research fellowships. Students also have the option to pursue a combined M.D.–Ph.D. curriculum either as a fellow in the Medical Scientist Training Program or as a graduate student in one of the basic science departments. Combined degrees with the School of Public Health (M.D./M.P.H.) and the School of Business Administration (M.D./M.B.A.) are available. Both programs are five years in length. Medical students typically apply to these two combined programs once they are enrolled in the medical curriculum.

The learning contexts, teaching methods, and expectations are designed to maintain the strengths of U-M's curriculum for the M.D. degree, and to enhance learning with the ultimate goal of graduating highly-qualified, compassionate, physician leaders who remain committed to excellence throughout their lives.

REQUIREMENTS FOR ENTRANCE

The MCAT and a minimum of 90 semester hours of university work are required. Grades below C in required courses are not acceptable. The specific course requirements are:

	Sem. hrs.
Biology (with lab)	6
General/Inorganic and Organic Chemistry (with lab)	8
Biochemistry	3
Physics (with lab)	6
English Composition and Literature	6
Nonscience/Humanities	18

SELECTION FACTORS

The Admissions Committee is dedicated to matriculating those individuals with the skills, intelligence, and personal attributes to become leaders in medicine. Although admitted students all have demonstrated the ability to succeed academically, other attributes such as compassion, empathy, altruism, leadership, honesty, and communication and interpersonal skills are viewed as being critical to future excellence. The Committee considers that all information pertaining to the ability, personality, and character of the applicant is relevant. Although a solid background in science is required, students with expertise in a wide variety of fields, including humanities, arts, and engineering, are encouraged to apply.

All applicants are requested to fill out a secondary application online, but only about 40 percent of applicants are asked to complete the application by submitting letters of reference. The mean undergraduate GPA for admitted students has been about 3.7 in recent years. Reports from college faculty, especially those who know the student best and have experience with pre-med students, are important. While only three years of undergraduate work are required, nearly all admitted students will have completed baccalaureate and more advanced degrees.

Interviews are offered to applicants based on review of submitted information and supporting documents. The interview is usually held in Ann Arbor. Applicants must have had at least one year, and preferably more, of their premedical training in the United States or Canada. Non-U.S. citizens must have a permanent resident visa in the United States. Any applicant who has been enrolled previously in a medical school in a program leading to the M.D. degree must be in good standing and eligible for re-entry to that school in order to be considered for admission to the University of Michigan Medical School. The medical school cannot accept transfer students from other medical schools or health care programs.

FINANCIAL AID

Application for financial aid may be initiated following acceptance to the medical school. Loan funds, grants and some scholarships are available to assist registered students with tuition expense and a share of their living expenses. It is the goal of the Financial Aid Office that no students should be required to interrupt their education solely for financial reasons.

INFORMATION ABOUT DIVERSITY PROGRAMS

The University of Michigan is committed to training a diverse cohort of physicians who are capable of caring for an increasingly diverse patient population. The university is one of the top ten U.S. medical schools in the number of physicians trained from groups underrepresented in medicine.

Medical students of color are very active in organizations such as LANAMA (Latino/a American/Native American Medical Association) and BMA (Black Medical Association). We have an alumni group that is very supportive and involved in the lives of our students from groups underrepresented in medicine. These students are also actively involved in setting the agenda for diversity and cultural competency programs, and participate in the Health System's Multi-cultural Community Health Alliance.

Institution Type: *Public*
Application Process: *AMCAS, see chapter 4.*

APPLICATION AND ACCEPTANCE POLICIES FOR 2005–2006 FIRST-YEAR CLASS

Filing of AMCAS application
  Earliest date: June 1, 2004
  Latest date: Dec. 15, 2004
M.D./Ph.D. latest date: Oct. 15, 2004
School application fee to all applicants: $60
Oldest MCAT scores considered: 2001
Does not have Early Decision Program (EDP)
Acceptance notice to regular applicants
  Earliest date: Oct. 15, 2004
  Latest date: Until class is filled
Applicant's response to acceptance offer
  Maximum time: n/a
Requests for deferred entrance considered: Yes
Deposit to hold place in class: None
Estimated number of new entrants: 170
Starting date: Aug. 2005

TUITION AND STUDENT FEES PER YEAR FOR 2003–2004 FIRST-YEAR CLASS

Tuition   Student fees: $818
  Resident: $19,708
  Nonresident: $30,708

INFORMATION ON 2003–2004 FIRST-YEAR CLASS

Number of	In-State	Out-of-State	Total
Applicants	815	3,952	4,767
Applicants Interviewed	180	492	672
New Entrants*	77	93	170

*All had baccalaureate degrees and 99% took the MCAT.

CHAPTER
11

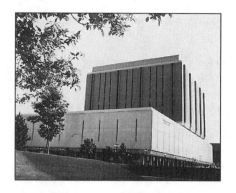

Wayne State University School of Medicine

Detroit, Michigan

Dr. John D. Crissman, *Dean*
Dr. Silas Norman, Jr., *Assistant Dean for Admissions*
Julia Simmons, *Director Diversity and Integrated Student Services Office*
Deirdre Moore, *Assistant Director, Financial Aid*

ADDRESS INQUIRIES TO:

Assistant Dean for Admissions
Wayne State University
School of Medicine
540 East Canfield
Detroit, Michigan 48201
(313) 577-1466; 577-9420 (FAX)
E-mail: admissions@med.wayne.edu
Web site: www.med.wayne.edu/admissions

MISSION STATEMENT

The mission of the Wayne State University School of Medicine is to provide the Michigan community with medical and biotechnical resources, in the form of scientific knowledge and trained professionals, so as to improve the overall health of the community.

GENERAL INFORMATION

The School of Medicine, which originated in 1868, is the oldest component of Wayne State University. It is located in the 236-acre Detroit Medical Center. The medical school is composed of a basic science building, Scott Hall (containing modern teaching facilities for the first two years of medical school), the Shiffman Medical Library, the Lande Medical Research Building, the Elliman Clinical Research Building, and the C. S. Mott Building. Harper University Hospital, Hutzel Women's Hospital, Children's Hospital of Michigan, Detroit Receiving Hospital, and University Health Center (an ambulatory care facility), the Rehabilitation Institute of Michigan, and the John Dingell Veterans Administration Medical Center, make up the Detroit Medical Center central campus. Grace-Sinai Hospital is located in NW Detroit. In addition, the WSU-OHEP Consortium brings together Wayne State University, the Detroit Medical Center and seven community-based teaching hospitals in the Detroit Metropolitan area.

CURRICULUM

The school's medicine curriculum employs a combination of traditional and newer approaches to the teaching of medical students. Year 1 begins with an introductory clinical course which runs through all four years including: Clinical Medicine, Human Sexuality, Medical Interviewing, Physical Diagnosis, Public Health and Prevention, and Evidence Based Medicine.

Year 1 is organized around the disciplines of structure (Anatomy, Histology, Embryology and Radiology) and function (Biochemistry, Physiology, Genetics and Nutrition), and ends with an integrated Neuroscience course. Second year is a completely integrated year focusing on pathophysiology, including Immunology/Microbiology and Pharmacology.

Year 3 is a series of clinical clerkships including Medicine, Surgery, Pediatrics, Family Medicine, Psychiatry, Neurology, and Obstetrics/Gynecology. During Year 3 all students have a six month Continuity clerkship. Year 4 is an elective year including Emergency Medicine, a subinternship and an ambulatory block month.

Students are required to pass the USMLE Step 1 before promotion to Year 3 and are required to pass the USMLE Step 2 before graduation.

The School of Medicine uses traditional lectures, small group and panel discussions, computer assisted instruction, and multimedia in our teaching program.

REQUIREMENTS FOR ENTRANCE

The MCAT is required in addition to a baccalaureate degree or its equivalent; however, the Committee on Admissions is prepared to review the records of third-year students with unusual academic attainment. The MCAT should be taken during the year of application, preferably in the spring. Required courses for medical school admission are:

Years
General Biology or Zoology (with lab) 1
Inorganic Chemistry (with lab) 1
Organic Chemistry (with lab) 1
General Physics (with lab) 1
English 1

Besides a strong preparation in the basic sciences, a broad educational background in a liberal arts-oriented program is desirable. Applicants are encouraged to select subjects that will contribute substantially to a broad cultural background.

Applicants must be U.S. or Canadian citizens or possess a U.S. permanent resident visa.

SELECTION FACTORS

The Committee on Admissions will select those applicants who, in its judgment, will make the best students and physicians. Consideration is given to the entire record, GPA, MCAT scores, recommendations, and interview results as these reflect the applicant's personality, maturity, character, and suitability for medicine. Additionally, the committee regards as desirable certain health care experiences, such as volunteering or working in hospitals, hospices, nursing homes, or doctor's offices. The committee also values experience in biomedical laboratory research. Following an initial screening process, students with competitive applications are selected to complete a secondary application. Special encouragement is given to candidates from medically underserved areas in Michigan.

As a state-supported school, the institution must give preference to Michigan residents; however, out-of-state applicants are encouraged to apply. An applicant's residency is determined by university regulations. Students whose educational backgrounds include work outside the United States must have completed two years of coursework at a U.S. or Canadian college. Interviews are required but scheduled only with those applicants who are given serious consideration. The Committee on Admissions meets on a weekly basis to evaluate candidates. Students are urged to apply by November 1.

FINANCIAL AID

Scholarships, loans, and grants are awarded on the basis of academic performance, financial need, and available funding. Students may borrow through various loan programs up to the amount of total school-related costs and living expenses. Loans not based on demonstrated financial need are also available. Although the primary responsibility for financing a medical education rests with the student and the student's family, the School of Medicine will assist students with unmet need as funds are available. Short-term loans may be made for emergency purposes after registration.

Financial aid awards administered by the School of Medicine are made by the financial aid officer based on federal guidelines and those established by the Committee on Financial Aid and Scholarships, which includes student representation.

The College Work-Study Program and other medically oriented jobs are generally available to eligible students for the summer break.

Financial aid seminars are held for incoming students and their families. Financial aid appointments and information are available by calling (313) 577-1039.

INFORMATION ABOUT DIVERSITY PROGRAMS

Wayne State University School of Medicine is committed to the recruitment and retention of disadvantaged applicants and applicants from groups underrepresented in medicine. The school supports a one-year postbaccalaureate program for disadvantaged medical school applicants from Michigan who have been denied admission, but who appear to have the potential for academic success. The program consists of premedical science courses, academic skills training, personal adjustment counseling, and academic tutoring. Successful

students are guaranteed admission to the School of Medicine. Through the Minority Recruitment office, the school also administers the Incoming Freshman Summer Program for students from groups underrepresented in medicine who are admitted to the first-year class. Additionally, college and high school premedical preparatory programs are offered. For information, write Julia Simmons, Director, Office of Diversity and Integrated Student Services.

Institution Type: *Public*
Application Process: *AMCAS, see chapter 4.*

APPLICATION AND ACCEPTANCE POLICIES FOR 2005–2006 FIRST-YEAR CLASS

Filing of AMCAS application
  Earliest date: June 1, 2004
  Latest date: Dec. 15, 2004
MD/PhD program: November 15, 2004
School application fee after screening: $50
Oldest MCAT scores considered: 2001
Does have Early Decision Program (EDP)
  EDP application period: June 1–Aug. 1, 2004
  EDP applicants notified by: Oct. 1, 2004
Acceptance notice to regular applicants
  Earliest date: October 20, 2004
  Latest date: varies
Applicant's response to acceptance offer
  Maximum time: 3 weeks
Requests for deferred entrance considered: Yes
Deposit to hold place in class (applied to tuition):
  $50, due with response to acceptance offer,
  nonrefundable
Estimated number of new entrants: 256 (15 EDP)
Starting date: August 2005

TUITION AND STUDENT FEES PER YEAR FOR 2003–2004 FIRST-YEAR CLASS

Tuition   Student fees: $855
  Resident: $16,873.20
  Nonresident: $35,114

INFORMATION ON 2003–2004 FIRST-YEAR CLASS

Number of	In-State	Out-of-State	Total
Applicants	1,082	1,640	2,722
Applicants Interviewed	571	213	784
New Entrants*	227	30	257

*All took the MCAT and had baccalaureate degrees.

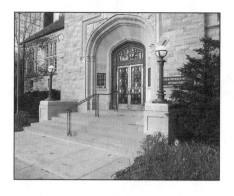

Mayo Clinic College of Medicine
Mayo Medical School

Rochester, Minnesota

Dr. Anthony J. Windebank, *Dean*
Dr. Patricia A. Barrier, *Associate Dean for Student Affairs*
Barbara L. Porter, *Assistant Dean for Student Affairs*
David L. Dahlen, *Director of Financial Aid and Registrar*

ADDRESS INQUIRIES TO:

Mayo Medical School
200 First Street, S.W.
Rochester, Minnesota 55905
(507) 284-3671; (507) 284-2634 (FAX)
Web site: www.mayo.edu/mms

MISSION STATEMENT

Mayo Medical School will be a national leader in medical education that graduates knowledgeable, skillful and compassionate physicians who will enter postgraduate training prepared to assume leadership roles in medical practice, education and research.

GENERAL INFORMATION

Mayo Medical School is an integral part of Mayo Clinic, the world's largest group practice of medicine.

Resources of MMS include a diverse patient population of more than 500,000 registrants annually, four affiliated hospitals with facilities for clinical and basic research, primary care facilities including several rural health centers, and affiliations with physicians who practice in surrounding communities and states. The faculty is drawn from the clinical and scientific staff of Mayo Clinic with locations in Rochester, Minnesota; Jacksonville, Florida; and Scottsdale, Arizona.

CURRICULUM

The curriculum is designed to emphasize the integration of basic and clinical sciences throughout all four years. Governance of the curriculum is centralized and structured around learning objectives such as the Scientific Foundations of Medical Practice; the Clinical Experiences; and the Patient, Physician, and Society. Through this mechanism, longitudinal oversight of teaching of the basic and clinical sciences can be assured and integration facilitated.

In the first year, basic sciences are taught with clinical correlation emphasizing the normal function of the cell and organ systems. Simultaneous with this learning is the introduction to clinical skills culminating in the ability to perform a history and examination on a Mayo patient by the end of the first year. Preceptor experiences throughout the first year in Continuity of Care keep the focus on the patient.

The second year is devoted to an introduction to the core clinical sciences while completing the introduction of the basic science of clinical practice. Emphasis here is on pathophysiology of the organ systems as students explore the use of basic clinical skills.

The third year is devoted to honing skills in all of the basic clinical clerkships, moving beyond the level of acquiring information to the level of synthesis and diagnosis. Clinical experiences at Mayo have always been both ambulatory and hospital based. Because of the small class size and more than 1,000 physician faculty, in most cases these experiences occur as one-on-one assignments with staff of the Mayo Clinic. One quarter of the third year is an opportunity to explore the realm of scientific investigation, as every Mayo student completes a research endeavor of his or her own choice under the mentorship of an experienced Mayo investigator. Approximately 175 Mayo scientists in 37 disciplines offer research experiences in which the students participate.

The fourth year has been carefully designed to produce students who have a well-structured completion of their undergraduate education leading to physician's who are prepared to enter any realm of medicine. Requirements include an internal medicine sub-internship and rotations in family medicine, pediatrics, surgery and emergency medicine. A social medicine elective to understand the role of community in the mission of medicine is also required. Integrated into the fourth-year curriculum is a three-week return to the classroom to explore issues in preventive medicine, biomedical ethics, palliative medicine, and clinical pharmacology. The remainder of the fourth year is fully elective to allow students to customize their learning to meet individual goals.

Formal evaluations are recorded as honors, high pass, pass, marginal pass, or fail, and are supplemented by narrative comments from the faculty. Individual support and tutoring are available to all students.

Six students are admitted to the Medical Scientist Training Program. These students pursue a combined-degree program leading to the M.D.-Ph.D. This joint effort with the Mayo Graduate School allows a student to be fully prepared for clinical practice as well as have all the tools for a career in scientific research. Another program in cooperation with the Mayo Graduate School of Medicine is available for two candidates with the D.D.S. degree who are seeking an M.D. degree and certification in oral and maxillofacial surgery. Stipend support and tuition waiver are included for these programs. A combined

M.D./M.S. degree in Clinical Research is offered in conjunction with the Mayo Graduate School. In addition, a combined M.D./M.P.H. program is available with the University of Minnesota School of Public Health. These programs require separate application **after** matriculation.

All students attending Mayo Medical School are supported by scholarship funds, which significantly reduce the tuition burden. Merit scholarship renewal is dependent upon achieving a grade of pass or higher in every course, but remediation is always available. In addition to participation in federal student assistance programs, Mayo has its own need-based grant program which is available to help offset educational expenses.

REQUIREMENTS FOR ENTRANCE

A baccalaureate degree from a U.S. or Canadian school is required, but no major field is preferred. The MCAT must have been taken within three years of application. College work must include:

	Years
Biology and/or Zoology	1
Inorganic Chemistry (with lab)	1
Organic Chemistry (with lab)	1
Physics (with lab)	1
Biochemistry (one course)	

Mayo Medical School seeks students with excellent academic records in a breadth of educational experiences. Valued highly are the diverse talents within the class, and candidates who have a lifelong commitment to service. Experiences that demonstrate unique personal characteristics along with a commitment to medicine are evaluated in the application process. Access to a personal computer is required of all matriculants.

SELECTION FACTORS

In evaluating candidates, the entire academic record, results of the MCAT, careful reading of the candidate's personal statement, and letters of recommendation are utilized in the initial steps. A standardized telephone interview is utilized in lieu of a secondary application for those candidates who have the academic credentials. A great deal of weight is placed on the personal interview in Rochester. Evidence of integrity, adaptability, maturity, leadership, and humanitarian concern is essential. Appointment notification occurs approximately every six weeks throughout the admissions process, though appointments may be given any time up to the time classes begin in August.

Applications are accepted from all U.S. citizens and those international students possessing a permanent resident visa. Transfers to Mayo Medical School are not accepted except under very unusual circumstances.

Some characteristics of the students accepted for the 2003 entering class were: *mean GPA,* 3.78; *mean MCAT scores,* above 10 in all categories; *gender,* 45 percent women, *students from groups underrepresented in medicine,* 23 percent.

Mayo does not discriminate on the basis of race, sex, creed, national origin, age, or handicap in its educational programs or activities.

FINANCIAL AID

An aggressive grant and scholarship program allows every student significant financial support. Forty-five percent of entering students receive a full-tuition scholarship. A merit scholarship program reduces the cost to all other students. All scholarships are forfeited by students holding appointments at other schools after May 15. Evidence of withdrawal from other institutions must be provided by that date. Comprehensive health care coverage is available. Further information may be obtained by telephoning the financial aid office at (507) 284-4839.

Institution Type: *Private*
Application Process: *AMCAS, see chapter 4.*

APPLICATION AND ACCEPTANCE POLICIES FOR 2005–2006 FIRST-YEAR CLASS

Filing of AMCAS application
    Earliest date: June 1, 2004
    Latest date: Nov. 1, 2004
School application fee to all applicants: $75
Oldest MCAT scores considered: 2002
Does have Early Decision Program (EDP)
    EDP application period: June 1–Aug. 1, 2004
    EDP applicants notified by: Oct. 1, 2004
Acceptance notice to regular applicants
    Earliest date: Oct. 15, 2004
    Latest date: Until class is filled
Applicant's response to acceptance offer
    Maximum time: 2 weeks
Requests for deferred entrance considered: Yes
Deposit to hold place in class:
    $100, due with response to acceptance offer
Deposit refundable prior to: May 16, 2005
Estimated number of new entrants: 42
Starting date: Aug. 2005

TUITION AND STUDENT FEES PER YEAR FOR 2003–2004 FIRST-YEAR CLASS

Tuition
    Resident: $11,250
    Nonresident: $22,500*

INFORMATION ON 2003–2004 FIRST-YEAR CLASS

Number of	*In-State*	*Out-of-State*	*Total*
Applicants	283	2,134	2,417
Applicants Interviewed	44	270	314
New Entrants†	11	33	44

*Mayo Scholarships and support from the state of Minnesota reduce tuition from $22,500 to $5,625 for residents of MN, AZ, and FL and $11,250 for nonresidents.

†All took the MCAT and had baccalaureate degrees.

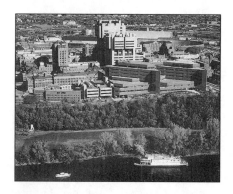

University of Minnesota
Medical School—Minneapolis

Minneapolis, Minnesota

Dr. Deborah Powell, *Dean*
Dr. Richard J. Ziegler, *Dean, Duluth Campus*
Dr. Marilyn J. Becker, *Director of Admissions, Twin Cities*
Dr. Lillian Repesh, *Associate Dean for Admissions and Student Affairs, Duluth*
Mary Tate, *Director of Minority Affairs and Diversity, Twin Cities*
Dr. Joy Dorscher, *Director of Center of American Indian and Minority Health*

ADDRESS INQUIRIES TO:

University of Minnesota Medical School
Twin Cities:
   (612) 625-7977; 625-8228 (FAX)
   E-mail: meded@umn.edu
   Web site: www.meded.umn.edu/
Duluth:
   (218) 726-8511; 726-6235 (FAX)
   E-mail: medadmis@d.umn.edu
   Web site: www.penguin.d.umn.edu/rhs/rhs.html

MISSION STATEMENT

The medical education mission at the University of Minnesota Medical School is to graduate physicians who serve the health needs of Minnesota, the nation, and the world through excellence in clinical medicine, research, education, and health care leadership. The specific educational mission of the U of MN School of Medicine Duluth is to educate students who will practice family medicine and other primary care specialties in rural Minnesota and American Indian communities.

GENERAL INFORMATION

Founded in 1888, the University of Minnesota Medical School is located on the Twin Cities campus of the University of Minnesota. A regional campus of the School of Medicine is located in Duluth. After two years, students transfer to the University of Minnesota Medical School on the Twin Cities campus. The medical programs are a unit of the multidisciplinary University of Minnesota Academic Health Center. Most major hospitals in the Minneapolis-St. Paul area are affiliated with the medical school. The School of Medicine Duluth has established agreements with the St. Mary's Duluth Clinic and St. Luke's Hospital of Duluth.

CURRICULUM

The first-year program in the Twin Cities consists of basic science courses that serve as a foundation for the study of medicine, with relevance of these areas reinforced through clinical correlations. Preceptorships enable students to acquire skills in interviewing, history taking, and physical diagnosis. A Physician and Society course in years one and two addresses topics related to the context of medical practice (i.e. professionalism, ethical issues, cultural diversity, medical law, health care systems). In the second year Twin Cities program, pathology and pharmacology are emphasized in organ system courses. Clinical skills are broadened through work in the primary care fields of medicine, pediatrics and family practice.

The two-year curriculum in Duluth is designed to prepare students for future medical practice through integrated instruction in basic, clinical, and behavioral sciences. Students have early exposure to patients, learning medical history-taking and physical examination skills. Ample time is also devoted to basic science-clinical correlations. In addition, each student is paired with a family physician in required preceptor arrangements in Year 1 and Year 2.

In the third and fourth years, the medical school program includes 52 weeks of required externships, 24 weeks of electives and 23 weeks of free time. Faculty advisors are selected during the second year to assist student in achieving their individual educational goals. Flexibility in scheduling in the third and fourth years provides the opportunity to pursue a wide range of clinical/academic interest.

The Combined M.D./Ph.D. Training Program (Twin Cities campus) is designed to train students for a career as academic physician scientists. This program is completed in approximately eight years and includes medical and graduate coursework, biomedical research and clinical training. Those accepted into the program receive a yearly stipend along with paid tuition and fees. Detailed information is available at ☞ http://mdphd.med.umn.edu.

M.D./M.B.A., M.D./M.P.H., M.D./M.H.I. and J.D./M.D. dual degree programs are also offered.

REQUIREMENTS FOR ENTRANCE

The MCAT and a bachelor's degree from an accredited U.S. or Canadian college or university are required.

Required courses are:

	Sem/Qtr
General Biology (with lab)	2/2
General or Inorganic Chemistry (with lab)	2/2
Organic Chemistry (with lab)	2/2
Biochemistry	1/1
General Physics (with lab)	2/3
English*	2/3
Calculus/Statistics*	1/1
Social and Behavioral Sciences and Humanities*	4/6

*Refer to Web sites for the specific course requirements at Twin Cities ☞ www.meded.umn.edu and Duluth ☞ http://penguin.d.umn.edu/.

SELECTION FACTORS

The Twin Cities medical school gives preference for admissions to legal residents of the state of Minnesota, but applicants from other states are encouraged to apply if they can demonstrate high level academic performance; have attained MCAT scores above the national mean; and demonstrate strength in personal qualities and attitudes. Although scholastic aptitude is essential, neither high grades alone or in combination are sufficient to gain admission. Evidence of personal integrity, maturity, problem-solving abilities, motivation for medicine, the ability to work cooperatively with others, cultural sensitivity, and a sense of dedication in service to others are factors that will be evaluated. These qualities and attitudes will be evaluated through letters of recommendation, the scope and nature of post-secondary experiences, the breadth of undergraduate education, responses to Committee questions on the supplemental application, and on-site interviews. Transfer students are rarely accepted due to limits on clinical training sites.

In keeping with the mandated goals of the Minnesota legislature for the School of Medicine in Duluth, the Committee on Admissions seeks persons with qualities as listed above but with personal and background traits that indicate a high potential for becoming a family physician or other primary care specialist in a small town or rural setting. Priority consideration will be given to in-state applicants who can demonstrate a high potential and motivation for practicing in Minnesota. Out-of-state applicants who also demonstrate interest in practicing in Minnesota will also be considered for admission. Applicants must be U.S. citizens or have permanent resident status. Transfer students are not admitted.

Students accepted to the Twin Cities and Duluth campuses enter a class of 165 and 53 students, respectively. With a variety of undergraduate majors, accepted students for the 2003 entering class have the following statistics. The following information pertains to the Twin Cities Medical School: *mean GPA, 3.67: mean MCAT*, Verbal Reasoning10.0, Physical Sciences 10.3, Biological Sciences 10.8; *mean age*, 24; 22% *multicultural*; 55% *women*; 45% *men*. A reapplication policy limits the number of times an applicant may reapply if not accepted. The following information pertains to the 2003 entering class in Duluth: *mean GPA, 3.67: mean MCAT*, Verbal Reasoning 8.9, Physical Sciences 9.4, Biological Sciences 9.6; *mean age*, 24; 40% *women*; 60% *men*; 98% *Minnesota residents*.

The University of Minnesota Medical School does not discriminate on the basis of race, gender, creed, sexual orientation, disability, or national origin.

FINANCIAL AID

Financial aid applicants must file the FAFSA. Loans and scholarship aid are available for students with demonstrated financial need. Approximately 95% of the students receive financial assistance. For information contact B.J. Gibson (Twin Cities, 612/625-4998) or Dinah Flaherty (Duluth, 218-726-6548).

INFORMATION ABOUT DIVERSITY PROGRAMS

The University of Minnesota Medical School is committed to the recruitment and education of students from groups underrepresented in medicine. The medical school is committed to students from disadvantaged backgrounds, those with high ability, and nonresidents. For more information, contact the Office of Minority Affairs (Twin Cities, 612/625-1494), or the Center for American Indian and Minority Health (one of the three Native American Centers of Excellence in the nation). CAIMH is headquartered in Duluth (218/726-7235) and also has a Twin Cities office (612/624-0465.

Institution Type: *Public*
Application Process: *AMCAS, see chapter 4.*

APPLICATION AND ACCEPTANCE POLICIES FOR 2005–2006 FIRST-YEAR CLASS

Filing of AMCAS application
    Earliest date: June 1, 2004
    Latest date: Nov. 15, 2004
School application fee after screening: $75
Oldest MCAT scores considered: 2001
Does have Early Decision Program (EDP)
    EDP application period: June 1–Aug. 1, 2004
    EDP applicants notified by: Oct. 1, 2004
Acceptance notice to regular applicants
    Earliest date: Oct. 15, 2004
    Latest date: Until class is filled
Applicant's response to acceptance offer
    Maximum time: 2 weeks
Requests for deferred entrance considered: Yes
Deposit to hold place in class (applied to tuition):
    $100, due with response to acceptance offer
Deposit refundable prior to: May 16, 2005
Estimated number of new entrants: 165 (15 EDP)
Starting date: Aug. 2005

TUITION AND STUDENT FEES PER YEAR FOR 2003–2004 FIRST-YEAR CLASS

Tuition   Student fees: $2,232
    Resident: $25,073
    Nonresident: $46,581

INFORMATION ON 2003–2004 FIRST-YEAR CLASS*

Number of	In-State	Out-of-State	Total
Applicants			
Twin Cities	581	1,406	1,987
Duluth	394	64	458
Applicants Interviewed			
Twin Cities	401	277	678
Duluth	126	13	139

*All had baccalaureate degrees and took the MCAT.

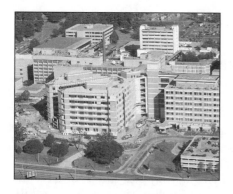

University of Mississippi
School of Medicine

Jackson, Mississippi

Dr. Daniel W. Jones, *Dean*
Dr. Steven T. Case, *Associate Dean for Admissions*
Dr. Jasmine P. Taylor, *Associate Dean for Multicultural Affairs*
Barbara M. Westerfield, *Registrar*

ADDRESS INQUIRIES TO:

Associate Dean for Admissions
University of Mississippi
School of Medicine
2500 North State Street
Jackson, Mississippi 39216-4505
(601) 984-5010; 984-5008 (FAX)
Email: admitmd@som.umsmed.edu
Web site: http://som.umc.edu

MISSION STATEMENT

The primary mission of the University of Mississippi School of Medicine is to offer an accredited program of medical education that will provide well-trained physicians and certain supporting health care professionals, in numbers consistent with the health care needs of the state, who are responsive to the health problems of the people and committed to medical education as a continuum, which must prevail throughout professional life. Related objectives are to (1) expand the body of basic and applied knowledge in biomedical sciences, (2) improve systems of health care delivery, (3) demonstrate model medical care for hospitalized and ambulatory patients, and (4) provide excellent programs of continuing education for the state's practicing physicians.

GENERAL INFORMATION

The School of Medicine, created by a special act of the Board of Trustees in June 1903, operated as a two-year school in Oxford until 1955, when it expanded to four years and moved to the University of Mississippi Medical Center in Jackson. The medical center complex includes the Schools of Medicine, Nursing, Health Related Professions, Dentistry, Graduate Studies in Health Sciences, and the 772-bed University Hospitals and Clinics. Newest campus facilities are the Guyton Research Building, the Blair E. Batson Hospital for Children, the Winfred L. Wiser Hospital for Women and Infants, the Wallace Conerly Hospital for Critical Care, and the Norman C. Nelson Student Center. A new 256-bed adult hospital is under construction. Clinical instruction is also carried out in the Veterans Administration Hospital and McBryde Rehabilitation Center for the Blind.

CURRICULUM

In the first year, the courses in anatomy, biochemistry, physiology, genetics, and psychiatry/behavioral science are reinforced with a program of clinical correlation that introduces the student to presentation of patients and clinical concepts. The second-year student has courses in biostatistics, epidemiology, microbiology, pathology, pharmacology, psychiatry/behavioral science, and the conjoint course introduction to clinical medicine. The third-year students rotate through family medicine, obstetrics-gynecology, pediatrics, psychiatry, medicine, and surgery for clinical instruction in these areas. The fourth year consists of a minimum of eight clinical clerkships (blocks), each one calendar month in length. Required blocks include core blocks in internal medicine, obstetrics-gynecology, pediatrics, and surgery. Of the required senior courses, internal medicine is largely an inpatient experience with an ambulatory component provided in medicine clinics at the Veterans Administration Medical Center or University Hospital. The required course in obstetrics-gynecology is largely ambulatory, but includes some inpatient experience in the labor and delivery suite. Of the core months required in pediatrics and surgery, one must be an inpatient clerkship. An additional ambulatory block is required. A fourth-year course in a senior seminar, which covers topics in medical ethics, medical economics and related issues, is required. The remaining months are available for elective experiences that the students select with the counsel of their advisor and the dean's office.

REQUIREMENTS FOR ENTRANCE

The MCAT and three years of college are required. Each applicant must have a minimum of 90 semester hours from an accredited college, excluding physical education, military training, and certain professional courses. However, preference is given to applicants who will have completed all requirements for a baccalaureate degree prior to matriculation.

The required courses are:

	Sem./Qtr. hrs.
General Biology or Zoology (with lab)	8/12
Inorganic or General Chemistry (with lab)	8/12
Organic Chemistry (with lab)	8/12
General Physics (with lab)	8/12
Advanced Science	6/9
Mathematics (Algebra and Trigonometry)	6/9
English	6/9

Science courses for nonscience majors, survey courses, and AP credits are not acceptable for fulfilling the science requirements. Two semesters of advanced science must be taken in a senior college.

Students who qualify by placement tests for a more advanced course in mathematics must take a semester course of calculus I rather than algebra and trigonometry.

The student is advised to develop proficiency in a specific area and acquire a background in the humanities and behavioral sciences in undergraduate school.

SELECTION FACTORS

Selection of applicants is made on a competitive basis without regard to age, sex, sexual orientation, race, creed, national origin, marital status, handicap, or veteran status. The Admissions Committee selects students who are best qualified on the basis of a demonstration of scholastic aptitude and personal achievement with due consideration of other factors. Major considerations are academic performance, MCAT results, motivation for medicine, and such personal characteristics as maturity, integrity, and stability. Additional factors are the recommendation of the premedical advisors or committee and the impression made on the personal interview. Strong preference is given to residents of Mississippi. Interviews are arranged at the discretion of the Admissions Committee.

The mean GPA for the 2003 entering class was 3.66.

Mississippi residents who are enrolled in other medical schools accredited by the Liaison Committee on Medical Education can be considered for transfer after successful completion of one or two years in another program. After completion of two years in another medical school, the transfer applicant must pass Step 1 of the United States Medical Licensure Examination before acceptance in this program.

FINANCIAL AID

Accepted students may apply for financial aid. The school participates in federal scholarship programs and federal loan programs, such as the Perkins Loan Program and the Stafford Student Loan Program. Eligible students may qualify for limited scholarship funds provided by private donors. Additional financial aid is available through the American Medical Association Education and Research Foundation loan program and the Mississippi State Medical Education Scholarship Loan Program, which was established by the state legislature. In the latter program, Mississippi resident medical students who contract to practice in Mississippi may borrow up to $6,000 per school year or $24,000 in four years. Students from groups underrepresented in medicine are assisted by the National Medical Fellowship, Inc., program. A limited number of prizes and scholarships are awarded to outstanding students. Four dean's awards, renewable annually, are awarded each year to the first-year students with the highest academic achievement at the end of the first year. Although the study of medicine is considered a full-time activity, students who maintain

satisfactory academic standing may apply for part-time jobs in the medical center.

INFORMATION ABOUT DIVERSITY PROGRAMS

The Admissions Committee encourages students from groups underrepresented in medicine to apply for admission. Further information on the various aspects of the program may be obtained by writing to the Associate Dean for Multicultural Affairs.

Institution Type: *Public*
Application Process: *AMCAS, see chapter 4.*

APPLICATION AND ACCEPTANCE POLICIES FOR 2005–2006 FIRST-YEAR CLASS

Filing of AMCAS application
  Earliest date: June 1, 2004
  Latest date: Oct. 15, 2004
School application fee: None
Oldest MCAT scores considered: 2001
Does have Early Decision Program (EDP)
  For Mississippi residents only
  EDP application period: June 1–Aug. 1, 2004
  EDP applicants notified by: Oct. 1, 2004
Acceptance notice to regular applicants
  Earliest date: Oct. 15, 2004
  Latest date: March 15, 2005
Applicant's response to acceptance offer
  Maximum time: Two weeks
Requests for deferred entrance considered: Yes
Deposit to hold place in class (applied to tuition):
  $50 for residents, due with response to
  acceptance offer
Deposit refundable prior to: May 16, 2005
Estimated number of new entrants: 100 (10 EDP)
Starting date: Aug. 2005

TUITION AND STUDENT FEES PER YEAR FOR 2003–2004 FIRST-YEAR CLASS

Tuition   Student fees: $1,650
  Resident: $6,938
  Nonresident: $13,298

INFORMATION ON 2003-2004 FIRST-YEAR CLASS

Number of	In-State	Out-of-State	Total
Applicants	239	0	239
Applicants Interviewed	159	0	159
New Entrants*	100	0	100

*All took the MCAT; 99% had baccalaureate degrees.

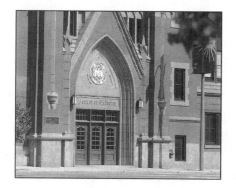

Saint Louis University School of Medicine

St. Louis, Missouri

Dr. Patricia Monteleone, *Dean*
Dr. L. James Willmore, *Associate Dean*
Mary B.W. Fenton, *Assistant Dean, Student Financial Planning*
Dr. George Rausch, *Associate Dean for Multicultural Affairs*

ADDRESS INQUIRIES TO:

Saint Louis University
School of Medicine
1402 South Grand Boulevard
St. Louis, Missouri 63104
(314) 977-9870; 977-9825 (FAX)
E-mail: slumd@slu.edu
Web site: http://medschool.slu.edu/admissions

MISSION STATEMENT

Beyond the important objective of training physicians who are scholars of human biology, the School of Medicine strives to graduate physicians who manifest in their personal and professional lives a special appreciation for what may be called humanistic medicine.

We regard humanistic medicine as a constellation of ethical and professional attitudes, which affect the physician's interactions with patients, colleagues, and society. Among these attitudes are concern for the sanctity of human life; commitment to dignity and respect in the provision of medical care to all patients; devotion to social justice, especially regarding inequities in the availability of health care; humility and awareness of medicine's limitations in the care of the sick; appreciation of the role of non-medical factors in a patient's state of well-being or illness; and mature, well-balanced professional behavior that derives from comfortable relationships with members of the human family and one's Creator.

GENERAL INFORMATION

Saint Louis University is a privately endowed, coeducational institution founded by the Jesuits in 1818. The first faculty of medicine was appointed in 1836, and the school assumed its general present form in 1903. Today the Saint Louis University School of Medicine includes the University Hospital, the School of Medicine (Schwitalla Hall, Caroline Bldg., Doisy Medical Research Facility, and Margaret McCormick Doisy Learning Resources Center), Desloge Towers, Bordley Pavilion, David P. Wohl Memorial Mental Health Institute, Cardinal Glennon Hospital for Children, SLU-Anheuser Busch Institute, University Medical Group, Orthopedic/Rehabilitation Center, Pediatric Research Institute, and the Institute of Molecular Virology. Major teaching affiliations include The University Hospital, Cardinal Glennon Hospital for Children, David P. Wohl Mental Health Institute, St. Elizabeth's Hospital, St. John's Mercy Medical Center, St. Mary's Hospital, and the St. Louis Veterans Affairs hospitals.

CURRICULUM

The M.D. degree program curriculum has undergone extensive changes in order to adapt to the needs of the evolving health care environment. All years have been reorganized. Distinctive aspects of the program are as follows:

1. Phase 1 (Year 1) consists of a Fundamentals of Biomedical Sciences course; a Health Information Resources course to develop computer skills and proficiency in gathering information on various aspects of human disease and patient care; and a Patient, Physician, and Society course that includes units such as ethics, communication skills, and physical diagnosis.

2. Phase 2 (Year 2) includes an organ and systems approach. Phase 3 incorporates Year 3 and Year 4, with a clerkship in Family Medicine and ample opportunities to design individualized programs including electives. Also, ambulatory care activities have been significantly expanded.

3. An Anesthesiology Laboratory and a Clinical Skills Center provide the latest methodology for instruction and evaluation using standardized patients and other devices to learn clinical skills, in addition to the regular training sites.

4. The opportunity exists to participate in a combined M.D./Ph.D. program, in which qualified medical students undertake graduate studies leading to the Ph.D. in one of the basic science disciplines. Students interested in research may opt to receive the M.D. with Distinction in Research Award.

5. The opportunity also exists to participate in a combined M.D.-M.P.H. and M.D./M.B.A. program.

6. The grade system consists of the following levels: honors, pass, and fail.

REQUIREMENTS FOR ENTRANCE

Saint Louis University School of Medicine encourages applications from students who have demonstrated a high level of academic achievement and who manifest in their personal lives those human qualities that are required for a career of service to society. Specific academic requirements include the MCAT and a minimum of 90 semester hours (135 quarter hours) in undergraduate arts and science courses. Most accepted applicants complete a baccalaureate degree of at least 120 semester hours (180 quarter hours) from an accredited college or university. Specific course requirements are:

Sem. hrs.

General Biology or Zoology (with lab) 8
Inorganic Chemistry (with lab) 8

Organic Chemistry (with lab). 8
Physics (with lab) 8
English 6
Other humanities and behavioral sciences 12

Biochemistry is strongly recommended.

Applicants are expected to have pursued one area of knowledge or discipline in depth. The Admissions Committee does not favor any specific major in its decisions.

SELECTION FACTORS

The selection of candidates is based upon demonstrated intellectual ability and personal qualifications, including motivation, character, emotional maturity, stability, and personality. There is no discrimination on the basis of race, color, sex, age, national origin, religion, sexual orientation, disability, or veteran status. All university policies, practices, and procedures are administered in a manner consistent with our Catholic Jesuit identity. There are no geographical restrictions or quotas for American citizens. All applicants receive serious consideration, and some additional attention is given to applicants from Saint Louis University.

Students for the 2003 entering class had the following average academic credentials: *Science GPA,* 3.55; *overall GPA,* 3.61; *mean MCAT Scores,* VR-9.82, PS-9.9, BS-10.27, WS-P; *sex,* 44 percent women; *residence,* 29 percent from Missouri, 31 states represented; *undergraduate major,* 60 percent in life sciences, 16 percent in chemistry.

Transfers into our School of Medicine are only possible at the beginning of the third year of studies. The only individuals who are eligible to apply for transfer are those who are currently enrolled in, and students in good standing at, other U.S. medical schools accredited by the Liaison Committee on Medical Education.

FINANCIAL AID

The Office of Student Financial Planning identifies a standard student budget and assists students in managing an aid plan to meet expenses for their directly related educational costs. Loan and scholarship aid is available and is awarded on the basis of financial need. It is absolutely necessary that an individual be "creditworthy" in order to qualify for financial assistance. Information on the financial status of parents is required of all students seeking University aid and some federal aid.

In 2003–04, 90 percent of the students received financial assistance from either school or noninstitutional sources.

Financial aid information is automatically sent upon acceptance to the School of Medicine. This information includes the need analysis document(s), descriptions of available aid sources, and the application form for financial assistance from the School of Medicine. Individuals in need of applying for financial aid may do so only after they have been accepted to the School of Medicine.

The Office of Student Financial Planning encourages financial aid applicants to contact it when questions arise regarding eligibility for aid and the financial aid process.

INFORMATION ABOUT DIVERSITY PROGRAMS

The School of Medicine is committed to diversity. There is an ongoing effort to increase the number of individuals from groups significantly underrepresented in the medical profession.

The Office of Multicultural Affairs (OMA) assists students from diverse backgrounds to be successful as they progress along the educational pathway in pursuit of a career as a physician.

Institution Type: *Private*
Application Process: *AMCAS, see chapter 4.*

APPLICATION AND ACCEPTANCE POLICIES FOR 2005–2006 FIRST-YEAR CLASS

Filing of AMCAS application
Earliest date: June 1, 2004
Latest date: Dec. 15, 2004
School application fee to all applicants: $100
Oldest MCAT scores considered: 2001
Does have Early Decision Program (EDP)
EDP application period: June 1–Aug. 1, 2004
EDP applicants notified by: Oct. 1, 2004
Acceptance notice to regular applicants
Earliest date: Oct. 15, 2004
Latest date: Until class is filled
Applicant's response to acceptance offer
Maximum time: 2 weeks
Requests for deferred entrance considered: Yes
Deposit to hold place in class (applied to tuition):
$100, due with response to acceptance offer
Deposit refundable prior to: May 16, 2005
Estimated number of new entrants: 150 (3 EDP)
Starting date: Aug. 2005

TUITION AND STUDENT FEES PER YEAR FOR 2003–2004 FIRST-YEAR CLASS

Tuition: $36,190   Student fees: $1,660

INFORMATION ON 2003–2004 FIRST-YEAR CLASS

Number of	In-State	Out-of-State	Total
Applicants	322	4,033	4,355
Applicants Interviewed	117	845	962
New Entrants*	46	112	158

*All took the MCAT and had baccalaureate degrees.

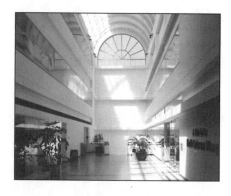

University of Missouri—Columbia School of Medicine

Columbia, Missouri

Dr. William Crist, *Dean*
Dr. Linda Headrick, *Senior Associate Dean for Medical Education*
Dr. Robert N. McCallum, *Associate Dean for Student Programs*
Dr. Michael Hosokawa, *Associate Dean for Curriculum*

ADDRESS INQUIRIES TO:

Judy Nolke, Admissions and Recruitment Coordinator
Office of Medical Education
MA215 Medical Sciences Building
University of Missouri—Columbia
School of Medicine
One Hospital Drive
Columbia, Missouri 65212
(573) 882-9219; 884-2988 (FAX)
E-mail: nolkej@health.missouri.edu
Web site: www.muhealth.org/~medicine

MISSION STATEMENT

MU's School of Medicine is committed to providing high-quality medical education and developing physicians who will meet the health-care needs of Missourians. To do so, it is committed to the following goals: *Content:* The MU School of Medicine will provide a series of learning experiences in the basic science curriculum and in the clinical clerkships to assure that graduates possess the knowledge and understanding of scientific principles and concepts essential to the practice of medicine, and master the scientific method and its application to the practice of medicine, while cultivating in them the qualities of integrity, respect, and compassion. *Application:* The MU School of Medicine will provide opportunities for students to attain skill in performance of a thorough medical history and a complete physical examination; to apply principles of diagnosis and treatment of major illnesses of patients; to incorporate the social, behavioral, and ethical aspects into their patient care; and to practice the principles of public health and preventive medicine. *Process:* The MU School of Medicine will provide an academic atmosphere emphasizing principles, independent thinking, and problem solving; a professional environment fostering and developing attitudinal and professional traits of a competent physician; and experiences for each student as a member of a health care team and a health care delivery system.

GENERAL INFORMATION

The University of Missouri—Columbia School of Medicine was established in 1872 as a two-year public medical school. In 1956 the curriculum was expanded to its present four-year program. The MU Health Sciences Center includes the University Hospital, Mid-Missouri Mental Health Center, Harry S. Truman Veterans Affairs Hospital, Medical Sciences Building, J. Otto Lottes Health Sciences Library, Howard A. Rusk Rehabilitation Center, Mason Institute of Opthalmology,

Cosmopolitan International Diabetes Center, and Ellis Fischel Cancer Center. Students have a total of 1,000 hospital beds available for patient care. Additional local outpatient clinics and rural primary care clinics within 35 miles of Columbia are available. The School of Medicine also maintains affiliations with various other health institutions across the state.

CURRICULUM

The educational program of the School of Medicine was completely revised in 1993 to emphasize a strong foundation in the basic sciences, problem solving, clinical skills, early experiences with patients and role-model physicians, self-directed learning/lifelong learning, and the attitudes essential to competent and compassionate patient care.

Each of the first two years has four 10-week blocks with two components—Basic Science/Problem-Based Learning and Introduction to Patient Care. Bsci/PBL focuses on eight patient cases per block integrating basic sciences, clinical concepts, and psychosocial aspects of medicine. Lectures and labs correlate with the cases. Students engage in collaborative learning and problem solving as they work in groups of eight with a faculty tutor. In IPC, students develop the clinical skills and critical thinking needed for third and fourth years clinical experiences.

The third year features six eight-week required clerkships in internal medicine, surgery, psychiatry/neurology, child health, obstetrics/gynecology, and family medicine. The fourth year has three eight-week required advanced clinical selectives from a surgical area, a medical area, and one other area; eight weeks of advanced biomedical science; and 12 years of general electives. Students with an interest in rural practice may elect to take some of their third- and fourth-year clinical experiences at a rural clinical center. Students with a special interest in biomedical research follow the physician-scientist tract by engaging in guided basic science research through summer experiences, post-sophomore fellowships, and fourth-year electives and selectives which could lead to a graduate degree.

A multilevel grading system is used, with satisfactory/unsatisfactory in the first year, honors/satisfactory/unsatisfactory in the second year, and honors/letter of commendation/satisfactory/unsatisfactory in the third and fourth years.

Students must pass the USMLE Step 1 prior to their fourth year, and Step 2 to graduate.

REQUIREMENTS FOR ENTRANCE

Applicants are required to take the MCAT (1999 or later) and to have earned a minimum of 90 semester hours (exclusive of physical education and military science) from a recognized college or university. All successful applicants will have completed a bachelor's degree. Specific courses required for admission are:

	Sem.
English Composition (or writing-intensive courses)	2
College-level math or calculus	1

	Hrs.
General Biology (with lab)	8
General Chemistry (with lab)	8
Organic Chemistry (with lab)	8
General Physics (with lab)	8

Only those courses required for science majors may be used to meet these requirements, not introductory survey courses. A course in biochemistry is strongly recommended. Applicants are also strongly urged to pursue a broad-based education which includes courses in the social sciences, humanities, and oral and written communication. The entering class typically shows a wide range of undergraduate majors.

SELECTION FACTORS

The Committee on Admissions is composed of faculty members, community physicians, and medical students. Strong selection preference is given to Missouri residents. Residents of states bordering Missouri may also gain acceptance.

On-campus personal interviews are required for admission. Selection for interview is based upon MCAT scores, academic performance, the AMCAS application, and letters of reference. Both academic qualifications and nonacademic attributes are important. The Committee assesses personal characteristics such as maturity, motivation, leadership, social concern, and commitment. Demographic factors may be considered.

Credentials of the members of the 2003 entering class: *mean science GPA,* 3.65; *mean GPA,* 3.71; *undergraduate major in sciences,* 81%; *gender,* 43% women; *mean MCAT,* 28.7; *Early Decision Program acceptance,* 2%; *overall acceptance rate,* 137 acceptances offered to complete a class of 96 students.

The School of Medicine participates in the Early Decision Program (EDP). Current requirements to apply are: Missouri resident with 3.75 overall GPA and MCAT sum of 30 with no individual score below 9. We occasionally accept transfer students in the third year from U.S. and/or foreign medical schools, primarily Missouri residents.

The School of Medicine does not discriminate on the basis of race, sex, creed, national origin, age, handicap, religion, or status as a Vietnam-era veteran in the admission or access to or treatment or employment in its programs and activities.

FINANCIAL AID

Students are admitted to the School of Medicine without regard to financial circumstances. After acceptance, prospective students are mailed the necessary forms to complete the financial aid process. The school participates in the federal scholarship and loan programs. The institutional scholarship program is primarily need-based. Institutional long-term loans

are available to third- and fourth-year students. The school also operates an emergency short-term loan program.

INFORMATION ABOUT DIVERSITY PROGRAMS

The University of Missouri is committed to the recruitment and education of disadvantaged and nontraditional applicants and those from groups underrepresented in medicine. The School of Medicine sponsors summer programs for rural and disadvantaged high school students and students from groups underrepresented in medicine interested in health care professions.

Institution Type: *Public*
Application Process: *AMCAS, see chapter 4.*

APPLICATION AND ACCEPTANCE POLICIES FOR 2005–2006 FIRST-YEAR CLASS

Filing of AMCAS application
  Earliest date: June 1, 2004
  Latest date: Nov. 1, 2004
School application fee after screening: $50
Oldest MCAT scores considered: 1999
Does have Early Decision Program (EDP)
  For Missouri residents only
  EDP application period: June 1–Aug. 1, 2004
  EDP applicants notified by: Oct. 1, 2004
Acceptance notice to regular applicants
  Earliest date: Oct. 15, 2004
  Latest date: until class is filled
Applicant's response to acceptance offer
  Maximum time: 30 days
Requests for deferred entrance considered: Yes
Deposit to hold place in class (applied to tuition):
  $100, due with response to acceptance offer
Deposit refundable prior to: May 16, 2005
Estimated number of new entrants: 96 (3 EDP)
Starting date: Aug. 2005

TUITION AND STUDENT FEES PER YEAR FOR 2003–2004 FIRST-YEAR CLASS

Tuition	Student fees: $780
Resident: $18,792	
Nonresident: $37,418	

INFORMATION ON 2003–2004 FIRST-YEAR CLASS

Number of	In-State	Out-of-State	Total
Applicants	389	433	822
Applicants Interviewed	207	44	251
New Entrants*	92	4	96

*All had baccalaureate degrees; 87% took the MCAT.

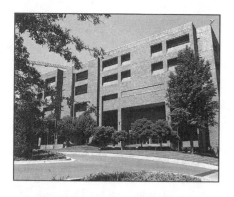

University of Missouri—Kansas City School of Medicine

Kansas City, Missouri

Dr. Betty Drees, *Dean*
Dr. Alan Salkind, *Assistant Dean and Chair Selection*
Jan Brandow, *Director of Student Financial Aid*
Dr. Reaner Shannon, *Associate Dean, Cultural Enhancement and Diversity*

ADDRESS INQUIRIES TO:

Council on Selection
University of Missouri—Kansas City
School of Medicine
2411 Holmes
Kansas City, Missouri 64108-2792
(816) 235-1870; 235-6579 (FAX)
Web site: http://research.med.umkc.edu

MISSION STATEMENT

The mission of the University of Missouri—Kansas City School of Medicine is to prepare graduates so they are able to enter and complete graduate programs in medical education, qualify for medical licensure, provide competent medical care, and have the educational background necessary for lifelong learning in order to address the health care needs of our state and nation.

GENERAL INFORMATION

The Board of Curators of the University of Missouri authorized the establishment of a medical school at the University of Missouri—Kansas City in 1969. Located on a 135-acre Hospital Hill campus, the medical school is near both the schools and colleges of the university and affiliated community hospitals.

CURRICULUM

The School of Medicine, in combination with the College of Arts and Sciences and the School of Biological Sciences, offers a year-round program leading to baccalaureate and M.D. degrees in six calendar years. The student is required to complete both degrees and has the freedom to major in any department of the School of Biological Sciences or the College of Arts and Sciences.

The program is designed primarily for high school seniors who are entering college. Students are permitted to obtain 30 semester hours of credit through the Advanced Placement program or the CLEP subject area examinations. To receive the baccalaureate degree, the student must complete 120 semester hours of credit.

The fundamental objective of the program is to provide students with a broad liberal arts education and to prepare physicians who are committed to providing comprehensive health care.

Under the guidance of a clinician-scholar, called a docent, small groups of first- and second-year students are introduced to medicine in several community hospitals where they can observe patients and their problems.

During the first two years of the program, the student is occupied predominantly with arts and sciences coursework, with about one-fourth of the time being devoted to introduction to medicine courses. After these two years the student advances, with the approval of the Council on Evaluation, to Year 3 of the six-year program.

During the last four years of the curriculum the student, with guidance from a docent and education assistant, plans a program for meeting the curriculum requirements. Two months of Years 4 through 6 are spent with the docent unit on an inpatient internal medicine rotation. The remaining months of each year are spent in a number of other required and elective course offerings in the basic and clinical sciences and the humanities and social sciences. Students spend two academic terms in arts and sciences coursework during the last four years of the program.

Basic, clinical, and behavioral science information is presented and emphasized throughout the six-year program. Thus, each student is expected to acquire a firm and broad base of information in each of these major content areas.

The academic program provides the medical student with a realistic working knowledge of community health problems and resources. The school provides an environment for learning medicine, which is enhanced by the strong student support system.

An alternative path is available for extended study.

REQUIREMENTS FOR ENTRANCE

Applicants for admission to Year 1 of the six-year baccalaureate-medical program must meet the admission requirements of both the University of Missouri—Kansas City and the School of Medicine. Applicants must graduate from an accredited U.S. high school and demonstrate the ability to perform successfully at the college level, based on a combination of high school rank and scores on the ACT (American College Testing Program) .

A student admitted to the combined program at UMKC is required to meet the following high school course requirements (one unit equals one year in class): four units of English; four units of mathematics; three units of science, including one unit of biology and one unit of chemistry; three units of social studies; one unit of fine arts; two units of a single foreign language. Applicants are strongly encouraged to pursue an extensive and challenging course of study.

Between the second and third years of the combined degree program, five to ten MD-only positions become available. Applicants for MD-only must have a baccalaureate or advanced degree and present MCAT scores.

SELECTION FACTORS

The criteria for selection are:

1. Applicant's academic potential as judged by quality of high school courses, rank in high school class, and scores on the ACT. In the 2003–2004 entering class, the average ACT score fell at the 90th percentile, and the average rank in class was at the 92nd percentile.

2. Personal qualities, including maturity, leadership, stamina, reliability, motivation for medicine, range of interests, interpersonal skills, compassion, and job experience.

The Council on Selection carefully reviews all applicants to this program. Applicants who appear to be well qualified are invited for interviews at the medical school campus. If invited, the applicant is notified in writing and will be required to be present at the scheduled date and time of the interview.

Students are considered on the basis of their individual qualifications without regard to race, creed, sex, or national origin. The program does not accept transfer students.

FINANCIAL AID

There is a variety of financial assistance available to all medical students. Further information and applications for financial aid may be obtained from: Student Financial Aid Office, University of Missouri—Kansas City, 5115 Oak, Kansas City, Missouri 64110. Application should be made prior to March 1 of the year for which the student is applying.

INFORMATION ABOUT DIVERSITY PROGRAMS

Information for students from groups underrepresented in medicine is available from Dr. Reaner Shannon, Associate Dean for Cultural Enhancement and Diversity, or Mary Anne Morgenegg, Coordinator of Admissions, Council on Selection, University of Missouri—Kansas City School of Medicine.

Institution Type: *Public*

APPLICATION AND ACCEPTANCE POLICIES FOR 2005–2006 FIRST-YEAR CLASS

Filing of application
  Earliest date: Aug. 1, 2004
  Latest date: Nov. 15, 2004
School application fee to all applicants: $35 (in-state)
  $50 (out-of-state)
Does not have Early Decision Program
Acceptance notice to regular applicants
  Earliest date: April 1, 2005
  Latest date: Varies
Applicant's response to acceptance offer
  Maximum time: 30 days
Requests for deferred entrance considered: No
Deposit to hold place in class (applied to tuition):
  $100, due with response to acceptance offer
  Deposit refundable prior to: May 16, 2005
Estimated number of new entrants: 100
Starting date: Aug. 2005

TUITION AND STUDENT FEES PER YEAR FOR 2003–2004 FIRST-YEAR CLASS

Tuition*   Student fees: $1,086
  Resident: $25,094
  Nonresident: $50,405

INFORMATION ON 2003–2004 FIRST-YEAR CLASS

Number of	In-State	Out-of-State	Total
Applicants	256	179	435
Applicants Interviewed	162	48	210
New Entrants	106	18	124

*These fees apply to Year 3 of the six-year program.

CHAPTER
11

Chapter 11: School Entries

227

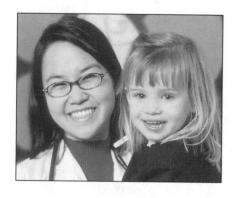

Washington University School of Medicine

St. Louis, Missouri

Dr. Larry J. Shapiro, *Dean and Executive Vice Chancellor for Medical Affairs*
Dr. W. Edwin Dodson, *Associate Vice Chancellor and Associate Dean for Admissions*
John F. Walters, *Assistant Dean and Director of Financial Aid*
Dr. Will Ross, *Associate Dean, Diversity Programs*

ADDRESS INQUIRIES TO:

Office of Admissions
Washington University
School of Medicine
660 South Euclid Avenue, #8107
St. Louis, Missouri 63110
(314) 362-6857; 362-4658 (FAX)
E-mail: wumscoa@msnotes.wustl.edu
Web site: http://medschool.wustl.edu/admissions/

MISSION STATEMENT

The mission of Washington University is the promotion of learning—learning by students and by faculty. Teaching, the transmission of knowledge, is central to our mission, as is research, the creation of new knowledge. Our goals are:
- to foster excellence in our teaching, research, scholarship, and service;
- to prepare students with attitudes, skills, and habits of lifelong learning and with leadership skills, enabling them to be useful members of a global society; and
- to be an exemplary institution in our home community, St. Louis, as well as in the nation and the world.

GENERAL INFORMATION

Washington University School of Medicine has a rich history of success in research, education, and patient care. It pioneered bedside teaching and led in the transformation of empirical knowledge into scientific medicine. From the earliest days, there has been an understanding that "investigation and practice are one in spirit, method, and object."

Responding to a national concern for improving doctors' training, Washington University in 1891 established a medical department. By 1900, scientific progress had accelerated the reform of medical education, and the medical department assumed new importance. In 1909, Robert Brookings, successful St. Louis businessman turned philanthropist, set about transforming the medical department into a modern medical school. Today, the medical school occupies more than 4 million gross square feet of space.

Washington University School of Medicine, Barnes-Jewish, St. Louis Children's, and Barnard hospitals, and Central Institute for the Deaf compose the 230-acre Washington University Medical Center. Barnes-Jewish Hospital is the largest hospital in the region. St. Louis Children's Hospital is one of the top pediatric health centers in the country, providing a full range of services throughout its 200-mile service area. Barnes-Jewish and St. Louis Children's hospitals have 1,620 beds and are members of BJC Health System, the largest academically linked health care system in the country.

A good doctor must be a compassionate and understanding human being as well as a good scientist. To this end, the School of Medicine has always selected applicants who, in addition to possessing keen minds, demonstrate an ability to perceive and serve their patients' interests. An education from Washington University School of Medicine provides graduates with solid opportunities for sought-after residencies and fellowships, challenging research endeavors, and rewarding medical careers.

CURRICULUM

The curriculum provides students with a stimulating education, in both the science and the art of clinical medicine. Instruction is by lecture, and small-group interactive sessions with faculty, and includes problem-based exercises and self-directed learning using computers and other resources led by faculty facilitators. Medical humanities and ethics are integrated into the four years of medical training. Throughout the curriculum, serious consideration is given to the sociological and cultural concerns of the patients and to the necessity of adapting medical care to their needs.

Patient contact begins in the first semester of the first year. Courses address the broad issues of normal structure and function of humans with emphasis on neuroscience, cell biology, and genetics. The effect of disease on bodily structure and function characterize the second-year curriculum. Expanded clinical experience is integrated with coursework in pathology, pathophysiology, and pharmacology. Core clinical clerkships occupy the entire third year with increasing emphasis on ambulatory medicine. The fourth year is a full year of electives planned and selected by the student with faculty guidance.

For students who care to participate, there are abundant opportunities to engage in basic and clinical research through summer research fellowships and research electives. A five-year M.A. and M.D. degree program is available for students desiring a full year of research training. A Medical Scientist Training Program permits students seeking a career in academic medicine to obtain both M.D. and Ph.D. degrees.

A tutorial program is available to any student in the school who needs academic assistance. A pass/fail grading system is used in the first year; an honors/high pass/pass/fail grading system is used thereafter.

REQUIREMENTS FOR ENTRANCE

Accepted applicants must present evidence of superior intellectual ability and achievement, completion of at least 90 semester hours of coursework in an approved college or university, satisfactory performance on the MCAT, and attributes necessary for a productive career in medicine.

Mathematics, physics, and chemistry provide the tools for modern biology, medicine, and the biological basis of patient care. Accordingly, premedical education should include a minimum of the following courses:

	Years
Biological Science	1
General or Inorganic Chemistry	1
Organic Chemistry	1
Physics	1
Mathematics (through differential and integral calculus)	1

Prerequisites are subject to waiver by the Committee on Admissions. The development of the intellectual talents of an individual often involves the in-depth pursuit of some areas of knowledge in humanities, social sciences, or natural sciences. A diversified background of cultural development is encouraged.

SELECTION FACTORS

Students are selected on the basis of character, attitude, interest, intellectual ability, motivation, maturity, and past achievement as indicated both by superior scholastic work and active participation in extracurricular activities prior to entering medical school. Washington University policies and programs are nondiscriminatory, and full consideration is given to all applicants without regard to sex, age, race, handicap, sexual preference, creed, or national or ethnic origin. Students from groups underrepresented in medicine are strongly encouraged to apply.

Students in the 2003 entering class had the following credentials: *mean science GPA,* 3.81; *mean nonscience GPA,* 3.83; *mean total GPA,* 3.82; *mean MCAT scores—VR*-11.3, *PS*-12.6, *BS*-12.5; *sex,* 46 percent women; *undergraduate major,* 44 percent in biological sciences or preprofessional studies, 32 percent in physical sciences, 8 percent in nonscience majors and 16 percent in all others including double majors.

Early submission of the AMCAS application permits its prompt evaluation by the Committee on Admissions. All applicants are invited to complete their application with letters of evaluation and additional personal information. Selected applicants are invited for interview. All accepted applicants are interviewed.

FINANCIAL AID

To facilitate financial planning, tuition is set for the first year and does not increase during the four years of medical school.

The financial resources of an applicant do not enter into the admission selection process. Need-based financial aid is awarded to accepted students who document financial need. An award decision is usually made within two weeks following receipt of completed financial aid application forms. Awards consist of both scholarships and loans. Merit-based full-tuition scholarships are awarded to multiple students in each entering class and are eligible for renewal each year of study for the M.D. degree. Application is by invitation of the Admissions Committee. For information contact: Committee on Student Financial Aid; 660 South Euclid Avenue, #8059; St. Louis, Missouri 63110; (314) 362-6845; 362-3045 (FAX); E-mail: money@msnotes.wustl.edu.

INFORMATION ABOUT DIVERSITY PROGRAMS

The school is committed to the recruitment, enrollment, education, and graduation of an increased number of individuals from groups underrepresented in medicine. For information contact: Will Ross, M.D., Associate Dean and Director of Diversity Programs; 660 South Euclid Avenue, #8023; St. Louis, Missouri 63110; (314) 362-6854; 747-3974 (FAX); E-mail:

Institution Type: *Private*
Application Process: *AMCAS, see chapter 4.*

APPLICATION AND ACCEPTANCE POLICIES FOR 2005–2006 FIRST-YEAR CLASS

Filing of AMCAS application
  Earliest date: June 1, 2004
  Latest date: Dec. 1, 2004
School application fee to all applicants: $50
Oldest MCAT scores considered: 2002
Does not have Early Decision Program
Acceptance notice to regular applicants
  Earliest date: Nov. 15, 2004
  Latest date: Until class is filled
Applicant's response to acceptance offer
  Maximum time: 2 weeks
Requests for deferred entrance considered: Yes
Deposit to hold place in class (applied to tuition):
  $100, due with response to acceptance offer
Deposit refundable prior to: May 16, 2005
Estimated number of new entrants: 120
Starting date: Aug. 2005

TUITION AND STUDENT FEES PER YEAR FOR 2003–2004 FIRST-YEAR CLASS

†Tuition: $37,032   Student fees: None

INFORMATION ON 2003–2004 FIRST-YEAR CLASS

Number of	In-State	Out-of-State	Total
Applicants	196	3,537	3,733
Applicants Interviewed	52	1,033	1,085
New Entrants*	15	107	122

*All took the MCAT and had baccalaureate degrees.
†Tuition is stabilized for four years.

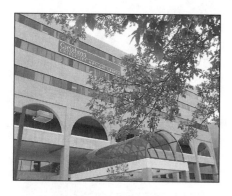

Creighton University
School of Medicine

Omaha, Nebraska

Dr. Cam E. Enarson, *Dean, School of Medicine and Vice President for Health Sciences*
Dr. Henry C. Nipper, *Assistant Dean for Admissions*
Tanya T. Avant, *Financial Aid Coordinator*
Dr. Sade Kosoko, *Associate Vice President for Multicultural and Community Affairs*

ADDRESS INQUIRIES TO:

Creighton University School of Medicine
Office of Admissions
2500 California Plaza
Omaha, Nebraska 68178
(402) 280-2799; 280-1241 (FAX)
E-mail: medschadm@creighton.edu
Web site: http://medicine.creighton.edu

MISSION STATEMENT

In the Catholic, Jesuit tradition of Creighton University, the mission of the School of Medicine is to improve the human condition through excellence in educating students, physicians and the public, advancing knowledge, and providing comprehensive patient care.

VISION STATEMENT

We will be a School of Medicine respected by our peers for excellence in teaching, research, and clinical care. We will be distinguished for preparing graduates who achieve excellence in their chosen fields and who demonstrate an extraordinary compassion and commitment to the service of others.

GENERAL INFORMATION

The Creighton University School of Medicine, a Jesuit institution, was opened over 100 years ago in October 1892, 14 years after the opening of the parent university. Its plant includes four units that provide all facilities for research, basic science, and preclinical teaching. The Medical Education Center offers over 12,000 sq. feet of newly remodeled space including state of the art small group classrooms, lecture halls, interactive space and a 60-seat computer classroom. Creighton University Medical Center, accommodating 404 patients, is the principal teaching hospital. Clinical instruction is also carried out in the Children's Memorial, Veterans Affairs, and Alegent Health System hospitals. Clinical services are also conducted at other area hospitals and clinics. The Bio-information Center, contains a multimedia self-instructional component, a biomedical communication center, an educational services unit, and the traditional library facilities.

CURRICULUM

Students participate in an integrated curriculum that incorporates basic and clinical science in all four years. The educational program has been divided into four components. Component One, Biomedical Fundamentals, serves as the foundation of the educational program followed by more complex basic science information presented in a clinically relevant context in Component Two. This component consists of a series of organ-based and disease-based courses. Component Three consists of required core clerkships emphasizing basic medical principles and acquisition of core clinical skills in a variety of inpatient and ambulatory settings. Component Four provides additional responsibilities for patient care including an eight-week block of critical care medicine, a four-week surgery selective, a four-week primary care sub-internship, and twenty-four weeks of elective study. Clinical experience is a prominent part of the curriculum in all components, beginning with the physical diagnosis instruction in the first year. Students interact with standardized patients in the first year and are assigned to longitudinal clinics during the second year. The curriculum also integrates ethical and societal issues into all four components. Instructional methodology utilizes case-based small-group sessions and computer-assisted instruction in all components. A close faculty/student relationship provides for mentoring and advising of students in choosing courses that will broaden their background for a career in medicine, as well as satisfying their special interests. Competency-based evaluation is used in all components, and the students are graded on a pass/fail/honors system. Students compete against standards and not each other.

STUDENT LIFE

"...service is a primary goal of education...our graduates and their mentors should be advocates of justice and crafters of a social order." —John Schlegel, S.J., President, Creighton University

The Creighton University School of Medicine is engaged in a myriad of programs, collaborations, and individual activities with the goal of serving the interests of those most in need. Our students are actively involved in programs such as our Institute for Latin American Concern where students provide health education and care in the Dominican Republic, Project CURE, Habitat for Humanity, Student Medical Outreach Clinic, Make-a-Wish, and many others. Although not required, 100% of our students participate in some form of community service.

In addition to their involvement in community service, students balance the rigors of academic study with a variety of wellness opportunities. Students are actively involved in the Wellness Council, which plans activities such as picnics, movie nights, golf outings, and stress management sessions, and publishes the *Wellness Chronicle*, a quarterly newsletter.

Our students participate in intramural sports, clubs, and other recreational activities available throughout the Omaha area.

REQUIREMENTS FOR ENTRANCE

The MCAT and three years (at least 90 semester hours) of accredited college work are mandatory. Preference is given, however, to holders of the baccalaureate degree. Applicants may take the MCAT in the fall of the year preceding their entry into medical school. All requirements for admission must be completed by June prior to entry. Coursework must include:

Sem. hrs.

General Biology (with lab) 8
Inorganic or General Chemistry (with lab). 8
Organic Chemistry (with lab) 8-10
General Physics (with lab) 8
English 6

Although no additional coursework is required, advanced study in human biology, especially biochemistry and/or genetics, is strongly encouraged. Any major in science or liberal arts (except military science) appropriate to their interests is acceptable. Non-science majors are expected to take advanced science study to the extent possible. Up to 27 semester hours of credit are accepted under CLEP and/or Advanced Placement programs.

SELECTION FACTORS

Consideration will be given to all of the qualities considered to be necessary in a physician. Intellectual ability and curiosity, emotional maturity, honesty, and proper motivation, in addition to proven scholastic ability, are of the utmost importance. Significant service to humanity and documented medical experience are deemed important. The preprofessional committee evaluations and letters of recommendation are equally important.

The school requires a formal interview on campus of every applicant selected before it finalizes the acceptance.

There are no restrictions placed on applicants because of race, religion, sex, national or ethnic origin, age, disability, or veteran status. Candidates are not restricted by state of residence. Creighton University values diversity in its medical classes. Not only is ethnic diversity encouraged, but Creighton considers the non-traditional applicant to be a positive influence on the school and its students. Advantage is given to applicants who have undertaken their preprofessional education at Creighton University.

Because the cumulative and science GPAs of the 120 candidates selected for the 2003 entering class were 3.65 and 3.70, respectively, it is suggested that no candidate apply whose GPA in either situation is below 3.2.

The AMCAS application is the principal source of information on the candidates. Additional (secondary) information is requested of all applicants upon receipt of AMCAS materials.

FINANCIAL AID

In addition to federally insured student loan programs and funds available from major foundation grants, a limited number of scholarships and fellowships are available for upperclassmen and for a few well-qualified entering students. Scholarship aid is awarded on the basis of overall qualifications and personal financial need.

Approximately 95 percent of the students receive some form of financial aid during a part or all of their four years of study. Students are discouraged from accepting outside employment. Spouses of students usually have no difficulty in finding employment in the Omaha metropolitan area.

INFORMATION ABOUT DIVERSITY PROGRAMS

Consideration is given to applications from candidates from groups underrepresented in medicine. The school application fee will be waived if AMCAS has first waived its charges. Financial aid in the form of grants and long-term loans is available on the basis of proven need.

Institution Type: *Private*
Application Process: *AMCAS, see chapter 4.*

APPLICATION AND ACCEPTANCE POLICIES FOR 2005–2006 FIRST-YEAR CLASS

Filing of AMCAS application
  Earliest date: June 1, 2004
  Latest date: Dec. 1, 2004
School application fee to all applicants: $75
Oldest MCAT scores considered: 2002
Does have Early Decision Program
  EDP application period: June 1—Aug. 1, 2004
  EDP applicants notified by: Oct. 1, 2004
  Acceptance notice to regular applicants
  Earliest date: Oct. 15, 2004
  Latest date: Until class is filled
Applicant's response to acceptance offer
  Maximum time: 2 weeks
Requests for deferred entrance considered: Yes
Deposit to hold place in class (applied to tuition):
  $100, due with response to acceptance offer
Deposit refundable prior to: May 16, 2005
Estimated number of new entrants: 120 (3 EDP)
Starting date: Aug. 2005

TUITION AND STUDENT FEES PER YEAR FOR 2003–2004 FIRST-YEAR CLASS

Tuition: $35,364   Student fees: $720

INFORMATION ON 2003–2004 FIRST-YEAR CLASS

Number of	*In-State*	*Out-of-State*	*Total*
Applicants	189	3,759	3,948
Applicants Interviewed	46	542	588
New Entrants*	14	106	120

*All had baccalaureate degrees and took the MCAT.

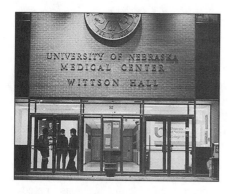

University of Nebraska College of Medicine

Omaha, Nebraska

Dr. John L. Gollan, *Dean*
Shirley Dohring, *Assistant Director of Financial Aid*
Dr. Jeffrey W. Hill, *Associate Dean, Office of Admissions and Students*
Dr. Kristie D. Hayes, *Assistant Dean for Student and Multicultural Affairs*

ADDRESS INQUIRIES TO:

Office of Admissions and Students
University of Nebraska College of Medicine
986585 Nebraska Medical Center
Omaha, Nebraska 68198-6585
(402) 559-2259; 559-6840 (FAX)
Web site: www.unmc.edu/UNCOM

MISSION STATEMENT

The mission of the University of Nebraska Medical Center is to improve the health of Nebraska through premier educational programs, innovative research, the highest quality patient care, and outreach to underserved populations.

GENERAL INFORMATION

Medical education has been continuous in Omaha since students first entered the Omaha Medical College in the fall of 1880. The University of Nebraska Medical Center includes colleges of dentistry, medicine, nursing, and pharmacy, a school of allied health, Nebraska Medical Center (University Hospital and Clarkson Hospital), University Outpatient Services, University Geriatric Center, Eppley Cancer Research Institute, and C. Louis Meyer Children's Rehabilitation Institute. These facilities are supplemented by direct teaching affiliations with the Veterans Affairs Hospital and eight private hospitals, two of which are on the medical center campus. Thus students have access to facilities with a total of approximately 2,800 teaching beds.

CURRICULUM

The goals of the College of Medicine are to provide the best possible training both in the science and art of medicine for students with the dedication and ability to become working practitioners of the healing arts. Education at the College of Medicine sets high standards for its students who, as a result, are recognized throughout the country as highly skilled practitioners with superior clinical ability. The college provides a sound basis for support of career choices in medical practice, teaching, research, or administration by stimulating students to obtain a background of basic information, a command of the language of biomedical science, a mastery of the skills necessary for clinical problem-solving, a habit of self-education, and a sympathetic understanding of the behavior of healthy and sick people. The college

is particularly oriented toward training physicians to meet all the health care needs of the citizens of Nebraska.

The curriculum ensures that students develop the understanding, clinical skills, and knowledge needed for residency training and practice. The Nebraska graduate develops superior skills in problem solving and clinical reasoning, extensive knowledge of the biomedical and psychosocial sciences, and the skills needed for lifelong learning of medicine. Courses in the first two years introduce students to the basic sciences of medicine: anatomy, behavioral science, biochemistry, microbiology, pathology, pharmacology, and physiology. Here students also begin to learn clinical skills and reasoning, through preceptorships and clinical case study in small groups.

In the third and fourth years students apply their knowledge on the hospital wards and clinical offices. Under faculty guidance students develop clinical diagnostic and management skills. They learn to select clinical tests and prescribe therapies. They learn to provide comprehensive care and learn the art of medicine. During the third year, students take clinical clerkships in Family Medicine, Internal Medicine, Obstetrics and Gynecology, Pediatrics, Psychiatry, and Surgery. In the fourth year, students select from a variety of clinical and basic science experiences.

At the beginning of medical school, students work in small groups with a faculty member to solve clinical cases. This initial exercise helps develop the library and information retrieval skills they will need in their medical studies. Case study and small-group teaching emphasizing problem-based learning are becoming more prominent features of all of the basic science courses. Since 1986, simulated patients have been used to supplement the clinical experience of medical students. These trained patient simulators are used to teach and evaluate history taking and physical examination skills. All these changes are making medical education more relevant to patient care and medical practice.

REQUIREMENTS FOR ENTRANCE

The MCAT and a minimum of 90 semester hours (three years of college work) in an accredited liberal arts and sciences college are required. The completion of a college major or baccalaureate degree is strongly recommended. The undergraduate program must include:

	Sem. hrs.
Biology (with lab)	8–10
General Chemistry (with lab)	8–10
Organic Chemistry (with lab)	8–10
Physics (with lab)	8–10
Humanities and/or Social Sciences	12–16
Calculus or Statistics	3
English Composition or writing course	3
Biochemistry	3
Genetics	3

In addition to meeting specific requirements, applicants are encouraged to adopt an educational goal that includes exploring areas of personal interest. In view of the rapidly broadening scope of medicine, a well-rounded education is considered optimum preparation. The requirements are consistent with that belief.

SELECTION FACTORS

Selection is based on a total assessment of each candidate's motivation, interests, character, demonstrated intellectual ability, previous academic record and its trends, personal interview, scores on the MCAT, and general fitness and promise for a career in medicine. Admission is based on individual qualifications without regard to age, sex, sexual preference, race, national origin, handicap, or religious or political beliefs. Academic credentials are evaluated on the basis of course level and load, involvement in cocurricular activities or employment, and other influential factors. Cutoff levels for GPAs or for scores on the MCAT are not utilized; however, applicants are reminded of the competition for entrance and are advised to be realistic. Personal attributes are assessed through letters of reference and in the interview.

Strong preference is given to residents of Nebraska, but a number of students from other states may be accepted. The University of Nebraska encourages, in particular, students from rural areas, small towns, or disadvantaged backgrounds to apply. The potential for service to underserved communities is taken into consideration during the preadmission evaluation.

Accepted students for the 2003 entering class had the following credentials: *mean GPA,* 3.65; *sex,* 40 percent women; *undergraduate major,* approximately 85 percent science majors.

FINANCIAL AID

Some scholarships are available each year. A few may be granted to entering first-year students. Several fellowships and assistantships are available to students who desire to take one or two years of graduate study or research in the basic sciences. Loan funds have been increased through efforts of physicians in Nebraska, fraternal organizations, and friends of the college. Approximately 98 percent of the students receive some financial aid.

INFORMATION ABOUT DIVERSITY PROGRAMS

The University of Nebraska College of Medicine is committed to increasing the number of physicians from groups currently underrepresented in the medical profession. Applications from members of these groups are encouraged. The accomplishments of applicants will be evaluated with due consideration given to their backgrounds. Specific information is available from the Office of Student Equity and Multicultural Affairs; 984275 Nebraska Medical Center, Omaha, NE 68198-4275; (402) 559-4437.

Institution Type: *Public*
Application Process: *AMCAS, see chapter 4.*

APPLICATION AND ACCEPTANCE POLICIES FOR 2005–2006 FIRST-YEAR CLASS

Filing of AMCAS application
  Earliest date: June 1, 2004
  Latest date: Nov. 1, 2004
School application fee to all applicants: $45
Oldest MCAT scores considered: 2002
Does have Early Decision Program (EDP)
  EDP application period: June 1–Aug. 1, 2004
  EDP applicants notified by: Oct. 1, 2004
Acceptance notice to regular applicants
  Earliest date: December 2004
  Latest date: Until class is filled
Applicant's response to acceptance offer
  Maximum time: 2 weeks
Requests for deferred entrance considered: No
Deposit to hold place in class (applied to tuition):
  $100, due with response to acceptance offer
Deposit refundable prior to: May 16, 2005
Estimated number of new entrants: 120 (25 EDP)
Starting date: Aug. 2005

TUITION AND STUDENT FEES PER YEAR FOR 2003–2004 FIRST-YEAR CLASS

Tuition	Student fees: $1,222
Resident: $16,640	
Nonresident: $39,020	

INFORMATION ON 2003–2004 FIRST-YEAR CLASS

Number of	In-State	Out-of-State	Total
Applicants	271	709	980
Applicants Interviewed	244	109	353
New Entrants*	104	14	118

*All took the MCAT; 100% had baccalaureate degrees.

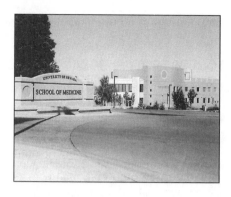

University of Nevada
School of Medicine

Reno, Nevada

Dr. Stephen McFarlane, *Dean*
Dr. Cheryl Hug-English, *Associate Dean for Admissions and Student Affairs*
Dr. Peggy Dupey, *Assistant Dean for Student Affairs*
Ann Diggins, *Director of Recruitment and Student Services, Las Vegas Campus*

ADDRESS INQUIRIES TO:

Office of Admissions and Student Affairs
University of Nevada
School of Medicine
Mail Stop 357
Reno, Nevada 89557-0129
(775) 784-6063; 784-6194 (FAX)
E-mail: asa@med.unr.edu
Web site: www.unr.edu/med

MISSION STATEMENT

To provide educational opportunities for Nevadans, to improve the quality of healthcare for citizens of Nevada, to create new biomedical knowledge through education, research, patient care and community service, and to provide continuing medical education.

GENERAL INFORMATION

The University of Nevada School of Medicine is a state-supported, community-based, university-integrated school which relies heavily on community physicians as teachers and community health facilities as sites for the majority of its clinical education. The school is dedicated to selecting individuals with diverse backgrounds who will learn to be compassionate and competent physicians. Students study comprehensive health care delivery considering the needs of the individual, the family, and the community.

CURRICULUM

The first two years of the program are concentrated in classrooms and laboratories on the Reno campus. The curriculum emphasizes biomedical and behavioral sciences basic to medicine. Basic science disciplines are integrated with each other and with clinical problems to promote the learning of problem-solving skills. A clinical correlation course, which explores the basics of biomedical ethics, is taught.

Early clinical training is provided for students to learn patient interviewing, doctor-patient relationship skills, and basics of physical examination and diagnosis. Throughout the first and second years, students spend time with a physician to observe medical practice in the office setting and clinic settings.

There are also opportunities to participate in basic and clinical science research throughout the curriculum. The third and fourth years emphasize a balance of ambulatory and inpatient medical education designed to better prepare students for

residency in all specialties and the practice of medicine in the twenty-first century. Third and fourth year students study clinical medicine throughout the state, including clinical campuses in Reno and Las Vegas and in rural Nevada.

Individualized M.D.-Ph.D. programs are offered to students, depending upon the specific interest area.

REQUIREMENTS FOR ENTRANCE

The MCAT and a minimum of three years of college work (90 semester hours) are required. The MCAT must be taken prior to the November 1 application deadline. (It is not necessary to wait for fall MCAT scores prior to applying.) The Admissions Selection Committee strongly recommends completion of a baccalaureate degree prior to matriculation in medical school.

Applicants are encouraged to have a broad educational background and to enroll in an in-depth curriculum that will lead to a discipline-oriented major, e.g., biology, chemistry, psychology. However, no specific major is favored over any other. In addition to academic coursework, people-oriented activities and health care exposure are important.

Coursework must include:

	Sem. hrs.
Biology	12
Must include 3 sem. hrs. of upper-division credit	
Inorganic Chemistry	8
Organic Chemistry	8
Physics	8
Behavioral Sciences	6
Must include 3 sem. hrs. of upper-division credit	

In fulfillment of the behavioral sciences requirement, students should take courses that deal with the psychological stages of the life cycle (e.g., human growth and development, adolescence, aging, human sexuality, abnormal psychology, family dynamics, or medically oriented sociology).

All required courses must be taken for a letter grade and in a classroom setting. Correspondence, on-line, graduate, CLEP, AP and/or pass/fail or audit in lieu of a letter or number grade is not acceptable.

A demonstrated competency in English composition and expression is required. Generally, students are expected to satisfy the English composition requirements of their undergraduate institution. Beyond these requirements, applicants are strongly encouraged to experience additional enrichment in the biological sciences (e.g., genetics, microbiology, immunology and biochemistry). Other important academic assets for the future physician rest on a solid base of general knowledge in the arts, humanities and social sciences which may include courses such as ethics, oral and written communication and computer sciences. Applicants are also encouraged to become exposed to people and their problems and to learn about the medical profession. Access to a personal computer is required of all matriculants. Accepted students are responsible for completing all prerequisite Coursework prior to matriculation.

Early submission of the AMCAS application permits its prompt evaluation during the process. Applicants are, therefore, urged to submit their applications and supporting credentials as early as possible.

Applicants educated abroad must have completed at least 2 years of study in an approved college or university in the United States or Canada before applying. Within those two years, the required courses must be completed.

SELECTION FACTORS

Candidates are evaluated on the basis of academic performance; results of the MCAT; the nature and depth of scholarly, extracurricular, and health care related activities during college years (excellence and balance of the natural sciences, social sciences, and humanities); academic letters of evaluation; and the personal interview. Select applicants are invited for interviews. Interviews are held in Reno and Las Vegas.

A high priority is given to residents of Nevada. A small number of nonresident applicants are considered each year who have strong residential ties to Nevada (that is, parents' residence, medical catchment area) or are residents of Alaska, Idaho, Montana, or Wyoming (western rural states without medical schools). Individuals who do not meet the residential requirements should not apply.

Matriculants for the 2003 entering class had the following profile: *average science GPA,* 3.5; *cumulative GPA,* 3.6; *average MCAT scores*—VR-9.1; PS-8.7; BS-9.3; 50 percent female; *average age,* 24.

Resident and nonresident applications for the Early Decision Program (EDP) are encouraged. It is suggested that EDP applicants call for updated requirements before application. Reapplicants are not eligible for EDP.

Only those students who are currently enrolled and in good academic standing at LCME-accredited medical schools and have a strong residential tie to Nevada are considered for transfer to the second and third years. The number of positions available for transfer is strictly limited by attrition and compatibility to the school's curriculum. Only U.S. citizens are considered. Applications from students attending foreign medical schools are not considered.

FINANCIAL AID

Every attempt is made to assist students and their families in meeting both their financial obligations to the School of Medicine and the student's essential personal needs. Financial status is not a determinant in selecting qualified applicants. A limited number of loans and scholarships are available to medical students on the basis of need and merit. Determination of financial aid award is made after acceptance. More than 80 percent of Nevada's medical students receive some type of financial assistance.

INFORMATION ABOUT DIVERSITY PROGRAMS

The School of Medicine is committed to the recruitment, selection, and retention of individuals who are members of groups traditionally underrepresented in American medicine. Residents of the state of Nevada and individuals who meet the nonresident criteria who are from such backgrounds are encouraged to apply.

The University of Nevada, Reno does not discriminate on the basis of race, color, religion, sex, age, creed, national origin, veteran status, physical or mental disability, and in accordance with university policy, sexual orientation, in any program or activity it operates.

Institution Type: *Public*
Application Process: *AMCAS, see chapter 4.*

APPLICATION AND ACCEPTANCE POLICIES FOR 2005–2006 FIRST-YEAR CLASS

Filing of AMCAS application
   Earliest date: June 1, 2004
   Latest date: Nov. 1, 2004
School application fee after screening: $45
Oldest MCAT scores considered: 2001
   Does have Early Decision Program (EDP)
   EDP application period: June 1–Aug. 1, 2004
   EDP applicants notified by: Oct. 1, 2004
Acceptance notice to regular applicants
   Earliest date: Jan. 15, 2005
   Latest date: Varies
Applicant's response to acceptance offer
   Maximum time: 2 weeks
Requests for deferred entrance considered: Yes
Deposit to hold place in class: None
Estimated number of new entrants: 52 (no more than 3 EDP)
Starting date: Aug. 2005

TUITION AND STUDENT FEES PER YEAR FOR 2003–2004 FIRST-YEAR CLASS

Tuition   Student fees: $2,375
   Resident: $9,232
   Nonresident: $26,810

INFORMATION ON 2003–2004 FIRST-YEAR CLASS

Number of	In-State	Out-of-State	Total
Applicants	176	117	293
Applicants Interviewed	n/a	n/a	n/a
New Entrants*	47	5	52

*All took the MCAT and had baccalaureate degrees.
n/a information not available

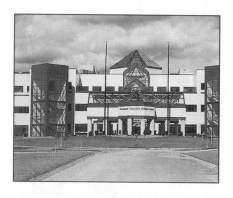

Dartmouth Medical School

Hanover, New Hampshire

Dr. Stephen P. Spielberg, *Acting Dean*
Andrew G. Welch, *Director of Admissions*
Nanci G. Cirone, *Director of Financial Aid*
Dr. Lori Alvord, *Associate Dean of Student and Multicultural Affairs*

ADDRESS INQUIRIES TO:

Dartmouth Medical School
Office of Admissions
3 Rope Ferry Rd.
Hanover, New Hampshire 03755-1404
(603) 650-1505; 650-1560 (FAX)
E-mail: dms.admissions@dartmouth.edu
Web site: www.dartmouth.edu/dms/

MISSION STATEMENT

Dartmouth Medical School is dedicated to advancing health through the dissemination and discovery of knowledge. Our chief responsibility is to select students of exceptional character and accomplishment and prepare them to become superb and caring physicians, scientists, and teachers.

We are committed to:

• education of health professionals in an environment of discovery;
• research that advances health;
• formulation of health policies in the interest of our citizens;
• service with our partners to maintain Dartmouth-Hitchcock Medical Center as a local, regional, and national resource for health care of the highest quality.

GENERAL INFORMATION

Dartmouth Medical School, the 4th oldest medical school in the United States, is a component of Dartmouth-Hitchcock Medical Center (DHMC), nationally recognized as one of the country's preeminent academic medical centers. DHMC, a modem, state-of-the-art facility located on a 230 acre campus, also includes Mary Hitchcock Memorial Hospital, the Dartmouth-Hitchcock Clinic, and the Veterans Affairs Hospital in White River Junction, VT. Centers of excellence within DHMC include the Norris Cotton Cancer Center (ranked one of the top 30 comprehensive cancer centers in the nation by U.S. News & World Report) and the Childrens Hospital at Dartmouth. Integrating quality care for its patient population of 1.6 million with advanced research taking place at the Cancer Center and in the Borwell Research Building, DHMC is the site of numerous clinical trials and a major force for medical treatment and medical discovery within the region. A major expansion of the 396 bed facility will be completed in 2006, adding 400,000 square feet of research labs, diagnostic and treatment space, and ambulatory care facilities. Supplementary teaching sites include the Brattleboro Retreat (VT), the Family Medical Institute of Augusta (ME), Hartford Hospital (CT), the Tuba City Indian Health Service Hospital (AZ), Children's Hospital of Orange County (CA), and numerous primary care sites in Maine, New Hampshire, and Vermont. The C. Everett Koop Institute at Dartmouth was founded in 1992. Dr. Koop serves as the institute's senior scholar. A faculty of approximately 1,000 offers all students the opportunity for individually based instruction.

CURRICULUM

Dartmouth's "New Directions" curriculum is designed to integrate the study of basic and clinical sciences throughout medical school. The curriculum's hallmarks are longitudinal experiences in both the basic and clinical sciences, introduction to the ambulatory care setting in the earliest weeks of study, extended participation in small-group learning, close working relationships with faculty members, and increased opportunities for independent learning. The first year includes On Doctoring, a course that pairs students with faculty practitioners in local communities. Clinical training in the course alternates with biweekly, small-group tutorials on the DMS campus. A major course in the second year is the Scientific Basis of Medicine, an interdisciplinary pathophysiology course that integrates, through lectures, seminars, and problem-based learning, the basic sciences with a broad introduction to the mechanisms of disease and the principles of clinical medicine. In the third year, students begin a series of clinical clerkships in: Internal Medicine Surgery; Obstetric Gynecology and Women's Health; Pediatrics, Psychiatry and Family Medicine, Ambulatory Medicine and Neurology. The fourth year includes a sub-internship and four short courses (Clinical Pharmacology, Advanced Medical Sciences, Health, Society and the Physician, and Advance Cardiac Life Support), but is largely tailored to students' individual needs and interests through substantial elective opportunities.

Entering class size at Dartmouth is approximately 80. Most students follow the four-year curriculum at DMS and receive the M.D. degree from Dartmouth. Approximately 15 students, admitted jointly by Dartmouth and the Brown University School of Medicine, spend the first two years at Dartmouth and the last two years studying at Brown. The Brown-Dartmouth students are awarded the M.D. from Brown.

DMS offers an M.D.-Ph.D. program that provides a comprehensive academic, intellectual, and financially supportive environment enabling highly qualified students to pursue an

M.D. and a Ph.D. in any of the degree-granting departments of the medical school and the college. A joint M.D.-M.B.A. program is offered through DMS and Dartmouth's Amos Tuck School of Business Administration. In addition, graduate degrees are available through Dartmouth's Center for the Evaluative Clinical Sciences, as well as an MPH.

REQUIREMENTS FOR ENTRANCE

Except in unusual circumstances, all candidates are expected to present MCAT scores. Where possible, the spring MCAT is recommended and helps the Admissions Committee to proceed expeditiously with the review of an application.

Specific courses required at college level are:

	Sem. hrs.
General Biology	8
Inorganic Chemistry	8
Organic Chemistry	8
Physics	8
Calculus	3

Proficiency in written and oral English is required. At least three years of study at a Canadian or American college or university is required. Also encouraged is a semester of biochemistry which is helpful preparation for medical school, though it is not required.

In general, the demonstration of excellence in an area of study is a more important criterion than the particular discipline. Hence, students are encouraged to major in the field of their special interest and, if possible, to pursue independent investigation in that field. Students majoring in nonsciences who have demonstrated ability in science are encouraged to apply.

SELECTION FACTORS

The decision of the Admissions Committee depends on appraisal of the entire application, including a thorough evaluation of personal, scholastic, and scientific qualifications. Rigid cutoff points and inflexible criteria are avoided. Dartmouth Medical School is a national institution enrolling students from across the country.

All candidates who apply to DMS through AMCAS receive a secondary application, and all applicants in the final group from which the class is chosen are interviewed in Hanover. A limited number of applicants are selected to interview and are invited throughout the academic year.

It is the long-standing policy of Dartmouth Medical School to support equality of opportunity for all persons regardless of race or ethnic background, and no student shall be denied admission or financial aid or be otherwise discriminated against because of age, disability, race, creed, religion, sex, sexual orientation, or national origin.

Application for the Brown-Dartmouth program is initiated at Dartmouth. All applicants invited for interviews receive a form on which to indicate their program choices. In selecting applicants for the joint program, the admission policies and standards of both institutions are observed. Successful applicants are offered acceptance to only one program at a time. Letters of acceptance state the program to which the student has been admitted and are binding.

FINANCIAL AID

Admission decisions are made without regard to financial need. All accepted U.S. citizens and permanent residents with documented need are offered financial aid packages. Approximately 80 percent of the students receive financial aid, usually as a combination of scholarship and loan or through federally supported service programs. Scholarships and loans are awarded on the basis of need as documented on the FAFSA, the Need Access form, and the DMS financial aid application and supporting documentation.

Application fee waiver is granted to individuals who have received an AMCAS fee waiver. Applicants who are neither U.S. citizens nor permanent residents should be aware that financial support for foreign students is extremely limited.

INFORMATION ABOUT DIVERSITY PROGRAMS

Applications from members of groups underrepresented in medicine are encouraged. Lori Alvord, M.D., is Associate Dean of Student and Multicultural Affairs.

Institution Type: *Private*
Application Process: *AMCAS, see chapter 4.*

APPLICATION AND ACCEPTANCE POLICIES FOR 2005–2006 FIRST-YEAR CLASS

Filing of AMCAS application
  Earliest date: June 1, 2004
  Latest date: Nov. 1, 2004
School application fee to all applicants: $75
Oldest MCAT scores considered: 2002
Does not have Early Decision Program
Acceptance notice to regular applicants
  Earliest date: Dec. 15, 2004
  Latest date: Until class is filled
Applicant's response to acceptance offer
  Maximum time: 2 weeks
Requests for deferred entrance considered: Yes
Deposit to hold place in class: None
Estimated number of new entrants: 80
Starting date: Aug. 2005

TUITION AND STUDENT FEES PER YEAR FOR 2003–2004 FIRST-YEAR CLASS

Tuition: $31,600   Student fees: $1,950

INFORMATION ON 2003–2004 FIRST-YEAR CLASS

Number of	In-State	Out-of-State	Total
Applicants	68	4,942	5,010
Applicants Interviewed	33	555	588
New Entrants*	12	66	78

*All had baccalaureate degrees; 95% took the MCAT.

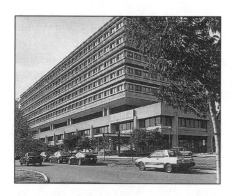

University of Medicine and Dentistry of New Jersey—New Jersey Medical School

Newark, New Jersey

Dr. Russell T. Joffe, *Dean*
Dr. George F. Heinrich, *Associate Dean for Admissions*
Michael Katz, *University Director of Student Financial Aid*
Dr. Maria Soto-Greene, *Senior Associate Dean for Education*

ADDRESS INQUIRIES TO:

Mercedes Lettman
Director of Admissions
University of Medicine and Dentistry of New Jersey
New Jersey Medical School
185 South Orange Avenue C-653
Newark, New Jersey 07103
(973) 972-4631; 972-7986 (FAX)
E-mail: njmsadmiss@umdnj.edu
Web site: http://njms.umdnj.edu

MISSION STATEMENT

The University of Medicine and Dentistry of New Jersey, the state's university of the health sciences, is the largest free-standing health sciences university in the United States. It has four main academic health center campuses in Newark, Camden, New Brunswick/Piscataway, and Stratford and also at educational and health care institutions in communities throughout the state.

The University of Medicine and Dentistry of New Jersey is dedicated to the pursuit of excellence in:

- the undergraduate, graduate, postgraduate, and continuing education of health professionals and scientists;
- the conduct of basic biomedical, psychosocial, clinical, and public health research;
- health promotion, and disease prevention,
- and the delivery of health care and service to our communities and the entire state.

The University of Medicine and Dentistry of New Jersey seeks to advance the health sciences; to prepare future health professionals for leadership roles; to respond to academic, health personnel, and service delivery needs, while recognizing the diversity of our constituencies; to provide educational opportunities to New Jerseyans; and to improve the health and quality of life of the citizens of New Jersey and society at large.

GENERAL INFORMATION

The New Jersey Medical School of the University of Medicine and Dentistry of New Jersey moved into facilities situated in Newark in 1977. A $350 million complex contains the teaching-research Biomedical Science Building, a hospital, an ambulatory care center, a library, a dental school, and a community mental health center.

Major clinical instruction is carried out at University Hospital, Hackensack University Medical Center, Veterans Affairs Medical Center in East Orange, Morristown Memorial Hospital, and Kessler Institute for Rehabilitation.

Major new facilities are being constructed on the Newark campus, including the $100 million new Cancer Center.

CURRICULUM

During the first two years, a thorough coverage of the basic medical sciences is implemented through a hybrid curriculum with departmental and integrated interdepartmental studies. There is substantial clinical exposure in the first year. A first-year course, The Art of Medicine, utilizes office–based preceptorships along with small group problem-based learning. Part of the second year is devoted to an introduction to the clinical sciences, during which the student receives instruction in history-taking, physical diagnosis, and pathophysiology. In addition, courses in preventive medicine and community health, behavorial science, and psychiatry are offered. The third year is spent in rotations through core clinical departments. This is a closely supervised, hands-on, comprehensive learning experience in which the student acquires the basic knowledge and techniques of clinical medicine. Instruction is carried out mainly in small groups and is individualized. The fourth year is devoted to advanced required work and elective programs. The required courses are emergency medicine, neurology, surgical subspecialties, physical medicine and rehabilitation, and an acting internship, all of which bring together the ethical, legal, and social factors that are part of total patient care. Sixteen weeks of electives are available.

An ongoing curriculum renewal process is aimed at achieving an organ-system approach in the preclinical years and strengthening clinical and professional skills in the clinical years.

REQUIREMENTS FOR ENTRANCE

The MCAT and a minimum of three years of college (90 credit hours) are required. Three-year applicants with good credentials are encouraged to apply.

The minimum requirements are:

	Sem. hrs.
Biology or Zoology (with lab)	8
Coursework must be exclusive of botany and invertebrate zoology.	
Organic Chemistry (with lab)	8
Other Chemistry (with lab)	8
Inorganic, physical, analytical chemistry or biochemistry will satisfy the requirement.	
General Physics (with lab)	8
English	6

A course in mathematics is recommended, but not required. Matriculants must be either U.S. citizens or permanent residents.

Specific requirements may be waived or imposed at the discretion of the Admissions Committee in any individual case.

The Admissions Committee urges all candidates to prepare themselves further by completing courses in social or cultural fields and generally broadening their academic backgrounds. Candidates who are not premedical or science majors are given equal consideration if they have demonstrated academic excellence in the course requirements listed above.

New Jersey Medical School offers a limited number of Academic Excellence Scholarships for entering first-year students.

Available combined degree programs are: M.D./Ph.D., M.D./J.D., M.D./M.P.H., and M.D./M.B.A.

Early Decision applications are encouraged from qualified applicants. There is also an Early Decision dual M.D./Ph.D. degree option.

SELECTION FACTORS

Students are selected on the basis of scholastic achievement, fitness, and aptitude for the study of medicine, and other personal qualifications. Since success in medicine depends on a number of related factors in a student's development, of which scholastic accomplishments are only a part, the Admissions Committee also gives consideration to the use of language, special aptitudes and motivation.

New Jersey Medical School applies no GPA or MCAT cut-off levels in its selection process. It must be remembered, however, that competition is very keen, and applicants who are high in all determinable categories often receive the highest priority for acceptance. There are no restrictions as to race, creed, sex, national origin, age, or handicap.

Accepted students in the 2003 entering class had the following profile: *average* GPA, 3.5; *gender,* 51 percent women; *minorities,* 27 percents.

Applications from nonresidents are encouraged.

The University of Medicine and Dentistry of New Jersey policy is that no program or activity administered by the University shall exclude from participation, admission, treatment or employment, or deny benefits to, or subject to discrimination any qualified individual solely by reason of his or her disability.

FINANCIAL AID

No questions of financial need are involved in the selection of students. All students who are accepted and wish to matriculate are advised to contact the financial aid officer immediately to discuss aid and fill out all necessary forms. All aid is given on the basis of financial need as assessed by an outside source. The needs analysis is usually adjusted upward to reflect costs in the northeastern United States. Approximately 70 percent of the students receive some form of financial aid. The Financial Aid Office extends itself to help all students in financial need.

INFORMATION ABOUT DIVERSITY PROGRAMS

NJMS has a long-standing strong commitment to the recruitment of applicants from groups underrepresented in medicine. A special summer program is open to economically and educationally disadvantaged students who have been accepted, as well as to other students in various stages of their undergraduate careers. Information is available from Lonnie Wright, Director of the Students for Medicine and Dentistry Program, at (973) 972-5433.

Institution Type: *Public*
Application Process: *AMCAS, see chapter 4.*

APPLICATION AND ACCEPTANCE POLICIES FOR 2005–2006 FIRST-YEAR CLASS

Filing of AMCAS application
  Earliest date: June 1, 2004
  Latest date: Dec. 15, 2004
School application fee to all applicants: $75
Oldest MCAT scores accepted: 2001
Does have Early Decision Program (EDP)
  EDP application period: June 1–Aug. 1, 2004
  EDP applicants notified by: Oct. 1, 2004
Acceptance notice to regular applicants
  Earliest date: Oct. 15, 2004
  Latest date: Until class is filled
Applicant's response to acceptance offer
  Maximum time: 2 weeks
Requests for deferred entrance considered: Yes
Deposit to hold place in class (applied to tuition):
  $100, due with response to acceptance offer
Deposit refundable prior to: May 16, 2005
Estimated number of new entrants: 170 (10 EDP)
Starting date: Aug. 2005

TUITION AND STUDENT FEES PER YEAR FOR 2003-2004 FIRST-YEAR CLASS

Tuition   Student fees: $2,391
  Resident: $19,776
  Nonresident: $30,947

INFORMATION ON 2003-2004 FIRST-YEAR CLASS

Number of	In-State	Out-of-State	Total
Applicants	930	2,010	2,940
Applicants Interviewed	502	177	679
New Entrants*	142	28	170

*All took the MCAT.

All out-of-state (non-resident) applicants who matriculated August 2003, qualified for in-state (resident) tuition.

CHAPTER
11

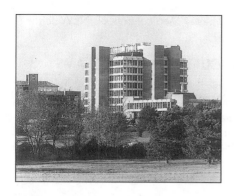

University of Medicine and Dentistry of New Jersey Robert Wood Johnson Medical School

Piscataway, New Jersey

Dr. Harold L. Paz, *Dean*
Dr. Carol A. Terregino, *Assistant Dean for Admissions*
Marshall Anthony, *Associate Director of Financial Aid*
Dr. Janice M. Johnson, *Assistant Dean for Multicultural Affairs*

ADDRESS INQUIRIES TO:

Mercedes Lettman
Director of Admissions
University of Medicine and Dentistry of New Jersey
Robert Wood Johnson Medical School
675 Hoes Lane
Piscataway, New Jersey 08854-5635
(732) 235-4576; 235-5078 (FAX)
E-mail: rwjapadm@umdnj.edu
Web site: http://rwjms.umdnj.edu

MISSION STATEMENT

The medical school is dedicated to the pursuit of excellence of health professionals, in the conduct of biomedical, clinical and public health research, in the delivery of health care and in the promotion of community health. Excellence in the educational programs is achieved through the work of a scholarly and creative faculty and a high-achieving and diverse student body.

GENERAL INFORMATION

Robert Wood Johnson Medical School, formerly known as Rutgers Medical School, was named after the former president and chairman of the board of Johnson & Johnson Company and the benefactor of the Robert Wood Johnson Foundation.

The Basic Science Building is located adjacent to the science campus of Rutgers University. University Behavorial Healthcare, which houses the Department of Psychiatry, adjoins the building. Facilities shared with Rutgers University include the Library of Science and Medicine, the Center for Advanced Biotechnology and Medicine, and the Environmental and Occupational Health Science Institute. New facilities on the Piscataway campus include the Robert Wood Johnson Medical School Research Building and the University of Medicine and Dentistry of New Jersey-School of Public Health.

Robert Wood Johnson University Hospital is the principal teaching hospital in New Brunswick. Cooper Hospital/University Medical Center is the principal teaching hospital in Camden. These two centers, supplemented by affiliations with university hospitals in central New Jersey, provide the medical school with a full complement of diverse clinical training facilities.

All students receive their basic education at the Piscataway campus. Students complete their clinical training on either the Piscataway/New Brunswick or Camden campus.

CURRICULUM

The curriculum is newly revised. It provides for an early introduction to patient care, an integration of clinical skills into the basic science curriculum, and the opportunity for self-directed learning within the context of a rigorous basic science education during the first two years. Multiple learning modalities are used including lectures, laboratory exercises, small-group discussions, and computer-assisted instruction. During the first two years, in addition to the traditional basic sciences, there are courses in ethics, introduction to the patient, physical diagnosis and clinical decision making, case-based learning, clinical prevention, clinical pathophysiology, human genetics, and community and environmental medicine, among others. The third-year curriculum consists of an introduction to the clinical experience followed by five eight-week clerkships in medicine, surgery, family medicine, obstetrics-gynecology, and pediatrics, and a six-week clerkship in psychiatry. Up to four weeks of elective time is available during the third year. There is also a formative clinical skills assessment at the beginning of the third year, with a summative clinical skills assessment at the end of the year. The fourth-year curriculum includes an advanced clerkship in ambulatory medicine, an advanced clerkship in surgery, neurology, a subinternship, and a minimum of 16 weeks of electives. Grades are reported as honors, high pass, pass, low pass, and fail. Students must pass USMLE Step 1 prior to completing the third year and must pass USMLE Step 2 prior to graduation.

There are a number of dual degree options available. In conjunction with the School of Public Health, a combined M.D.-M.P.H. program is available with tuition support during the M.P.H. phase for selected students. Combined M.D.-Ph.D. programs are available in the medical school and in conjunction with the Graduate School of Biomedical Sciences and Rutgers University. Financial support that includes both tuition remission and stipends is available throughout the seven-year program. A new combined M.D.-J.D. program, in conjunction with Rutgers Law School or Seton Hall Law School; a combined M.D.-M.S. in Jurisprudence, in conjunction with Seton Hall Law School; a combined M.D.-M.S. in Medical Informatics, in conjunction with the New Jersey Institute of Technology; and a combined M.D.-M.B.A. in conjunction with Rutgers Business School are also available with tuition support during the M.B.A. phase for selected students.

REQUIREMENTS FOR ENTRANCE

The MCAT and a minimum of three years of college consisting of 90 semester hours of college work (exclusive of military and physical education) are required. The MCAT must be taken within the four years preceding application and no later than the fall of the year of application. The following undergraduate courses are required:

	Semesters
Biology or Zoology (with lab)	2
Inorganic Chemistry (with lab)	2
Organic Chemistry (with lab)	2
Physics (with lab)	2
College Mathematics	1
English	2

Must include one semester of a college writing course College-approved "writing intensive courses" may substitute for English.

Robert Wood Johnson Medical School places high value on a balanced undergraduate education. While this balance will vary with the background and interests of the individual, it is expected that applicants will have exposed themselves to coursework in the humanities, the behavioral sciences, and liberal arts as well as the premedical sciences.

Students capable of superior performance in any academic field, whether in the sciences or humanities, should feel free to pursue their intellectual interests in depth, provided only that they can do well in the required courses mentioned above. The Admissions Committee may waive or impose specific requirements at its discretion. We encourage students in post-baccalaureate programs to apply. We have linkage agreements with a number of post-baccalaureate programs. Applicants must be U.S. citizens or permanent residents to be eligible for admission.

SELECTION FACTORS

Preference for admission is given to residents of New Jersey. However, we recognize the importance of geographic diversity among our students and encourage out of state applicants with outstanding credentials to apply. 12-15% of our student body are out of state residents.

Admission is determined on the basis of academic achievement in a balanced undergraduate education, results of the MCAT, preprofessional committee evaluations, other recommendations, character, motivation, and personal interview. Applications from members of groups underrepresented in medicine are encouraged. Interviews are arranged by invitation.

Accepted students for the 2003 entering class had a *mean GPA* of 3.63 (10 percentile-3.24, 90 percentile-3.91). Women represented 54 percent of the class.

FINANCIAL AID

Accepted students who believe they will need financial aid are encouraged to request information and application forms from the Financial Aid Office. About 80 percent of the student body received some sort of financial assistance during the 2001–02 academic year. Financial aid is awarded on the basis of evaluated need computed by an approved needs analysis method. All awards consist of a package of loans and grants when funds are available. Funds have been allocated for scholarships.

INFORMATION ABOUT DIVERSITY PROGRAMS

University of Medicine and Dentistry of New Jersey—Robert Wood Johnson Medical School is committed to the education and training of physicians from groups underrepresented in medicine. Applications from both in-state and out-of-state candidates are welcome, and ample financial aid assistance is offered. Numerous support services are available, including a pre-enrollment summer program for accepted students. A summer Biomedical Careers Program for undergraduates interested in health care careers is also offered. Further information is available from Betty Treadwell-Oglesby, (oglesby@umdnj.edu).

Institution Type: *Public*
Application Process: *AMCAS, see chapter 4.*

APPLICATION AND ACCEPTANCE POLICIES FOR 2005–2006 FIRST-YEAR CLASS

Filing of AMCAS application
    Earliest date: June 1, 2004
    Latest date: Dec. 1, 2004
School application fee to all applicants: $75
Oldest MCAT scores considered: 2001
Does have Early Decision Program (EDP)
    EDP application period: June 1–Aug. 1, 2004
    EDP applicants notified by: Oct. 1, 2004
Acceptance notice to regular applicants
    Earliest date: Oct. 15, 2004
    Latest date: Until class is filled
Applicant's response to acceptance offer
    Maximum time: 2 weeks
Requests for deferred entrance considered: Yes
Deposit to hold place in class (applied to tuition):
    $50, due with response to acceptance offer
Deposit refundable prior to: May 16, 2005
Estimated number of new entrants: 142 (5 EDP)
Starting date: Aug. 2005

TUITION AND STUDENT FEES PER YEAR FOR 2003–2004 FIRST-YEAR CLASS

Tuition   Student fees: $2,291
    Resident: $19,776
    Nonresident: $30,947

INFORMATION ON 2003–2004 FIRST-YEAR CLASS

Number of	In-State	Out-of-State	Total
Applicants	945	1,553	2,498
Applicants Interviewed	469	156	625
New Entrants*	137	19	156

*All took the MCAT and had baccalaureate degrees.

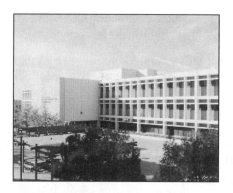

University of New Mexico
School of Medicine

Albuquerque, New Mexico

Dr. Paul B. Roth, *Dean*
Dr. Roger J. Radloff, *Assistant Dean for Admissions*
Dr. Valerie Romero-Leggott, *Director, Office of Cultural and Ethnic Programs*
Ed Wyckoff, *Supervisor, Financial Aid*

ADDRESS INQUIRIES TO:

University of New Mexico
Health Sciences Center
School of Medicine
Office of Admissions
MSC084690
Basic Medical Sciences Building, Room 106
Albuquerque, New Mexico 87131-0001
(505) 272-4766; 272-6857 (FAX)
Web site: http://hsc.unm.edu/som/admissions

MISSION STATEMENT

The mission of the University of New Mexico School of Medicine is to educate physicians, scientists, and allied health professionals through the transmission of biomedical knowledge acquired from research and patient care. The school is dedicated to the creation, evaluation, transmission, and application of biomedical knowledge to be applied directly for the improvement of the health of the public. Our primary focus is on the unique health needs of New Mexico's culturally and ethnically diverse populations. The environment in which we work recognizes and respects all who make up the community and those we serve.

GENERAL INFORMATION

The establishment of a school of the basic medical sciences was authorized by the regents and the faculty of the University of New Mexico (UNM) in 1961. The first entering class of 24 students was enrolled in September 1964, and progress to the full four-year program was approved by the New Mexico State Legislature in 1966.

The medical school facilities are located on the north campus of the university and include a basic medical sciences building, biomedical research facility, Health Sciences Library and, UNM Mental Health Center, UNM Children's Psychiatric Center, family practice center, Center for Non-Invasive Diagnosis, and an international cancer center. The 379-bed University Hospital serves as the major teaching hospital of the medical school, with additional teaching at the 165-bed New Mexico Veterans Administration. The faculty numbers 694, with 593 full-time appointments.

The School of Medicine is a professional and graduate school of the university. In addition to providing education in the basic and clinical sciences for the doctor of medicine

degree, opportunities are available for work leading to a doctor of philosophy degree as well as for a combined MD/PhD degree. Medical education at the resident and postgraduate levels is offered through the university's teaching hospitals.

CURRICULUM

The University of New Mexico School of Medicine implemented a new curriculum in the fall of 1993, which incorporated aspects of its prior educational innovations from the Conventional Curriculum Track, Primary Care Curriculum, and Health of the Public Program.

The goals of the new curriculum are to graduate physicians who: are excited and enthusiastic about learning; have assumed a major responsibility for their continued learning; have the ability to define problems, formulate questions, and carry out scholarly inquiry; are skilled in self and peer assessment; have a broad perspective on the importance of human biology, behavior, environment, culture and social setting, in the health of individuals and of populations.

Educational innovations include the following: the integration of the basic and clinical sciences throughout undergraduate medical education, early clinical skills training and community-based learning, the incorporation of a population and behavioral perspective into the clinical years, and peer teaching and computer-assisted instruction.

Student assessment will value mastery of knowledge, writing skills, critical appraisal, interpersonal and clinical skills, teaching ability, and peer and self-assessment. Assessment will be competency-based and cumulative.

REQUIREMENTS FOR ENTRANCE

The MCAT and three years of college are required. A college program leading to the bachelor's degree from an accredited college of arts and sciences is ordinarily recommended.

Minimum course requirements are:

	Sem. hrs.
General Biology (with lab)	8
General or Inorganic Chemistry (with lab)	8
Organic Chemistry (with lab)	8
General Physics	6
Biochemistry	3

The following courses are strongly recommended: anatomy/physiology, microbiology, and Spanish.

SELECTION FACTORS

All applicants for first-year positions must apply through AMCAS. All New Mexico applicants will be sent additional application materials upon receipt of their application from AMCAS. Nonregional applicants, including WICHE and former New Mexico residents, must apply through the Early Decision Program to receive any consideration for admission. Those who pass an initial screening process will be sent full application materials and invited for interviews.

Selection is based upon scholastic achievement, performance on the MCAT, personal interviews with members of the Admissions Committee, and recommendations of a college professional advisory committee. The University of New Mexico is committed to providing equal educational and employment opportunities regardless of sex, marital or parental status, race, religion, age, or physical handicap. Preference is given to residents of New Mexico and to those applicants who are residents of western states that participate in the WICHE program.

To guide applicants in considering application to the School of Medicine, the following information is provided on the 2003 applicant pool: 578 total applicants, 99 accepted, 75 matriculated; 224 New Mexico applicants, 93 accepted, 72 matriculated; 3 WICHE applicants, 0 accepted, 0 matriculated; 339 nonregional applicants, 3 accepted, 3 matriculated. Some characteristics of the 2003 entering class were *average GPA*, 3.51 (93 percent above 3.0); *average MCAT* 28.2; sex, 58.7 percent *women*; *ethnic minorities*, 20 percent. All students offered acceptance were interviewed at this school.

TRANSFER

Applications for transfer into Phase II of the curriculum will be considered from New Mexico and WICHE residents attending four-year U.S. medical schools or American Osteopathic Association schools approved either by the Liaison Committee on Medical Education (LCME) or by the American Osteopathic Association, respectively. New Mexico and WICHE residents in approved World Health Organization foreign schools who have completed the equivalent of the first two years of basic science coursework will also be considered for transfer. Applicants will be accepted on a space-available basis, and all acceptances will be contingent upon passing the USMLE Step 1. Criteria for acceptance will be based on medical school academic performance, residency considerations, and a compelling need to transfer to this school.

FINANCIAL AID

The school makes available financial aid in the form of loans and scholarships to those students with demonstrated financial need. The amount of award varies according to the student's need and the level of funding available. A short-term, no-interest loan fund is available to all students in need of immediate financial help. The Student Affairs Office assists all students in locating necessary funds to support their medical education.

INFORMATION ABOUT DIVERSITY PROGRAMS

The School of Medicine is committed to the recruitment, selection, and retention of qualified residents of New Mexico and American Indian residents of New Mexico, from groups underrepresented in medicine, and the Navajo Nation. The Office of Cultural and Ethnic Programs, directed by Dr. Valerie Romero-Leggott, offers several programs to support the above commitment. Additional information may be obtained by contacting the Office of Cultural and Ethnic Programs at (505) 272-2728.

Institution Type: *Public*
Application Process: *AMCAS, see chapter 4.*

APPLICATION AND ACCEPTANCE POLICIES FOR 2005–2006 FIRST-YEAR CLASS

Filing of AMCAS application
   Earliest date: June 1, 2004
   Latest date: Nov. 15, 2004
School application fee after screening: $50
Oldest MCAT scores considered: 2001
Does have Early Decision Program
Nonresidents must apply through EDP
   EDP application period: June 1–Aug. 1, 2004
   EDP applicants notified by: Oct. 1, 2004
Acceptance notice to regular applicants
   Earliest date: Oct. 15, 2004
   Latest date: March 15 or until class is filled
Applicant's response to acceptance offer
   Maximum time: 2 weeks
Requests for deferred entrance considered: Yes
Deposit to hold place in class: None
Estimated number of new entrants: 75 (25 EDP)
Starting date: Aug. 2005

TUITION AND STUDENT FEES PER YEAR FOR 2003-2004 FIRST-YEAR CLASS

Tuition   Student fees: $1,749
   Resident: $10,369
   Nonresident: $29,805

INFORMATION ON 2003-2004 FIRST-YEAR CLASS

Number of	In-State	Out-of-State	Total
Applicants	239	339	578
Applicants Interviewed	224	26	250
New Entrants*	72	3	75

*All took the MCAT and had baccalaureate degrees.

CHAPTER

11

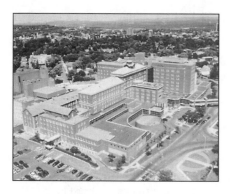

Albany Medical College

Albany, New York

Dr. Vincent Verdile, *Dean*
Sara J. Kremer, *Assistant Dean for Admissions and Student Records*
Assie Bishop, *Assistant Dean for Student and Minority Affairs*
Dr. I. Thomas Cohen, *Associate Dean for Academic and Student Affairs*

ADDRESS INQUIRIES TO:

Office of Admissions, Mail Code 3
Albany Medical College
47 New Scotland Avenue
Albany, New York 12208
(518) 262-5521; 262-5887 (FAX)
E-mail: admissions@mail.amc.edu
Web site: www.amc.edu/academic

MISSION STATEMENT

The goal of the admissions process is to recruit, select, and enroll a class of students who have the potential to develop into excellent physicians. Excellence is broadly defined as pertaining to a range of competencies that will enable physicians to meet the needs of the "total patient" and to contribute in constructive and important ways to the profession of medicine and health care systems.

Therefore, we seek students who are academically qualified and exhibit high moral character, demonstrate the potential for professional growth and development, and can make significant and unique contributions to the Albany Medical College community and to medical science and clinical practice. Accordingly, the ideal candidate for admission will hold clear promise of developing competencies in all dimensions of patient care, including scientific, technical, psychosocial, interpersonal, and ethical.

GENERAL INFORMATION

Founded in 1839, the Albany Medical College is one of the oldest medical schools in the country. The college is coeducational, nondenominational, and privately supported.

The college buildings and those of the 650-bed Albany Medical Center Hospital are physically joined in one large complex that comprises Albany Medical Center. The hospital is one of the largest teaching hospitals in New York State. A wide range of patient care, from primary to tertiary, is provided for over 2^1/$_2$ million residents of eastern New York and western New England. Additional clinical facilities are provided by the Albany Veterans Affairs Medical Center, the Capital District Psychiatric Center, and other affiliated hospitals located nearby.

CURRICULUM

Basic and clinical sciences are integrated into themes (primarily organ systems) stressing normal function in Year 1 and pathological processes in Year 2. There are also 4 longitudinal

themes that are integrated throughout the curriculum: clinical skills, ethical and health systems issues, evidence-based medicine and nutrition. In every theme, student learning is focused on clinical presentations. Year 1 students learn to interview patients by interacting with standardized patients and interviewing independently living elderly. The first year students also learn physical exam techniques appropriate to each organ system theme. Basic science seminars reinforce the importance of the basic sciences in years 3 and 4. Emphasis is placed on primary care throughout the four years, with an increased emphasis on care in ambulatory settings in the clinical rotations of Year 3. Year 4 emphasizes specialty care in various required rotations. Additional electives are available in Year 4 at Albany Medical Center Hospital, other affiliated hospitals, and at other institutions in the United States and abroad. Senior students may plan programs with their advisors that provide opportunities to explore career possibilities.

SPECIAL PROGRAMS

The Albany Medical College provides various pathways for admission including several combined-degree programs offered conjointly with Rensselaer Polytechnic Institute, Union College, and Siena College. Information on these programs is included in Chapter 10.

REQUIREMENTS FOR ENTRANCE

Applicants for admission must have completed at least three years of study at an accredited college preferably in the United States or Canada. Most students admitted, however, will have earned the bachelor's degree.

Minimal course requirements for admission are:

	Sem./Qtr. hrs.
Biology or Zoology (with lab)	6/9
Inorganic Chemistry (with lab)	6/9
Organic Chemistry (with lab)	6/9
General Physics (with lab)	6/9

Proficiency in oral and written English is required.

When achievement in the required science courses is less than optimal, augmenting the minimum requirements with additional experience in the fields of chemistry, embryology, genetics, and mathematics should be considered. Ideally a physician's education should also rest on a base of general knowledge that includes a broad liberal arts education. Accordingly, students who have majored in the arts or humanities are considered on an equal basis with those who have majored in the sciences, provided that these students have demonstrated good capability in the required science studies.

The MCAT is also required and must be taken no later than August of the year prior to the intended date of matriculation.

SELECTION FACTORS

In selecting students, emphasis is placed upon integrity, character, academic achievement, motivation, emotional stability, and social and intellectual suitability. The Albany Medical College is committed to the belief that educational opportunities should be available to all eligible persons without regard to race, creed, age, gender, religion, marital status, handicap, national origin or sexual orientation. Admission is not restricted to New York State residents. Although preference is usually given to U.S. citizens, the committee will occasionally admit outstanding applicants who are citizens of other countries.

For the 2003 entering class, all matriculants had a *mean cumulative undergraduate GPA* of 3.5.

All applications are reviewed in the order in which they are received and are given equal consideration. Applications are individually reviewed by admission committee members, who are looking for qualities other than, and in addition to, the MCAT scores and GPA. Invitations for interview are made at the discretion of the Committee and all interviews are conducted on campus. Preapplication inquiries or questions from applicants concerning the status of their application are welcome at any time.

A transfer admission program is no longer offered.

FINANCIAL AID

Albany Medical College's Financial Aid Office attempts to secure financial assistance by providing the necessary information and application forms, by determining eligibility for Albany Medical College scholarship funds and Federal Work-Study and by certifying loans. Eighty-seven percent of the student body receives some scholarship and/or loan assistance. Applicants who are offered admission are automatically sent financial aid application materials. Scholarships are awarded on the basis of need until the funds are expended. Students are encouraged to apply as early as January of each year and applications for financial aid are accepted throughout the year. The Financial Aid Office offers general financial counseling as well as debt management strategies to assist in planning your future. You are welcome to contact the Financial Aid Office at any time throughout the year at (518) 262-5435 to obtain specific information about financing your medical school education.

INFORMATION ABOUT DIVERSITY PROGRAMS

The Office of Minority Affairs is actively involved in the recruitment and retention of qualified applicants from groups underrepresented in medicine. We also host a high school program for promising junior high and high school students.

Because of our firm commitment to educating and graduating a diverse group of students, guidance is offered to students from

the application stage forward. The Assistant Dean for Student and Minority Affairs is available for counseling and assistance at any time. Our Admissions Committee is sensitized to important factors in the selection of a diverse student body. Albany Medical College has graduated an impressive number of culturally diverse students who are practicing in a wide variety of specialties across the nation.

This office also coordinates academic, social, and cultural support services for students. More information may be obtained by calling (518) 262-5824.

Institution Type: *Private*
Application Process: *AMCAS, see chapter 4.*

APPLICATION AND ACCEPTANCE POLICIES FOR 2005–2006 FIRST-YEAR CLASS

Filing of AMCAS application
  Earliest date: June 1, 2004
  Latest date: Nov. 15, 2004
School application fee to all applicants: $100
Oldest MCAT scores considered: 2001
Does not have Early Decision Program
Acceptance notice to regular applicants
  Earliest date: Oct. 15, 2004
  Latest date: Until class is filled
Applicant's response to acceptance offer
  Maximum time: 2 weeks
Requests for deferred entrance considered: Yes
Deposit to hold place in class (applied to tuition):
  $100, due with response to acceptance offer
Deposit refundable prior to: May 16, 2005
Estimated number of new entrants: 128
Starting date: Aug. 2005

TUITION AND STUDENT FEES PER YEAR FOR 2003–2004 FIRST-YEAR CLASS

Tuition: $38,860   Student fees: $1,599

INFORMATION ON 2003–2004 FIRST-YEAR CLASS

Number of	In-State	Out-of-State	Total
Applicants	1,325	4,778	6,103
Applicants Interviewed	201	555	756
New Entrants*			
(Regular Program)	25	64	89
(Special Programs and deferred)	20	24	44

*67% took the MCAT; 90% had baccalaureate degrees.

(NOTE: Students applying through AMCAS must take the MCAT; those matriculating through Albany's combined degree programs have not earned their baccalaureate degree prior to enrolling and are not required to take the MCAT.)

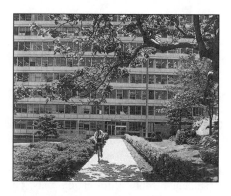

Albert Einstein College of Medicine of Yeshiva University

Bronx, New York

Dr. Dominick P. Purpura, *Dean*
Noreen Kerrigan, *Assistant Dean for Student Admissions*
Lloyd Greenberg, *Financial Aid Officer*
Dr. Milton A. Gumbs, *Associate Dean for Minority Affairs*

ADDRESS INQUIRIES TO:

Office of Admissions
Albert Einstein College of Medicine
of Yeshiva University
Jack and Pearl Resnick Campus
1300 Morris Park Avenue
Bronx, New York 10461
(718) 430-2106; 430-8840 (FAX)
E-mail: admissions@aecom.yu.edu
Web site: www.aecom.yu.edu

MISSION STATEMENT

To conduct educational programs of the highest quality in the biomedical and clinical sciences. To conduct fundamental biomedical and clinical research related to health and disease and health policy. To maintain excellent patient care in association with the education and training of medical students and postgraduate physicians. To conduct collaborative educational, research, and training programs with affiliated institutions. To provide, sustain, and improve health care in our community. To encourage widespread participation in the evolution of public policy in biomedical science, education, and health care.

GENERAL INFORMATION

The Albert Einstein College of Medicine is a privately endowed, coeducational, and nondenominational institution situated on a 17-acre site in a residential area of the northeast Bronx. Clinical education takes place in affiliated acute care hospitals, long-term care and skilled nursing facilities, hospices, and neighborhood health centers that serve the health care needs of a very diverse population of patients in the boroughs of the Bronx, Queens, and Manhattan. These institutions include Jacobi Medical Center, which is a municipal hospital, and four private voluntary hospitals—Beth Israel Medical Center, Montefiore Medical Center, Bronx Lebanon Hospital Center, and Long Island Jewish Medical Center. In addition to these clinical sites, there are extensive facilities devoted to biomedical research and teaching.

Apartments for students are located on and close to the campus, and a recreational sports center with a swimming pool is located on the grounds of the main apartment building complex.

CURRICULUM

Students in the first two years participate in an innovative interdisciplinary series of biomedical science courses in which there are abundant opportunities for self-directed learning and application of basic science knowledge to clinical problems. Most basic science courses are interdisciplinary, integrating different basic science disciplines with each other and with clinical sciences. Running parallel to the biomedical science courses is the Introduction to Clinical Medicine program in which students encounter patients in various hospital and non-hospital settings, learn and practice the basic skills of communication and the clinical examination, and discuss psychosocial, cultural and ethical aspects of the doctor-patient relationship in small-group conferences. A one-year period of clerkship rotations in the third year enables students to acquire clinical skills and knowledge while working with patients at various health care sites in inpatient and outpatient settings. The senior year provides extensive experience in ambulatory care as well as additional responsibilities for the care of hospitalized patients during a subinternship. Special senior elective opportunities include overseas exchange programs, international health fellowships, and a research program that leads to the M.D. degree with distinction in the student's research discipline. Evaluation of performance is on a pass/fail basis in Year 1 and 2, supplemented by Honors and detailed narrative reports in clinical courses.

A fully funded M.D.-Ph.D. program is offered to students at the end of Year 1 or 2. It is a requirement that all students pursue an in-depth study of an area of interest and prepare a written, referenced report of scholarly substance prior to graduation. There is an extensive program of activities and projects in community and population health, including volunteer work in a free clinic in the South Bronx. Different levels of Medical Spanish courses are offered as electives.

Tutoring in most basic science courses is available, and individual counseling is provided to students in need of long-term assistance to assure retention.

REQUIREMENTS FOR ENTRANCE

The MCAT and a minimum of three years of full-time undergraduate study are required; four years are preferred. The minimum course requirements are:

	Sem. hrs.
Biology (with lab)	8
General Chemistry (with lab)	8
Organic Chemistry (with lab)	8
Physics (with lab)	8
College Mathematics	6
(May include statistics and computer science)	
English	6

The undergraduate major is not an important selection factor, and the scholarly pursuit of a broad liberal arts education, including the study of humanities and social sciences, is strongly recommended.

Applicants should provide evidence of participation in intra- or extramural activities that serve to enhance one's communication and interpersonal skills. Such activities may include tutoring, counseling, and community service, as well as experience in the health care system.

SELECTION FACTORS

Students are carefully selected on the basis of academic performance, letters of recommendation, MCAT scores, potential for professional achievement, and motivation and evidence of other personal qualities deemed essential for the study and practice of medicine. Letters of recommendation from commercial educational consultants will not be considered. Applicants are considered without regard to race, religion, creed, color, national origin, sex, age, disability, veteran or disabled veteran status, marital status, sexual orientation or citizenship status as those terms are used in the law. Students who do not gain admission are discouraged from reapplying the subsequent year or until such time as they can present new data to warrant a more favorable decision. Applicants may only apply twice.

The 2003 entering class represented 23 states, 64 undergraduate colleges, and is 59 percent female. The entering class had an average undergraduate GPA of 3.64; the average combined MCAT score was 31. Receipt of the application will be acknowledged, and the applicant will be requested to submit letters of recommendation and the college application fee. A decision regarding a formal interview is made upon receipt of all supporting documents. Interviews are required of all applicants under serious consideration.

FINANCIAL AID

Every attempt is made to assist students and their families in meeting both their financial obligations to the college and the student's essential personal needs. Financial status is not a determinant in selecting among qualified applicants. Awards and loans from the college are available after all other means of financial assistance have been exhausted. Financial aid applications are available only after acceptance. Advice on financial assistance and applications is available from the Student Finance Office. About 50 percent of the students receive institutional loans and/or scholarships, and about 75 percent of them qualify for outside loans and/or grants.

The application fee may be waived upon written request from the applicant only after a fee waiver from AMCAS has been granted.

INFORMATION ABOUT DIVERSITY PROGRAMS

The College of Medicine is actively seeking and welcomes applications from students from groups underrepresented in medicine. The college's Office of Minority Student Affairs provides abundant opportunities for medical students to participate in special programs for high school and college students.

Institution Type: *Private*
Application Process: *AMCAS, see chapter 4.*

APPLICATION AND ACCEPTANCE POLICIES FOR 2005–2006 FIRST-YEAR CLASS

Filing of AMCAS application
    Earliest date: June 1, 2004
    Latest date: Nov. 1, 2004
School application fee to all applicants: $95
Oldest MCAT scores considered: 2001
Does have Early Decision Program (EDP)
    EDP application period: June 1–Aug. 1, 2004
    EDP applicants notified by: Oct. 1, 2004
Acceptance notice to regular applicants
    Earliest date: Jan. 15, 2005
    Latest date: Until class is filled
Applicant's response to acceptance offer
    Maximum time: 2 weeks until May 1, 2005
        1 week thereafter
Requests for deferred entrance considered: Yes
Deposit to hold place in class (applied to tuition):
    $100, due with response to acceptance offer
Deposit refundable prior to: June 1, 2005
Estimated number of new entrants: 180 (EDP varies)
Starting date: Aug. 2005

TUITION AND STUDENT FEES PER YEAR FOR 2003–2004 FIRST-YEAR CLASS

Tuition: $34,375   Student fees: $2,050

INFORMATION ON 2003–2004 FIRST-YEAR CLASS

Number of	In-State	Out-of-State	Total
Applicants	1,445	4,312	5,757
Applicants Interviewed	477	1,049	1,526
New Entrants*	84	96	180

*All took the MCAT and 99% had baccalaureate degrees.

CHAPTER

11

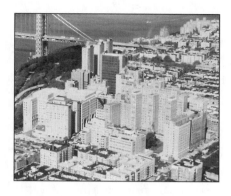

Columbia University
College of Physicians and Surgeons

New York, New York

Dr. Gerald D. Fischbach, *Executive VP for Health and Biomedical Sciences and Dean of the Faculty of Medicine*
Dr. Andrew G. Frantz, *Associate Dean for Admissions*
Ellen Spilker, *Director, Office of Student Affairs (Financial Aid)*
Dr. Hilda Y. Hutchenson, *Associate Dean, Office of Minority Affairs*

ADDRESS INQUIRIES TO:

Columbia University
College of Physicians and Surgeons
Admissions Office, Room 1-416
630 West 168th Street
New York, New York 10032
(212) 305-3595; 305-3601 (FAX)
E-mail: psadmissions@columbia.edu
Web site: http://cpmnet.columbia.edu/dept/ps/

MISSION STATEMENT

The mission of Columbia is to produce physicians who excel in both the science and art of medicine, and who will become leaders in their fields. It seeks to do this by providing an atmosphere that is collegial rather than competitive, and by offering students opportunities to express their interests in a wide variety of humanistic as well as scientific activities.

GENERAL INFORMATION

The College of Physicians and Surgeons originated in 1767 as the Medical Faculty of King's (later Columbia) College and was the first school to award an earned doctor of medicine degree in the American colonies. The college is now a part of the Columbia-Presbyterian Medical Center. Clinical teaching is provided at the Medical Center; Roosevelt-St. Luke's Hospital Center and Harlem Hospital Center in Manhattan; Bassett Hospital in Cooperstown, New York; and Overlook Hospital in New Jersey.

University housing is available for unmarried and married students.

CURRICULUM

Our curriculum aims to prepare students with a solid foundation in basic sciences, as well as in the art and practice of clinical medicine, that will equip them for a wide range of careers. Recent revision of our curriculum has been carried out to develop an interdisciplinary and integrative approach to the basic science subjects taught in the first two years, and which intertwines basic science and clinical education throughout the four years. Teaching in small groups is emphasized. Patient contact begins in the first year and is maintained throughout the year by means of selective clinical courses in which students participate with physicians in a variety of settings involving community clinics and doctors' offices. Clinical correlation with basic sciences is emphasized, and, in the second year, all topics in pathophysiology are studied by means of case-based histories led by preceptors in small-discussion groups. In addition to the evaluation of scientific data, the program is designed to inculcate the school's attitudes about patient care, which include the attitude that the patient is not simply a disease entity and is being improperly cared for if treated as such. The concept of the patient as a whole person is fostered by means of a variety of teaching experiences, including an interdisciplinary course in the first year entitled Introduction to Clinical Practice. Ethical problems as well as topics in health care are discussed in this course, which continues in the second year. Student participation in research is encouraged, and many opportunities for laboratory and clinical clinical research under faculty guidance are available. These take place principally during the summer between the first and second years, as well as in the fourth year.

In early July after the second year, students begin a full year of clerkships in which they participate in all of the clinical services. From July after the third year until graduation, the student follows an individually selected program of studies. A great variety of elective courses are offered, including research electives and opportunities for study abroad. Courses also may be taken in other branches of the university. In cooperation with 14 of the university's departments and programs, an M.D./Ph.D. program is offered for which a maximum of eight openings are usually available annually.

An M.D./M.P.H. program also is offered in conjunction with our School of Public Health, and M.D./M.B.A. and M.D./J.D. programs are offered as well.

Courses are graded on the basis of honors, pass, and fail.

REQUIREMENTS FOR ENTRANCE

The MCAT and a minimum of three years of full-time study in an accredited college are required; four years are recommended. The undergraduate program must include the following courses:

Years

Biology (with lab) 1
    Mammalian Biology preferred.
General Chemistry (with lab). 1
Organic Chemistry (with lab). 1
Physics 1
English 1

Applicants who have more than one of the required courses to complete are at a disadvantage in the competition for admission.

SELECTION FACTORS

Admission is offered to those applicants who have shown the greatest evidence of excellence and leadership potential in both the science and the art of medicine. For classes entering in the last few years the mean GPA has been 3.79, and the mean total MCAT score between 35 and 36. Beyond academic ability, the art of medicine also demands personal qualities of integrity, the ability to relate easily to other people, and concern for their welfare. These qualities are evaluated by several means: the tenor of letters of recommendation, the extent of participation in extracurricular and summer activities, breadth of interests and undergraduate education (the choice of field of concentration is not an important consideration), and the personal interview.

Each year, some applicants are accepted who display extraordinary promise with regard to either the science or the art of medicine, even though they do not meet, in optimal measure, all of the criteria described above.

The Admissions Committee seeks diversity of background among its applicants, geographical and otherwise; no preference is given to state of residence. Admission is possible for all qualified applicants regardless of sex, race, age, religion, sexual orientation, national origin, or handicap.

FINANCIAL AID

Admission is not based on an applicant's ability to pay for medical school. We make every effort to help accepted students finance their medical education. Federal and private student loan programs are available to cover educational expenses that cannot be met by family resources. We also award more than $6.5 million in need-based grants and low-cost loans annually. To be considered for our need-based funds, you must provide financial data for yourself and your parents. After subtracting "calculated family resources" from the student budget, remaining need is met first with a package of low-cost loans, then with school grants and scholarships. Students who do not qualify for need-based funds from the school can access Federal Stafford and private loans. Approximately 80% of our student body receives some type of need-based assistance annually.

INFORMATION ABOUT DIVERSITY PROGRAMS

The college has a strong commitment to increase the numbers of medical students from groups underrepresented in medicine. There is a highly diverse student body and faculty. Applications from students from groups underrepresented in medicine are welcomed. Additional information can be sought from Hilda Y. Hutchenson, associate dean, Office of Minority Affairs, (212) 305-4158.

Institution Type: *Private*
Application Process: *AMCAS, see chapter 4.*

APPLICATION AND ACCEPTANCE POLICIES FOR 2005–2006 FIRST-YEAR CLASS

Filing of application
    Earliest date: June 1, 2004
    Latest date: Oct. 15, 2004
School application fee to all applicants: $75
Oldest MCAT scores considered: 2000
Does not have Early Decision Program
Acceptance notice to regular applicants
    Earliest date: Feb. 20, 2005
    Latest date: Varies
Applicant's response to acceptance offer
    Maximum time: 3 weeks
Requests for deferred entrance considered: Yes
Deposit to hold place in class: None
Estimated number of new entrants: 150
Starting date: Aug. 2005

TUITION AND STUDENT FEES PER YEAR FOR 2003–2004 FIRST-YEAR CLASS

Tuition: $35,036   Student fees: $2,828

INFORMATION ON 2003–2004 FIRST-YEAR CLASS

Number of	*In-State*	*Out-of-State*	*Total*
Applicants	475	2,069	2,544
Applicants Interviewed	269	976	1,245
New Entrants*	49	101	150

*All took the MCAT and had baccalaureate degrees.

CHAPTER

11

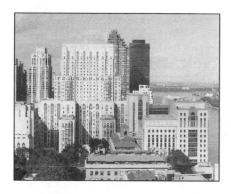

Weill Medical College of Cornell University

New York, New York

Dr. Antonio M. Gotto, *Dean*
Dr. Charles L. Bardes, *Associate Dean and Chair,*
   Committee on Admissions
Gladys Laden, *Director of Financial Aid*
Dr. Bruce L. Ballard, *Associate Dean for Student Affairs*

ADDRESS INQUIRIES TO:

Office of Admissions
Weill Medical College of Cornell University
445 East 69th Street
New York, New York 10021
(212) 746-1067; 746-8052 (FAX)
Web site: www.med.cornell.edu
E-mail: cumc-admissions@med.cornell.edu

GENERAL INFORMATION

Cornell University Medical College was established in 1898. In 1998, the name was changed to the Weill Medical College of Cornell University. Although the university is situated in Ithaca, the medical college was opened in New York City to take advantage of the facilities of a large urban area. Clinical instruction is carried on in the New York–Presbyterian Hospital; Memorial Sloan-Kettering Cancer Center; the Hospital for Special Surgery; the New York Hospital Medical Center of Queens; the New York Methodist Hospital; Brooklyn Hospital Medical Center; Flushing Hospital Medical Center in Queens; the New York Community Hospital; St. Barnabas Hospital; Lincoln Medical and Mental Health Center; Wyckoff Heights Medical Center in Brooklyn; the Burke Rehabilitation Hospital in White Plains, New York; United Hospital Medical Center in Port Chester, New York; and the Cayuga Medical Center in Ithaca, New York.

CURRICULUM

Medical education at Weill Cornell aims to develop individuals who not only recognize and are dedicated to the highest quality patient care, but who also understand their responsibility for contributions through continuing personal scholarship. Many Weill Cornell alumni pursue academic and research careers in addition to the clinical practice of medicine. The education process at Weill Cornell integrates the teaching of the basic and clinical sciences throughout the four years of study and emphasizes problem-solving in the context of scientific inquiry and clinical care.

Core basic science materials are presented during Years 1 and 2, and advanced basic science courses are offered during Years 3 and 4. Learning during the first two years occurs in the setting of problem-based tutorials, small-group conferences, laboratories, lectures, and a journal club. Information is presented in a series of highly integrated, multi-disciplinary block courses: Molecules to Cells, Genes and Development, Human Structure and Function, Host Defenses, Brain and Mind, and Basis of Disease.

Clinical instruction begins in Year 1 with a full day-a-week course, Medicine, Patients, and Society I, during which the student acquires early clinical skills in an ambulatory setting and studies the doctor-patient relationship and socioeconomic, behavioral, and public health issues. This course continues as Medicine, Patients, and Society II in Year 2 with the student gaining experience in the physical examination of patients and clinical problem solving and medical ethics. In Year 3, the focus of Medicine, Patients, and Society III is on student experience with patients, clinical dilemmas, and multiculturalism. Clinical clerkships begin during the later third of Year 2 and include a primary care clerkship, which, in conjunction with the Medicine, Patients, and Society sequence, constitutes the central feature of the primary care curriculum. The clinical clerkships include rotations in medicine, neurology, obstetrics and gynecology, pediatrics, psychiatry, and surgery. Year 4 provides the major time block for electives in clinical medicine, research, and international health experiences. Performance is graded by an honors/pass/fail system during the basic science curriculum and an honors/high pass/pass/fail system during the core curriculum.

For students interested in teaching and research careers in the medical sciences, Weill Cornell offers a fully funded Tri-Institutional M.D.-Ph.D. Program, which is coordinated with the Cornell University Graduate School of Medical Sciences, Memorial Sloan-Kettering Cancer Center, and Rockefeller University. Applicants interested in applying to this program should contact the Tri-Institutional M.D.-Ph.D. Program, 1300 York Avenue, Room D-115, or telephone (212) 746-6023. The deadline to apply is October 15.

REQUIREMENTS FOR ENTRANCE

A minimum of three years in an accredited college and the MCAT are required; most students have completed four years of undergraduate work and hold a baccalaureate degree. The Committee on Admissions considers a strong foundation in the sciences a fundamental requirement but does not wish to establish rigid guidelines for admission. Therefore, Weill Cornell requires satisfactory completion of at least 24 semester hours in science courses including biology or zoology, general chemistry, organic chemistry, and physics. In addition, six semester hours are required in English literature or composition. For nonscience majors, at least two terms of biology beyond the introductory course are suggested. Weill Cornell regards a broad liberal arts education as fundamental for the making of a good physician. The Committee on Admissions will review and evaluate achievement in the humanities and social sciences.

SELECTION FACTORS

Students are selected for their leadership potential in various areas of medicine. There is an attempt to select the best qualified students from various academic, geographic, and social backgrounds. Maturity, stability, motivation, academic achievement, and other qualities are evaluated. Recent preparation for the study of medicine, particularly in the sciences, is preferred.

The 2003 entering class had the following characteristics: 54 percent, *women; mean science GPA 3.73; average MCAT scores,* VR-10.6, PS-11.7, BS-11.7; *science majors,* 70 percent. *Students from groups underrepresented* constituted 20 percent of the class.

Weill Cornell's policy actively supports equality of education and employment opportunity and is committed to the maintenance of affirmative action programs, which will assure the continuation of such equality of opportunity.

Students who are unsuccessful in gaining acceptance to Weill Cornell are rarely successful on reapplication unless there has been substantial improvement in their qualifications.

FINANCIAL AID

Admission decisions are made without regard to financial need. Every effort is made to assist students to finance their medical education without incurring unreasonable debt. Substantial institutional grants and subsidized loans are available and are allocated according to need after an analysis of student and family resources. Fifty percent of the students receive medical college support, and 80 percent receive grants or loans from some source. Since subsidized housing is available for all students at the medical college and cars are not necessary, living costs and transportation expenses are reasonable. Support for community service, summer research, and international electives is available for all students. The application fee will be waived if it represents a hardship to the applicant.

Unfortunately, students who are not citizens or permanent residents of the United States are not eligible for medical college financial aid, institutional grants, or loans. Any one not a U.S. citizen or permanent resident who is accepted for admission to Weill Cornell will be expected to comply with one of the two requirements listed below on or before July 1 of the year of matriculation:

1. The accepted student must deposit in an escrow account (to be established under terms acceptable to the medical college) funds sufficient to meet tuition charges for the total period of enrollment.
2. The accepted student must pre-pay his or her four years of tuition by multiplying the current tuition at the time of matriculation by four.

Details of the agreements and/or requirements listed above are available in the Office of Admissions. *In all cases, students are responsible for any and all fees and other expenses.*

INFORMATION ABOUT DIVERSITY PROGRAMS

The medical college makes a nationwide effort to enroll qualified students from groups underrepresented in medicine, and we have one of the best records in recruitment and retention of such students among private U.S. medical schools.

Weill Cornell conducts a summer research fellowship program for about 25 premedical students who have a major interest in the health problems of underserved populations. The program consists of research activities with faculty members of the medical center and brief coursework in cardiovascular physiology, which provides a preview of the basic science years of medical school. The participants are housed in the medical students' residence.

Institution Type: *Private*
Application Process: *AMCAS, see chapter 4.*

APPLICATION AND ACCEPTANCE POLICIES FOR 2005–2006 FIRST-YEAR CLASS

Filing of AMCAS application
  Earliest date: June 1, 2004
  Latest date: Oct. 15, 2004
School application fee to all applicants: $75
Oldest MCAT scores considered: 2002
Does have Early Decision Program (EDP)
  EDP application period: June 1–Aug. 1, 2004
  EDP applicants notified by: Oct. 1, 2004
Acceptance notice to regular applicants
  Earliest date: December 15, 2004
  Latest date: Until class is filled
Applicant's response to acceptance offer
  Maximum time: 2 weeks
Requests for deferred entrance considered: Yes
Deposit to hold place in class (applied to tuition):
  $100, due May 15, 2005
Deposit refundable prior to: May 16, 2005
Estimated number of new entrants: 101 (2 EDP)
Starting date: Aug. 2005

TUITION AND STUDENT FEES PER YEAR FOR 2003–2004 FIRST-YEAR CLASS

Tuition: $30,170   Student fees: $915

INFORMATION ON 2003–2004 FIRST-YEAR CLASS

Number of	In-State	Out-of-State	Total
Applicants	1,200	4,107	5,307
Applicants Interviewed	200	512	712
New Entrants*	39	62	101

*All took the MCAT and had baccalaureate degrees.

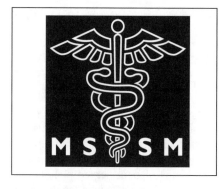

Mount Sinai School of Medicine of New York University

New York, New York

Dr. Kenneth Davis, *Dean*
Dr. Scott H. Barnett, *Associate Dean for Admissions*
Glenda Palmer, *Director of Student Financial Services*
Dr. Gary C. Butts, *Associate Dean for Multicultural and Community Affairs*

ADDRESS INQUIRIES TO:

Office of Admissions
Mount Sinai School of Medicine
Annenberg Building, Room 5-04
One Gustave L. Levy Place-Box 1002
New York, New York 10029-6574
(212) 241-6696; 828-4135 (FAX)
Web site: www.mssm.edu
E-mail: admissions@mssm.edu

MISSION STATEMENT

The School is committed to serving science and society through outstanding research, education, patient care, and community service. We strive to develop new approaches to teaching, translate scientific discoveries into improvements in patient care, and identify new ways to enhance the health and educational opportunities of our neighbors.

GENERAL INFORMATION

Mount Sinai School of Medicine is privately endowed, coeducational, and nondenominational. Developed from the 150-year tradition of patient care, professional education, and research of the Mount Sinai Hospital, it enrolled its first students in 1968 and is officially affiliated with New York University.

The campus's 22 buildings include a hospital, numerous research and service laboratories, teaching facilities, the Postgraduate School of Medicine, and the Graduate School of Biological Sciences.

The Mount Sinai Hospital, a 1,200-bed facility with a clinical research center, constitutes the basic resource for clinical training. Additional clinical training sites in our health system extend throughout New York City, New Jersey, Westchester County, and Long Island. They include municipal hospitals, a Veteran's Affairs Medical Center, and private community hospitals, as well as private practitioners' offices.

CURRICULUM

Mount Sinai School of Medicine has completely revised its curriculum to give our graduates a core knowledge of the biological basis of human function in health and disease, skills in critical thinking, dedication to lifelong learning, professional and humanistic attitudes, a scientific approach to medicine, and an appreciation of their obligation to society and the community in which they live. Our curriculum emphasizes the interdisciplinary nature of the various basic sciences, clinical sciences, as well as the interface between the two. Lecture, small group seminars, problem-based learning, and independent study complement laboratory-based instruction. Courses are graded pass/fail during the first two years, and honors/high pass/pass/fail in the last two.

Student–patient interactions begin in the first month of school with The Art and Science of Medicine. The first year focuses on an integrated approach to the study of Molecules and Cells, Structure and Function, and Pathogenesis and Host Defense Mechanisms. The year ends with a block of Bench to Bedside selectives, linking the contributions of bench research to patient care. The Art and Science of Medicine continues in the second year, accompanied by a year-long study of Mechanisms of Disease, Pharmacology, and Epidemiology and Biostatistics.

Clinical rotations include new and innovative clerkships which combine the disciplines of Medicine and Geriatrics, and Pediatrics and Obstetrics/Gynecology. An integrated seminar series spans the entire third year.

The fourth year provides the student an increasing degree of patient care responsibility, and allows for extended electives. An Emergency Medicine rotation and a subinternship in Medicine or Pediatrics immerses students in the care of the acutely ill patient. A Clinical Translational Fellowship combines the clinical practice of medicine with the relevant basic science. Our year-end Post-match Integrated Selective focuses on mastering the skills that are necessary to ensure a productive and educational internship experience.

One of our unique educational resources is the Morchand Center for Clinical Competence, the first media training facility of its kind in New York. Here, with the aid of state-of-the-art audiovisual systems and standardized patients, students develop the interpersonal communication, history taking, and physical exam skills essential to a successful physician-patient relationship.

The Medical Scientist Training Program (MSTP) was developed for students interested in a career in medical research and academic medicine. This M.D.-Ph.D. program is funded by a training grant from the NIH as well as by other extramural and intramural awards. Students may apply for the combined program at the time of application for admission or during the second year of medical school.

A Master of science degree in community medicine is available, and is designed to produce a new generation of leaders in preventive medicine while providing advanced training in the population-based medical sciences.

REQUIREMENTS FOR ENTRANCE

A minimum of three years of college and the MCAT are required. Most students admitted have earned the bachelor's degree. The prospective student should have basic knowledge of the biological and physical sciences and mathematics, plus an appreciation of the social forces influencing man. Students majoring in nonscience disciplines who meet all admission requirements will be given consideration on an equal basis with those having specific scientific backgrounds.

Admission requirements include accredited college work in the following subjects:

	Years
Biology (with lab)	1
Inorganic Chemistry (with lab)	1
Organic Chemistry (with lab)	1
Physics	1
Mathematics	1
English	1

Biology and chemistry courses must be accompanied by laboratory experience. Courses in statistics or computer science may fulfill the mathematics requirements.

SELECTION FACTORS

The school is keenly interested in a total appraisal of a student's potential for a career in medicine. Excellence in scholarship, personal maturity, integrity, intellectual creativity, and motivation for medicine are important factors. A personal interview is required, and all interviews are conducted at Mount Sinai. The interview is given considerable weight; premedical advisory committee letters of recommendation and MCAT scores are criteria for evaluation. All applicants, regardless of race, sex, color, creed, age, national origin, handicap, veteran status, marital status, or sexual orientation, are given serious and thorough consideration by the Admissions Committee.

Transfer students are accepted into the third year. They will be considered on a space available basis for the second year.

Accepted students for the 2003 entering class had the following characteristics: *mean GPA,* 3.66; *mean MCAT,* 10.83; *sex,* 58 percent women. Distribution of undergraduate major reflects the distribution in the applicant pool.

FINANCIAL AID

It is the policy of the school to provide as much financial assistance as possible to students who require such assistance in order to maintain attendance. Students who are accepted for admission are provided financial assistance applications on which they may document their request for financial aid. Applications are treated confidentially, and awards are made by a faculty committee on financial aid. Each applicant is considered on an individual basis so that the greatest support for the most needy students can be distributed.

Financial aid may be offered in the form of a scholarship, a loan, or both, in accordance with the requirements of the individual situation and the availability of funds in the various categories. Over 85 percent of the students receive financial assistance; 65 percent receive direct institutional support. Students who are not citizens or permanent residents of the United States are not eligible for financial assistance.

INFORMATION FOR MINORITY APPLICANTS

Strongly motivated students from groups underrepresented in medicine are actively sought and encouraged to apply. A pre-entrance summer enrichment program is available for students who are accepted to the first-year class. Tutorial assistance is available for all students.

The school's Office of Multicultural and Community Affairs serves to support its commitment to cultural and ethnic diversity within the school. This office provides leadership and coordination for minority affairs activities, multicultural diversity program activities, and a variety of enrichment programs. In addition, this office assists in providing advisory and career counseling services for all students.

Institution Type: *Private*
Application Process: *AMCAS, see chapter 4.*

APPLICATION AND ACCEPTANCE POLICIES FOR 2005–2006 FIRST-YEAR CLASS

Filing of AMCAS application
    Earliest date: June 1, 2004
    Latest date: Nov. 1, 2004
School application fee to all applicants: $100
Oldest MCAT scores considered: 2002
Does have Early Decision Program (EDP)
    EDP application period: June 1–Aug. 1, 2004
    EDP applicants notified by: Oct. 1, 2004
Acceptance notice to regular applicants
    Earliest date: Nov. 1, 2004
    Latest date: Varies
Applicant's response to acceptance offer
    Maximum time: 2 weeks
Requests for deferred entrance considered: Yes
Deposit to hold place in class: None
Estimated number of new entrants: 120 (1 EDP)
Starting date: Aug. 2005

TUITION AND STUDENT FEES PER YEAR FOR 2003–2004 FIRST-YEAR CLASS

Tuition: $31,250   Student fees: $2,670

INFORMATION ON 2003–2004 FIRST-YEAR CLASS

Number of	*In-State*	*Out-of-State*	*Total*
Applicants	1,103	3,099	4,202
Applicants Interviewed	248	478	726
New Entrants*	46	74	120

*All Entrants had baccalaureate degrees, 92% took the MCAT.

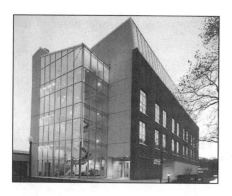

New York Medical College

Valhalla, New York

Dr. Ralph A. O'Connell, *Provost and Dean, School of Medicine*
Dr. Fern R. Juster, *Associate Dean and Chair, Committee on Admissions*
Anthony M. Sozzo, *Associate Dean and Director of Student Financial Planning*
Dr. Gladys M. Ayala, *Associate Dean, Student and Minority Affairs*

ADDRESS INQUIRIES TO:

Office of Admissions
Administration Building
New York Medical College
Valhalla, New York 10595
(914) 594-4507; 594-4976 (FAX)
E-mail: mdadmit@nymc.edu
Web site: www.nymc.edu

MISSION STATEMENT

New York Medical College, a health sciences university in the Catholic tradition, exists to advance your health. We educate physicians, scientists and healthcare professionals. We conduct research and provide service. We have one goal: your well-being.

Our academic community provides programs that improve the health of the population. We join with many partners, among them people like you whom we educate and encourage to adopt healthier lifestyles, whom we treat during times of illness and who benefit from our scientific progress. We are a university with a special responsibility to the underserved and with a deep awareness and recognition of the sacredness of all human life. Our programs are vital to the quality of health care throughout the Hudson Valley and the New York metropolitan area.

GENERAL INFORMATION

New York Medical College is located in Valhalla, N.Y., in suburban Westchester County, within the nation's largest metropolitan region. The college is committed to educating individuals for careers in the medical, science and health professions. The university comprises three schools—a School of Medicine, conferring the M.D. degree, and two graduate schools—the Graduate School of Basic Medical Sciences and the School of Public Health, which together offer advanced degrees in 39 program areas and an enrollment exceeding 1,500. Founded in 1860, the School of Medicine has a longstanding reputation for producing superior clinicians, both generalists and specialists. The university's wide range of affiliated hospitals, which include large urban medical centers, small suburban hospitals and technologically advanced regional tertiary care facilities, provide extensive resources and educational opportunities.

CURRICULUM

Though centered on the basic sciences, the curriculum of the first two years maintains a consistent clinical focus. The program

was revised and expanded to bring clinical relevance and small-group teaching into all courses. The core of the first-year curriculum—anatomy, histology, biochemistry, physiology, neural science, and behavioral science—is supplemented by clinical case correlations and courses in epidemiology and biostatistics. All first-year students have regular patient contact working in the office of a primary care physician. The Introduction to Primary Care course allows students to work one-on-one with a physician preceptor, examining patients and focusing on issues such as health maintenance, ethics, and cultural perspectives of health care in an ambulatory setting.

The redesigned second-year curriculum, with its strong focus on pathology/pathophysiology, pharmacology, and medical microbiology emphasizes small-group discussion, problem-based learning, and self-study. The clinical skills course provides students with a variety of learning opportunities to master essential communication and physical diagnosis skills preparing students for full entry into the clerkship experience of the next two years.

The third year runs for a full calendar year. Students complete clerkships in seven disciplines—medicine, neurology, obstetrics and gynecology, pediatrics, psychiatry, surgery, and family medicine. Because of the medical school's unique location just outside New York City, students can choose from demographically and clinically diverse settings which extend from the city to suburban and rural Hudson Valley sites. About half the third-year class moves into New York City for their clinical years, and many live in college-owned housing in Manhattan.

The fourth year comprises required clinical rotations taken at affiliated hospitals and electives at medical institutions across the country and around the world. Approximately 15 percent of the fourth-year students take international electives each year.

Special programs are available through the college's two graduate schools. Medical students can simultaneously pursue an M.P.H. degree through the Graduate School of Public Health. The dual degree can be finished within the four years of medical school or can be extended to five years. Similarly, the Graduate School of Basic Medical Sciences affords the opportunity for joint M.D.–Ph.D. degrees, which typically require six to seven years to complete. These programs do not have a separate application process; applicants apply first to the School of Medicine.

REQUIREMENTS FOR ENTRANCE

It is strongly recommended that the applicant complete undergraduate work leading to a baccalaureate degree from an accredited college of arts and sciences in the United States or Canada. All courses offered in satisfaction of the requirements for admission must be taken in or accepted as transfer credit by an accredited college in the United States or Canada and must be acceptable to that institution toward a baccalaureate degree in general arts or sciences. The Committee on Admissions has no preference for a major field of undergraduate study, but any college work submitted must include the specified credits below.

Sem. hrs.

Biology (with lab) 8
Inorganic Chemistry (with lab) 8
Organic Chemistry (with lab). 8
Physics (with lab) 8
English 6

All candidates are required to take the MCAT.

SELECTION FACTORS

The Committee on Admissions selects students after carefully considering all those factors of intellect, character, and personality that point toward their ability to become informed and caring physicians. This basic platform must include a history of academic excellence. Although the majority of students have had undergraduate majors in the sciences, it is not at all a requirement or a factor in selection. We welcome applicants with a broad education in the humanities who have completed their premed requirements in a postbaccalaureate program.

In addition to purely academic factors, we look for students who show clear evidence through their activities of strong motivation toward medicine and a sense of dedication to the service of others. Personal qualities of character and personality are evaluated from letters of recommendation, from the personal statement, and from the interview. New York Medical College does not deny admission to any applicant on the basis of race, gender, religion, national origin, age, or handicap.

All AMCAS applicants are requested to complete an online secondary application. After the completed secondary application and all letters of recommendation have been processed, the applicant's file is reviewed for consideration. Interviews are by invitation and are conducted on campus. We generally interview from October through April and decisions are made on a rolling basis.

In the most recent entering first-year class, the class of 2007, students had the following credentials: *mean GPA, 3.5; mean total MCAT, 30; gender, 50* percent women.

FINANCIAL AID

Approximately 85 percent of the student body receives some financial assistance. Financial aid is awarded on the basis of need; limited grants and scholarships are available; and Trustee Scholarships, based on academic merit and need, are also available to entering students. The college provides services including debt management and loan counseling. Students are discouraged from seeking outside employment during the academic year. All invited students will receive an informational financial aid packet. For further information call the Office of Student Financial Planning at (914) 594-4491 or email bello@nymc.edu.

INFORMATION ABOUT DIVERSITY PROGRAMS

New York Medical College seeks to admit a diverse class; including diversity of gender, race, ethnicity, cultural and economic background and life experience. A diverse student body provides a valuable educational experience that prepares medical students for the real world of medical practice in a multicultural society. Diversity in medicine has been shown to improve access to healthcare for underserved populations.

Institution Type: *Private*
Application Process: *AMCAS, see chapter 4.*

APPLICATION AND ACCEPTANCE POLICIES FOR 2005–2006 FIRST-YEAR CLASS

Filing of AMCAS application
  Earliest date: June 1, 2004
  Latest date: Dec. 15, 2004
School application fee to all applicants: $100
Oldest MCAT scores considered: 2001
Does have Early Decision Program (EDP)
  EDP application period: June 1–Aug. 1, 2004
  EDP applicants notified by: Oct. 1, 2004
Acceptance notice to regular applicants
  Earliest date: Dec. 6, 2004
  Latest date: Until class is filled
Applicant's response to acceptance offer
  Maximum time: 2 weeks
Requests for deferred entrance considered: Yes
Deposit to hold place in class (applied to tuition): $100
Deposit refundable prior to: May 16, 2005
Estimated number of new entrants: 190 (2 EDP)
Starting date: Aug. 2005

TUITION AND STUDENT FEES PER YEAR FOR 2003–2004 FIRST-YEAR CLASS

Tuition: $34,040   Student fees: $700

INFORMATION ON 2003–2004 FIRST-YEAR CLASS

Number of	In-State	Out-of-State	Total
Applicants	1,586	6,729	8,315
Applicants Interviewed	359	973	1,332
New Entrants*	65	124	189

*All took the MCAT and had baccalaureate degrees.

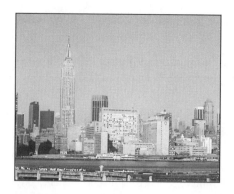

New York University
School of Medicine

New York, New York

Dr. Robert M. Glickman, *Dean*
Raymond J. Brienza, *Associate Dean for Admissions and Director of Financial Aid*

ADDRESS INQUIRIES TO:

Office of Admissions
New York University
School of Medicine
P.O. Box 1924
New York, New York 10016
(212) 263-5290
Web site: www.med.nyu.edu/admissions

MISSION STATEMENT

The mission of the medical school is threefold: the education and training of physicians and scientists, the search for new knowledge, and the care of the sick. The three are inseparable. Medicine can be handed on to succeeding generations only by long training in the scientific methods of investigation and by the actual care of patients. Progress in medicine, which is medical research, must look constantly to the school for its investigators and to the patient for its problems, whereas the whole future of medical care rests upon a continuing supply of physicians and upon the promise of new discovery. The purpose of medical school, then, can only be achieved by endeavor in all three directions—medical education, research, and patient care—and they must be carried on simultaneously for they are wholly dependent upon each other, not only for inspiration, but for their very means of success.

GENERAL INFORMATION

The New York University School of Medicine was founded in 1841 when it admitted a class of 239 students to a four-month course of lectures conducted by six professors on the faculty. The medical school is a constituent of New York University (NYU), one of the oldest and largest private universities in the United States.

CURRICULUM

Several changes in the curriculum have been implemented in the past few years, culminating in the launching of Curriculum 2003. The innovations within the basic science curriculum are designed to promote independent, interdisciplinary learning through an increase in small-group seminars, problem-solving activities, and computer-assisted instruction exercises. Interdepartmental faculty collaborate in instructing and precepting students in thematic curricular modules during the first two years. The broad educational goal of this segment of the curriculum is to provide students with the essential information base, concepts, and critical skills necessary to understand, apply, and continually build upon the principles that are the foundation of clinical medicine. Study of the clinical sciences begins in the first year of training and continues longitudinally though the third and forth years; advanced biomedical concepts are brought forward into the clerkship years through palindromic case studies that stress the translation of molecular biological and molecular genetic knowledge into rational decision making and clinical care. Flexibility in the scheduling of required clerkships and electives throughout the third and fourth years permits students to design a course of study specific to their educational and career goals. The training program is enriched by the Honors research program, opportunities for independent study projects, and the Masters Scholars program, through which students forge mentored relationships and cultivate their interests in public health, bioethics and human rights, biomedical health sciences, medical informatics, and arts and literature in medicine.

REQUIREMENTS FOR ENTRANCE

The requirements for admission are as follows: the MCAT; a minimum of three years of college work; and the following courses plus an acceptable concentration in any of these fields, or in any other field, at the college level:

	Sem. hrs.
Biology (with lab)	6
Inorganic Chemistry (with lab)	6
Organic Chemistry (with lab)	6
General Physics (with lab)	6
English	6

Biochemistry is strongly recommended for all students.

Molecular biology and genetics are recommended for students who select extra work in biology.

It is strongly recommended that candidates complete their college work for the baccalaureate degree.

To achieve an earlier processing of their applications in the fall applicants should take the MCAT in the spring of the year in which they are applying to medical school. In no case should the MCAT be taken later than August of the application year.

SELECTION FACTORS

The selection process involves judging the applicant from several viewpoints, among them the following: excellence in coursework at the college level; evaluation of the student by college instructors, premedical committees, and other similar mechanisms provided by the colleges; an interview at NYU; and the results of the MCAT. The Committee on Admissions does not computerize the candidate's profile in terms of MCAT scores and GPAs because qualitative considerations, such as college evaluation and interview impression, are also given great weight in the final evaluation. The Committee on Admissions does lend some weight to trends in the student's college progress. Students who may, for one reason or another, get off to a slow start in college and then show that they are capable of honors work in later years are given sympathetic consideration. NYU is a private institution and has no geographical or other quotas. It should be noted, however, that international applicants who do not hold a permanent resident visa have only a slight chance of being admitted.

Volunteer activities, independent research, and accomplishments in the humanities and liberal arts fields are strongly considered by the Admissions Committee when evaluating candidates.

Women have constituted 51 percent of recent entering classes.

FINANCIAL AID

The Financial Aid Office reviews all applications for financial assistance. The school's resources are drawn from scholarships and loan programs. Enrolled students and those students accepted for admission to the school are eligible to file applications for assistance. The School of Medicine participates in the Primary Care Loan and the Perkins Loan Program, which provide low-interest support for deserving students. Federal Stafford loans are also available through the New York Higher Education Assistance Corporation. New York State Tuition Assistance Program Awards are available to many residents of New York who are degree candidates.

INFORMATION ABOUT DIVERSITY PROGRAMS

The medical school is committed to admitting a diverse entering class each year. Every effort is made in the case of all candidates, including those from groups underrepresented in medicine, to reach some determination on motivation, character, and capacities of the candidate, regardless of such standard measures as test scores and college performance. Considerable reliance is placed on the evaluation of students by their college teachers. This is particularly important in terms of the candidate's motivation under adverse circumstances. It is possible to have application fees waived in cases of demonstrated need.

Institution Type: *Private*
Application Process: *AMCAS, see chapter 4.*

APPLICATION AND ACCEPTANCE POLICIES FOR 2005–2006 FIRST-YEAR CLASS

Filing of AMCAS application
    Earliest date: June 1, 2004
    Latest date: Nov. 1, 2004
School application fee to all applicants: $85
Oldest MCAT scores considered: 2001
Does not have Early Decision Program
Acceptance notice to regular applicants
    Earliest date: Dec. 1, 2004
    Latest date: Until class is filled
Applicant's response to acceptance offer
    Maximum time: 2 weeks
Requests for deferred entrance considered: Yes
Deposit to hold place in class (applied to tuition):
    $100, due with response to acceptance offer
Deposit refundable prior to: May 16, 2005
Estimated number of new entrants: 160
Starting date: Aug. 2005

TUITION AND STUDENT FEES PER YEAR FOR 2003-2004 FIRST-YEAR CLASS

Tuition: $26,750   Student fees: $6,750*

INFORMATION ON 2003-2004 FIRST-YEAR CLASS

Number of	In-State	Out-of-State	Total
Applicants	N/A	N/A	3,178
Applicants Interviewed	N/A	N/A	854
New Entrants†	68	92	160

*Includes $3,000 Health Insurance fee.

†All took the MCAT and had baccalaureate degrees.

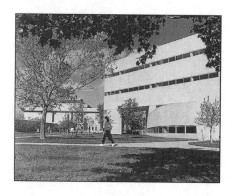

State University of New York at Buffalo
School of Medicine and Biomedical Sciences

Buffalo, New York

Dr. Margaret W. Paroski, *Interim Vice President Health Affairs and Dean*
Dr. Nancy Nielsen, *Interim Senior Associate Dean of Medical Education*
Dr. Charles M. Severin, *Interim Associate Dean for Medical Education and Admissions*
Dr. David A. Milling, *Assistant Dean, Multicultural Affairs*

ADDRESS INQUIRIES TO:

Office of Medical Admissions
University at Buffalo
131 Biomedical Education Building
Buffalo, New York 14214-3013
(716) 829-3466; 829-3849 (FAX)
E-mail: jjrosso@acsu.buffalo.edu
Web site: www.smbs.buffalo.edu/ome

MISSION STATEMENT

- To provide well-trained physicians and other health care professionals who will attend to the health needs of citizens.
- To offer a source of continuing education to the community of health care providers,
- To provide a center of research and scholarship that will advance and promote health-related services

As a public institution, the mission places particular emphasis on diversity, inclusion, and the special needs of New York State such as minority recruitment and retention, and the underserved urban and rural health populations.

GENERAL INFORMATION

The School of Medicine was founded by Millard Fillmore and a group of physicians in 1846. It was a privately supported school until the University of Buffalo joined the State University of New York (SUNY) system in 1962. The University at Buffalo has the most comprehensive campus in the SUNY system and was honored in 1989 with election to the Association of American Universities. The preclinical campus and library are located on the Main Street Campus at the northeastern corner of the city. The clinical education program is conducted in cooperation with nine area hospitals.

CURRICULUM

The curriculum is designed to emphasize the relevance of medical education to the practice of medicine, demonstrate the relevance of basic science to clinical practice, introduce patient contact and patient-centered learning in the first year of medical school, and increase the experience in ambulatory care in the clinical years. An integrated curriculum, including Introduction to Clinical Medicine, will be taught throughout the first two years and is designed to prepare students in the

knowledge, skills, and attitudes required to successfully enter the clinical clerkships in the third year and provide the foundation for their medical careers. Ethics, the doctor-patient relationship, principles of health promotion, disease prevention, and promotion of self-learning and inquiry are emphasized, in addition to extensive education in the skills basic to medical practice and patient care. All students must pass Step 1 of the USMLE within three attempts before being allowed to matriculate in the clinical years. The clinical years include required clerkships in internal medicine, surgery, pediatrics, obstetrics and gynecology, psychiatry, neurology, family medicine, and surgical specialties. There is ample free time in the senior year for electives here or away. UB's goal is to prepare its graduates to enter and complete graduate education, qualify for licensure, provide excellence in medical care, and have the educational background for continued learning.

REQUIREMENTS FOR ENTRANCE

An MCAT taken within three (3) years of applying and a minimum of 60 credit hours of higher education in the U.S. or Canada is required. Courses required for admission:

	Semesters
Biology (with lab)	2
With not more than one semester of Botany.	
General Chemistry (with lab)	2
Organic Chemistry (with lab)	2
General Physics	2
English	2

The choice of undergraduate concentration is optional. The prerequisites for admission reflect the need for a basic preparation in the sciences and are meant to encourage student's to develop a foundation in the social sciences and in the humanities.

MEDICAL SCIENTIST TRAINING PROGRAM

The Medical Scientist Training Program (MSTP) is a seven- to eight-year program designed for preparation for careers in biomedical sciences and combines the training for both the M.D. and Ph.D. degrees. Interested applicants should request an application from the MSTP Office, University at Buffalo, 128 Biomedical Education Building (BEB), Buffalo, NY 14214; (716) 829-3398.

EARLY ASSURANCE PROGRAM

Undergraduate sophomores can apply to this program if they have demonstrated a high level of academic competence by attaining around a 3.75 GPA in science and nonscience courses and have completed at least half of the premedical course requirements. Persons from groups underrepresented in medicine with competitive records are especially encouraged to apply. Application deadline is February 1, 2005. Submission of SAT scores is required. Accepted candidates are not required to take the MCAT, are encouraged to pursue their intellectual interests in their remaining college years, and will commence their medical education in August 2007. Approximately 15 applicants are accepted each year.

SELECTION FACTORS

The Admissions Committee seeks to identify and select students who display favorable qualities deemed important for the pursuit of a career in medicine. In making its assessments and determinations, the committee relies on information contained in the application and in documents submitted in support of the applicant. Based on careful screening, applicants are invited to appear for an interview. Reapplications are treated no differently than initial applications. Rejected applicants should seek the advice and counsel of their premedical advisor.

Students are accepted without regard to race, sex, creed, national origin, age, or handicap. All applicants will receive the *Essential Functions of the Medical School Curriculum* including technical standards with our secondary application. Some preference is given to qualified residents of New York State. Competitive out-of-state applicants are encouraged to apply. Applications are not accepted from foreign nationals. The present freshman class has an average GPA of 3.54 and an average MCAT of 9.5 with a composition of 56 percent female and 12.6 percent students from groups underrepresented in medicine. Transfers are considered only into the third-year class, and only from U.S. Citizens or permanent residents who are presently enrolled in an LCME approved U.S. medical school or in a foreign medical school not disapproved by the New York State Education Department. Transfers must have passed Step 1 of the USMLE to be considered.

FINANCIAL AID

The FAFSA should be received at the Federal Student Aid Office by May 15, 2005, for all students applying to the 2005 entering class. Forms received after the deadline are subject to funds available. Requests for financial aid are considered after admission, and awards are made based on the student's need as estimated by the university's Office of Financial Aid. In most financial aid requests, parental income information is required regardless of dependency status. All financial aid is need based. A limited number of scholarships based on academic merit and financial need are provided each year.

INFORMATION ABOUT DIVERSITY PROGRAMS

A Summer Enrichment and Support Program is available to facilitate students' retention in medical school. The enrichment program, designed for first-year educationally and socio-economically disadvantaged students admitted to SUNY-Buffalo, offers a review of the integrated curriculum, and small group learning skills development. The program begins June 1 and runs through July. Tutorial and counseling services are offered during the summer and throughout the academic year. The School of Medicine has a strong retention program; however, each student must meet the academic standards established by the faculty.

Institution Type: *Public*
Application Process: *AMCAS, see chapter 4.*

APPLICATION AND ACCEPTANCE POLICIES FOR 2005–2006 FIRST-YEAR CLASS

Filing of AMCAS application
  Earliest date: June 1, 2004
  Latest date: Nov. 15, 2004
School application fee to all applicants: $65
Oldest MCAT scores considered: 2001
Does have Early Decision Program (EDP)
  EDP application period: June 1–Aug. 1, 2004
  EDP applicants notified by: Oct. 1, 2004
Acceptance notice to regular applicants
  Earliest date: Oct. 15, 2004
  Latest date: Until class is filled
Applicant's response to acceptance offer
  Maximum time: 2 weeks
Requests for deferred entrance considered: Yes
Deposit to hold place in class (applied to tuition):
  $100, due with response to acceptance offer
Deposit refundable prior to: May 16, 2005
Estimated number of new entrants: 135 (3 EDP)
Starting date: Aug. 2005

TUITION AND STUDENT FEES PER YEAR FOR 2003–2004 FIRST-YEAR CLASS

Tuition   Student fees: $1,184
Resident: $16,800
Nonresident: $29,900

INFORMATION ON 2003–2004 FIRST-YEAR CLASS

Number of	In-State	Out-of-State	Total
Applicants	1,517	546	2,063
Applicants Interviewed	397	67	464
New Entrants*	116	19	135

*All had baccalaureate degrees, and all, except EAP, took the MCAT.

CHAPTER

11

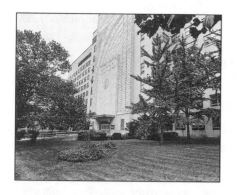

State University of New York
Downstate Medical Center College of Medicine

Brooklyn, New York

Dr. Eugene B. Feigelson, *Senior Vice President for Biomedical Education and Research and Dean, College of Medicine*
Dr. Constance Hill, *Associate Dean for Minority Affairs*

ADDRESS INQUIRIES TO:

Admissions Office
State University of New York
Downstate Medical Center
450 Clarkson Avenue-Box 60
Brooklyn, New York 11203-2098
(718) 270-2446; 270-7592 (FAX)
E-mail: admissions@downstate.edu
Web site: www.downstate.edu

MISSION STATEMENT

Our primary mission is to make high quality education available to New York's next generation of health professionals. Integral to our concept of professional education are both a commitment to confront the health problems of urban communities and a responsibility to advance the state of knowledge and practice in the health disciplines through basic and applied clinical research.

GENERAL INFORMATION

The College of Medicine of the State University of New York Downstate Medical Center traces its roots to the founding in 1860 of the Long Island College Hospital, the first hospital-based medical school in the country. In 1950, the College of Medicine joined the State University of New York system and developed into a major center for health sciences. The University Hospital, a 376-bed teaching hospital, opened in 1966. In addition to its own hospital, Downstate uses several major affiliated community hospitals in the clinical years. In 1992, the campus' new Health Science Education Building opened. It houses state-of-the-art classrooms, laboratories, a 500-seat auditorium, and the Medical Research Library of Brooklyn. Current information about the college, curriculum and admissions is available on the Web site.

CURRICULUM

In preparing physicians to practice in the future health care system, the medical education process is under constant evaluation. The main goals of the curriculum at the Downstate Medical Center are: to improve the integration of basic and clinical science throughout the four years of medical school; to provide earlier exposure to patient care by introducing a weekly clinical experience in the first and second years of medical school; to provide for a more small-group, self-directed and case-based learning; and to foster lifelong learning skills through the introduction of new applications of information science, outcome studies, and evidence-based medicine. An organ system approach is followed, with first-year topic areas such as genes to cells, skin and connective tissue, musculoskeletal, lymphoid/head and neck, cardiovascular, respiratory, gastrointestinal/nutrition, urinary, endocrine/reproduction, and neuroscience. The emphasis is on the development of clinical reasoning and problem-solving skills. During the first year, attention is focused on the basic components of human biology and behavior, as well as on the essential aspects of physician-patient relationship. The second year begins the study of human disease, its diagnosis, prevention, and treatment. All students are required to pass Step 1 of the USMLE at the end of their second year. The third year and fourth years are integrated clerkships and electives. See Web site for more details.

All courses are graded fail, conditional, pass, high pass, and honors.

The College of Medicine and the School of Graduate Studies sponsor a combined M.D./Ph.D. program designed for students who are interested in academic medicine involving a combination of research, teaching, and clinical activities. A concurrent Master in Public Health is also available.

A B.A./M.D. Honors program is offered in conjunction with Brooklyn College of the City University of New York. Information on special admission and matriculation criteria is available from the Office of Admissions at Brooklyn College. An Early Assurance Program is offered with the College of Staten Island.

REQUIREMENTS FOR ENTRANCE

Admission policies are posted on our Web site and applicants should review them for additional information.

Applicants must have taken the new MCAT and completed a minimum of 90 semester credits of undergraduate work at an accredited college. Courses required for admission are:

	Semester Credits
General Biology (with lab)	8
Inorganic Chemistry (with lab)	8
Organic Chemistry (with lab)	8
General Physics (with lab)	8
English	6

If first-year English is exempted, a more advanced course is required.

The remainder of the courses should be in the liberal arts curriculum and credited toward a bachelor's degree. At least one year of college mathematics, one in an advanced scientific subject, and a course in biochemistry are recommended. Students educated abroad must complete a minimum of one year of full-time college study in an accredited college or university in the United States or Canada.

Applicants are urged to take the MCAT in the spring of the year of application and to have completed the premedical requirements at the time of application.

SELECTION FACTORS

The Committee on Admissions considers the total qualifications of each applicant without regard to sex, sexual orientation, race, color, creed, religion, national origin, age, or disability. Women and groups underrepresented in medicine are encouraged to apply. Decisions are based on a number of factors, including prior academic performance; completion of required courses; the potential for academic success including performance on the MCAT; communication skills, character, and personal skills; demonstrated commitment to community-social service outreach activities; and motivation for medicine. Preference is given to qualified New York State residents. Reapplicants adhere to the same procedures, policies, and deadlines as first-time applicants.

A secondary application is available on the Web site. Applications are screened when all of the required information has been submitted (AMCAS application, secondary application, MCAT scores, and recommendations).

The 2003 entering class attended 69 different colleges and universities. It was 49 percent women and 11 percent students from groups underrepresented in medicine; age ranged from 20 to 37, with the mean on matriculation being 23.

Admission to advanced standing is limited to U.S. citizens or permanent residents who are matriculated, in good standing, and in attendance as second-year medical students in an LCME-accredited college of medicine in the United States. Applications are accepted to the third-year class on a space available basis, and admissions preference is given to New York State residents.

FINANCIAL AID

The college is committed to help students meet their educational expenses through various types of financial assistance. Aid is granted on the basis of need (determined in accordance with federal regulations), and for some scholarships, on academic achievement. The major portion of our assistance is derived from federal and state allocations: grants, scholarships, loans and/or college work study. Loans are the most common form of assistance. Financial aid application materials are sent to all accepted applicants, and students' financial aid needs are reviewed annually.

INFORMATION ABOUT DIVERSITY PROGRAMS

The SUNY Downstate Medical Center maintains a tradition of commitment to the enrollment of students from groups underrepresented in medicine. The Office of Minority Affairs directs several programs targeted to furnish information and support to students from underrepresented and disadvantaged backgrounds. Operation Success is an eight-week elective summer enrichment program designed to provide first-year students from groups underrepresented in medicine with a head start on the first-semester medical curriculum. Entering students from groups underrepresented in medicine are matched with a faculty mentor. The Daniel Hale Williams Society, the primary voice of students from groups underrepresented in medicine on campus, provides peer support.

Institution Type: *Public*
Application Process: *AMCAS, see chapter 4.*

APPLICATION AND ACCEPTANCE POLICIES FOR 2005–2006 FIRST-YEAR CLASS

Filing of AMCAS application
    Earliest date: June 1, 2004
    Latest date: Dec. 15, 2004
School application fee to all applicants: $80
Oldest MCAT scores considered: 2002
Does have Early Decision Program (EDP)
    Non-residents must apply through the EDP Program
    EDP application period: June 1–Aug. 1, 2004
    EDP applicants notified by: Oct. 1, 2004
Acceptance notice to regular applicants
    Earliest date: Oct. 15, 2004
    Latest date: Until class is filled
Applicant's response to acceptance offer
    Maximum time: 2 weeks
Requests for deferred entrance considered: Yes
Deposit to hold place in class (applied to tuition):
    $100, due within two weeks of acceptance;
    refundable upon written request prior to
    May 16, 2005
Estimated number of new entrants: 185
Starting date: Aug. 2005

TUITION AND STUDENT FEES PER YEAR FOR 2003–2004 FIRST-YEAR CLASS

Tuition   Student fees: $2,193
    Resident: $16,800
    Nonresident: $29,900

INFORMATION ON 2003–2004 FIRST-YEAR CLASS

Number of	In-State	Out-of-State	Total
Applicants	1,941	1,054	2,995
Applicants Interviewed	691	143	834
New Entrants*	160	20	180

*All had baccalaureate degrees; and took the MCAT.

CHAPTER

11

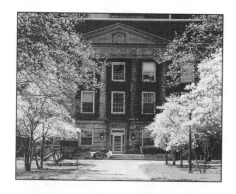

State University of New York
Upstate Medical University College of Medicine

Syracuse, New York

Dr. Steven J. Scheinman, *Dean, College of Medicine*
Dr. E. Gregory Keating, *Dean, Student Affairs*
Jennifer Welch, *Director of Admissions*
Barbara Hamilton, *Assistant Dean, Multicultural Resources*

ADDRESS INQUIRIES TO:

Admissions Committee
State University of New York
Upstate Medical University
College of Medicine
766 Irving Ave.
Syracuse, New York 13210
(315) 464-4570; 464-8867 (FAX)
Web site: www.upstate.edu

MISSION STATEMENT

The central mission of the SUNY Upstate Medical University is the education of professionals in health care and biomedical research. Excellence in patient care and the generation of new knowledge including understanding of disease, technology, and therapy are intrinsic to this mission. To this end, Upstate Medical University clinical faculty members and health care professionals commit themselves not only to their educational activities but also to patient care, demonstrating, in both areas, excellence and compassion. Similarly, a large segment of the faculty and staff must engage in research, both basic and applied, to acquire and generate new knowledge and technologies in the effort to promote health and provide a stimulating environment for the training of future scientists. In pursuing its mission, the Upstate Medical University provides its family of faculty, staff, students, and volunteers an environment of mutual trust and respect with opportunities to grow personally and professionally and to make a positive difference in the lives of others.

GENERAL INFORMATION

Upstate Medical University was established in 1834 as the Geneva Medical College. The college joined Syracuse University in 1872 and was transferred to the State University of New York (SUNY) in 1950 as the Upstate Medical Center. Since 1986, the university has been known as the SUNY Health Science Center at Syracuse. In 1999, our name was changed to SUNY Upstate Medical University to best reflect our academic mission in medical care and research, nursing, health professional training, and graduate education.

CURRICULUM

The curriculum integrates the basic and clinical sciences, with basic science courses teaching the clinical implications of the material, and provides clinical experience starting in the first semester. All courses are aligned by organ systems. The curriculum also addresses the humanistic aspects of medicine, including its ethical, legal and social implications. Students acquire the knowledge, skills and attitudes necessary to become competent, caring physicians throughout the four-year curriculum. During the third year, the students apply the principles of basic science to clinical problem-solving. Clinical clerkships in pediatrics, neurosciences, family medicine, medicine, surgery, obstetrics-gynecology, psychiatry, and radiology constitute the core of the third year. Clerkships in subspecialty services are required for all students. Thereafter, each student has the opportunity to attain individual educational objectives during 22–24 weeks of available elective time.

The clinical campus at Binghamton provides a core curriculum with programs in internal medicine, growth and development, perinatology, child and adolescent health, geriatrics, ambulatory surgery, neuropsychiatry, and primary care. A community orientation fosters a close working relationship between the campus and practicing physicians and other health care professionals.

A medical student research track is available, as are other research opportunities. Students who wish to develop skills in research may elect a special course of study. After selecting a project advisor, these students spend the first two summers as well as elective time on an independent research project.

Early assurance and deferred matriculation programs are available for qualified candidates. The M.D.-Ph.D. program is designed for those interested in investigating fundamental and applied issues of human health and disease. The central goal is to emphasize the best training in contemporary science in combination with the most practical experience in patient care. The Rural Medical Education Program places students in rural communities for nine consecutive months of clinical and didactic education, including a community project.

A modified pass/fail grading system is used; however, students may earn honors for outstanding performance in their courses.

REQUIREMENTS FOR ENTRANCE

Applications are accepted from U.S. citizens and from permanent residents who have completed at least three years of college study (90 semester hours) in the United States or Canada at an accredited institution of higher education. International applicants and individuals from foreign schools must complete at least two years of study, which include all course requirements, at an accredited American or Canadian college or university prior to application and demonstrate competency in English composition and expression. Preference is also given to those applicants who have completed the courses required for admission at the time of application. Reapplicants are discouraged unless their qualifications have significantly improved.

The MCAT and satisfactory completion of the following courses are required:

Sem. hrs.

Inorganic Chemistry (with lab) 6–8
Organic Chemistry (with lab) 6–8
Biology or Zoology (with lab) 6–8
Physics (with lab) 6–8
English 6

Choice of major should be determined by the student's primary interests. Achieving excellence in the basic sciences is essential; however, academic work in the humanities and social sciences is equally important, and are meaningful experiences in relating to people.

SELECTION FACTORS

The Admissions Committee endeavors to take into consideration as much information as possible that delineates an applicant's total qualifications for the study and practice of medicine, without regard to race, creed, religion, national origin, age, sex, marital status, or degree of physical handicap. Several application forms are used in the medical school admission process. Each form collects information appropriate to the program an applicant may be seeking. Preadmission inquiries, which relate to gender, age, ethnicity, veteran status, or other characteristics, are collected for statistical purposes only. This information has no bearing on the selection process or final decisions regarding admission to the college.

Major factors in selection of applicants include: review of college records, which include scholastic aptitude and science aptitude; MCAT scores; letters of recommendation from premedical advisory committees; communication skills; character; motivation; and an evaluation of the personal interview.

FINANCIAL AID

Accepted applicants are eligible to apply for financial aid to the Office of Admissions and Student Affairs. Financial need is determined by the ACT needs analysis system (see Part 1). The Financial Aids Committee generally makes awards in July. The major portion of financial aid for each student is in loans. Scholarships are not readily available except for those state residents who qualify for the Tuition Assistance Program Awards.

INFORMATION ABOUT DIVERSITY PROGRAMS

The SUNY Upstate Medical University is committed to making student enrollment reflective of the diverse population in New York state. Disadvantaged students and students from groups underrepresented in medicine are actively sought. A matriculation summer program is available. Premed counseling, application fee waivers, and off-campus interview programs are available. Program descriptions and further information can be obtained from either the Admissions Office or the Office of Multicultural Resources.

Institution Type: *Public*
Application Process: *AMCAS, see chapter 4.*

APPLICATION AND ACCEPTANCE POLICIES FOR 2005–2006 FIRST-YEAR CLASS

Filing of AMCAS application
   Earliest date: June 1, 2004
   Latest date: Nov. 1, 2004
School application fee to all applicants: $100
Oldest MCAT scores considered: 2001
Does have Early Decision Program (EDP)
   EDP application period: June 1–Aug. 1, 2004
   EDP applicants notified by: Oct. 1, 2004
Acceptance notice to regular applicants
   Earliest date: Oct. 15, 2004
   Latest date: Varies
Applicant's response to acceptance offer
   Maximum time: 2 weeks
Requests for deferred entrance considered: Yes
Deposit to hold place in class: $100, (applied to
   tuition), due with response to acceptance offer
Deposit refundable prior to: May 16, 2005
Estimated number of new entrants: 152 (less than 4)
Starting date: Aug. 2005

TUITION AND STUDENT FEES PER YEAR FOR 2003–2004 FIRST-YEAR CLASS

Tuition   Student fees: $781
   Resident: $16,800
   Nonresident: $29,900

INFORMATION ON 2003–2004 FIRST-YEAR CLASS

Number of	In-State	Out-of-State	Total
Applicants	1,687	754	2,441
Applicants Interviewed	575	145	720
New Entrants†	130	21	151

†All had baccalaureate degrees 76% took the MCAT.

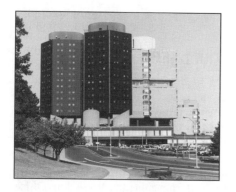

Stony Brook University School of Medicine

Stony Brook, New York

Dr. Norman H. Edelman, *Vice President, Health Sciences Center and Dean, School of Medicine*
Dr. Jack Fuhrer, *Associate Dean for Admissions*
Dr. Aldustus E. Jordan, *Associate Dean for Student and Minority Affairs*

ADDRESS INQUIRIES TO:

Committee on Admissions
Level 4 Health Sciences Center
Stony Brook University
School of Medicine
Stony Brook, New York 11794-8434
(631) 444-2113; 444-6032 (FAX)
E-mail: somadmissions@stonybrook.edu
Web site: www.hsc.sunysb.edu/som/

MISSION STATEMENT

The mission of the School of Medicine is to improve the quality of health care available to the citizens of New York and the nation by demonstrating national leadership in education, research, patient care, and community service.

To this end, the School of Medicine aims to achieve excellence in the preparation of students for careers in medical practice or research through its curriculum, and through activities that are designed to provide students with the skills that are appropriate for success in all fields of medicine.

GENERAL INFORMATION

Stony Brook University's School of Medicine accepted its first class in 1971. It is part of the Stony Brook Health Sciences Center, which includes the 540-bed University Hospital.

CURRICULUM

The curriculum of the School of Medicine is designed to provide the opportunity for extensive training in the basic medical sciences and teaching in the clinical disciplines of medicine. The curriculum requires the acquisition and utilization of a variety of skills in basic and clinical sciences. The faculty has determined that a successful candidate for the M.D. degree must pass each unit of curriculum and that waiver of units of curriculum is offered only to those who because of prior experience are able to place out through examination. The grading system is honors/pass/fail.

The first year of the curriculum consists of integrated instruction in the basic sciences and introductions to clinical skills, human behavior, nutrition, and preventive medicine. The second-year curriculum includes microbiology, pharmacology, and an interdisciplinary course in pathophysiology of the different organ systems. In both the first and second years,

students participate in the introduction to clinical medicine and medicine in contemporary society courses.

In the third year, students move to a series of clinical clerkships in medicine, surgery, pediatrics, obstetrics and gynecology, psychiatry, and family medicine, where opportunities for problem solving and patient responsibility are presented. Additional experiences are provided in radiology and emergency medicine. Clinical teaching in the introduction to clinical medicine course, in the systems program, and in the clinical clerkships takes place at the University Hospital and various clinical facilities affiliated with the School of Medicine. The clerkship program is followed by selectives and electives in the fourth year. The curriculum emphasizes social issues in medicine and bioethics at each level of medical training.

In addition, four-year programs leading to the M.D. with recognition in research, M.D. with recognition in humanities, and a six- to eight-year federally funded MSTP (M.D./Ph.D. program) are available.

REQUIREMENTS FOR ENTRANCE

Candidates for admission to the 2005 entering class are required to take the MCAT no later than August 2004 and have official scores sent to Stony Brook. Because of the rigorous competition, candidates are advised to submit applications early in the application period. All applications must be submitted through AMCAS. Prospective applicants should be aware that those who successfully applied to us in the past represent an exceptional, able, and diverse group.

Specific minimum course requirements are:

	Years
Biology (with lab)	1
Inorganic Chemistry (with lab)	1
Organic Chemistry (with lab)	1
Physics (with lab)	1
English	1

A basic course in biochemistry is strongly recommended for all students.

This minimum of preparation should be completed prior to filing the application. The Committee on Admissions makes a careful examination of the candidate's preparation and promise for creative work in medicine, regardless of the area of concentration prior to medical school.

SELECTION FACTORS

Grades, MCAT scores, letters of evaluation, and extracurricular and work experiences are carefully examined. Motivational and personal characteristics as indicated in the application, letters of evaluation, and a personal interview are also a major part of the admissions assessment. There is no discrimination in the admissions review and selection process on the basis of sex, race, religion, national origin, age, marital status, or handicap.

Students learn from each other as well as from their teachers, their textbooks, and their patients; therefore, the school attempts to acquire a class representative of a variety of backgrounds and academic interests. Indeed, given the demands on physicians in the twenty-first century, breadth of individual background is particularly important. Stony Brook hopes to attract a significant representation of groups that have historically been underrepresented in medicine. Applicants from foreign schools must have completed at least one year in an American college or university. Residents of New York constitute the majority of the applicants and entrants; however, out of state applicants will be given due consideration, particularly to special programs, e.g. MSTP (M.D./Ph.D.).

Required supporting documentation includes official transcripts of all college work and a letter of official evaluation from the applicant's premedical advisor (or, when no advisor exists at the applicant's college, from two instructors, one of whom must be from a science field). If there are other individuals who also may be in a position to provide important information, the school would be happy to receive letters from them. Personal interviews will be arranged at the initiative of the school for candidates who appear to be serious contenders for admission.

The 2003 entering class was 52 percent *women*, 33 percent *Asian/Pacific Islander*, and 17 percent *students from groups underrepresented in medicine*. The *mean GPA* of this class was 3.65; *MCAT scores averaged:* Verbal Reasoning, 10; Physical Sciences, 10; Writing Sample, P; and Biological Sciences, 11. It must be emphasized, however, that these numbers represent a range of scores, and that Stony Brook does not utilize a "cutoff" in grades or MCATs in making admission decisions.

The school is committed to giving all applicants the individualized attention that they merit.

FINANCIAL AID

Stony Brook participates in all financial aid programs available at the medical schools of the SUNY system. Financial aid and counseling are available through the Office of Student Affairs, as is assistance in securing housing and in meeting other personal needs. On-campus housing is available. Students are advised to have transportation available because there is no public transportation to the outlying clinical facilities.

The secondary application fee of $75 will be waived for those who forward a copy of the AMCAS fee waiver. Other students who believe they are eligible for a fee waiver must present supporting documentation from the financial aid advisor at their institution.

INFORMATION ABOUT DIVERSITY PROGRAMS

Stony Brook encourages applications from students from groups underrepresented in medicine, and the school makes a detailed review of these applications. The School of Medicine is in the process of initiating the Minority Access to Medicine (MAccsMed) Program to enhance interest in medicine among undergraduate students who reside or attend college on Long Island (including Brooklyn and Queens) and who are members of groups underrepresented in medicine.

Institution Type: *Public*
Application Process: *AMCAS, see chapter 4.*

APPLICATION AND ACCEPTANCE POLICIES FOR 2005–2006 FIRST-YEAR CLASS

Filing of AMCAS application
   Earliest date: June 1, 2004
   Latest date: Dec. 15, 2004
School application fee to all applicants: $75
Oldest MCAT scores considered: 2000
Does have Early Decision Program (EDP)
   EDP application period: June 1–Aug. 1, 2004
   EDP applicants notified by: Oct. 1, 2004
Acceptance notice to regular applicants
   Earliest date: Oct. 15, 2004
   Latest date: Until class is filled
Applicant's response to acceptance offer
   Maximum time: 15 days, unless otherwise specified
Requests for deferred entrance considered: Yes
Deposit to hold place in class: $100, applied to
   tuition, and due with response to acceptance offer
Deposit refundable prior to: May 16, 2005
Estimated number of new entrants: 100 (3 EDP)
Starting date: Aug. 2005

TUITION AND STUDENT FEES PER YEAR FOR 2003–2004 FIRST-YEAR CLASS

Tuition   Student fees: $766
   Resident: $16,800
   Nonresident: $29,900

INFORMATION ON 2003–2004 FIRST-YEAR CLASS

Number of	In-State	Out-of-State	Total
Applicants	1,880	643	2,523
Applicants Interviewed	549	15	564
New Entrants*	99	2	101

*All took the MCAT and had baccalaureate degrees.

CHAPTER

11

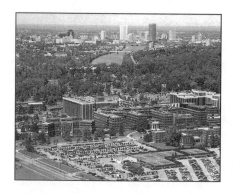

University of Rochester
School of Medicine and Dentistry

Rochester, New York

Dr. David S. Guzick, *Dean*
Dr. John T. Hansen, *Associate Dean for Admissions*
Patricia Samuelson, *Director of Admissions*
Dr. Nathaniel Holmes, *Director, Office for Ethnic and Multicultural Affairs*

ADDRESS INQUIRIES TO:

Director of Admissions
University of Rochester
School of Medicine and Dentistry
Medical Center Box 601A
Rochester, New York 14642
(585) 275-4539; 756-5479 (FAX)
E-mail: mdadmish@urmc.rochester.edu
Web site: www.urmc.rochester.edu/smd/admiss

MISSION STATEMENT

As the home of the biopsychosocial model, Rochester offers a student-centered educational program that prepares physicians for the twenty-first century. Our curriculum fosters knowledge, skills, attitudes, and behaviors of the physician/scientist/humanist by combining cutting-edge, evidence-based medical science with the relationship-centered art that is medicine's distinctive trademark.

GENERAL INFORMATION

The School of Medicine and Dentistry was established in 1920 as an academic division of the University of Rochester, a privately endowed institution founded in 1850. The university was one of the first to combine a medical school and a teaching hospital within the same facility. The original medical center has been greatly expanded to include a new medical education wing, new research facilities and clinical centers, the Strong Memorial Hospital, and a recently completed Ambulatory Care Center. Clinical teaching also is conducted at five affiliated hospitals within the community. Opportunities for independent work include summer and full-year fellowships and a wide selection of elective offerings.

CURRICULUM

Rochester's Double Helix Curriculum represents a major revision, beginning with the entering class of 1999, that captures the integrated strands of basic science and clinical medicine as they are woven throughout the four-year curriculum. The focus of our educational program is not merely the transfer of information but the transformation of the learner in a culture providing that ingenious combination of support and challenge, which leads to education. Every course is interdisciplinary and, unlike most medical schools, clinical skills training from day one leads not to shadowing or preceptor experiences but to the start of real clinical work as part of the health care team.

Students' actual clinical cases drive the learning of science, and students return to increasingly advanced basic science in the second, third, and fourth years through an integrated series of problem-based learning (PBL) exercises. Clinical exposure begins during the first week of school with an introduction to clinical medicine in the fall semester and the start of the ambulatory care clerkship beginning during the first spring semester. This experience, unlike any other in the country, includes the ambulatory components of family medicine, pediatrics, internal medicine, women's health, psychiatry, and ambulatory surgery, and is completed by the end of the second year.

Years 2 and 4 conclude with case seminars that present basic and clinical science with increasing levels of depth. Inpatient clerkships focus on acute care experiences in adult medicine, women's and children's health, mind/brain/behavior, and urgent/emergent care.

A formal tutoring system and assistance programs are available to all students with special academic needs.

A rich and diverse menu of opportunities is available to students, including a strong M.D.-Ph.D. program and a year-long research fellowship program, reflecting the institution's commitment to research and the preparation of medical scientists and academicians. Master's programs are offered in public health, business, and in several other disciplines. Opportunities to participate in volunteer service to the Rochester community and to experience medicine through our international medicine program reflect the school's commitment to providing the broadest possible educational experience.

REQUIREMENTS FOR ENTRANCE

All entering students usually have completed the baccalaureate degree. Rochester utilizes the AMCAS application and requires the MCAT examination.

Satisfactory completion of the following premedical coursework is required:

	Sem. Hr.
Biology (with lab)	6-8
General or Inorganic Chemistry	6-8

Organic Chemistry 6-8
  One semester of biochemistry may be substituted
  for a semester of organic chemistry. Within the
  two-year chemistry sequence, one year of laboratory
  is required.
Physics (with lab) 6-8
Expository Writing 6-8
  May be met with writing, English, or nonscience
  courses that involve expository writing
Humanities and/or social or behavioral sciences 12-16

The requirements above are designed with the expectation that students will enter with a liberal and diversified education. Courses in Calculus and Statistics, Biochemistry, and experience in research, clinical practice, public health, or health policy issues are strongly recommended.

Advanced Placement (AP) credit may not be used to satisfy the biology, English, or nonscience requirements. AP credit may substitute for one semester of general chemistry and/or one semester of physics only.

SELECTION FACTORS

Evaluation of applicants includes a careful examination of the entire academic record, letters of recommendation, and the candidate's personal statement. Candidates who show particular promise of achievement are invited for interviews at the medical school.

Demonstrated excellence in a demanding academic program, including a high level of achievement in the natural sciences, is an absolute requirement for acceptance. Evidence of intrinsic intellectual drive and curiosity is highly valued since the program at Rochester emphasizes independent opportunities for individual students. Particular attention is given to achievements that demonstrate breadth and commitment. The school is characterized by an atmosphere in which students and faculty work closely together toward the attainment of knowledge and understanding and in which patients are treated with compassion and sensitivity. Students are sought who will contribute to this climate for learning.

Selections are made without regard to gender, sexual orientation, race, religion, national origin, age, or handicap. State residency is not a factor in selection. Transfer applicants are not accepted.

All applicants must have completed at least two years of undergraduate college study in the United States, including all premedical requirements. Only citizens or permanent residents of the U.S. are eligible to apply, unless they are Rochester graduates.

Applicants who have not been accepted may reapply in a subsequent year, but applicants who twice have been unsuccessful in gaining admission are discouraged from reapplying.

The 2003 entering class came from 29 different states and attended 57 different colleges and universities. The *mean age* of the class was 24 years (range 20-38), 54 percent were women, and 12 percent students from groups underrepresented in medicine. The *mean GPA* was 3.67, and the *average MCAT scores* were VR-10.1, PS-10.5, and BS-10.6.

FINANCIAL AID

The medical school offers scholarships and long-term loans to those students who demonstrate financial need. Decisions concerning admission are made independently of financial circumstances.

In 2003–2004, 85 percent of the enrolled students received financial assistance from either school or noninstitutional sources. Entering students applying for institutional financial aid are required to provide a FAFSA, a more detailed financial statement including parent information, and the School of Medicine's financial aid application.

INFORMATION ABOUT DIVERSITY PROGRAMS

The Office of Ethnic and Multicultural Affairs represents a serious commitment on the part of the University of Rochester School of Medicine and Dentistry to meet the urgent need for diverse physicians in all aspects of the medical profession. An active recruitment program seeks applicants for both the M.D. and M.D.-Ph.D. programs.

Institution Type: *Private*
Application Process: *AMCAS, see chapter 4.*

APPLICATION AND ACCEPTANCE POLICIES FOR 2005–2006 FIRST-YEAR CLASS

Filing of application
  Earliest date: June 1, 2004
  Latest date: Oct. 15, 2004
School application fee to all applicants: $75
Oldest MCAT scores considered: 2001
Does not have Early Decision Program
Acceptance notice to regular applicants
  Earliest date: Oct. 15, 2004
  Latest date: Until class is filled
Applicant's response to acceptance offer
  Maximum time: 2 weeks
Requests for deferred entrance considered: Yes
Deposit to hold place in class (applied to tuition): $100,
  due with response to acceptance offer
Deposit refundable prior to: May 16, 2005
Estimated number of new entrants: 100
Starting date: Aug. 2005

TUITION AND STUDENT FEES PER YEAR FOR 2003–2004 FIRST-YEAR CLASS

Tuition: $31,500   Student fees: $2,818

INFORMATION ON 2003–2004 FIRST-YEAR CLASS

Number of	In-State	Out-of-State	Total
Applicants	1,050	2,913	3,963
Applicants Interviewed	211	445	656
New Entrants*	42	58	100

*100% had baccalaureate degrees; 86% took the MCAT.

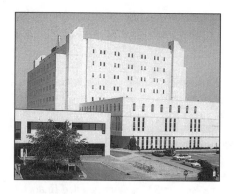

The Brody School of Medicine at East Carolina University

Greenville, North Carolina

Dr. Cynda A. Johnson, *Dean*
Dr. James G. Peden, Jr., *Associate Dean for Admissions*
Vickie Ogden, *Director of Financial Aid and Student Services*
Dr. Virginia D. Hardy, *Assistant Dean for Intercultural Academic Affairs*

ADDRESS INQUIRIES TO:

Associate Dean
Office of Admissions
The Brody School of Medicine
 at East Carolina University
Greenville, North Carolina 27858-4354
(252) 744-2202
E-mail: somadmissions@mail.ecu.edu
Web site: www.ecu.edu/bsomadmissions

MISSION STATEMENT

Simply stated, our goal at the Brody School of Medicine at East Carolina University is to provide students with the knowledge and clinical experience needed to attain successful careers in medicine. Our mission is threefold: educating primary care physicians, making medical care more readily available to the people of eastern North Carolina, and providing opportunities for disadvantaged students. Among the most important elements making up the educational approach at the School of Medicine are the relatively small class sizes, a highly competent and concerned faculty, and exceptional facilities.

GENERAL INFORMATION

In 1972 East Carolina University enrolled students in the First-Year Program in Medical Education. The Board of Governors of the University of North Carolina system and the General Assembly of North Carolina authorized East Carolina University to expand the First-Year Program and establish a degree-granting School of Medicine. The School of Medicine enrolled the first class of students in August 1977.

The school's educational facilities are located on the 100-acre Health Sciences Center campus. Preclinical instruction is offered in the nine-story Brody Medical Sciences Building, which is contiguous to the Pitt County Memorial Hospital. Comprehensive clinical instruction is offered in the hospital (731 beds). Other clinical settings, either adjacent to or near the Health Sciences Center, include the Leo W. Jenkins Cancer Center, Heart Center, Mental Health Center, Rehabilitation Center, Area Health Education Center, and the Intensive/Intermediate Care Neonatal Unit.

CURRICULUM

The first year of the four-year curriculum is devoted to the study of the anatomy and functions of the body through courses in gross and microscopic anatomy, biochemistry, physiology, microbiology/immunology, and genetics. Correlative clinical lectures in these as well as courses in psychosocial basis of medical practice, ethical and social issues in medicine, and Doctoring I are presented. A primary care preceptorship is mandatory.

The second-year curriculum is directed toward clinical medicine. Courses include Doctoring II, pathogenic microbiology, pharmacology, pathology, and introduction to medicine. Also included in the second-year curriculum are courses in psychiatry, human sexuality, life-style abuse, ethical and social issues in medicine, and a primary care preceptorship.

The third year is composed of six required clerkships: 8 weeks each in family medicine, internal medicine, obstetrics and gynecology, pediatrics, psychiatry, and surgery. At least 10 weeks of ambulatory care are included in the third year.

The fourth year is composed of 36 weeks of clinical and basic science electives, which must include blocks in primary care, medicine, and surgery. Students select an individualized curriculum after consulting with faculty advisors.

Student performance is evaluated by letter grade, and promotion to the next year's class is recommended to the dean by the Promotions Committee of the respective year.

A combined M.D.-M.B.A. program is available to students. Coursework in the School of Business is completed in 12 months, usually taken between the second and third years of the medical curriculum. Both the M.D. and M.B.A. degrees are awarded after five years of study.

Students may also apply at any time after their enrollment in the M.D. program for a combined M.D.-Ph.D. option, which they begin after successful completion of the USMLE Step I exam. Accepted students can take up to four years to complete the Ph.D. requirements, and participate in a clinical skills component during the year prior to their reentry into the M.D. curriculum.

REQUIREMENTS FOR ENTRANCE

The MCAT and a minimum equivalent of three undergraduate years of preparation are required. Minimum coursework requirements are:

Semester Hour

General Biology or Zoology (with lab) 8
Inorganic Chemistry (with lab) 8
Organic Chemistry (with lab). 8

Physics (with lab) 8
English 6

Additional courses in biostatistics, English, humanities and social sciences are recommended.

SELECTION FACTORS

Factors considered in the selection process encompass the social, personal, and intellectual development of each applicant. All available application data are evaluated: MCAT scores; academic performance; comments contained in letters of reference/recommendation; and the results of two personal interviews, conducted only at the medical school campus, with two members of the Admissions Committee.

The Brody School of Medicine at East Carolina University seeks competent students of diverse personalities and backgrounds, and all applicants are evaluated without regard to race, religion, sex, age, national origin, or handicap. Very strong preference is given to qualified residents of North Carolina.

In conjunction with the undergraduate Office of Admissions, the Brody School of Medicine offers an Early Assurance Program for highly qualified high school seniors. Selected scholars enroll in the University and are assured of a spot in the medical school class after receiving their baccalaureate degree (provided certain academic standards are maintained).

Characteristics of the 2003 entering class of 72 students were: *mean GPA,* 3.6; *sex,* 37 women; *students from groups underrepresented in medicine,* 18 students. *MCAT scores* (mean): *VR*-8.7; *PS*-8.5; *WS*-0; *BS*-8.9.

Qualified North Carolina residents from schools with similar medical curricula may be considered for transfer into the second- or third-year classes. Advanced standing positions are dependent on the very limited number of seats that become available through attrition. Interested students should send letters describing their circumstances to the Office of Admissions for further information.

FINANCIAL AID

Resources are available for loans and scholarships. The Financial Aid Office will make every effort to provide information and financial aid to those students who demonstrate need for financial assistance in order to meet the costs of their educational and living obligations. Awards are based on need as determined by confidential information supplied by the students merit awards are also available. Sixty-five percent of the student body receive some financial assistance.

INFORMATION ABOUT DIVERSITY PROGRAMS

Persons from groups underrepresented in medicine who hold residence in North Carolina are encouraged to apply. There is diverse membership on the Admissions Committee, and the Academic Support and Enrichment Center offers a wide range of services to students desiring assistance or guidance.

Institution Type: *Public*
Application Process: *AMCAS, see chapter 4.*

APPLICATION AND ACCEPTANCE POLICIES FOR 2005–2006 FIRST-YEAR CLASS

Filing of AMCAS application
  Earliest date: June 1, 2004
  Latest date: Nov. 15, 2004
School application after screening: $50
Oldest MCAT scores considered: 2001
Does have Early Decision Program (EDP)
  For North Carolina residents only
  EDP application period: June 1–Aug. 1, 2004
  EDP applicants notified by: Oct. 1, 2004
Acceptance notice to regular applicants
  Earliest date: Oct. 15, 2004
  Latest date: Class matriculation date
Applicant's response to acceptance offer
  Maximum time: 3 weeks
Requests for deferred entrance considered: No
Deposit to hold place in class (applied to tuition):
  $100, due with response to acceptance offer
Deposit refundable prior to: May 16, 2005
Estimated number of new entrants: 72 (9 EDP)
Starting date: Aug. 2005

TUITION AND STUDENT FEES PER YEAR FOR 2003–2004 FIRST-YEAR CLASS

Tuition   Student fees: $1,313
  Resident: $3,609
  Nonresident: $28,524

INFORMATION ON 2003–2004 FIRST-YEAR CLASS

Number of	In-State	Out-of-State	Total
Applicants	671	228	899
Applicants Interviewed	453	0	453
New Entrants†	72	0	72

†96% took the MCAT; all had baccalaureate degrees.

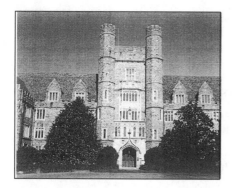

Duke University School of Medicine

Durham, North Carolina

Dr. R. Sanders Williams, *Vice Chancellor for Academic Affairs and
    Dean, School of Medicine*
Dr. Brenda E. Armstrong, *Associate Dean and Director of Admissions*
Stacey R. McCorison, *Director of Financial Aid*
Dr. Delbert R. Wigfall, *Associate Professor of Pediatrics and
    Associate Dean, Medical Education*

ADDRESS INQUIRIES TO:

Committee on Admissions
Duke University
School of Medicine
Duke University Medical Center
P.O. Box 3710 DUMC
Durham, North Carolina 27710
(877) 684-2985 (toll free); (919) 684-8893 (FAX)
E-mail: medadm@mc.duke.edu
Web site: http://dukemed.duke.edu

MISSION STATEMENT

Duke University School of Medicine is a community of scholars devoted to understanding the causes, prevention and treatment of human disease. The missions of the School of Medicine, to train scholars and leaders across a broad spectrum of career paths in medicine, are undertaken by women and men unswervingly committed to the highest of academic goals: the generation, conservation, and dissemination of knowledge leading to the prevention and eradication of human disease. Through innovative curricula and outstanding resources in education, clinical care and basic and clinical research and in the context of a diverse community, Duke University School of Medicine prepares students for roles of scholarly endeavor, leadership and innovation for healthcare into the new millennium.

GENERAL INFORMATION

The Duke University Medical Center is located on the campus of Duke University in Durham, North Carolina. A hospital was opened for patients in July 1930, and the first medical students were admitted in October of that year. The first doctor of medicine degrees were conferred in June 1932. Duke Hospital (1,000 beds) is supplemented by the Durham Veterans Affairs Hospital (489 beds) for clinical teaching.

CURRICULUM

The curriculum has been designed to provide the flexibility to encompass the rapid expansion of medical knowledge as well as the broad range of individual student interests and talents. First-year students receive instruction in the basic science principles of modern medicine. A two-year introduction to clinical medicine complements instruction in each of the first two years of the medical school curriculum. The second year is the clinical clerkship year. The third and fourth years are elective; with the guidance of an advisory dean and several senior faculty advisors, students design their programs to include half basic science and half clinical coursework. In the third year students may participate in a mentored research project enabling them to learn basic principles of research and to critically evaluate the research of others. Having completed the required courses in the first and second years, students may explore relevant areas of basic science in more depth and complement their first-year acquisition of science knowledge. Students who elect dual-degree programs (M.D./M.P.H., M.D./M.P.P., M.D./M.B.A., M.D./J.D., and M.D./M.A./Ph.D. in medical history) begin their respective curricula during the third year. In the fourth year, clinical courses may be elected to enhance general medical education in more depth and breadth. Students graduate prepared to pursue careers in community practice, academic medicine, or public health and to contribute expertise in health policy and medical ethics issues.

The Medical Scientist Training Program is designed to provide both the M.D. and Ph.D. degrees over a six- to seven-year period of study. The first two years are spent in the medical school program, followed by a three- to four-year period of graduate study. Upon completion of the Ph.D. degree, the last year is spent in the clinical sciences. It is expected that candidates for this combined degree plan to have careers in academic medicine.

REQUIREMENTS FOR ENTRANCE

The MCAT and three years of college are required. The spring MCAT is preferred and advantageous. A minimum of 90 semester hours of approved college credit is also required. Prerequisite courses must be taken within seven years before application. Coursework must include:

	Years
Biology	1
Inorganic Chemistry	1
Organic Chemistry	1
General Physics	1
Calculus	1
English	1

An introductory course in biochemistry is suggested during the senior year.

Premedical students should be aware of the importance of a well-rounded general education as preparation for the study of medicine and not limit themselves to scientific courses. The Committee on Admissions places more importance on the way applicants handle their undergraduate work than on the subject matter taken.

SELECTION FACTORS

The selection of students is based upon the quality rather than the quantity of preparation and upon demonstrated evidence of personal attributes of intelligence, character, and general fitness for the study and practice of medicine. In considering an applicant, many sources of information may be consulted: curricular and extracurricular college record; fitness as reflected by carefully prepared, confidential appraisals by teachers who know the individual well; MCAT scores; and the applicant's showing in the interview that is held with members of the Committee on Admissions or one of its regional representatives.

Accepted students for the 2003 entering class had high GPAs and MCAT scores, were active in campus and community service, represented 50+ collegiate institutions, 27 states and 4 countries. 51% of the students in the class of 2003 were women. The Committee on Admissions does not discriminate on the basis of race, sex, sexual preference, creed, age, handicap, or national origin.

FINANCIAL AID

The Office of Financial Aid asks that students who wish to be considered for institutional funds complete the *Need Access* diskette and the federal government's Free Application for Federal Student Aid (FAFSA). These may be obtained via Internet or the Office of Financial Aid. Students seeking to apply for only Federal Stafford Loans need to complete the FAFSA. We urge that students complete and submit the applications as soon as possible. Accepted students will receive an award notice once we have received the FAFSA and the *Need Access* computations.

Students applying for institutional funds who demonstrate need as determined by both the FAFSA and the *Need Access* analysis will receive approximately 40 percent Stafford and/or Duke loans and 60 percent institutional grants. While more than 80 percent of currently enrolled medical students receive some type of scholarship, grant, or loan, their financial circumstance has no bearing on the admissions process.

Eight Nanaline H. Duke Scholarships in the amount of current tuition are awarded each year by the Dean to academically excellent first-year students. Seven Dean's Tuition Scholarships in the amount of current tuition are awarded each year by the Dean to academically excellent students from groups underrepresented in medicine.

Financially needy and disadvantaged students, and students from groups underrepresented in medicine selected for the North Carolina Board of Governors Medical Scholarship will receive full tuition, fees, and a stipend.

Students who enter the Medical Scientist Training Program receive full tuition, fees, and a stipend.

INFORMATION ABOUT DIVERSITY PROGRAMS

An aggressive effort to identify and recruit talented students from groups underrepresented in medicine is in place, supported by significant members of house staff and faculty from these groups, resulting in the consistent enrollment of significant numbers of students from these groups in the School of Medicine. Medical students from groups underrepresented in medicine have access to a dean/faculty/student group that supports first-year students and meets regularly to discuss common issues pertinent to the experience of these students. These efforts are supplemented by multiple departmental and medical school-wide programs to address cross-cultural issues in medicine.

Institution Type: *Private*
Application Process: *AMCAS, see chapter 4.*

APPLICATION AND ACCEPTANCE POLICIES FOR 2005–2006 FIRST-YEAR CLASS

Filing of AMCAS application
    Earliest date: June 1, 2004
    Latest date: Nov. 15, 2004
School application fee to all applicants: $85
Oldest MCAT scores considered: 2001
Does not have Early Decision Program
Acceptance notice to regular applicants
    Earliest date: March 1, 2005
    Latest date: Until class is filled
Applicant's response to acceptance offer
    Maximum time: 2 weeks
Requests for deferred entrance considered:
    Yes, prior to June 1st
Deposit to hold place in class (applied to tuition):
    $100, due May 16, 2005; nonrefundable
Estimated number of new entrants: 100
Starting date: Aug. 2005

TUITION AND STUDENT FEES PER YEAR FOR 2003–2004 FIRST-YEAR CLASS

Tuition: $31,194   Student fees: $3,807

INFORMATION ON 2003–2004 FIRST-YEAR CLASS

Number of	In-State	Out-of-State	Total
Applicants	365	4,838	5,205
Applicants Interviewed	76	731	807
New Entrants†	9	91	100

†All took the MCAT and had baccalaureate degrees.

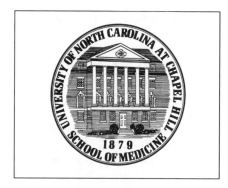

University of North Carolina at Chapel Hill School of Medicine

Chapel Hill, North Carolina

Dr. Jeffrey L. Houpt, *Dean and Vice Chancellor for Medical Affairs*
Dr. Axalla J. Hoole, *Associate Dean for Admissions*
Larry D. Keith, *Assistant Dean for Admissions, Director of Recruitment/ Special Programs*
Sheila M. Graham, *Financial Aid Officer*

ADDRESS INQUIRIES TO:

Admissions Office
CB# 1500 121 MacNider Hall
University of North Carolina at Chapel Hill
School of Medicine
Chapel Hill, North Carolina 27599-9500
(919) 962-8331; 966-9930 (FAX)
E-mail: admissions@med.unc.edu
Web site: www.med.unc.edu/

MISSION STATEMENT

The School of Medicine of the University of North Carolina at Chapel Hill exists to educate students and professionals of the health and biomedical sciences, to conduct scholarly investigation in biomedical, behavioral, and social sciences, and to render service to the people and institutions of the state, the region, the nation, and, as appropriate, throughout the world.

GENERAL INFORMATION

The School of Medicine of the University of North Carolina (UNC) at Chapel Hill was established in 1879 and expanded to a four-year school in 1952. Other schools of health sciences are adjacent, allowing easy interaction and collaboration. The School of Medicine is continuing a major expansion and renovation of teaching and clinical facilities. Among other projects, two hospitals, Women's and Children's, were completed September, 2001. Additional educational and clinical facilities are available throughout the state in Area Health Education Centers (AHEC) established in 1972 to provide clinical experience and educational opportunities in community settings.

CURRICULUM

The curriculum offers an education that reflects our mission. The first year presents courses in basic biomedical science. Presentation is largely through lectures; problem-based and case-based small group sessions are increasingly being used. Introduction to the profession of medicine begins in the first week of the first year through Introduction to Clinical Medicine (ICM). ICM provides a two-year continuum of weekly small-group seminars and experience with simulated and real patients. Local sessions are supplemented by five one-week immersion experiences in a community in North Carolina which allow students to apply clinical skills and gain understanding of the context of patient care. A weekly seminar, Medicine and Society, focuses on health care issues. The second year presents the pathophysiology of disease in organ based courses. Clinical skills development continues through the second year of ICM, and issues in social aspects of health care are presented through selectives offered by the Department of Social Medicine. A course in clinical epidemiology gives students tools to evaluate research and literature and to apply evidence based medicine to patient care. Third year core clinical experiences include internal medicine, surgery, family medicine, obstetrics and gynecology, pediatrics, and psychiatry. Some rotations are at AHEC sites. The fourth year is made up of four required clinical selectives and three electives, which are typically used by students to explore areas of interest and make internship decisions. Rotations may be off campus, including international programs. Students conduct research with faculty mentorship support by school or grant funding, or through selection to the Distinguished Medical Scholars or Doris Duke programs (a year of funded study and research). Students pursue interest in rural and community medicine, public policy, or public health through Social Medicine selectives, fourth year Ambulatory Care Selectives, and Community Health Projects. Students interested in combined degrees may be admitted to the MSTP funded M.D./Ph.D. program or obtain an M.Ph. through the School of Public Health. The grading system is Honors/Pass/Fail and passing USMLE Step I is required to enter the third year and USMLE Step II for graduation.

REQUIREMENTS FOR ENTRANCE

A minimum of 96 semester hours of accredited college work and the MCAT are required. Students may take the MCAT no later than the August prior to the year of matriculation and scores from an MCAT administered more than five years before the projected date of matriculation are not accepted. Students may choose any field of major study, but must demonstrate proficiency in the natural sciences. Appreciation of the core principles in biochemistry, molecular and cellular biology, and genetics is expected. Work in the humanities and social sciences is valued and proficiency in the English language is essential.

Minimum Sem. hrs.

English 6
Biology (including at least one course with lab). It is
   strongly suggested that students take at least
   one course in cell and molecular biology or genetics 7
General and Organic Chemistry (with labs). One semester

of biochemistry may be substituted for one semester of
Organic Chemistry. 16
Physics (with labs). 8

SELECTION FACTORS

The Committee on Admissions evaluates the qualifications
of all applicants to select those with the greatest potential for
accomplishment in one of the many careers open to medical
graduates. Preference is given to North Carolina residents. The
University of North Carolina does not discriminate on the
basis of race, national origin, religion, sex, age, or handicap.

The AMCAS application is used for initial screening.
Qualified North Carolina applicants and selected nonresidents
are sent a supplementary application. Following receipt of a supplementary application, applicants are invited for an interview.
In making its final selections from the group of qualified applicants, the committee considers evidence of each candidate's
motivation, maturity, leadership, integrity, and a variety of other
personal qualifications and accomplishments in addition to the
scholastic record. All information available about each applicant
is considered without assigning priority to any single factor. No
special admission tracks or quotas are applied among applicants. The undergraduate major is not an important consideration, but excellence in the chosen field is expected. Previously
rejected applicants are considered without prejudice, but reapplications are compared to those previously submitted to
assess changes in the applicants qualifications.

FINANCIAL AID

Grants and low-interest, long-term loans are available to
students with financial need, determined through an evaluation
of the total resources available to the student. Awards are based
on information obtained from the Free Application for Federal
Student Aid (FAFSA) submitted by the student. At last calculation, 85 percent of the student body applied for aid from
funds for which eligibility is certified by the university.
Financial need will not adversely affect a student's chances of
admission, and no student, once admitted, should have to leave
for personal financial need. Part-time employment is discouraged. A few scholarships are awarded for academic achievement and promise; there is no separate application for these.

Economically or environmentally disadvantaged students
admitted to the School of Medicine are eligible for nomination
to the Board of Governors' Medical Scholars Program. Those
students who are selected receive annual stipends of $5,000
plus tuition and fees. Recipients must be residents of North
Carolina who demonstrate exceptional financial need and are
enrolled in one of the schools of medicine on a full-time basis.

For additional information, contact the Student Aid Section
at (919) 962-6118.

INFORMATION FOR DISADVANTAGED STUDENTS

Disadvantaged students are urged to apply, and there is an
active recruitment program for students from groups underrepresented in medicine. The Medical Education Development

Program is available to premedical disadvantaged students to
acquaint them with the medical school curriculum and faculty and to assist them with learning skills development for
medical school.

The Office of Student Affairs provides academic counseling
after admission. Academic assistance is provided through tutorial programs, the Learning and Assessment Laboratory, and
other resources within the university. Faculty members are available to assist students, and students are encouraged to see them
for specific curricular problems. For students who have significant problems mastering the curriculum, a reduction in courses
can be considered. A review program during the summer is provided for students with limited academic deficiencies. Students
are reexamined at the end of the review period and promoted
upon successfully passing the reexamination.

Institution Type: *Public*
Application Process: *AMCAS, see chapter 4.*

APPLICATION AND ACCEPTANCE POLICIES FOR 2005–2006 FIRST-YEAR CLASS

Filing of AMCAS application
  Earliest date: June 1, 2004
  Latest date: Nov. 15, 2004
School fee for supplement application: $65
Oldest MCAT scores considered: 2000
Does have Early Decision Program (EDP)
  EDP application period: June 1–Aug. 1, 2004
  EDP applicants notified by: Oct. 1, 2004
Acceptance notice to regular applicants
  Earliest date: Oct. 15, 2004
  Latest date: Until class is filled
Applicant's response to acceptance offer
  Maximum time: 3 weeks
Requests for deferred entrance considered: Yes
Deposit to hold place in class (applied to tuition):
  $100, due with response to acceptance offer
Deposit refundable prior to: May 16, 2005
Estimated number of new entrants: 160 (7 EDP)
Starting date: Aug. 2005

TUITION AND STUDENT FEES PER YEAR FOR 2003–2004 FIRST-YEAR CLASS

Tuition   Student fees: $1,110
  Resident: $7,385
  Nonresident: $33,001

INFORMATION ON 2003–2004 FIRST-YEAR CLASS

Number of	In-State	Out-of-State	Total
Applicants	744	2,280	3,024
Applicants Interviewed	435	103	538
New Entrants*	143	17	160

*All took the MCAT and had baccalaureate degrees.

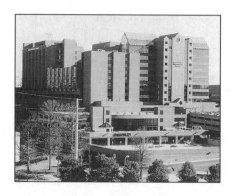

Wake Forest University School of Medicine

Winston-Salem, North Carolina

Dr. William B. Applegate, *Senior Vice President and Dean*
Dr. Lewis H. Nelson, III, *Associate Dean for Admissions*
Melissa Stevens, *Financial Aid Director*
Dr. Brenda Latham-Sadler, *Assistant Dean for Student Services*

ADDRESS INQUIRIES TO:

Office of Medical School Admissions
Wake Forest University School of Medicine
Medical Center Boulevard
Winston-Salem, North Carolina 27157-1090
(336) 716-4264; 716-9593 (FAX)
E-mail: medadmit@wfubmc.edu
Web site: www.wfubmc.edu/school/

MISSION STATEMENT

The Medical Center is committed to serving society by providing a superior education; by rendering exemplary and efficient patient care; by fostering the discovery and application of new knowledge through research; and to improve the health and well-being of the nation.

GENERAL INFORMATION

The School of Medicine was established in 1902 at Wake Forest, North Carolina, and of the existing 166 medical schools, it was one of 11 that required college preparation. Patient care, research, education, and community service remain the fourfold mission of the school as part of Wake Forest University. The name of the medical school was changed from The Bowman Gray School of Medicine to Wake Forest University School of Medicine, the Bowman Gray Campus, in 1997.

The main teaching hospital of the medical school is the 880-bed North Carolina Baptist Hospital. Affiliated institutions include the 896-bed Forsyth Memorial Hospital, the Downtown Health Plaza of Baptist Hospital, and Northwest Area Health Education Center.

CURRICULUM

The curriculum, Prescription for Excellence: A Physician's Pathway to Lifelong Learning, is organized to meet the seven goals of the undergraduate medical education program: self-directed learning and life-long learning skills, core biomedical science knowledge, clinical skills, problem solving/clinical reasoning skills, interviewing and communication skills, information management skills, and professional attitudes and behavior.

Students study the basic and clinical sciences in an integrated fashion throughout the four-year curriculum utilizing small-group problem-based learning and other educational methods which are closely integrated through the computer network. Early community-based clinical experience, as well as a focus on population health are hallmarks of the curriculum. Professionalism issues are addressed longitudinally across the curriculum in formats designed to provide students with a clear understanding of the role and responsibilities of physicians within society. Information technology has been integrated into the curriculum to a considerable degree, and all incoming students are provided with an IBM ThinkPad laptop computer.

A foundation in core biomedical science is provided by the Human Structure and Development and the Cellular and Subcellular Processes courses in Phase I of the first year. Interviewing and physical examination skills are taught through patient contact beginning in the first week of school in the Foundation of Clinical Medicine (FCM) course. Pharmacology, pathology, and radiology topics are integrated with clinical topics within the organ system-based topics in the Systems Pathophysiology courses. Evidence-based decision making is the focus of the Evidence-Based Medicine course. Issues, such as genetic engineering, culture and medicine, and death and dying, related to the practice of medicine, are discussed within the Medicine as a Profession (MAAP) course, which extends across the first two phases. Topics relating to population health and epidemiology are presented in the first year Population Health-Epidemiology course. The third phase consists of clerkships in medicine, surgery and anesthesiology, pediatrics, psychiatry, obstetrics and gynecology, family medicine, neurology/rehabilitation medicine, and women's health. The fourth phase consists of 11 four-week rotations: two advanced in-patient management clerkships, intensive care and emergency medicine. The remainder are electives. The fifth phase completes the fourth year with an emphasis on preparation for the challenges of internship and residency. Performance is evaluated on a zero-to-three scale across the four-year curriculum.

EARLY ASSURANCE PROGRAM (EAP)

Well-qualified college students, upon completion of the sophomore year, at very competitive schools may apply for acceptance to the class entering two years later. Eligibility requires an overall GPA of 3.5, a science GPA of 3.5, and completion of half of the required prerequisites. The MCAT will not be required.

A student applies early in the junior year through the AMCAS process (November 1 deadline), asking consideration for the EAP. The applicant must agree to complete requisite courses, to continue academic excellence, to demonstrate high ethical conduct, and not to apply to any other medical school. Non-acceptance by the EAP does not influence future applications. The EAP should not be confused with the Early Decision Program.

JOINT-DEGREE PROGRAMS

The Wake Forest University School of Medicine offers three five-year joint-degree programs and the M.D.-Ph.D. The M.D.–M.B.A. program is offered in conjunction with the Babcock Graduate School of Management. The five-year M.D.-Master of Arts in Intercultural Studies is offered in conjunction with the Southeastern Theological Seminary.The M.D.-M.S. and the M.D.-Ph.D. are offered in conjunction with the Graduate School of Wake Forest University.

The M.D.-M.B.A. program responds to the growing need for professionals who are trained in both medicine and management. The M.D.-Masters of Arts in Intercultural Studies is designed for students with an interest in medical missions. The M.D.-M.S. in Clinical Epidemiology and Health Services Research provides a combination of coursework in epidemiology and health services research and is designed for students with an interest in clinical research. The M.D.-Ph.D. program is expected to be completed within seven years. All joint degrees require completion of all requirements of both programs before degrees are awarded.

Applicants for the joint-degree programs must be accepted via a separate admissions process to the business and graduate schools. The Babcock School of Management requires applicants to take the GMAT; the Graduate School accepts the MCAT.

REQUIREMENTS FOR ENTRANCE

The MCAT is required except for the EAP. The minimum requirement for admission is 90 semester hours of college work, although most candidates benefit from a well-rounded four-year college curriculum. Required courses should be completed by the time of application. Generally, prerequisites are:

	Sem. hrs.
General Biology	8
General or Inorganic Chemistry	8
Organic Chemistry	8
General Physics	8

SELECTION FACTORS

Candidates are selected on the basis of the quality of their academic records, MCAT scores, and general qualifications. North Carolina residents and nonresidents are given equal and careful consideration. There are no restrictions because of race, creed, sex, religion, age, physical disadvantages, marital status, or national origin.

The Committee on Admissions (COA) and/or the Associate Dean for Admissions will evaluate each application. Applicants whose performance suggests they would have difficulty in handling the curriculum are notified. All other applicants are sent a supplemental application. Applicants who have completed files are considered for local interviews at the discretion of the COA. No regional interviews are conducted.

The School of Medicine may be able to accept an application for transfer from a student who is currently enrolled, and in good standing, in a medical school accredited by the Liaison Committee on Medical Education and who meets the prerequisite requirements.

Characteristics of the 2003 entering class are students from 28 states and 58 colleges and universities; *gender*, 44 percent women;

acceptance rate, 10 percent of all applicants were interviewed and 49 percent of those interviewed offered acceptance for 108 places.

FINANCIAL AID

Loans and scholarships are awarded to qualified applicants on the basis of financial need and academic standing. Applicants must complete required application forms prior to the April 1 deadline. Students receive a significant amount of their funding from federal student loan programs. Eighty percent of the student body receive financial assistance. Students should not work part-time because of the demands of the study of medicine.

INFORMATION ABOUT DIVERSITY PROGRAMS

The Office of Minority Affairs actively recruits students from groups underrepresented in medicine and has developed programs for academic enrichment, academic reinforcement, tutorial, and counseling services for enrolled students. Address inquiries to the Office of Minority Affairs.

Institution Type: *Private*
Application Process: *AMCAS, see chapter 4.*

APPLICATION AND ACCEPTANCE POLICIES FOR 2005–2006 FIRST-YEAR CLASS

Filing of AMCAS application
   Earliest date: June 1, 2004
   Latest date: Nov. 1, 2004
School application fee after screening: $55
Oldest MCAT scores considered: 2001
Does have Early Decision Program (EDP)
   EDP application period: June 1–Aug. 1, 2004
   EDP applicants notified by: Oct. 1, 2004
Acceptance notice to regular applicants
   Earliest date: Oct. 15, 2004
   Latest date: Until class is filled
Applicant's response to acceptance offer
   Maximum time: 2 weeks
Requests for deferred entrance considered: Yes
Deposit to hold place in class (applied to tuition):
$100, due with response to acceptance offer
Deposit refundable prior to: May 1, 2005
Estimated number of new entrants: 108 (2 EDP)
Starting date: July 25, 2005

TUITION AND STUDENT FEES PER YEAR FOR 2003–2004 FIRST-YEAR CLASS

Tuition: $32,056   Student fees: None

INFORMATION ON 2003–2004 FIRST-YEAR CLASS

Number of	In-State	Out-of-State	Total
Applicants	580	4,572	5,152
Applicants Interviewed	155	417	572
New Entrants*	40	68	108

*All had baccalaureate degrees; 97% took the MCAT.

CHAPTER

11

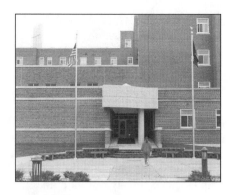

University of North Dakota
School of Medicine and Health Sciences

Grand Forks, North Dakota

Dr. H. David Wilson, *Dean*
Judy L. DeMers, *Associate Dean, Student Affairs and Admissions*
Sandra K. Elshaug, *Financial Aid Administrator*
Eugene DeLorme, *Director, INMED Program*

ADDRESS INQUIRIES TO:

Secretary, Committee on Admissions
University of North Dakota
School of Medicine and Health Sciences
501 North Columbia Road, Box 9037
Grand Forks, North Dakota 58202-9037
(701) 777-4221; 777-4942 (FAX)
E-mail: jdheit@medicine.nodak.edu
Web site: www.medicine.nodak.edu/admissions.html

MISSION STATEMENT

The mission of the University of North Dakota School of Medicine and Health Sciences is to educate and prepare physicians, medical scientists, and other health professionals for service to North Dakota and the nation, and to advance medical and biomedical knowledge through research.

GENERAL INFORMATION

The School of Medicine was established in 1905 as a basic science school offering the first two years of medical education. In 1973, legislative action created an expanded curriculum and in 1981, the legislature approved a full four-year medical school program within the state of North Dakota. The School of Medicine is university-based but utilizes community physicians, clinics, and hospitals for the clinical education.

CURRICULUM

The School of Medicine emphasizes the training of primary care physicians. The first-year and second-year years are spent at the University of North Dakota (UND) in Grand Forks. Beginning with the 1998-99 academic year, the school initiated a new curriculum, utilizing a "patient-centered learning" (PCL) approach. The number of traditional lecture hours is reduced significantly and greater emphasis is placed on small-group teaching and learning, active student participation, and early clinical experience. The curriculum is integrated across disciplines and consists of four 10-week blocks of instruction during each of the first and second years. Students are assigned to either the Bismarck, Fargo or Grand Forks campuses for the third year and the Minot campus is added as a fourth site for the senior year. A student also may participate in the ROME (Rural Opportunities in Medical Education) program during the third year, completing seven months of clinical experience in a rural community. Comprehensive and continuing assessment of student learning is stressed throughout the four years of medical education.

The School of Medicine offers accredited undergraduate degrees in the allied health fields of clinical laboratory science, cytotechnology, and sports medicine. Graduate degrees in anatomy and cell biology, biochemistry and molecular biology, microbiology and immunology, clinical laboratory science, occupational therapy, physician assistant, physical therapy, physiology, and pharmacology also are offered. Information on these programs may be obtained from the UND undergraduate and graduate catalogs.

A student, additionally, may apply for a combined M.D.-Ph.D. program once accepted for admission to the School of Medicine.

The school utilizes a grading system of honors, satisfactory, or unsatisfactory.

REQUIREMENTS FOR ENTRANCE

The MCAT and the equivalent of three academic years or a minimum of 90 semester hours from an approved college are required for admission. Preference is given to applicants who will have completed an undergraduate degree and who are broadly educated in the sciences and the humanities.

Coursework must include the following:

Sem. hrs.

General Biology or Zoology (with lab) 8
Inorganic and Qualitative Chemistry (with lab) 8
Organic Chemistry* (with lab). 8
General Physics (with lab) 8
College Algebra 3
Psychology or Sociology 3
English Composition and Literature. 6

*A semester or quarter of biochemistry may be substituted for the final semester/quarter of organic chemistry.

It also is highly recommended that students be computer literate.

SELECTION FACTORS

A student should have maintained a GPA of 3.0 or better (A=4.0) to be considered for admission. Selection is based upon the scholastic record, letters of recommendation, MCAT scores, and a personal interview. Interviews are conducted only at the medical school.

In addition to high academic achievement, selection is based on a number of factors, including the demonstration of such qualities as motivation and commitment to a medical career, empathy, compassion in interpersonal relationships, problem solving, and the ability to work well in small groups.

Qualified North Dakota residents are given preference in admission. Almost all accepted students in recent classes have been residents of North Dakota. The only exceptions for non-North Dakota residents include a limited number of Minnesota residents or admission through either the Indians into Medicine (INMED) Program or through WICHE participation. Only persons who are U.S. citizens or legal permanent residents of the United States are eligible for consideration for admission.

The School of Medicine participates in the Professional Students Exchange Program administered by WICHE, under which legal residents of western states without a medical school may receive preference in admission. Certified WICHE students pay resident tuition. To be certified as eligible for this program, students must write to the WICHE certifying officer in their state of legal residence for the program application form. The number of students to be supported in each state in the field of medicine depends upon state appropriations. Addresses of state certifying officers are available from the Office of Student Affairs at the UND School of Medicine and Health Sciences or from WICHE.

The School of Medicine and Health Sciences does not utilize AMCAS. Once applications are received, they are ranked based on a combination of state residency, grade-point average, and MCAT scores. The top ranking candidates are automatically invited to interview. The records of all other candidates are reviewed by the Admissions Committee. A majority vote is required to issue an invitation to interview. The School of Medicine is unable to accept transfer students from other medical schools.

The fall 2003 entering class had the following profile: *GPA mean*: overall undergraduate, 3.71; science, 3.65. *The mean MCAT scores were as follows*: VR-8.6; PS-8.4; BS-9.0. The MCAT writing score was O. *Gender*, 54 percent female; students from groups underrepresented in medicine, 6 students (9.9 percent).

It is the policy of the University of North Dakota that there shall be no discrimination against persons because of race, religion, age, creed, color, sex, disability, sexual orientation, national origin, marital status, veterans' status, or political belief or affiliation, and that equal opportunity and access to facilities be available to all.

FINANCIAL AID

The financial resources of applicants are not considered in the selection process. Immediately after acceptance into the School of Medicine, the applicant is sent all available financial aid information and may make application for financial aid.

The awarding of financial aid is based on documented need. Loans and a limited number of scholarships and prizes are available. Some awards and scholarships are based on scholarship as well as need. Approximately 85 percent of the students receive some form of financial aid. Students are discouraged from working. The financial aid office may be reached at (701) 777-2849.

INFORMATION ABOUT DIVERSITY PROGRAMS

The INMED Program is a recruitment and retention program for American Indian students. It is a federally funded program that provides educational opportunities for fully qualified members of U.S. recognized tribes. State residency is not a consideration for admission through the INMED Program.

Institution Type: *Public*

APPLICATION AND ACCEPTANCE POLICIES FOR 2005–2006 FIRST-YEAR CLASS

Earliest date: July 1, 2004
Latest date: Nov. 1, 2004
School application fee to all applicants: $50
Oldest MCAT scores considered: August 2001
Does not have Early Decision Program
Acceptance notice to regular applicants
  Earliest date: January 10, 2005
  Latest date: Until class is filled
Applicant's response to acceptance offer
  Maximum time: 4 weeks
Requests for deferred entrance considered: Yes
Deposit to hold place in class (applied to tuition):
  $100, due with response to acceptance offer
Deposit refundable prior to: May 16, 2004
Estimated number of new entrants: 62
Starting date: Aug. 2005

TUITION AND STUDENT FEES PER YEAR FOR 2003–2004 FIRST-YEAR CLASS

Tuition   Student fees: $1,040
  Resident: $15,343
  Nonresident: $40,963

INFORMATION ON 2003–2004 FIRST-YEAR CLASS

Number of	In-State	Out-of-State	Total
Applicants	145	104	249
Applicants Interviewed	99	47	146
New Entrants*	47	14	61

*All took the MCAT and had baccalaureate degrees.

CHAPTER
11

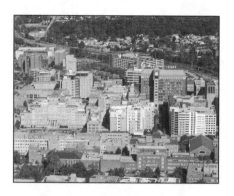

Case Western Reserve University School of Medicine

Cleveland, Ohio

Dr. Ralph I. Horwitz, *Dean, School of Medicine and Vice President for Medical Affairs*
Dr. Albert C. Kirby, *Associate Dean for Admissions and Student Affairs*
Wanda L. Rollins, *Director, Financial Aid*
Joseph T. Williams, *Director of Minority Programs*

ADDRESS INQUIRIES TO:

Associate Dean for Admissions and Student Affairs
Case Western Reserve University
School of Medicine
10900 Euclid Avenue
Cleveland, Ohio 44106-4920
(216) 368-3450; 368-6011 (FAX)
Web site: http://mediswww.cwru.edu

MISSION STATEMENT

The mission of the Case Western Reserve University School of Medicine is to advance the health of humankind through three interrelated components: Education. Research. Service.

CURRICULUM

CWRU School of Medicine offers two programs leading to the M.D. degree — the 4-year University program based primarily at the main University campus during the first two years, and the 5-year Cleveland Clinic Lerner College of Medicine program (the College program) based primarily at The Cleveland Clinic. The goal of the University program is to provide a broad education, preparing students to pursue the full array of medical careers including primary care, research, and specialization. The goal of the College program is to educate a limited number of students who wish to become physician investigators; the College curriculum will include education and practical experience in basic, translational and clinical research integrated throughout the 5-year continuum and a research thesis will be required for graduation. 145 students are admitted to the University program each year; among these up to 15 students are admitted to the Medical Scientist Training Program (MSTP) to pursue a combined M.D.-Ph.D. 32 additional students will be admitted to the College program each year. Applications to the University program, the College program, and the Medical Scientist Training Program are initiated through the AMCAS process by applying to Case Western Reserve University School of Medicine.

Basic science teaching in both programs is organ-system based, with integrated teaching by multidisciplinary faculty teams. In the University program, the basic science courses are lecture-based, supported by an extensive electronic curriculum and supplemented by case-oriented problem solving and laboratories. In the College program, research and basic science courses will use a problem-based learning approach emphasizing small group tutorials and self-directed learning supplemented by laboratories and interactive seminars. The University program features an extensive electives program (the Flexible Program) in all four years, pre-clinical years and clinical, with an opportunity to focus on a specific area of concentration or to sample widely, including taking graduate courses at CWRU. The first two years of the College program are structured with in-depth exposures to research in the summers and ample time for independent study in which some students may pursue additional research or graduate coursework leading to a master's degree. The Office of International Health provides opportunities for students to study outside the United States, typically in the fourth year of the University program or years 3 to 5 of the College program.

Both programs introduce clinical education early in the first year; in the University program, each student is responsible for a patient in the family care clinic, while in the College program each student will have a weekly continuity experience with a faculty preceptor. Required core clerkships include family medicine, internal medicine, neurosciences, obstetrics-gynecology, pediatrics, psychiatry and surgery in both programs. In the University program, most core clerkships are taken during the third year and the fourth year is available for electives. In the College program, the curriculum for the last 3 years will be unique for each student, based on his/her research project, clinical interest, and other individual educational goals, and will be developed in consultation with the student's M.D and research advisors.

In addition to the MSTP program, which offers a Ph.D. in all the basic science departments in the School of Medicine, joint degree programs are offered with the Schools of Law, Management, and Engineering. An M.D.-Ph.D. is available in Health Services Research. Several special Master's programs are offered including Applied Anatomy, Biomedical Ethics, and Public Health. Students interested in these degrees must apply independently to those schools or programs and the School of Medicine and satisfy the admissions requirements of both.

REQUIREMENTS FOR ENTRANCE

Only three years of college are required, but in practice, few students without the baccalaureate degree have ever been admitted. All candidates are expected to take the MCAT. The quality of work done is much more important than the field in which the student has majored. Specific requirements are minimal and include:

Biology: A one-year course in modern biology that emphasizes biochemical and quantitative concepts. Courses in anatomy, botany, ecology, and taxonomy will not fulfill this requirement.

Chemistry: Two years of chemistry including organic. Courses with an organic/biological chemistry content are acceptable. A biological chemistry course is required for the College program.

Physics: A one-year course in introductory physics.

Demonstration of writing skills: This can be met by a course in freshman expository writing; however, other courses with significant writing content are acceptable.

SELECTION FACTORS

The Admissions Committee selects students without regard to age, national origin, race, religion, sex, or sexual orientation. With respect to disability, technical standards for admission are available upon request. The School of Medicine deliberately seeks a diverse student body. Over 20 states of residence and 70 to 80 undergraduate colleges are represented in a typical entering class.

While the Committee does not rely on grades and MCAT scores alone in the selection process, all students have demonstrated exceptional academic strength. Completed secondary applications are reviewed with great attention given to the candidate's written statements and letters of recommendation in the decision to invite an applicant for an interview.

Some characteristics of the 2002 class entering the University program include: 49 percent *women*; 12 percent *students from groups underrepresented in medicine*; 60 percent legal residents of Ohio; undergraduate major, 65 percent in the sciences. The *average GPA* was 3.6 and the *average MCAT* was 10.6.

CWRU School of Medicine rarely accepts transfer students and then only from LCME-accredited schools and when the transfer will alleviate an extreme hardship situation. Students wishing to transfer must submit their requests in writing.

FINANCIAL AID

Financial aid is based on demonstrated need of the student. All applicants for aid must submit data for an analysis of need by NEED ACCESS. This requires complete disclosure of resources available to the student from all sources. Students are also required to submit income and asset information from parents. Approximately 75 percent of the students receive financial aid. Applications for financial aid are sent to accepted students in January, with awards being made by May 15. Because of the earlier matriculation date for the College program, financial aid awards will be made by April 1 for that program. Funds from the University are limited; consequently students have to rely on other sources of support including the Stafford Student Loan Program and alternative loan programs. Aid available from CWRU is a combination of loan and scholarship with the proportion of each being dependent upon total need.

Up to 21 merit scholarships can be awarded each year to students in the University program displaying outstanding personal and academic achievement. The Cleveland Clinic Lerner College of Medicine program will provide separate merit and needs-based scholarships and stipends for research.

INFORMATION ABOUT DIVERSITY PROGRAMS

The Office of Minority Programs and the Office of Student Services offer a wide variety of academic and personal support programs for all students from groups underrepresented in medicine. These include special speakers, mentoring with faculty, a tutoring program, and counseling.

Two summer programs are sponsored for college students interested in careers in medicine. The Health Career Enhancement Program is a rigorous six-week enrichment program for highly motivated and capable students. Review of the sciences and MCAT preparation are major components. Part of the program includes medical apprenticeships with working physicians. A research program is also available for students from groups underrepresented in medicine interested in careers in biomedical research.

There is an active Student National Medical Association chapter, which sponsors many activities including tutoring and community projects. The Latino Organization of Medical Students is especially interested in health care in Cleveland's Latino community.

More information, including applications for the summer program, may be obtained from the Office of Minority Programs at the address at the top of this entry or call (216) 368-2212.

Institution Type: *Private*
Application Process: *AMCAS, see chapter 4.*

APPLICATION AND ACCEPTANCE POLICIES FOR 2005–2006 FIRST-YEAR CLASS

Filing of AMCAS application
    Earliest date: June 1, 2004
    Latest date: Nov. 1, 2004
School application fee to all applicants: $85
Oldest MCAT scores considered: 2001
Does not have Early Decision Program (EDP)
Acceptance notice to regular applicants
    Earliest date: Oct. 15, 2004
    Latest date: Until class is filled
Applicant's response to acceptance offer
    Maximum time: 4 weeks
Requests for deferred entrance considered: Yes
Deposit to hold place in class: None
Estimated number of new entrants: 177
Starting date: July-August 2005

TUITION AND STUDENT FEES PER YEAR FOR 2003–2004 FIRST-YEAR CLASS

Tuition: $36,500   Student fees: $1,404

INFORMATION ON 2003–2004 FIRST-YEAR CLASS

Number of	In-State	Out-of-State	Total
Applicants	771	3,733	4,504
Applicants Interviewed	317	464	781
New Entrants*	74	72	146

*All had baccalaureate degrees; 97% took the MCAT.

CHAPTER

11

Medical College of Ohio

Toledo, Ohio

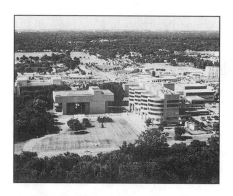

Dr. Amira F. Gohara, *Executive Vice President and Provost*
  Dean, School of Medicine
Dr. Mary Ann Myers, *Associate Dean for Admissions*
Dr. Robert A. Burns, *Assistant Dean for Admissions*
Dr. Barry L. Richardson, *Assistant Vice President of Multicultural Affairs*

ADDRESS INQUIRIES TO:

Admissions Office
School of Medicine
Medical College of Ohio
3045 Arlington Avenue
Toledo, Ohio 43614
(419) 383-4229; 383-4005 (FAX)
Web site: www.mco.edu

MISSION STATEMENT

The mission of the Medical College of Ohio shall be the creation and maintenance of an academic environment that attracts the most highly qualified students and faculty and fosters the pursuit of excellence in health education, research and service.

GENERAL INFORMATION

The Medical College of Ohio graduated its first students in June 1972. The academic medical center is located on 475 acres in a residential/commercial area of south Toledo. The center has almost 400 faculty members and 1,100 volunteer faculty members. The faculty is dedicated to establishing a learning atmosphere through balanced teaching, research, and patient care.

The Medical College of Ohio has five endowed chairs and conducts biomedical research in many areas, including genetics of hypertension, autoregulation of blood pressure, genetics of carcinogenesis, mechanism of fungi formation, role of immunophilius in steroid action carcinogenesis, and environmental microbiology.

In this medical school setting, the entering student is considered a graduate scholar by faculty members at all levels of seniority. The Medical College of Ohio seeks students who can grow intellectually and personally in this academic atmosphere.

CURRICULUM

The curriculum of the Medical College of Ohio is composed of an integrated basic science/clinical science four-year approach to medical education with emphasis on clinically

oriented objectives and problem-based learning. The first year is devoted to integrated blocks of cellular and molecular biology, growth and development, human structure and neuroscience, and behavioral science. Each of these sections will have a corresponding integrated clinical applied component. Also included will be Introduction to Primary Care (IPC), which runs concurrently throughout the first two years. The basic and clinical sciences are more intently brought together by the Pathophysiology course, which acts as a conduit between the basic sciences and the IPC experience.

The second year is composed of immunity and infection, an integrated systems course involving pathology, pharmacology, and physiology. Each section will have an appropriate integrated clinical component. There is continuation of IPC and pathophysiology. During the first two years, approximately 45 percent of the student's time will be spent in a non-lecture format with emphasis placed on small-group interaction. Students will be required to pass Step 1 of the USMLE before beginning their third year, and pass Step 2 prior to graduation.

The last two years of the curriculum are devoted to mandatory clerkships in internal medicine, surgery, pediatrics, obstetrics and gynecology, psychiatry, and family practice; neurology; and electives. All students are required to rotate through a clinical Area Health Education Center (AHEC) comprising 10 percent of their total clerkship time. Most components of the curriculum are evaluated on an honors, high pass, pass, fail system. The Medical College of Ohio also has an M.D.-Ph.D. and M.D.-M.S. program. Additionally, there is a five-year curriculum for disadvantaged students.

During the clinical phase, each student is exposed to one or two months of internal medicine in generalist settings. One of these months is spent in an area health education center so that the student will see health care delivery in a rural setting. Additionally there is a four week exposure to family medicine.

Our third- and fourth-year students are also offered a separate two-year clinical track at the Henry Ford Health System, which is designed to attract those students with a long term interest in the practice of primary care medicine in a managed care environment. This is a competitive program, and 10 students are selected for this unique educational opportunity.

The Medical College of Ohio School of Medicine offers a substantial amount of required generalist physician educational experiences and a wide variety of electives to enhance experiences in the specialist areas, which provide our students with a well-rounded basic medical education.

REQUIREMENTS FOR ENTRANCE

The MCAT is required unless the student is accepted through the MEDStart program. A baccalaureate degree is required.

Students must plan their educational sequence with due appreciation for the biologically oriented, psychologically sensitive task that they are undertaking for their life's work. The minimal premedical course requirements are:

	Years
Biology	1
Inorganic Chemistry	1
Organic Chemistry	1
Physics	1
College Mathematics	1
College English	1

Additional upper-level biology courses are recommended. A comprehensive command and understanding of the English language are essential.

Beyond these requirements, concentration in humanities, sciences, or other areas is viewed with equal favor. Close attention will be paid to the general scope of the applicant's academic background and to whether or not there is an adequate general understanding of the physical, biological, chemical, and social sciences and some reasonable sensitivity to the humanities.

SELECTION FACTORS

In selecting applicants, the Medical College of Ohio looks more for evidence of general competence and capability than for specific areas of study. Students are admitted on the basis of individual qualifications, regardless of sex, religion, race, age, or handicap.

Students in the 2002 entering class had the following credentials: *mean science GPA,* 3.5; *mean total GPA,* 3.6; *mean MCAT scores,* VR-9.5, PS-9.6, BS-10; *sex,* 43 percent women; *students from groups underrepresented in medicine,* 4 percent; *undergraduate major,* 88 percent in science. Interviews are by invitation only. Reapplicants are not penalized. Preference is given to Ohio residents.

FINANCIAL AID

Financial aid is awarded on the basis of demonstrated financial need according to federal methodology. Applicants for financial aid must file the FAFSA. Several scholarships are available on a competitive basis. These scholarships are funded by the Office of the Dean, the MCO Foundation, and the Associated Physicians of MCO. Approximately 50 students are employed during the academic year in the Federal Work-Study Program. Summer employment opportunities also exist with the Summer Research Program, the Community Health Project, and the Preceptorships in Family Practice Program.

INFORMATION ABOUT DIVERSITY PROGRAMS

The Medical College of Ohio is committed to increasing opportunities for individuals from traditionally underrepresented groups, as well as those from economically disadvantaged backgrounds. The Office of Multicultural Affairs works in cooperation with the Admissions Committee, the Office of Student Affairs, and all other campus departments in the recruitment, selection, and retention of qualified students. For more information write, Dr. Barry Richardson, assistant vice president for multicultural affairs.

Institution Type: *Public*
Application Process: *AMCAS, see chapter 4.*

APPLICATION AND ACCEPTANCE POLICIES FOR 2005–2006 FIRST-YEAR CLASS

Filing of AMCAS application
  Earliest date: June 1, 2004
  Latest date: Dec. 1, 2004
School application fee after screening: $50
Oldest MCAT scores considered: 2002
Does have Early Decision Program (EDP)
  For Ohio residents only
  EDP application period: June 1–Aug. 1, 2004
  EDP applicants notified by: Oct. 1, 2004
Acceptance notice to regular applicants
  Earliest date: Oct. 15, 2004
  Latest date: Until class is filled
Applicant's response to acceptance offer
  Maximum time: 2 weeks
Requests for deferred entrance considered: Yes
Deposit to hold place in class: None
Estimated number of new entrants: 135 (10 EDP)
Starting date: Aug. 2005

TUITION AND STUDENT FEES PER YEAR FOR 2003–2004 FIRST-YEAR CLASS

Tuition   Student fees: $4,289
  Resident: $16,800
  Nonresident: $36,500

INFORMATION ON 2003–2004 FIRST-YEAR CLASS

Number of	In-State	Out-of-State	Total
Applicants	873	1,568	2,441
Applicants Interviewed	273	164	437
New Entrants*	117	39	156

*All had baccalaureate degrees; 86% took the MCAT.

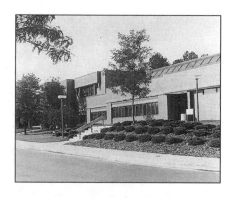

Northeastern Ohio Universities College of Medicine

Rootstown, Ohio

Dr. Lois Margaret Nora, *President and Dean*
Dr. R. Stephen Manuel, *Director of Admissions*
Yvonne Mathis, *Director of Diversity Affairs*

ADDRESS INQUIRIES TO:

Office of Admissions
Northeastern Ohio Universities
College of Medicine
P.O. Box 95
Rootstown, Ohio 44272-0095
(330) 325-6270; 325-8372 (FAX); 1(800) 686-2511
E-mail: admission@neoucom.edu
Web site: www.neoucom.edu
E-mail: admission@neoucom.edu

MISSION STATEMENT

The mission of the Northeastern Ohio Universities College of Medicine (NEOUCOM) is to graduate qualified physicians oriented to the practice of medicine at the community level, with an emphasis on primary care: family medicine, internal medicine, pediatrics, and obstetrics/gynecology.

GENERAL INFORMATION

NEOUCOM is a state medical school consisting of a basic medical sciences campus in Rootstown, a consortium of three major public universities and 17 community hospitals with more than 6,500 teaching beds in the greater Akron, Canton, and Youngstown areas. The faculty numbers more than 1,800.

CURRICULUM

NEOUCOM offers a combined B.S.-M.D. degree curriculum for honors-level high school graduates who have not begun college study and, supplementarily, a four-year program leading to the M.D. degree. NEOUCOM also conducts an Advanced Standing admission program for students seeking transfer from U.S. and/or foreign medical schools.

B.S.-M.D. degree students spend their first two or three years at either The University of Akron, Kent State University or Youngstown State University studying the sciences, mathematics and humanities while in the process of completing the required courses for the baccalaureate degree.

NEOUCOM's education of physicians is oriented to the practice of medicine at the community level. The first year medical student concentrates on the basic medical sciences during the nine months spent on the Rootstown campus. The curriculum and educational activities for the second year correlate body system learning and concentrate on basic pathophysiologic processes and mechanisms underlying clinical signs and symptoms of disease. During the first and second years, part of the teaching is done at the ambulatory care teaching centers of the major associated teaching hospitals. In the Ambulatory Care Experience course in the M1 and M2 years, students are exposed to the ways in which various health and human service professionals provide medical, nursing, social service, educational and biopsychological care for people in manifold settings. Students continue their clinical education through the core clerkships (internal medicine, surgery, pediatrics, psychiatry, obstetrics-gynecology and family medicine) during the third year at hospitals on the Akron, Canton or Youngstown clinical campuses. There is an expanding problem-based learning (PBL) program across the first three years of the curriculum, both as a stand-alone course and within core clerkships. In three of the core clerkships (internal medicine, Ob/Gyn and psychiatry), M3 students work with standardized patients in NEOUCOM's Center for Studies of Clinical Performance and get an objective measure of their clinical skills. The fourth medical school year includes electives and specially designed selectives in the medical humanities as well as a community medicine clerkship and a primary care preceptorship. All students are required to pass Step 1 and Step 2 Clinical Knowledge and Clinical Skills of the USMLE.

REQUIREMENTS FOR ENTRANCE

Admission to the combined B.S./M.D. degree program is restricted to students who have taken no college coursework following high school graduation. Applicants should take the full science-oriented college preparatory sequence which their high school offers. The American College Test (ACT) or Scholastic Aptitude Test (SAT) must be taken, the early action deadline is October 1st, and the regular application deadline is December 15 of the year preceding anticipated entrance. Applications may be requested after August 1. Each year 105 students are chosen for the B.S./M.D. degree program.

Persons who have completed the equivalent of at least three years of undergraduate study may be admitted to the M.D. degree program. These applicants are required to have completed at least one year each of university-level organic chemistry and physics. All students seeking direct entry into the M.D. degree program are required to take the MCAT no later than the fall prior to the year of anticipated enrollment. The number of spaces available for M.D. degree program candidates varies with the amount of attrition from Year 2 or Year 3 of the B.S.-M.D. degree program. If an applicant (for the 4-year M.D. program) possessing the equivalent of three years of study shows unusual promise, is considered and subsequently accepted, NEOUCOM requires the student to complete the baccalaureate degree before the M.D. degree will be granted.

SELECTION FACTORS

Applicants must demonstrate strong academic preparation as measured by GPAs and entrance examination scores. In addition, they must show appropriate personal characteristics and motivation for the practice of medicine. Selection interviews are by invitation only.

Admissions preference is given to Ohio residents. Typically, no more than 10 percent of students are non-Ohio residents.

While all applicants are considered and no formulas are used for the selection process, applicants who are sent supplementary applications are generally competitive, have 3.25 overall GPA's, a 3.10 BCPM, MCAT scores of 8 and higher, and who have taken the required coursework. Only those who complete supplementary applications are given full consideration by the Admissions Committee. Early submission of application materials is strongly encouraged, particularly through the Early Decision Program if the applicant is competitive.

The Northeastern Ohio Universities College of Medicine (NEOUCOM) is an equal opportunity/affirmative action educator and employer.

NEOUCOM is committed to preparing students for the practice of medicine in a multicultural environment by increasing the diversity of the student body, faculty and staff and by enhancing policies, procedures and practices that support a collaborative environment.

FINANCIAL AID

Campus-based financial aid is awarded on the basis of demonstrated need. In general, students apply for this aid by completing the FAFSA application (see Part 1) and the NEOUCOM financial aid application, and by submitting copies of federal income tax forms and financial aid transcripts. The awards are made through the Student Aid and Awards Committee after a thorough analysis of the student's financial situation.

Long-term federal educational loans are a major part of the aid program. A limited number of need-based scholarships are available, as well as other limited scholarship funds for disadvantaged and/or medical students from groups underrepresented in medicine. About 80 percent of enrolled students receive some form of financial aid. Financial need is not a factor in admissions considerations.

INFORMATION ABOUT DIVERSITY PROGRAMS

It is one of the goals of the Admissions Committee to seek out, recruit and support qualified nontraditional applicants (members of groups underrepresented in medicine and disadvantaged rural students). Students interested in further information should contact the admissions office or the Diversity and Multicultural Affairs Office.

Institution Type: *Public*
Application Process: *AMCAS, see chapter 4.*

APPLICATION AND ACCEPTANCE POLICIES FOR 2005–2006 FIRST-YEAR CLASS

Filing of AMCAS application
    Earliest date: June 1, 2004
    Latest date: Nov. 1, 2004
School application fee after screening: $30
Oldest MCAT scores considered: 2002
Does have Early Decision Program (EDP)
    EDP application period: June 1–Aug. 1, 2004
    EDP applicants notified by: Oct. 1, 2004
Acceptance notice to regular applicants
    Earliest date: Oct. 15, 2004
    Latest date: Until class is filled
Applicant's response to acceptance offer
    Maximum time: 2 weeks
Requests for deferred entrance considered: No
Deposit to hold place in class: None
Estimated number of new entrants: 25 (5 EDP)
Starting date: Aug. 2005

TUITION AND STUDENT FEES PER YEAR FOR 2003–2004 FIRST-YEAR CLASS

Tuition   Student fees: $738
    Resident: $18,255
    Nonresident: $36,510

INFORMATION ON 2003–2004 FIRST-YEAR CLASS

Number of	In-State	Out-of-State	Total
Applicants	521	346	867
Applicants Interviewed	104	8	112
New Entrants*	33	4	37

NOTE: Figures do not include combined B.S.-M.D. degree program students.

*All took the MCAT and had baccalaureate degrees.
** Data not available.

CHAPTER

11

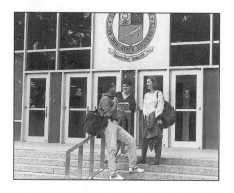

Ohio State University
College of Medicine and Public Health

Columbus, Ohio

Dr. Fred Sanfilippo, *Vice President of Health Sciences and Dean,*
College of Medicine and Public Health
Dr. Mark Notestine, *Assistant Dean, Admissions*
Dr. William Lush, *Financial Aid Director*
Dr. Leon McDougle, *Assistant Dean, Minority Affairs*

ADDRESS INQUIRIES TO:

Admissions Committee
The Ohio State University
College of Medicine and Public Health
209 Meiling Hall
370 West Ninth Avenue
Columbus, Ohio 43210-1238
(614) 292-7137; 247-7959 (FAX)
E-mail: medicine@osu.edu
Web site: http://medicine.osu.edu

MISSION STATEMENT

It is the mission of the College to achieve distinction in education, scholarship and public service; to educate skilled professionals in the basic and clinical medical sciences, public health and allied medical professions; to create, evaluate and disseminate knowledge and technology; and, to provide innovative solutions for improving the health of our people.

GENERAL INFORMATION

Established in 1914, The Ohio State University College of Medicine blends traditional medical education, innovative learning opportunities, and a strong reputation in the preparation of students for primary care and specialized residencies. As part of one of the largest public universities in the country, the College of Medicine provides an environment that encourages the research interests of students. Strong emphasis is placed on medical humanities and a biopsychosocial approach to patient care.

The College of Medicine is on the south edge of the main university campus, located in metropolitan Columbus. Medical center facilities include university hospitals, the Arthur G. James Cancer Hospital and Richard J. Solove Research Institute, the Dorothy M. Davis Heart and Lung Research Institute, and a network of outpatient facilities and affiliated small-town and rural hospitals and clinics. In addition, students can spend part of their clinical clerkships in other hospitals in Columbus and throughout the state.

CURRICULUM

Following an intensive initial 12-week course in anatomy, there are two different pre-clinical tracks for the first two years: the Integrated Pathway; and an Independent Study Pathway. Choice of curricula allows students to self-select into

the method of learning that works best for them, a special option that attracts top students from around the nation.

The Integrated Pathway features body systems-oriented content that fuses the basic and clinical sciences. It combines the proven educational methods of student-centered active learning, small group case-based discussion, and lectures.

In the Independent Study Pathway (ISP) students use highly structured objectives, resource guides, and Web and computer-based materials to read, review, and learn on their own. They proceed through the curriculum at their own pace within certain time limits. Faculty are available to coach students through difficult concepts and materials. It is possible to complete the ISP program over a three-year period, an option that may interest non-traditional students with family obligations.

Students enter into the clinical setting beginning in the first year with Patient Centered Medicine and Physician Development, spending time with a community health organization and learning how to evaluate patients. This is a gradual process and increases as history taking, interviewing, physical exam, and psycho-social skills mature. These courses take place during the pre-clinical years, combining small group role-playing settings, lectures, and experiences with senior citizens and physicians in the community. This lays the building blocks of how to do a thorough patient interview.

Ohio State's Standardized Patient Program allows students to build clinical proficiency in a low-pressure setting that includes patient actors.

The third year includes foundation clerkships in family medicine, general internal medicine, internal medicine, obstetrics and gynecology, pediatrics, psychiatry, neurology, and surgery. The fourth-year requirements include the Differentiation of Care Selectives. The selectives are a series of four clerkships, each of which focuses on the care of patients at various stages of illness and wellness: the undifferentiated patient; the patient with chronic care needs; subinternship in internal medicine, and a sub-internship in surgical care. With the exception of the subinternship, all required clerkships include ambulatory experiences, with some done entirely in outpatient settings. Students have great flexibility in the fourth year, with four months of elective rotations and three months of vacation.

A common thread through all experiences is physician educators in Columbus and around Ohio who mentor, support and prepare College of Medicine students. Ohio State has funded a state-of-the-art Clinical Skills facility that will be used year-round by students and medical residents. This center provides opportunities to learn and to measure ability to gather information, perform physical examinations, practice common procedures, and effectively communicate with patients.

Many opportunities exist at Ohio State to explore research interests through fellowships, scholarships, basic science, clinical and translational research symposia.

The M.D.-Ph.D. Medical Scientist program, M.D.-M.B.A., M.D.-M.P.H., M.D.-M.H.A. and M.D.-J.D. programs are also available.

REQUIREMENTS FOR ENTRANCE

The MCAT and a bachelor's degree or certified eligibility for a degree in absentia are required. No specific undergraduate curriculum or major is required or preferred. A medical school candidate should follow an undergraduate program that is as broad and comprehensive as possible in order to prepare best for a career in a people-oriented profession in a changing society. Candidates are urged to take advantage of the undergraduate opportunity to study history, art, literature, creative writing, philosophy, social sciences, and communication skills.

The minimum course requirements are:

	Years
Biology	1
Inorganic Chemistry (with lab)	1
Organic Chemistry (with lab)	1
General Physics	1

SELECTION FACTORS

First consideration is given to applicants whose academic record and MCAT scores predict a high degree of academic accomplishment in medical school.

Successful candidates have had the following general profile of characteristics: *mean GPA,* 3.65; *mean MCAT* composite of 31.

Applicants who have returned completed secondary applications are carefully reviewed by the Admissions Committee. All completed applications are given thorough review to be certain that excellent candidates who do not fit the general profile are not overlooked.

In addition to strong academic performance, factors that lend significant weight in further consideration are clinical and shadowing experiences, community service and leadership activities, research experience, academic recommendations, and personal information in the application itself. Nonacademic accomplishments and evidence of suitability for the study of medicine are carefully considered.

FINANCIAL AID

The Ohio State University College of Medicine and Public Health values the ability to offer need-based financial aid assistance for its students. Every year, students are given the opportunity to participate in various scholarship and low-interest loan programs. All accepted candidates are mailed financial aid materials prior to entering to be considered with students already in school. Financial need is not a deterrent to acceptance. Every effort is made to assist each student with securing sufficient resources for continuing their education.

INFORMATION FOR DISADVANTAGED STUDENTS

Students whose previous educational and economic deprivation warrant special consideration are carefully evaluated and are offered special help in the acquisition of additional resources. Special programs, such as the MedPath Medical Careers Pathway, are provided to enhance students' educational development.

The Medpath Medical Careers Pathway is a postbaccalaureate program aimed at developing the academic knowledge-base and skills of students enhancing their preparation for medical school.

Institution Type: *Public*
Application Process: *AMCAS, see chapter 4.*

APPLICATION AND ACCEPTANCE POLICIES FOR 2005–2006 FIRST-YEAR CLASS

Filing of AMCAS application
    Earliest date: June 1, 2004
    Latest date: Dec. 15, 2004
School application fee after screening:
    $60 domestic, $70 international
Oldest MCAT scores considered: 2002
Does have Early Decision Program (EDP)
    EDP application period: June 1–Aug. 1, 2004
    EDP applicants notified by: Oct. 1, 2004
Acceptance notice to regular applicants
    Earliest date: Oct. 15, 2004
    Latest date: Varies
Applicant's response to acceptance offer
    Maximum time: 2 weeks
Requests for deferred entrance considered: Yes
Deposit to hold place in class: None
Estimated number of new entrants: 210 (10 EDP)
Starting date: Aug. 2005

TUITION AND STUDENT FEES PER YEAR FOR 2003–2004 FIRST-YEAR CLASS

Tuition   Student fees: $396
    Resident: $18,927
    Nonresident: $43,485

INFORMATION ON 2003–2004 FIRST-YEAR CLASS

Number of	In-State	Out-of-State	Total
Applicants	1,001	2,275	3,276
Applicants Interviewed	368	315	683
New Entrants*	130	80	210

*All took the MCAT and had baccalaureate degrees.

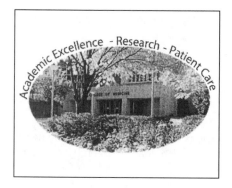

University of Cincinnati College of Medicine

Cincinnati, Ohio

Dr. William J. Martin II, *Dean*
Dr. Laura Wexler, *Associate Dean for Student Affairs/Admissions*
Clarice P. Fooks, *Assistant Dean for Admissions*
Dr. Daniel Burr, *Director of Financial Aid*

ADDRESS INQUIRIES TO:

Office of Student Affairs/Admissions
University of Cincinnati
College of Medicine
P.O. Box 670552
Cincinnati, Ohio 45267-0552
(513) 558-7314; 558-1165 (FAX)
Web site: www.med.uc.edu/

MISSION STATEMENT

The University of Cincinnati College of Medicine envisions medical education as an integrated, systematic, and student-centered learning process. As graduates, each student will possess an excellent conceptual knowledge base, critical lifelong learning and thinking skills, outstanding interpersonal and clinical abilities, and an understanding of and commitment to the physician's role and responsibility in society.

GENERAL INFORMATION

The College of Medicine provides both outstanding research facilities and superb clinical and teaching experiences. Graduates, ranked highly competitive by national residency program directors, choose careers in a broad range of specialty areas. Approximately 47 percent of the 2003 graduating class chose residency programs in family medicine, internal medicine, obstetrics/gynecology, or pediatrics.

Research opportunities for students are extensive. Nationally, the College of Medicine is ranked in the top 26 percent among all public medical schools in National Institutes of Health research funding.

CURRICULUM

The focus of the first year is on the normal structure, function, and development of the human body using an integrated systems approach to basic and clinical science topics. It includes an introduction to doctor/patient relationships, interviewing skills and physical diagnosis skills. The second year continues the integrated systems approach focusing on the disease processes, prevention, and the further development of physical diagnosis skills.

Third-year clerkships include 8-week rotations each in internal medicine, obstetrics-gynecology, pediatrics, and surgery; a 6-week rotation in psychiatry; a 4-week rotation in family medicine, a 2-week rotation in radiology; and 4 weeks of selectives.

The fourth-year requirements include an 8-week acting internship in internal medicine, a 4-week clinical neuroscience selective; and 24 weeks of electives. Portions of the elective time may be taken at other U.S. medical centers or abroad. The Department of Family Medicine maintains an extensive network of clinical opportunities all over the world. Students are encouraged to participate.

Evaluation of students is by an honors, high pass, pass, remediate, and fail grading system. Students are required to take and pass Step 1 and Step 2 of the USMLE examinations. All students are required to pass Step 1 prior to promotion into Year 3.

A state-of-the-art Center for Competency Development and Assessment is utilized for formative and summative evaluation including a required Clinical Competency Exam (CCX).

SUMMER PREMATRICULATION PROGRAM

A Summer Prematriculation Program (SPP) is offered to any accepted student. The program provides exposure to actual first year lectures, labs, course-related discussion groups, and tests. There are also sessions on study strategies, test taking skills, stress management, and leadership skills.

REQUIREMENTS FOR ENTRANCE

Applicants must complete a minimum of 90 semester hours at a U.S. accredited, four-year, degree-granting institution of higher education. Students who have attended an undergraduate college outside of the United States should have a graduate degree or a minimum of 20 hours of science coursework from a U.S. college or university.

Students currently in a professional school or a degree-granting graduate program must complete all degree requirements and show documentation of graduation or completion of requirements *prior to matriculation*.

A baccalaureate degree is encouraged but not required. MCAT scores received within the past three years are required.

All majors are valued. Students are expected to engage in a rigorous academic program that enables them to understand the basic principles of the sciences fundamental to medicine and to appreciate the psychosocial nature of man. *All* applicants are expected to have the knowledge usually obtained in one-year courses in biology, general and organic chemistry, physics, and mathematics. In addition, the undergraduate program should provide an understanding of the basic social, cultural, and behavioral factors that influence individuals, families, and communities. Regardless of the area of concentration, the applicant should have acquired effective learning, communication, and problem-solving skills. A knowledge of the basic principles of statistics and computer literacy are strongly recommended.

As a state-supported university, priority will be given to Ohio residents.

All applicants must meet the College of Medicine Admissions and Graduation Standards (technical standards) with or without reasonable accommodations.

SELECTION FACTORS

In addition to the AMCAS application, the University of Cincinnati asks all perspective students to complete an on line supplementary form. Applicants are directed to our Web site to complete this secondary process. Once the secondary application and letters of recommendation are received, the applicant will be evaluated for an interview. In addition to the online application, the Web site provides information about the progress of each applicant in the admissions process.

The interview day program is designed to present a brief description of the college and student services. It will include: one interview; presentations on the admissions process, the curriculum, and student services; lunch, and a tour.

Notification of final decisions will be made on or near the 15th of each month. Prior to January, acceptances may be sent on a weekly basis.

Offers of acceptance are based upon the overall evaluation of academic and personal qualities. Postbaccalaureate and graduate coursework will be considered. Personal characteristics include demonstrated motivation, maturity, coping skills, interpersonal skills, sensitivity and tolerance toward others, communication and critical-thinking skills. Students are admitted on the basis of individual qualifications, regardless of age, sex, sexual orientation, race, color, national origin, or physical or mental disabilities. Please view our Web site (✍ www.med.uc.edu) for current application status.

FINANCIAL AID

The college provides students with information about options for funding a medical education and counseling to help them make sound financial decisions. Over 85 percent of enrolled students receive some type of financial assistance. A financial aid packet is mailed to accepted applicants in February. Students who wish to be considered for need-based funds administered by the college must submit the Need Access application.

The current level of indebtedness for graduates is below the national mean for public medical schools. For further information, please contact the Financial Aid Office at (513) 558-6797.

INFORMATION FOR MINORITY AND NONTRADITIONAL STUDENTS

The College of Medicine is pleased to announce a new Office of Cultural Diversity. Two Associate Deans will work to ensure that the University of Cincinnati will include both students and faculty from diverse backgrounds, and that the curriculum will prepare all students to meet the needs of a diverse patient population upon graduation.

PHYSICIAN SCIENTIST TRAINING PROGRAM

The Physician Scientist Training Program (PSTP) of the College is a rigorous and prestigious integrated program that leads to the M.D.-Ph.D. combined degree. PSTP students are provided full financial support, including stipend ($20,000 in 2003), tuition and health insurance. For more detailed information, visit the PSTP Web site at ✍ www.med.uc.edu/pstp.

Institution Type: *Public*
Application Process: *AMCAS, see chapter 4.*

APPLICATION AND ACCEPTANCE POLICIES FOR 2005–2006 FIRST-YEAR CLASS

Filing of AMCAS application
  Earliest date: June 1, 2004
  Latest date: Dec. 15, 2004
School application fee to all applicants: $25
Oldest MCAT scores considered: 2002
Does have Early Decision Program (EDP)
  EDP application period: June 1–Aug. 1, 2004
  EDP applicants notified by: Oct. 1, 2004
Acceptance notice to regular applicants
  Earliest date: Oct. 15, 2004
  Latest date: Until class is filled
Applicant's response to acceptance offer
  Maximum time: 2 weeks
Requests for deferred entrance considered: Yes
Deposit to hold place in class: None
Estimated number of new entrants: 160
Starting date: Aug. 2005

TUITION AND STUDENT FEES PER YEAR FOR 2003–2004 FIRST-YEAR CLASS

Tuition   Student fees: $2,157
  Resident: $18,630
  Nonresident: $33,159

INFORMATION ON 2003–2004 FIRST-YEAR CLASS

Number of	In-State	Out-of-State	Total
Applicants	833	1,393	2,226
Applicants Interviewed	390	244	634
New Entrants*	122	39	161

*All took the MCAT and had baccalaureate degrees.

CHAPTER

11

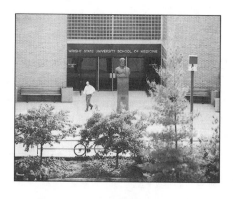

Wright State University School of Medicine

Dayton, Ohio

Dr. Howard Part, *Dean*
Dr. Paul G. Carlson, *Associate Dean for Student Affairs/Admissions*
Dr. Gwen Sloas, *Director of Financial Aid*
Dr. Alonzo Patterson III, *Assistant Dean for Minority Affairs*

ADDRESS INQUIRIES TO:

Office of Student Affairs/Admissions
Wright State University
School of Medicine
P.O. Box 1751
Dayton, Ohio 45401-1751
(937) 775-2934; 775-3322 (FAX)
E-mail: som_saa@desire.wright.edu
Web site: www.med.wright.edu/

MISSION STATEMENT

The mission of the school is to provide for the general professional education of students with an emphasis on primary care preparation in an environment that advances medical knowledge and is responsive to lifelong learning, research, and the community we serve. These goals and objectives are achieved through an educational program with the following core components:

- opportunities to learn in clinical settings beginning in the first quarter;
- integration of basic and clinical science knowledge throughout a four-year curriculum;
- instruction in community-based, in-patient, and out patient settings;
- utilization of diverse learning strategies and training methods;
- interaction with faculty in an atmosphere that fosters teamwork, camaraderie, and collegiality; and
- diversity in the student body and patient population, reflecting many ethnic, racial, social, age, lifestyle, and gender differences.

GENERAL INFORMATION

The Wright State University School of Medicine was established in 1973 and enrolled its first class of students in 1976. It is located on the university campus in Fairborn, a suburb of Dayton. Clinical facilities associated with the medical school include six major teaching hospitals with over 3,500 patient beds. These hospitals emphasize and provide experience with modern scientific technology. A faculty of over 1,000 provides students with the opportunity for individualized attention. The school has a strong interest in preparing students for careers in primary care as family practitioners, general internists, and

general pediatricians. The educational program emphasizes early patient exposure, humanistic and compassionate care, outpatient experiences, health promotion and disease prevention, the provision of care to underserved populations, and cultural diversity.

CURRICULUM

The primary goal of the educational program is to educate students to provide comprehensive care to patients and their families. During the first two years, students are taught in an interdisciplinary fashion using large-group lectures, small-group discussions, computer-based instruction, and case-based/problem-based learning. The curriculum introduces students to normal structure and functioning in an integrated fashion. Instruction progresses through various organizational levels from molecular to organ. The basic principles and mechanisms of disease are taught in the first year.

Throughout the first two years, the curriculum integrates the behavioral sciences, humanities, wellness, and disease prevention. Regular didactic instruction by clinical faculty is provided. Students are taught medical history taking and physical examination skills and evaluation of patients' concerns, and they are provided with an understanding of catastrophic illnesses. Students meet regularly with preceptors to develop clinical skills. To provide additional opportunities for clinical expo-sure and enrichment, clinically based electives are offered as immersion experiences between academic periods in the first two years.

In the third year, students are exposed to the basic disciplines of medicine through six clerkship rotations. Primary care clerkships are offered as part of a block rotation to coordinate instruction among the three disciplines. The fourth year includes clerkship rotations, time for board study, and junior internships, and students may choose from over 140 elective offerings.

REQUIREMENTS FOR ENTRANCE

The MCAT and three years (90 semester hours or 135 quarter hours) of collegiate preparation in an approved college or university in the United States or Canada are required. Applicants must be U.S. citizens or possess a permanent resident visa. Applicants are expected to present the equivalent of the usual premedical preparation. Coursework must include:

	Years
Biology	1
Chemistry	2
Must include Organic Chemistry.	
Physics	1
College Mathematics	1
English	1

Courses in calculus and biochemistry are strongly recommended. The Admissions Committee is interested in students with broad education in the humanities, and the biological and social sciences. Each applicant's credentials for admission will be individually reviewed and evaluated. The MCAT should be taken in the spring of the year in which the application is filed and no more than three years prior to making application. Only those MCAT scores available at the time of review will be considered by the Admissions Committee.

A minimum MCAT score or GPA is not required by the Admissions Committee.

SELECTION FACTORS

It is the philosophy of the School of Medicine to seek a student body of diverse social, ethnic, and educational backgrounds. Women, students from groups underrepresented in medicine, and applicants from rural Ohio are particularly encouraged to apply. However, applicants are admitted solely on the basis of individual qualifications without regard to race, religion, gender, sexual orientation, disability, veteran status, national origin, age, or ancestry. Dedication to human concerns, compassion, intellectual capacity, and personal maturity in the applicant are of greater importance to the Admissions Committee than specific areas of preprofessional preparation. The Admissions Committee, which is broadly based, also seeks positive evidence of motivation, altruism, selflessness, and human empathy in the prospective medical student. The committee carefully reviews the completed application, the academic record, MCAT performance, letters of recommendation, and the results of a personal interview (by invitation only) in making its final selection. Ohio residents are given preference, but some nonresidents are accepted.

Upon receipt of the AMCAS application, all applicants will be invited to submit a supplementary application and letters of evaluation. After review of all submitted material, applicants are selected for interviews.

FINANCIAL AID

Financial aid in the form of scholarships, grants, loans, and various work opportunities is available to assist students in financial need. The Office of Student Affairs/Admissions offers financial counseling services and assists students in obtaining needed support. An emergency loan fund for students in good academic standing is also available through this office. The financial status of applicants has no effect whatever on their acceptance to the School of Medicine.

INFORMATION ABOUT DIVERSITY PROGRAMS

The Wright State University School of Medicine and its faculty have a stated policy of providing educational opportunities to disadvantaged applicants and applicants from groups underrepresented in medicine. The school is in the top 15 percent of the U.S. medical schools in the enrollment of students from such groups. Special support services that meet the needs of students from groups underrepresented in medicine include a prematriculation program, a mentoring program in which students are paired with physicians in the community, a big brother/big sister program, tutoring, board preparation courses, and assistance in development of skills in critical thinking and learning. The admissions process gives careful consideration to all applicants. Both resident and nonresident students from groups underrepresented in medicine are strongly encouraged to apply.

Institution Type: *Public*
Application Process: *AMCAS, see chapter 4.*

APPLICATION AND ACCEPTANCE POLICIES FOR 2005–2006 FIRST-YEAR CLASS

Filing of AMCAS application
  Earliest date: June 1, 2004
  Latest date: Nov. 15, 2004
School application fee to all applicants: $45
Oldest MCAT scores considered: 2001
Does have Early Decision Program (EDP)
  EDP is for residents of Ohio only.
  EDP application period: June 1–Aug. 1, 2004
  EDP applicants notified by: Oct. 1, 2004
Acceptance notice to regular applicants
  Earliest date: Oct. 15, 2004
  Latest date: Until class is filled
Applicant's response to acceptance offer
  Maximum time: 2 weeks
Requests for deferred entrance considered: Yes
Deposit to hold place in class: None
Estimated number of new entrants: 90 (5 EDP)
Starting date: Aug. 2005

TUITION AND STUDENT FEES PER YEAR FOR 2003–2004 FIRST-YEAR CLASS

Tuition	Student fees: $930
Resident: $16,602	
Nonresident: $23,496	

INFORMATION ON 2003–2004 FIRST-YEAR CLASS

Number of	*In-State*	*Out-of-State*	*Total*
Applicants	886	1,888	2,774
Applicants Interviewed	343	66	409
New Entrants†	80	11	91

† All took the MCAT and had baccalaureate degrees.

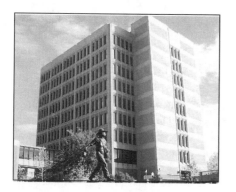

University of Oklahoma College of Medicine

Oklahoma City, Oklahoma

Dr. Nancy K. Hall, *Associate Dean for Academic Affairs*
Dotty Shaw Killam, *Director of Admissions*
Anthony Spano, *Director of Financial Aid*
Rennie Cook, *Executive Director for ITSC Student Affairs*

ADDRESS INQUIRIES TO:

Dotty Shaw Killam
University of Oklahoma
College of Medicine
P.O. Box 26901
Oklahoma City, Oklahoma 73190
(405) 271-2331; 271-3032 (FAX)
E-mail: Dotty-Shaw@ouhsc.edu
Web site: www.medicine.ouhsc.edu

MISSION STATEMENT

The mission of the University of Oklahoma is to provide the best possible educational experience for our students through excellence in teaching, research and creative activity, and service to the state and society.

New structures, new facilities, and new technology—plus an internationally prominent faculty—will undoubtedly make the University of Oklahoma Health Sciences Center and the O.U. College of Medicine one of the next century's regional leaders in education, research, and patient care. OUHSC is ideally positioned to meet the demands of a rapidly changing health care system and to provide a model environment for medical education.

GENERAL INFORMATION

The University of Oklahoma College of Medicine offers students a quality education with added advantages. Access to modern patient care facilities and an aggressive research program are provided at a reasonable cost with a proven record of choice residency placement.

Students gain experience in a variety of settings. The college is part of a modern health sciences complex that serves as the state's principal education and research facility for physicians, dentists, nurses, biomedical scientists, pharmacists, public health administrators, and a wide range of allied health professionals.

Seven colleges—medicine, dentistry, nursing, pharmacy, public health, allied health, and the graduate college—educate more than 3,000 graduate and undergraduate students through programs offering degrees at several levels from baccalaureate through doctorate. The College of Medicine offers programs in Oklahoma City and Tulsa. The Health Sciences Center in Oklahoma City is part of a 200-acre complex of 28 public and private institutions known as the Oklahoma Health Center.

CURRICULUM

The four-year curriculum consists of two years of study in the basic sciences and two in the clinical sciences. Letter grades are awarded for all coursework on a course-hour basis rather than a credit-hour basis. The first two years are complemented by a Web-based on-line curriculum. All students are required to have a computer.

There are 17 required courses in the basic science portion of the curriculum. They account for 1,677 hours of instruction or 33 percent of the total. First-year courses provide a strong basic science foundation, and second-year classes form a bridge leading directly into the clinical portion of the curriculum. A significant feature of this portion of the curriculum is early exposure to patients through the continuum courses: Principles of Clinical Medicine I and II. The bioethical and legal issues in medicine courses are also offered.

The clinical program provides training at two sites. "The Tulsa Option" offers third- and fourth-year students the opportunity to complete their clinical training in the setting of a community-based educational program. Approximately 25 percent of the class will complete their education in several community hospitals in the Tulsa area. The clinical curriculum consists of 3,440 hours of instruction representing 67 percent of the total curriculum. A unique feature of the fourth year is a required rural preceptorship experience under the guidance of a physician in an Oklahoma community of less than 10,000 people.

Dual-degree programs are offered by the College of Medicine with full funding in place for the M.D./Ph.D. program.

REQUIREMENTS FOR ENTRANCE

The MCAT is required and should be taken the year in which the application is filed. Applicants who have completed only 90 semester hours of college work may be considered; however, the college discourages such applications except from students who have demonstrated personal and intellectual maturity.

The following courses are required:

Semesters

General Zoology or General Biology
(with lab) 1

Cell Biology, Embryology, Histology, Genetics,
  or Comparative Vertebrate Anatomy. 1
Inorganic (General) Chemistry. 2
Organic Chemistry. 2
General Physics 2
English 3
Psychology, sociology, anthropology,
  philosophy, humanities, or foreign
  language (any combination). 3

Additional coursework in the social sciences is suggested.

Pass/fail grading, Advanced Placement, and CLEP courses are accepted. It is required that higher courses be taken for a grade.

No particular major is given preference; however, applicants must provide evidence of their capability of understanding and utilizing scientific methods.

The University of Oklahoma has an October 15 deadline for applications to be submitted to AMCAS. A request for supplemental information is sent upon notification from AMCAS of a candidate's interest. The supplemental information consists of a filing fee, a premedical advisory committee letter of recommendation, plus an additional faculty recommendation, or three faculty letters. Applicants must have a complete file by November 1.

SELECTION FACTORS

Acceptance into the College of Medicine is based on GPA, MCAT scores, letters of evaluation from faculty and premedical committees, and personal interviews conducted on campus by members of the Admissions Board. Emphasis is placed on self-awareness, self-discipline, empathy, personal competence, social competence, and an over-all evaluation of character. Non-residents can represent up to 15% of the student body.

In the 2003 entering class there were 55 *women*, the *mean GPA* of the class was 3.68, and the *MCAT average* was 9.27.

The University of Oklahoma College of Medicine does not discriminate on the basis of race, sex, creed, national origin, age, or handicap.

FINANCIAL AID

The College of Medicine offers a number of financial assistance opportunities in addition to the federally sponsored programs. The most prominent scholarships are the Regents' Scholarship Fee Waiver, the Oklahoma Rural Medical Education Loan Scholarship Fund designed for residents wishing to practice in rural communities, and the Oklahoma Tuition Aid Grant. The loan funds established by the Shepherd Foundation, Inc., and the Lew Wentz Foundation, along with over 20 other scholarships, also aid many students annually. Additional support for students from groups underrepresented in medicine is available through the State Regents for Higher Education, the Ungerman Trust, and the Belknap, Culpeper, Maurer, and Reid-Winnie scholarships.

About 94 percent of all students receive some form of assistance through the Office of Financial Aid.

In a need or merit-based application process, the College of Medicine awards approximately $350,000.00 in scholarships to over 150 medical students.

INFORMATION ABOUT DIVERSITY PROGRAMS

The University of Oklahoma has a strong commitment to identify, recruit, and educate qualified students from groups underrepresented in medicine. Applications are strongly encouraged from these groups as well as from any candidate with a disadvantaged background.

Institution Type: *Public*
Application Process: *AMCAS, see chapter 4.*

APPLICATION AND ACCEPTANCE POLICIES FOR 2005–2006 FIRST-YEAR CLASS

Filing of AMCAS application
  Earliest date: June 1, 2004
  Latest date: Oct. 15, 2004
School application fee to all applicants: $50
Oldest MCAT scores considered: 2001
Does not have Early Decision Program (EDP)
Acceptance notice to regular applicants
  Earliest date: Dec. 1, 2004
  Latest date: Until class is filled
Applicant's response to acceptance offer
  Maximum time: 2 weeks
Requests for deferred entrance considered: No
Deposit to hold place in class (applied to tuition):
  $100, due with response to acceptance offer
Deposit refundable prior to: May 16, 2005
Estimated number of new entrants: 150
Starting date: Aug. 2005

TUITION AND STUDENT FEES PER YEAR FOR 2003–2004 FIRST-YEAR CLASS

Tuition   Student fees: $1,902
  Resident: $13,234
  Nonresident: $33,611

INFORMATION ON 2003–2004 FIRST-YEAR CLASS

Number of	In-State	Out-of-State	Total
Applicants	309	539	848
Applicants Interviewed	210	32	242
New Entrants*	135	7	142

*All took the MCAT; 95% had baccalaureate degrees.

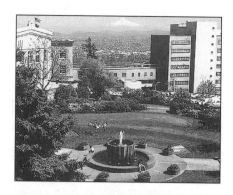

Oregon Health & Science University School of Medicine

Portland, Oregon

Dr. Joseph E. Robertson, Jr., *Dean*
Dr. Stephanie Anderson, *Assistant Dean for Minority Affairs*
Dr. Cynthia Morris, *Assistant Dean for Admissions*
Debbie Melton, *Director of Admissions*

ADDRESS INQUIRIES TO:

Oregon Health & Science University
Office of Education and Student Affairs, L102
3181 S.W. Sam Jackson Park Road
Portland, Oregon 97239-3098
(503) 494-2998; 494-3400 (FAX)
Web site: www.ohsu.edu/som/dean/md

MISSION STATEMENT

A fundamental priority throughout Oregon Health & Science University (OHSU) is to enable each student to fulfill his or her potential as a human being and as a health care professional. It is the mission of the School of Medicine to enhance human health through programs of excellence in education, research, health care and public service. In achieving these goals, the OHSU School of Medicine challenges students to strive for academic excellence and fosters the development of compassion, humanism and professionalism in the care of patients from their first days in the classroom to their final rotation in the hospitals and clinics.

GENERAL INFORMATION

The University of Oregon Medical School was established by charter from the Board of Regents of the University of Oregon in 1887. The name was changed in November 1974 when the School of Medicine and the Schools of Nursing and Dentistry reorganized as the University of Oregon Health Sciences Center, subsequently the Oregon Health Sciences University. In 2001, it was renamed Oregon Health & Science University (OHSU) with the addition of the School of Science and Engineering. OHSU occupies a 101-acre site and 31 buildings in Sam Jackson Park overlooking the city of Portland, but within one and a half miles of the business center. Campus physical facilities include basic science, research and laboratory buildings; two hospital units with a licensed capacity of 509 beds; an outpatient clinic; Child Development and Rehabilitation Center; hearing and speech center; library and auditorium, and a student activities building. The School of Medicine is affiliated with the 563-bed Veterans Affairs Medical Center and Shriner's Hospital for Crippled Children located on the campus.

The School of Medicine provides educational programs for medical students, graduate students in basic medical sciences, interns, residents and faculty as well as programs for physician assistants, radiological technologists, medical technologists and dietitians. An extensive postgraduate program exists.

CURRICULUM

The first two years of the integrated curriculum are primarily devoted to the sciences basic to medicine, focusing initially on the normal structure and function of the human body and continuing with the study of the pathophysiological basis of disease and its treatment. An early clinical experience is afforded through the Principles of Clinical Medicine course, which is presented concurrently during the first and second years to develop fundamental clinical knowledge and skills in patient interviewing, physical diagnosis and reinforcement of these skills through a continuity clinical preceptorship experience. The socioeconomic, behavioral and population health issues are also introduced during this period. Core clinical clerkship experiences constituting the third and fourth years of the curriculum are undertaken at OHSU Hospital and Clinics as well as at affiliated hospitals in the Portland area. During the clinical phase of the curriculum, a six-week community-based primary care experience is provided in a medically underserved region of the state and opportunities are available to pursue elective courses in clinical and basic sciences in order to individualize and enhance the educational experience.

The MD/PhD combined degree program in the School of Medicine at OHSU provides an opportunity for students to experience the rewards of research and graduate study, while at the same time pursuing a medical education. PhD degrees may be obtained in a variety of basic science disciplines. This combined degree program is designed for superior students with a strong basic science background. Prior research experience is essential. Full funding is provided for up to four students per year.

The MD/MPH combined degree program is administered jointly by the School of Medicine and the Department of Public Health & Preventive Medicine and is a component of the Oregon MPH Program. It is specifically designed for students who demonstrate the potential for a career in public health policy or research. The MPH program at OHSU emphasizes training in epidemiology and biostatistics.

REQUIREMENTS FOR ENTRANCE

All applicants must meet the requirements listed below: A Bachelor of Arts or Bachelor of Science degree, or its equivalent, from an accredited college or university is required prior to matriculation in medical school. No particular major is preferred, but a broad educational background is encouraged.

The following are the minimum acceptable college-level courses for admission:

Biology—One academic year of general biology to include one genetics course. Laboratories are recommended.

Chemistry—One course each of general chemistry, organic chemistry and biochemistry. Laboratories are recommended. (Since undergraduate curricula vary from school to school, in fulfilling this requirement it is implied that the required prerequisite sequences in general and organic chemistry will have been completed in order to take the biochemistry course.)

Physics—One academic year of general physics. Laboratories are recommended.

Mathematics—One mathematics course (not including statistics). A course in statistics is strongly recommended.

Humanities, Social Sciences and English—Two academic years of humanities and/or social sciences to include one course in English composition (or equivalent writing emphasis).

(Note: One academic year is equivalent to two semesters or three academic quarters.)

An eligible MCAT is required. For the 2005 cycle, eligible MCAT scores are those recorded in 2002, 2003 or 2004.

All applicants must have United States citizenship or resident alien status with a current green card indicating they are a permanent resident of the United States.

SELECTION FACTORS

The Admissions Committee seeks students who have demonstrated academic excellence and who have demonstrated readiness for the profession of medicine. Applicants are selected on the basis of demonstration of motivation for medicine, humanistic attitudes, and a realistic understanding of the role of the physician in health care. The ideal student will demonstrate evidence of strong communication skills; altruism, empathy, personal integrity; self-appraisal and emotional maturity; and an ability to make a positive contribution to society and the profession. Attention is paid to achievements that demonstrate applicants' breadth of interests, commitment to others, and leadership among their peers. Evaluation of applicants includes the academic record as demonstration of scholarship; the MCAT; recommendations from undergraduate or graduate school faculty and employers; experiences in health care settings and in other volunteer commitments; and the personal interview.

The Admissions Committee embraces diversity in the student body and adheres to a policy of equal opportunity in considering applicants without regard to sex, age, race, ethnic origin, religion, or sexual orientation. Preference is given to residents of Oregon, members of underrepresented ethnic/racial groups, WICHE-certified residents of Montana and Wyoming, MD/PhD and MD/MPH candidates, and nonresident applicants with superior achievements in academics and related experiences. The entering class of 2003 graduated from 66 different undergraduate schools. Characteristics of the entering class include: 63% women, 8% students from groups underrepresented in medicine and 51% residents of Oregon. The mean GPA was 3.65 and the mean MCAT composite score was 31.

FINANCIAL AID

Financial aid in the form of scholarships, grants, and loans is available based upon the demonstrated need of the student. Consideration of financial status has no bearing upon the admissions process. About 92% of the student body receives some type of financial assistance. For more information please review the Web site at www.ohsu.edu/finaid/.

INFORMATION ABOUT DIVERSITY PROGRAMS

The School of Medicine Admissions Committee fully recognizes the importance of diversity in the physician workforce in providing for the health of the public. Accordingly, the OHSU School of Medicine strongly encourages applications from persons from all socioeconomic, racial, ethnic, religious, and educational backgrounds. More information may be obtained by contacting the office of Dr. Stephanie Anderson, Assistant Dean for Minority Affairs at (503) 494-1608.

Institution Type: *Public*
Application Process: *AMCAS, see chapter 4.*

APPLICATION AND ACCEPTANCE POLICIES FOR 2005–2006 FIRST-YEAR CLASS

Filing of AMCAS application
  Earliest date: June 1, 2004
  Latest date: Oct. 15, 2004
School application fee after preliminary screening: $75
Oldest MCAT scores considered: 2002
Does not have Early Decision Program
Acceptance notice to regular applicants
  Earliest date: Oct. 15, 2004
  Latest date: Until class is filled
Applicant's response to acceptance offer
  Maximum time: 2 weeks
Requests for deferred entrance considered: No
Deposit to hold place in class: None
Estimated number of new entrants: 108
Starting date: August 2005

TUITION AND STUDENT FEES PER YEAR FOR 2003–2004 FIRST-YEAR CLASS

Tuition   Student fees: $3,462
  Resident: $21,000
  Nonresident: $31,500

INFORMATION ON 2003–2004 FIRST-YEAR CLASS

Number of	In-State	Out-of-State	Total
Applicants	316	2,424	2,740
Applicants Interviewed	178	290	468
New Entrants*	55	52	107

*All took the MCAT and had baccalaureate degrees.

CHAPTER

11

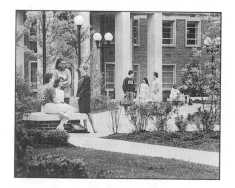

Drexel University College of Medicine
(Formerly MCP Hahnemann University School of Medicine)

Philadelphia, Pennsylvania

Dr. Stephen Klasko, *Dean*
Dr. Allan R. Tunkel, *Associate Dean for Admissions*
Cynthia A. DeLone, *Associate Director for Student Financial Aid*
Dr. Emily Pollard, *Associate Dean for Minority Affairs*

ADDRESS INQUIRIES TO:

Admissions Office
Drexel University College of Medicine
2900 Queen Lane
Philadelphia, Pennsylvania 19129
(215) 991-8202; 843-1766 (FAX)
E-mail: medadmis@drexel.edu
Web site: www.drexel.edu/med/

MISSION STATEMENT

At Drexel University College of Medicine, we are committed to providing our students with the finest possible medical education. Academic instruction in basic and clinical sciences, utilizing state-of-the-art technology, is enriched by an emphasis on compassionate patient care and community service.

GENERAL INFORMATION

The Medical College of Pennsylvania (MCP) was founded in 1850 as the first medical school in the nation for women. Coeducational since 1969, the college continues to live up to its rich history, actively seeking students with diverse backgrounds and experiences. Hahnemann University, a private nondenominational institution, was founded in 1848. These two institutions have come together as part of Drexel University College of Medicine, melding their rich histories and many resources to provide diversity, strength, and excellence in medical education. The medical school has a supportive environment that fosters a spirit of teamwork and personal interaction. It draws on its strengths as the academic medical anchor in a multihospital system.

Medical students have the opportunity for clinical training in the extensive, integrated network of hospitals of the Tenet system and at a large number of affiliated hospitals and clinics. In 1992 the School of Medicine opened a new education and research facility on a 15-acre site. This facility is the home of the first and second years of medical education.

CURRICULUM

The College of Medicine medical students are trained to consider each patient's case and needs in a comprehensive, integrated manner, taking into account many more factors than the presenting physiological condition. Because of this tradition, the school is dedicated to preparing "physician healers," doctors who practice the art, as well as the science and skill, of medicine.

Recognizing that different students have different ways of learning, Drexel University College of Medicine offers a choice between two innovative academic curricula for their first two years of study. Interdisciplinary Foundations of Medicine (IFM) integrates basic-science courses and presents them through clinical symptom-based modules. IFM is faculty-driven; students learn in lectures, labs, and small groups. The Program for Integrated Learning (PIL), a problem-based curriculum, is student-driven, supervised and facilitated by faculty. Students learn in small groups, labs, and resource sessions by focusing on case studies.

Both options focus on professional medical education, preparing students to pursue careers in either a generalist or a specialty discipline. Both stress problem solving, lifelong learning skills, and the coordinated training of basic science with clinical medicine. Both curricula also include the introduction of clinical skills training very early in the first year.

The basic clinical clerkships are offered in the third year and include experiences in all major disciplines of medical practice. The pathway program in the fourth year includes a balance of four week-long required and elective clinical experiences arranged by students with the pathway advisors to be consistent with general medical training and the student's ultimate career goals.

Drexel University College of Medicine has joint accelerated, early assurance and post-baccalaureate programs with several colleges and universities. Combined M.D.-M.P.H., M.D.-M.B.A., and M.D.-Ph.D. programs are available for qualified students.

REQUIREMENTS FOR ENTRANCE

The MCAT, a minimum of 90 semester hours from an accredited college and a baccalaureate degree are required. To expedite the processing of applications, the MCAT and the required coursework should be completed prior to the time of application.

The required courses are:

	Semesters
Chemistry (with lab)	2
Organic Chemistry (with lab)	2
Biology (with lab)	2

Physics (with lab) 2
English 2

Biochemistry should not be counted in this total but may be taken in addition. A course in molecular and cell biology is recommended.

SELECTION FACTORS

In accord with the historical commitment of this institution, applications from women, students brought up in small towns or rural areas, those who come from Pennsylvania, students interested in a career as a generalist physician, and those underrepresented in medicine are particularly encouraged.

Matriculated students had an average GPA of 3.44 and MCAT scores at or above the 75th percentile level. In addition to academic criteria, the interviews, which are conducted by a faculty member and a current student, are used in selecting our students.

Administrative regulations relative to the application of Public Law 93-380 (Family Educational Rights and Privacy Act) shall govern.

The medical school reserves the right to change, without notice, degree requirements, curriculum, courses, teaching personnel, rules, regulations, tuition, fees, and any other information published herein.

The medical school actively supports equality of educational opportunity. The school does not discriminate on the basis of race, color, national origin, gender, sexual preference, age, religion, creed, or handicap in admission or access to, or treatment or employment in, its programs or faculties activities. The compliance coordinator in the Office of Student Affairs is the senior associate dean.

All students must be able to meet the essential functions of the medical school. Applicants must be U.S. citizens or permanent residents.

STUDENT FINANCIAL AID

In addition to the Federal Stafford Student Loan Program, the Primary Care Loan Program, other federally funded aid programs, and assistance in obtaining money from foundation sources, the Office of University Student Financial Affairs has at its disposal limited private grant and loan funds. A College Work-Study Program for qualified students is also available. Money allocated by the school is awarded on the basis of financial need and merit. Information and applications are available from the Office of University Student Financial Affairs. Please review our Web site for more information: www.drexel.edu/med/medsfa.

INFORMATION ABOUT DIVERSITY PROGRAMS

Applications are actively encouraged from students from groups underrepresented in medicine and disadvantaged backgrounds.

Institution Type: *Private*
Application Process: *AMCAS, see chapter 4.*

APPLICATION AND ACCEPTANCE POLICIES FOR 2005–2006 FIRST-YEAR CLASS

Filing of AMCAS application
    Earliest date: June 1, 2004
    Latest date: Dec. 15, 2004
School application fee to all applicants: $75
Oldest MCAT scores considered: 2002
Does have Early Decision Program (EDP)
    EDP application period: June 1–Aug. 1, 2004
    EDP applicants notified by: Oct. 1, 2004
Acceptance notice to regular applicants
    Earliest date: Oct. 15, 2004
    Latest date: Until class is filled
Applicant's response to acceptance offer
    Maximum time: 6 weeks
Requests for deferred entrance considered: Yes
Deposit to hold place in class (applied to tuition):
    $100, due two weeks from acceptance offer
Deposit refundable prior to: May 16, 2005
Estimated number of new entrants: 250 (15 EDP)
Starting date: Aug. 2005

TUITION AND STUDENT FEES PER YEAR FOR 2003–2004 FIRST-YEAR CLASS

Tuition: $33,100   Student fees: $1,000

INFORMATION ON 2003–2004 FIRST-YEAR CLASS

Number of	In-State	Out-of-State	Total
Applicants	846	6,497	7,434
Applicants Interviewed	284	1,354	1,638
New Entrants*	71	179	250

*All took the MCAT; 98% had baccalaureate degrees.

CHAPTER
11

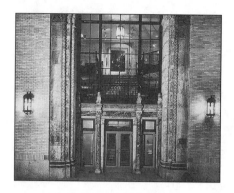

Jefferson Medical College of Thomas Jefferson University

Philadelphia, Pennsylvania

Dr. Thomas J. Nasca, *Senior Vice President and Dean*
Dr. Clara Callahan, *Vice Dean of Academic Affairs*
Susan Batchelor, *Director of Student Financial Aid*
Dr. Edward Christian, *Associate Dean for Diversity and Minority Affairs*

ADDRESS INQUIRIES TO:

Grace Hershman, Director of Admissions
Jefferson Medical College
of Thomas Jefferson University
1015 Walnut Street, Suite 110
Philadelphia, Pennsylvania 19107-5099
(215) 955-6983; (215) 955-5151 (FAX)
E-mail: jmc.admissions@jefferson.edu
Web site: www.jefferson.edu

MISSION STATEMENT

Jefferson's teaching mission centers on the education of outstanding individuals in the art and science of medicine. By helping these individuals to develop their medical knowledge, clinical and research skills, and professional values, attitudes and behaviors, we strive to provide outstanding physicians for the United States and, indeed, the world.

GENERAL INFORMATION

As one of the oldest institutions of higher education in the nation, Thomas Jefferson University has, since its founding as the Jefferson Medical College in 1824, emphasized the attainment of clinical excellence in its educational programs. A recent significant expansion of the research programs has created a better balanced institutional mission and has enhanced the clinical instruction at Thomas Jefferson University Hospital and 19 affiliated hospitals.

CURRICULUM

The curriculum at Jefferson Medical College has been developed to enable students to acquire basic knowledge and skills in the biomedical sciences as well as to develop appropriate professional behaviors. The curriculum also allows students to pursue some of their special interests throughout their medical training. The tradition of providing a clinically balanced medical education, encouraged by the faculty, is that students support, and cooperate with, each other.

During the first year, students focus on the function of the human organism in its physical and psychosocial context. Coursework includes human gross and microscopic anatomy, biochemistry and human genetics, neuroscience, and physiology. Other fundamental courses such as medical informatics, biostatistics and ethics are also introduced during the first year.

Clinical coursework focuses on the doctor-patient relationship, medical interviewing and history-taking, human development, behavioral science principles, and core clinical skills and reasoning. In addition to increasing emphasis on the study of clinical skills, the curriculum shifts in the second year to the study of pathophysioiogy and disease. Immunology, microbiology, pharmacology, pathology and clinical medicine are presented as an interdisciplinary curriculum. The curriculum includes small group sessions focusing on problem-solving, evidence-based medicine and service-based learning.

The clinical program consists of two 42-week phases. Phase I covers required clerkships, including family medicine, general surgery, internal medicine, pediatrics, psychiatry, and obstetrics and gynecology. Advanced basic science, rehabilitation medicine, the medical and surgical subspecialties and inpatient and outpatient subinternships in medicine or surgery are usually included in the second clinical phase.

Jefferson Medical College and the Pennsylvania State University select highly qualified high school seniors to earn both the B.S. and M.D. degrees in six or seven years. The Medical Scholars Program involving the University of Delaware and Jefferson Medical College allows highly qualified students a coordinated program of education for the baccalaureate and medical degrees. The Physician Shortage Area Program serves to recruit selected students who agree to practice family medicine in physician shortage areas (especially in rural communities of Pennsylvania). Residents of the state of Delaware are admitted to Jefferson Medical College through a program involving the Delaware Institute of Medical Education and Research. Jefferson offers a fully funded with stipend M.D./Ph.D. program for students interested in research and academic medicine, as well as an M.D./M.B.A. and M.D./M.H.A. program. An M.D./M.Ph. program is offered in cooperation with Johns Hopkins School of Public Health. Opportunities in basic science research and in clinical research are also available to students.

REQUIREMENTS FOR ENTRANCE

A baccalaureate degree from an accredited U.S. or Canadian college or university, a personal on-site interview (by invitation), and the MCAT are required. It is recommended that, regardless of major, each student acquire a baccalaureate education, which includes broad study in the natural and social sciences and in the humanities. The undergraduate program should include a strong preparation in the sciences and mathematics basic to medical school studies. Courses taken to meet the basic requirements should be rigorous and, in general, comparable to courses accepted for concentration in these disciplines.

Coursework must include:

	Years
General Biology (with lab)	1
Inorganic Chemistry (with lab)	1
Organic Chemistry (with lab)	1
General Physics (with lab)	1

In individual cases, specific requirements may be modified at the discretion of the admissions committee.

Students are encouraged to take additional upper-level science courses out of interest or to fulfill requirements of their major.

If Advanced Placement credits in required subjects are submitted, additional courses in similar subjects are encouraged.

All academic requirements must be completed prior to the date of matriculation.

Students are advised to take the MCAT in the spring prior to the year of application.

SELECTION FACTORS

Jefferson, in accordance with local, state, and federal law, is committed to providing equal educational and employment opportunities for all persons, without regard to race, color, national and ethnic origin, religion, sexual orientation, age, handicap, or veteran's status. Jefferson complies with all relevant ordinances and state and federal statutes in the administration of its educational and employment policies and is an affirmative action employer. The selection of students is made after careful consideration of many factors, including the college attended, the academic record, the letters of recommendation, the MCAT scores, and the interview results of the Committee on Admissions and their opinion of the applicant's personal qualities, motivation, interpersonal skills, and achievement in nonacademic areas. Jefferson Medical College traditionally has given special consideration to offspring of alumni and faculty, groups underrepresented in medicine, applicants to Jefferson's special programs and, in the past, residents of Pennsylvania. Foreign applicants must have a degree from an accredited U.S. or Canadian college or university.

The 229 members of the 2003 entering class came from 92 different undergraduate schools, 26 different states, and 4 foreign countries; United Kingdom, Canada, Nigeria, and United Arab Emirates. A profile of the matriculated students includes the following: *mean science GPA,* 3.51; *mean MCAT score,* 10.3; *sex,* 51 percent women; *mean age,* 22.8 (range 18–35) and 26 percent groups underrepresented in medicine.

Each year several applicants are accepted who display extraordinary personal qualities and promise in regard to medicine, even though they do not meet all of the criteria described above.

FINANCIAL AID

Financial aid awards are based on need determined by a confidential analysis of information that is provided by the student and the student's family to the designated needs analysis service. If need is established, the student is directed to obtain a federally subsidized Stafford loan. If need exists beyond this program, Jefferson will try to meet a portion of this need from loan and grant funds. Applications for financial aid are available after December 18 from the Office of Student Financial Aid. Completed financial aid applications for the next academic year must be submitted before April 1 or within two weeks of the date of acceptance. Eighty-four percent of the 2003 entering class received financial assistance.

INFORMATION ABOUT DIVERSITY PROGRAMS

Applications from qualified students from groups underrepresented in medicine are encouraged.

Institution Type: *Private*
Application Process: *AMCAS, see chapter 4.*

APPLICATION AND ACCEPTANCE POLICIES FOR 2005–2006 FIRST-YEAR CLASS

Filing of AMCAS application
    Earliest date: June 1, 2004
    Latest date: Nov. 15, 2004
School application fee to all applicants: $75
Oldest MCAT scores considered: 2001
Does have Early Decision Program (EDP)
    EDP application period: June 1–Aug. 1, 2004
    EDP applicants notified by: Oct. 1, 2004
Acceptance notice to regular applicants
    Earliest date: Oct. 15, 2004
    Latest date: Until class is filled
Applicant's response to acceptance offer
    Maximum time: 2 weeks
Requests for deferred entrance considered: Yes
Deposit to hold place in class (applied to tuition):
    $100, due by May 15, 2005
Deposit refundable prior to: May 16, 2005
Estimated number of new entrants: 228 (10 EDP)
Starting date: Aug. 2005

TUITION AND STUDENT FEES PER YEAR FOR 2003–2004 FIRST-YEAR CLASS

Tuition: $34,565   Student fees: None

INFORMATION ON 2003–2004 FIRST-YEAR CLASS

Number of	In-State	Out-of-State	Total
Applicants	960	6,539	7,499
Applicants Interviewed	204	540	744
New Entrants*	102	127	229

*100% took the MCAT; 93% had baccalaureate degrees; 8% were in the B.S.-M.D. program.

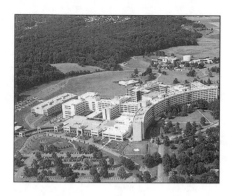

Pennsylvania State University College of Medicine

Hershey, Pennsylvania

Dr. Darrell G. Kirch, *Senior Vice President for Health Affairs,*
  Dean and Chief Executive Officer
Dr. Dwight Davis, *Associate Dean for Admissions and Student Affairs*
Marc Lubbers, *Assistant Director for Admissions*
Dr. Alphonse E. Leure-duPree, *Associate Dean for Academic Achievement*

ADDRESS INQUIRIES TO:

Office of Student Affairs
Pennsylvania State University
College of Medicine
500 University Drive H060
Hershey, Pennsylvania 17033
(717) 531-8755; 531-6225 (FAX)
E-mail: StudentAdmissions@hmc.psu.edu
Web site: www.hmc.psu.edu/md/

MISSION STATEMENT

The Pennsylvania State University College of Medicine is strongly committed to the education and training of medical students, basic science graduate students, medical residents, sub-specialty fellows, other students in health-related professions, and practicing health professionals.

We seek to enroll exceptional students from all regions of the United States and to provide them with an education based on present and future national health care needs. Students will be exposed to a medical environment of active basic science and clinical research where patient medical care is provided in a humanistic fashion.

Our objective is to provide a full range of patient care services, which extend from prevention of illness and maintenance of health through primary care to highly sophisticated tertiary care.

We strive to be a national leader in pursuing scientific investigation and developing programs to advance medical and scientific knowledge.

GENERAL INFORMATION

In 1963, the M.S. Hershey Foundation offered $50 million to the Pennsylvania State University to establish a medical school in Hershey. With this grant and $21.3 million from the U.S. Public Health Service, the University built a medical school, teaching hospital, and research center. Penn State's Milton S. Hershey Medical Center opened its doors to the first class of students in 1967 and became the first College of Medicine in the nation to establish a Department of Humanities, introducing humanistic disciplines into the required medical curriculum. It also was the first to start an independent Department of Family and Community Medicine. From its beginning, medical education and patient care have been guided by the institution's commitment to provide humane, compassionate, and expert care, emphasizing individual dignity.

The 550-acre medical campus is located in the rolling hills of southeastern Pennsylvania approximately eight miles from the state capital, Harrisburg, PA. The main facility houses the School of Medicine, the 504-bed University Hospital and Children's Hospital, the Rehabilitation Center, the Biomedical Research Building, and the Center for Emergency Medical Services. We also serve as the Level 1 Regional Resource Trauma Center with additional qualifications in pediatric trauma for South Central Pennsylvania.

The George T. Harrell Library is symbolically located in the center of the complex, housing 125,000 volumes, 1,800 periodicals, and the latest on-line research technology. The library also contains a computer learning center and individual student study carrels, and is open 24 hours each day.

Surrounding the main facility are the outpatient physicians center, a magnetic resonance imaging building, a heliport for LIFE LION-the University aeromedical service, an animal research farm, the Penn State Center for Sports Medicine, the University fitness center, student apartments, a child care center, and outdoor recreational facilities including a walk/jogging track, a baseball diamond, and a soccer field.

CURRICULUM

In recent years the practice of medicine has undergone major changes. Many of these changes are part of a transformation that will significantly alter the way health care is organized and delivered for many years in the future. Therefore, the curriculum is learner-centered and has been designed to prepare our students for the challenges of a restructured medical environment and for work in a more integrated health care system.

A single integrated curriculum for Years 1 and 2 has been developed, which combines elements of traditional medical teaching and case-based learning. The first-year curriculum and courses are interdisciplinary rather than departmental or discipline based, combining case-based, student-centered learning with strategic lectures, laboratories, and small-group discussions. A parallel course during Years 1 and 2 entitled Physicians, Patients, and Society provides students with a core background in the important areas of humanistic medicine, psychosocial aspects of illness, epidemiology, medical ethics, and the physician-patient relationship. The second-year curriculum is more heavily oriented to case-based learning in an organ-system approach to human health, pathophysiology, and disease.

Years 3 and 4 are considered a single academic unit with Year 3 having a sequence of required core clinical clerkships in internal medicine, general surgery, pediatrics, obstetrics and gynecology, psychiatry, family and community medicine, and primary care supplemented by two selectives. Year 4 consists of a minimum of four elective rotations and four required advanced experiences, including acting internships in a medical and a surgical discipline, a primary care area, and the humanities. The College of Medicine offers a wide variety of both clinical and research electives. Students may select outpatient clinical rotations at the teaching hospitals or in university-affiliated physician offices located in a variety of rural and metropolitan communities across Pennsylvania. In addition, there are many opportunities for clinical experiences in other regions of the country and abroad.

All students must complete a medical student research project and pass USMLE Steps 1 and 2 to earn the M.D. degree.

There is an honors, high pass, pass, and fail grading system in all four years.

REQUIREMENTS FOR ENTRANCE

The MCAT and the baccalaureate degree are required for admission.

The following subjects are considered by the Medical Student Selection Committee to be required:

Years

Biology (with lab) 1
General or Inorganic Chemistry (with lab). 1
Organic Chemistry (with lab). 1
Physics (with lab) 1
Mathematics 1
Humanities 1/2
Behavioral Science 1/2

Other recommended courses are calculus, statistics, psychology, sociology, radiobiology, genetics, and anthropology.

Students should be exposed to a broad background in the humanities and social sciences. Studies that develop verbal competence and enlarge perspectives and capacities for critical, historical, and moral judgments are especially encouraged.

Students are urged to take the MCAT in the spring of the year they expect to apply. Taking the MCAT in August will delay consideration of the application. It is recommended that basic science courses be completed before applying. All requirements must be met prior to matriculation.

SELECTION FACTORS

Applicants must show evidence of superior undergraduate achievement and outstanding personal characteristics. Each application is considered individually; a decision is reached after thorough evaluation of the applicant's academic record, letters of assessment, extracurricular activities MCAT scores, and personal interview. Since the practice of medicine requires a lifelong devotion to self-education, emphasis is placed on the excellence of the individual scholar no matter what the student's previous area of study.

Applicants admitted to the College of Medicine have a *mean GPA* of 3.62 and *mean MCAT scores* of 10 on each section.

FINANCIAL AID

Financial aid is granted based upon need as determined by federal methodology. Parental income information is required for University scholarship and loan consideration as well as some other financial assistance programs. Approximately 89 percent of the student body receives financial assistance from some source. Additional financial aid information is available on the school's Web site.

INFORMATION ABOUT DIVERSITY PROGRAMS

Applications from students underrepresented in medicine are encouraged. Faculty members, with student support, are active in the recruitment of students from groups underrepresented in medicine.

Institution Type: *Public*
Application Process: *AMCAS, see chapter 4.*

APPLICATION AND ACCEPTANCE POLICIES FOR 2005–2006 FIRST-YEAR CLASS

Filing of AMCAS application
  Earliest date: June 1, 2004
  Latest date: Dec. 15, 2004
School application fee to all applicants: $60
Oldest MCAT scores considered: 2002
Does have Early Decision Program (EDP)
  EDP application period: June 1–Aug. 1, 2004
  EDP applicants notified by: Oct. 1, 2004
Acceptance notice to regular applicants
  Earliest date: Oct. 15, 2004
  Latest date: Until class is filled
Applicant's response to acceptance offer
  Maximum time: 2 weeks
Requests for deferred entrance considered: Yes
Deposit to hold place in class (applied to tuition):
  $100, due May 15, 2005
Deposit refundable prior to: May 16, 2005
Estimated number of new entrants: 135
Starting date: Aug. 2005

TUITION AND STUDENT FEES PER YEAR FOR 2003–2004 FIRST-YEAR CLASS

Tuition	Activity fees: $360
Resident: $26,062	
Nonresident: $36,232	

INFORMATION ON 2003–2004 FIRST-YEAR CLASS

Number of	*In-State*	*Out-of-State*	*Total*
Applicants	839	4,391	5,230
Applicants Interviewed	248	592	840
New Entrants*	51	74	125

*All took the MCAT and had baccalaureate degrees.

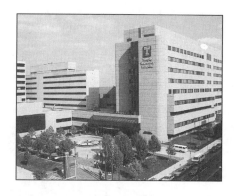

Temple University School of Medicine

Philadelphia, Pennsylvania

Dr. John M. Daly, *Dean*
Dr. Audrey B. Uknis, *Associate Dean for Admissions*
Dr. Raul De La Cadena, *Assistant Dean for Recruitment, Admissions, and Retention*

ADDRESS INQUIRIES TO:

Office of Admissions
Temple University
School of Medicine
3340 N. Broad Street
SFC, Suite 305
Philadelphia, Pennsylvania 19140
(215) 707-3656; 707-6932 (FAX)
E-mail: medadmissions@temple.edu
Web site: www.medschool.temple.edu

MISSION STATEMENT

The mission of Temple University School of Medicine is to educate qualified individuals in the art and science of medicine, preparing them to be the leaders in fields of patient care and research. In so doing, the school will give admissions preference to those who are residents of the Commonwealth of Pennsylvania, and will maintain a strong effort to recruit underrepresented minorities. The school will also recruit qualified students for its Master's and doctoral level degree programs in the biomedical sciences, based upon the capacity of the graduate faculty and apparent workforce need. The School will maintain high quality programs in basic science and clinical research and in patient care, both to support its educational needs and to generate new knowledge necessary for the advancement of medical science. The school, in order to enhance its own resources and fulfill its educational obligations, will affiliate with selected institutions which share Temple's goals and commitment.

GENERAL INFORMATION

The Temple University School of Medicine opened as a college of Temple University in 1901. The School of Medicine shares a campus with Temple Hospital, Temple University Children's Medical Center, other health-related schools of the university, and the Student/Faculty Center. Clinical experience and instruction are given at Temple University Hospital, Temple University Children's Medical Center, Crozer-Chester Medical Center, Fox Chase Cancer Center, Abington Memorial Hospital, and 17 other affiliated hospitals, in both Philadelphia and other Pennsylvania cities. A clinical campus has been established in Pittsburgh at the Western Pennsylvania Hospital.

CURRICULUM

The curriculum is designed to prepare students for graduate medical education by providing them with a background of basic factual knowledge and concepts, a command of the language of biomedical science, a mastery of the skills necessary for clinical problem solving and therapy, and a habit of continued self-education.

In the first two years, although primary emphasis is on the basic sciences taught in part in a small-group format, attention is also given to the clinical application of this material. In addition, courses on clinical medicine and primary care concepts prepare the students to assume initial clinical responsibilities. The third year includes clerkships in family practice, internal medicine, obstetrics-gynecology, pediatrics, psychiatry, and surgery, which provide experience in clinical diagnosis, problem solving, therapeutic planning, and patient relationships. In the fourth year, there are required rotations in emergency medicine, neuroscience, and a subinternship and 20 weeks of individually planned electives that permit students to explore career choices, correct deficits, and expand clinical knowledge.

There is an honors/high pass/pass/conditional/fail grading system. M.D.-Ph.D., M.D.-M.P.H., and M.D.-M.B.A. programs are available.

REQUIREMENTS FOR ENTRANCE

The MCAT and a minimum of 90 semester hours in an accredited college or university are required for admission. Applicants need not major in science, and a strong background and preparation in the humanities with particular emphasis on expository writing are essential. Students who have not completed the baccalaureate degree but who have demonstrated exceptional academic capability and evidence of unusual maturity may apply. The undergraduate program must include:

Sem. hrs.

Biology (with lab) 8
Inorganic Chemistry (with lab) 8
Organic Chemistry (with lab). 8
General Physics (with lab). 8
Humanities 6

Applicants are asked to have recommendations sent from their undergraduate premedical committee or faculty with whom they have completed coursework in two of the following three subjects: biology, chemistry, and physics.

It is suggested that the MCAT be taken in the spring of the calendar year of application and that all courses required for medical school be completed by the time of application.

SELECTION FACTORS

A variety of objective and subjective factors are considered in making decisions. Among these are the academic record and the college attended, MCAT scores, recommendations from faculty, extracurricular activities, and work experience. Those candidates who are to be given very serious consideration are invited for personal interviews with a member of the Admissions Committee.

As a state-related school, Temple shows preference to residents of Pennsylvania; however, a significant percentage of matriculants may be residents of other states. Nonresidents with a particular interest in Temple and strong credentials are encouraged to apply. Foreign nationals without permanent resident status are ineligible for consideration.

Temple University School of Medicine does not discriminate on the basis of race, sex, creed, national origin, age, or handicap.

Selected characteristics of the 2003 entering class are as follows: *average GPA,* 3.5; *average MCAT:* 29; *sex,* 46 percent women; *underrepresented minorities,* 12 percent.

FINANCIAL AID

Students wishing to apply for any type of student assistance (loans, scholarships or grants) must file a Free Application for Federal Student Aid (FAFSA). The FAFSA form helps to determine a student's ability to contribute to the cost of his/her education. Please be advised that students wishing to be considered for Temple University funding will also be required to have their parents fill out the parental section of the FAFSA form. Combined, the student's and parental information forms the basis for determining which students will qualify for need-based Temple University scholarships and low-interest loans. Approximately 86% of all students received some form of financial assistance.

The majority of loan funding for students is secured through the Federal Stafford Loan program. Through this source, students may borrow up to $38,500 per year ($8,500 subsidized, $30,000 unsubsidized). Should additional funding be necessary, students may apply for funding through an alternative loan program. Such programs are administered by private lenders and require that a student not have an adverse credit history.

Students are also encouraged to explore other funding options including those from medical societies, fraternal organizations, church groups and other organizations. Students wishing to research scholarship opportunities on the Internet can do so by visiting www.fastweb.com or www.wiredscholar.com. The National Health Service Corps (www.bphc.hrsa.dhhs.gov/nhsc) and Armed Forces scholarships (see your local recruiter) are also options for interested students.

Please visit the Temple University Office of Student Financial Services Web site at www.temple.edu/sfs/med for additional regarding financial assistance programs at the university.

INFORMATION ABOUT DIVERSITY PROGRAMS

An active program, Recruitment, Admission, and Retention (RAR), meets the special needs of disadvantaged applicants and those from groups underrepresented in medicine. RAR provides exceptional resources for professional academic guidance and personal counseling. Participation in the Summer Educational Reinforcement Activity is encouraged for accepted disadvantaged students and students from groups underrepresented in medicine.

Institution Type: *Private*
Application Process: *AMCAS, see chapter 4.*

APPLICATION AND ACCEPTANCE POLICIES FOR 2005–2006 FIRST-YEAR CLASS

Filing of AMCAS application
  Earliest date: June 1, 2004
  Latest date: Dec. 15, 2004
School application fee to all applicants: $55
Oldest MCAT scores considered: 2002
Does have Early Decision Program (EDP)
  EDP application period: June 1–Aug. 1, 2004
  EDP applicants notified by: Oct. 1, 2004
Acceptance notice to regular applicants
  Earliest date: Oct. 15, 2004
  Latest date: Varies
Applicant's response to acceptance offer
  Maximum time: 2 weeks
Requests for deferred entrance considered: Yes
Deposit to hold place in class (applied to tuition):
  $100, due with response to acceptance offer
Deposit refundable prior to: May 16, 2005
Estimated number of new entrants: 180 (5 EDP)
Starting date: Aug. 2005

TUITION AND STUDENT FEES PER YEAR FOR 2003–2004 FIRST-YEAR CLASS

Tuition   Student fees: $645
  Resident: $30,020
  Nonresident: $36,766

INFORMATION ON 2003–2004 FIRST-YEAR CLASS

Number of	In-State	Out-of-State	Total
Applicants	913	6,326	7,239
Applicants Interviewed	388	382	770
New Entrants*	107	70	177

*All took the MCAT and had baccalaureate degrees.

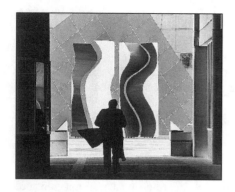

University of Pennsylvania School of Medicine

Philadelphia, Pennsylvania

Dr. Arthur H. Rubenstein, *Dean*
Dr. Gail Morrison, *Vice Dean for Education*
Gaye W. Sheffler, *Director of Admissions and Financial Aid*
Dr. Karen Hamilton, *Assistant Dean for Student Affairs, Director of Minority Affairs*

ADDRESS INQUIRIES TO:

Office of Admissions and Financial Aid
Suite 100, Edward J. Stemmler Hall
University of Pennsylvania School of Medicine
3450 Hamilton Walk
Philadelphia, Pennsylvania 19104-5065
(215) 898-8001; 573-6645 (FAX)
E-mail: admiss@mail.med.upenn.edu
Web site: www.med.upenn.edu

MISSION STATEMENT

Our mission is to create the future of medicine through:
Patient Care and Service Excellence
Educational Pre-eminence
New Knowledge and Innovation
National and International Leadership

GENERAL INFORMATION

The School of Medicine, the first in the United States, was founded in 1765 and is a private, nondenominational school located on the urban campus of the University of Pennsylvania.

As part of the one university concept, medical students participate throughout their enrollment as members of the university as well as the School of Medicine communities. In their clinical years, medical students receive their education mostly in the Hospital of the University of Pennsylvania and the Children's Hospital of Philadelphia, the Veterans Administration of Philadelphia hospitals, Presbyterian Medical Center of Philadelphia, Pennsylvania Hospital, and Phoenixville Hospital. Student housing, both on and off campus, is plentiful.

CURRICULUM

To prepare students with diverse talents and interests for a range of career paths, the objective of Curriculum 2000 is to facilitate the development of skills, competencies, and professional attitudes, which will help all students, as future physicians, master the challenges that they will face in an ever-changing practice environment. Across the six modules of the curriculum, concepts in basic science and clinical medicine are integrated in order to emphasize the intrinsic inextricability of these disciplines. Professional attitudes and communication abilities are fostered and invaluable skills for lifelong learning are developed.

Module 1: Core Principles. The first four months of Year 1 provide the student with fundamental concepts in basic science that underlie the biomedical basis of disease.

Module 2: Integrative Systems and Diseases. The latter six months of Year 1 and the first four months of Year 2 are organized along organ system blocks each of which, through the integration of anatomy, histology, physiology, pathophysiology, pathology, microbiology, and pharmacology, provides the student with an all-encompassing picture of each organ system in normal and abnormal states.

Concurrent with Modules 1 and 2 is Module 3: The Art and Practice of Medicine. Module 3 facilitates development of competencies and attitudes in history-taking, physical exam administration, differential diagnosis, clinical epidemiology, and managed care policies and practices. Mini-courses comprising Module 3 are coordinated with subject matter addressed in Modules 1 and 2 expanding upon and providing clinical relevance to basic science concepts. A component of Module 3 is open time for students to explore individual interests through elective coursework in other schools of the university as well as projects in the community.

Module 4: Core Clinical Clerkships. One year of required clinical experiences, begins January of Year 2. While primary emphasis is upon the development of clinical skills, re-emphasis of basic science concepts and formal attention to professionalism, humanism, and ethics are ensured through symposia and interdisciplinary problem-based learning sessions based upon cases of clinical significance. The curricula of all required clerkships include ambulatory and inpatient experiences.

The final 16 months of Curriculum 2000 are occupied by Module 5: Electives, Selectives, and Scholarly Pursuit. Students are encouraged to explore individual interests and to prepare for future career paths. Required experiences include advanced clinical electives, "Frontiers in Medical Science" mini-courses and a "scholarly pursuit" of at least three months in length. Module 6 runs throughout the entire curriculum focusing on professionalism, humanism and ethical issues related to patient care and collegiality.

Many opportunities exist for students of the School of Medicine to become involved in both basic science and clinical research, to study medicine through international exchange programs, and to participate in study and special projects through other schools of the university. Long-term opportunities are available through dual-degree programs. Students interested in pursuing careers in academic medicine or research and possessing strong science backgrounds and research experience may apply to the M.D./Ph.D. program, while students who are interested in careers that include responsibilities as community leaders may augment their qualifications through combined-degree programs offering graduate degrees in business/health care economics, government administration, clinical epidemiology, and education.

REQUIREMENTS FOR ENTRANCE

The MCAT and a baccalaureate degree from an accredited U.S. college or university are required. Students with degrees from foreign institutions must have completed one year of coursework in the sciences in a U.S. college or university.

Students are encouraged to obtain a broad education in the liberal arts while undertaking rigorous preparation in the sciences. Science courses should include laboratory experience, which enables students to become active participants in problem solving.

Because the content of courses varies among different educational institutions, the School of Medicine does not have specific course requirements. Students are expected to acquire appropriate competence in English and communication, biology, chemistry, physics, and mathematics. The school has developed general outlines of the requisite knowledge and skills in these disciplines.

In addition, students should carry out additional work in accordance with their own interests and curiosity. They should attempt to develop, through their formal coursework and other educational experiences, an appreciation of the basic social, cultural, and behavioral factors that influence both individuals and communities in their approach to health and disease.

SELECTION FACTORS

The School of Medicine will emphasize those qualities of motivation, intellect, and character essential to the physician. Consideration also will be given to special features of background and experience, which may contribute to a candidate's potential for a medical career. Applicants should give evidence of their capacity to deal effectively with other people, organize their own activities, set priorities, accept responsibility, and function under stress.

While the Committee on Admissions has no preference regarding the area of concentration, applicants are expected to have approached their chosen field in a scholarly fashion and to have demonstrated excellence in whatever courses of study they have pursued.

In evaluating candidates, the Committee on Admissions reviews the academic record, recommendations from college premedical committees, scores on the MCAT, quality of and commitment to extracurricular activities, and strength of personal qualifications. Interviews are required for admission and are arranged by invitation of the Committee on Admissions. Applicants from all sections of the country are invited to apply, although some preference is given to Pennsylvania residents.

In recent years, applicants granted admission have had a *mean GPA* of 3.78 and *mean MCAT scores* of 11.4.

The class entering in September 2003 was composed of 55 percent *women;* 32 percent *Pennsylvania residents;* 19 percent *groups underrepresented in medicine* and 31 percent *nonscience majors.*

The University of Pennsylvania does not discriminate on the basis of race, sex, sexual preference, age, religion, national or ethnic origin, or physical handicap. There is no transfer admissions program.

FINANCIAL AID

Approximately 45% of the matriculated students receive school scholarship/grant/loan support through the financial aid programs of need and/or merit. In addition, all combined degree students (approximately 17 per year) are fully funded by the school. The ability of students to pay for their medical education does not affect the admission process.

INFORMATION ABOUT DIVERSITY PROGRAMS

Penn's mission fosters diversity and the curriculum teaches cultural competence.

Detailed information for students from groups underrepresented in medicine can be obtained at (215) 898-4409.

Institution Type: *Private*
Application Process: *AMCAS, see chapter 4.*

APPLICATION AND ACCEPTANCE POLICIES FOR 2005–2006 FIRST-YEAR CLASS

Filing of AMCAS application
   Earliest date: June 1, 2004
   Latest date: Oct. 15, 2004
School application fee to all applicants: $65
Oldest MCAT scores considered: 2001
Does Have Early Decision Program
   EDP application period: June 1–Aug. 1, 2004
   EDP applicants notified by: Oct. 1, 2004
Acceptance notice to regular applicants
   Earliest date: March 1, 2005
   Latest date: Until class is filled
Applicant's response to acceptance offer
   Maximum time: May 16, 2005
Requests for deferred entrance considered: Yes
Deposit to hold place in class (applied to tuition):
   $100, due on May 16, 2005
Deposit refundable prior to: May 16, 2005
Estimated number of new entrants: 145 (5 EDP)
Starting date: August 2005

TUITION AND STUDENT FEES PER YEAR FOR 2003–2004 FIRST-YEAR CLASS

Tuition: $34,482   Student fees: $2,180

INFORMATION ON 2003–2004 FIRST-YEAR CLASS

Number of	In-State	Out-of-State	Total
Applicants	596	4,370	4,966
Applicants Interviewed	118	698	816
New Entrants*	47	100	147

*All took the MCAT and had baccalaureate degrees.

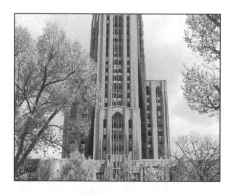

University of Pittsburgh
School of Medicine

Pittsburgh, Pennsylvania

Dr. Arthur S. Levine, *Senior Vice Chancellor for Health Sciences and Dean, School of Medicine*
Dr. Edward I. Curtiss, *Associate Dean of Admissions and Financial Aid*
Linda A. Berardi-Demo, *Director of Admissions and Financial Aid*
Paula K. Davis, *Assistant Dean, Office of Student and Minority Affairs*
Dr. Beth Piraino, *Assistant Dean of Admissions*

ADDRESS INQUIRIES TO:

Office of Admissions and Financial Aid
518 Scaife Hall
University of Pittsburgh
School of Medicine
Pittsburgh, Pennsylvania 15261
(412) 648-9891; 648-8768 (FAX)
E-mail: admissions@medschool.pitt.edu
Web site: www.medschool.pitt.edu

MISSION STATEMENT

The principal goal of the University of Pittsburgh School of Medicine remains the education of scholarly physicians. This goal is to be achieved by emphasizing the centrality of the patient as the focus of health care, by providing a firm understanding of the sciences basic to medicine, and by fostering the application of principles of biomedical problem solving to the care of patients. We feel that students must develop an understanding of ethical principles in medicine and share in the application of these principles to specific problems. Development, early in the student's career, of habits of self-education by methods that include problem-based and self-directed learning, communication skills, and computer-assisted education is critical to the learning process, which must occur throughout the professional life of a physician.

GENERAL INFORMATION

Drawing patients from all over the nation and from more than 30 foreign countries, UPMC is one of the largest non-profit academic health systems in the nation. UPMC sites and affiliations on the main campus in Oakland, or nearby, include Western Psychiatric Institute and Clinic, the University of Pittsburgh Cancer Institute, UPMC Presbyterian Hospital, UPMC Montefiore Hospital, Magee Women's Hospital, Eye and Ear Institute, the Benedum Geriatric Center, Children's Hospital of Pittsburgh and the University Drive and Highland Drive VA Medical Centers. UPMC also has 11 additional primary care hospitals throughout the region, 9 additional regional hospital affiliations, more than 24 surgical centers and satellites, more than 65 rehabilitation centers and facilities, and 10 long-term/retirement residences. UPMC Presbyterian is also home to Pittsburgh's EMS/Medic Command which provides physician oversight for 95 percent of the ambulance traffic in Pittsburgh.

CURRICULUM

The School of Medicine has initiated extensive curricular revisions that were implemented in the fall of 1992. The goal-oriented, integrated, and centrally governed new curriculum emphasizes general principles and encourages student self-learning based on actual clinical cases. In the first two years, the curriculum employs a multidisciplinary approach organized by organ systems (such as the heart, lungs, and kidneys) rather than by individual disciplines (e.g., physiology and biochemistry). It emphasizes problem-solving skills and learning in smaller groups. The curriculum mainstreams social, cultural, and ethical issues and introduces the student to clinical medicine during the first year. The final several weeks of the second year are devoted to an Integrated Case Studies course. This course emphasizes data acquisition, problem solving, and communication skills. It is intended to help the student actively review the material presented during the first two years and serves as a bridge to the patient-care responsibilities assumed in the third-year clinical clerkships. In the third year of medical school, all students have required rotations in family medicine, internal medicine, obstetrics-gynecology, pediatrics, psychiatry, surgery, as well as ambulatory subspecialties. Some students rotate through anesthesia during the third year, while others take it during the fourth year. All fourth-year students rotate through both neurology and diagnostic imaging clerkships. Some students have one elective scheduled during the third year, and all students have extensive elective time during the fourth year.

In addition to the curricular offerings, there are opportunities for students to interact with community physicians through the Western Pennsylvania Health Preceptorship Program.

An honors/pass/fail system is used for grading.

The M.D./Ph.D. Program of the University of Pittsburgh and Carnegie Mellon University offers exceptionally talented students the opportunity to undertake a physician-scientist training program tailored to their specific research interests. Over a period of seven or eight years, these individuals meet the degree requirements of both a graduate school and the medical school. Information may be obtained from the M.D./Ph.D. office in 526 Scaife Hall. The telephone number is (412) 648-2324.

The School of Medicine offers two other combined-degree programs where the course of study is five years—M.D/M.P.H. and M.D/M.A. in Ethics.

REQUIREMENTS FOR ENTRANCE

The faculty of the School of Medicine consider currently enrolled students and graduates of accredited collegiate institutions for admission. Only under exceptional circumstances are students accepted to the School of Medicine with fewer than 120 hours of undergraduate work or without an undergraduate degree. The MCAT is required, and must be taken within 3 years of application.

Specific minimum admission requirements include:

	Years
Biology, exclusive of Botany (with lab)	1
General or Inorganic Chemistry (with lab)	1
Organic Chemistry (with lab)	1
Physics (with lab)	1
English	1

English courses must engender effective writing skills as well as familiarity with the great works of literature. A strong background in mathematics is highly recommended. Studies in social and behavioral sciences and humanities are strongly encouraged.

Acceptance of course requirements taken at foreign universities is determined on an individual basis at the discretion of the Dean of Admissions.

Applicants should have completed most premedical requirements to receive serious consideration. All requirements must be met prior to matriculation.

Students whose applications have been refused by us in three prior submissions will not be considered.

In order to apply, foreign nationals must have permanent resident visas and have completed at least one full year of undergraduate education in the United States, preferably including the premedical requirements.

SELECTION FACTORS

Applicants are chosen on the basis of intellect, integrity, maturity, and the ability to interact sensitively with people. In the competitive evaluation of applicants, consideration is given to the past academic record and MCAT scores; evaluations of college preprofessional committees; letters of recommendation, preferably from faculty members with whom the student has interacted in scholarly pursuits; extracurricular activities; and personal interviews. No one is accepted without an interview. Interviews are conducted only at the medical school campus. All applicants are considered without regard to race, color, religion, ethnicity, national origin, age, sex, sexual orientation, marital, veteran, or handicap status. Some preference is given to Pennsylvania residents since the university is a state-related school. We accept four students through our Early Assurance Program. For the entering class of 2003, matriculated students had an *average science GPA* of 3.70 and a *mean MCAT* score of 10.9.

The School of Medicine is committed to increasing the number of students from groups underrepresented in medicine, and thus actively recruits and strongly encourages applications from students from these groups. The school hosts premedical summer enrichment programs, as well as a prematriculation program for admitted students. Following admission, a broad range of support services are available to ensure retention. Specific information on the services provided to applicants from groups underrepresented in medicine can be obtained by contacting the Office of Student Affairs/Minority Programs at (412) 648-8987.

FINANCIAL AID

All loans and scholarships are awarded on the basis of financial need as documented by the FAFSA. Students demonstrating financial need are expected to obtain the first $25,000 from the Federal Stafford Student Loan.

Institution Type: *Private*
Application Process: *AMCAS, see chapter 4.*

APPLICATION AND ACCEPTANCE POLICIES FOR 2005–2006 FIRST-YEAR CLASS

Filing of AMCAS application
  Earliest date: June 1, 2004
  Latest date: Dec. 1, 2004
School application fee after screening: $60
Oldest MCAT scores considered: 2001
Does not have Early Decision Program
Acceptance notice to regular applicants
  Earliest date: March 2005
  Latest date: Until class is filled
Applicant's response to acceptance offer
  Maximum time: 2 weeks
Requests for deferred entrance considered: Yes, until April 15, 2005
  Deposit to hold place in class: $100, (which must reach our office between May 16–23, 2005); non-refundable
Estimated number of new entrants: 148
Starting date: Aug. 2005

TUITION AND STUDENT FEES PER YEAR FOR 2003–2004 FIRST-YEAR CLASS

Tuition   Student fees: $2,511
  Resident: $30,084
  Nonresident: $35,876

INFORMATION ON 2003–2004 FIRST-YEAR CLASS

Number of	In-State	Out-of-State	Total
Applicants	775	4,067	4,842
Applicants Interviewed	196	722	918
New Entrants*	52	93	145

*97% took the MCAT; 100% had baccalaureate degrees.

CHAPTER 77

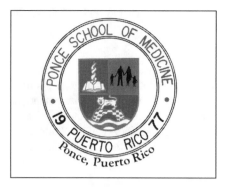

Ponce School of Medicine

Ponce, Puerto Rico

Dr. Manuel Martinez-Maldonado, *President and Dean*
Dr. Carmen M. Mercado, *Assistant Dean for Admissions*
Rosalia Martinez, *Financial Aid Director*
Arvin Baez, *Assistant Dean for Student Affairs*

ADDRESS INQUIRIES TO:

Admissions Office
Ponce School of Medicine
P.O. Box 7004
Ponce, Puerto Rico 00732
(787) 840-2575; 842-0461 (FAX)
E-mail: mis@psm.edu
Web site: www.psm.edu

MISSION STATEMENT

Ponce School of Medicine has as its mission the provision of high quality education and graduate training, which shall strengthen students' character, moral fiber and ethics, and prepare physicians and scientists for a fast changing world in the area of healthcare delivery and research.

GENERAL INFORMATION

The Ponce School of Medicine of the Ponce Medical School Foundation, Inc., formerly Catholic University of Puerto Rico School of Medicine, took over the operations on July 1, 1980, under the government of a board of trustees. The school graduated its first class in June 1981.

Clinical training is offered at the following facilities in Ponce: Damas Hospital, a private institution with 356 beds; La Playa Diagnostic Center, which serves as the main training area for community and family practice; Ponce District Hospital with 550 beds; Dr. Pila Hospital with 160 beds; and St. Luke's Hospital with 160 beds. Clinical training is also offered at the Concepción Hospital with 188 beds, located in San Germán, and at Yauco Regional Hospital with 140 beds.

CURRICULUM

The medical program's basic objective is to provide the Commonwealth of Puerto Rico, especially the southern region of the island, with ethically motivated, professionally competent primary care physicians. The curriculum provides students with an early experience in family and community health needs. During the first two years the basic medical sciences are thoroughly emphasized. Clinical experience takes precedence during the third and fourth years. The correlation between the basic and clinical sciences is achieved in a multidisciplinary

program. Throughout the four-year program great emphasis is placed on the student's contact with patients and their families, as a complement to the student's academic-hospital experience.

Every academic semester contains, in addition to the regular curriculum, a series of supplementary seminars dealing with the ethical and social components of medical practice and with additional specific subjects that are incidental and relevant to the profession. A problem-based learning program has been introduced in clinical correlation sessions in the first year of medical studies and in the Pathophysiology course, in which it is presented as a student-centered integrative exercise. Subject oriented small group discussions are included in the Basic Sciences courses.

The Program seeks to develop well-balanced, mature general practitioners, equally well qualified in the professional ethical aspects of Medicine.

Students must pass USMLE Step 1 before being promoted to the third year and USMLE Step 2 for graduation.

Students' work is graded according to Honor/Pass/Fail.

REQUIREMENTS FOR ENTRANCE

The MCAT and a minimum of three years (90 semester hours) of accredited college work are required. Accredited courses should include the following minimum requirements:

Sem. hrs.

Biology 8
Inorganic Chemistry 8
Organic Chemistry. 8
Physics 8
College Mathematics or Trigonometry. 6
Humanities*. 12
English 12
Spanish 6

*Coursework must be in sociology, psychology, political science, economics, or anthropology.

Academic requirements should be met not later than during the academic year immediately preceding the applicant's anticipated entrance to the school. Applicants are required to submit written evaluations from three faculty members of the institution where they have recently studied or one from their premedical advisory committee.

SELECTION FACTORS

Selection of applicants is made by the Admissions Committee on the basis of academic achievement, MCAT scores, evaluation letters, and personal interviews. The interviews are used to determine the motivation and character of the applicants. Only those who pass a preliminary screening, based on MCAT scores and college grades, are interviewed. Careful consideration is given to all applicants regardless of racial or ethnic background, religious affiliation, sex, or national origin. Residents of Puerto Rico are given preference, although a limited number of applicants who live in the United States is accepted. Candidates who do not have a functional knowledge of both English and Spanish are not encouraged to apply, since instruction is given in both languages.

The 2003 entering class had the following profile: *average GPA*, 3.40 (91 percent above 3.0); *sex*, 45 percent women; *residence*, 70 percent from Puerto Rico, 30 percent from the continental United States; *undergraduate major*, 83 percent in biology and general science.

FINANCIAL AID

Students are admitted to Ponce School of Medicine without regard to financial circumstances. After acceptance, prospective students are informed of the necessary forms they must submit in order to complete the financial aid process. All students must process, preferably electronically, the U.S. Department of Education — "Free Application for Federal Student Aid" (FAFSA), and submit an approved response to the school. Upon review of the results of the federal analysis, and determination of the cost of education, the school awards the aid.

Approximately 89 percent of the new MD entrants in July 2002 were recipients of some sort of student financial aid: federal/private loans, scholarships and or grants.

Upon receiving the financial aid package of instruction, we highly recommend submitting all documents as quickly as possible before the deadline date.

E-mail any question to: psmfinstu@psm.edu.

Institution Type: *Private*
Application Process: *AMCAS, see chapter 4.*

APPLICATION AND ACCEPTANCE POLICIES FOR 2005–2006 FIRST-YEAR CLASS

Filing of AMCAS application
    Earliest date: June 1, 2004
    Latest date: Dec. 15, 2004
School application fee to all applicants: $100
Oldest MCAT scores considered: 2001
Does have Early Decision Program (EDP)
    EDP is for residents of Puerto Rico only.
    EDP application period: June 1–Aug. 1, 2004
    EDP applicants notified by: Oct, 1, 2004
Acceptance notice to regular applicants
    Earliest date: Nov. 15, 2004
    Latest date: Until class is filled
Applicant's response to acceptance offer
    Maximum time: 20 days
Requests for deferred entrance considered: No
Deposit to hold place in class (applied to tuition):
    $1,000, due with response to acceptance offer;
    nonrefundable
Estimated number of new entrants: 62 (3 EDP)
Starting date: July 2005

TUITION AND STUDENT FEES PER YEAR FOR 2003–2004 FIRST-YEAR CLASS

Tuition   Student fees: $3,553
    Resident: $17,836
    Nonresident: $26,590

INFORMATION ON 2003–2004 FIRST-YEAR CLASS

Number of	In-State	Out-of-State	Total
Applicants	321	408	729
Applicants Interviewed	147	39	186
New Entrants*	45	21	66

*All took the MCAT; 98% had baccalaureate degrees.

CHAPTER
11

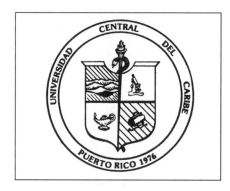

Universidad Central del Caribe
School of Medicine

Bayamón, Puerto Rico

Dr. Jose Ginel Rodriguez, *Acting Dean of Medicine*
Dr. Nereida Díaz-Rodriguez, *Dean of Admissions and Student Affairs*
Dr. Pedro L. Barnes, *Financial Aid Director*

ADDRESS INQUIRIES TO:

Office of Admissions
Universidad Central del Caribe
School of Medicine
P.O. Box 60-327
Bayamón, Puerto Rico 00960-6032
(787) 740-1611 Ext. 210; 269-7550 (FAX)
Web site: www.uccaribe.edu

MISSION STATEMENT

The mission of the UCC is "to prepare high-quality and committed health professionals to meet the health needs of the community in its biological, physical and social context with a human focus and high sense of moral obligation. It is characterized by its emphasis on the excellence of its educational programs and services in health maintenance, prevention, and, and early detection of illnesses."

GENERAL INFORMATION

The Universidad Central del Caribe School of Medicine was founded in 1976 as a nonprofit private institution chartered under the laws of the Commonwealth of Puerto Rico. The new building for the basic sciences, library, animal house, and central administration was inaugurated in 1990 adjacent to Dr. Ramón Ruíz Arnau University Hospital, which serves as the principal teaching hospital. The school facilities are located in a 56-acre academic health center in the city of Bayamón.

CURRICULUM

The educational goal of the medical school is to develop an individual who is oriented toward the provision of primary health care. In line with this goal, the medical school experience emphasizes community health, family medicine, and primary medical care aspects of internal medicine, surgery, pediatrics, obstetrics and gynecology, and psychiatry.

· The medical curriculum is organized in two years of preclinical and two years of clinical experiences. Clinical correlations are included in the basic science courses. Introduction to clinical medicine has as its foundation the biopsychosocial model. This is a problem-based course structured around prevalent problems encountered in primary care. The third-year learning experience evolves around the required clerkships in internal medicine, pediatrics, obstetrics-gynecology, general surgery, and family and community medicine. The latter takes place in the ambulatory setting. Also, during the third year, students enroll in the surgical subspecialties and psychiatry clerkships. Sixteen weeks of electives are provided in the fourth year, plus three months in required courses in Neurology, Primary Care, and Bioethics and Humanistics in Medicine.

Individual student evaluation in all requisite basic science and clinical science courses is based on letter grade and pass/fail systems. Student evaluation in all elective courses is based on an honors/pass/fail system.

REQUIREMENTS FOR ENTRANCE

The MCAT and a minimum of 90 credits of satisfactory work in an accredited undergraduate institution are required. A baccalaureate degree is highly recommended. All premedical course requirements must either be completed or be in progress prior to consideration for admission.

Required premedical courses and minimum required credits are:

Sem. hrs.

General Biology or Zoology 8
General Chemistry (with lab). 8
Organic Chemistry (with lab). 8
General Physics (with lab). 8
College Mathematics 6
English 12
Spanish 6
Behavioral/Social Sciences* 12

*Coursework must be in sociology, psychology, political science, economics, or anthropology.

The applicant must demonstrate proficiency in both Spanish and English. Teaching in basic sciences and clinical sciences is conducted mainly in Spanish.

A strong background and preparation in the humanities and behavioral sciences is highly encouraged so that the applicant may obtain a well-rounded undergraduate education. This background should provide the applicant with a broad cultural foundation, and it will allow our institution to produce physicians with a humanistic approach to the practice of the profession. As long as students fulfill the basic requirements for admission, they may obtain a baccalaureate degree in any field of learning.

Applicants are strongly urged to take the MCAT in the spring prior to application and to have completed the required courses by the time of application since applications are not reviewed by the Admissions Committee until the MCAT scores and grades are available. Taking the fall MCAT or having required courses in process may delay consideration of an application, thus reducing the applicant's chances of acceptance.

SELECTION FACTORS

The selection of candidates for admission is made exclusively by the Admissions Committee. The admission process does not discriminate against any individual on the basis of sex, age, race, religion, economic status, political ideology, or national origin. Major factors considered in the selection of candidates for admission include undergraduate academic record, overall GPA and science GPA, performance in all areas of the MCAT, results of a personal interview, and letters of recommendation. A personal interview is required prior to consideration for admission. All interviews are arranged by the Office of Admissions and are conducted at the medical school facilities in Bayamón. Rejected applicants are given the opportunity to reapply for admission.

For the 2001 entering class the *mean undergraduate general GPA* was 3.31, and 47 percent of the entering students were women.

FINANCIAL AID

The Office of the Dean for Student Affairs provides financial aid counseling to all prospective students. Incoming students qualify for application to all pertinent federal and commonwealth scholarship and loan programs. Economic status of the applicant is not a consideration during the selection of candidates for admission.

Institution Type: *Private*
Application Process: *AMCAS, see chapter 4.*

APPLICATION AND ACCEPTANCE POLICIES FOR 2005–2006 FIRST-YEAR CLASS

Filing of AMCAS application
    Earliest date: June 1, 2004
    Latest date: Dec. 15, 2004
School application fee to all applicants: $50
Oldest MCAT scores considered: 2001
Does not have Early Decision Program
Acceptance notice to regular applicants
    Earliest date: Dec. 15, 2004
    Latest date: Until class is filled
Applicant's response to acceptance offer
    Maximum time: 2 weeks
Requests for deferred entrance considered: No
    Deposit to hold place in class: $500, due with
    response to acceptance offer (of which $400 is
    applicable to tuition); nonrefundable
Estimated number of new entrants: 60
Starting date: Aug. 2005

TUITION AND STUDENT FEES PER YEAR FOR 2003–2004 FIRST-YEAR CLASS

Tuition   Student fees: $3,455
   Resident: $18,000
   Nonresident: $25,000

INFORMATION ON 2003–2004 FIRST-YEAR CLASS

Number of	In-State	Out-of-State	Total
Applicants	340	385	726
Applicants Interviewed	108	20	128
New Entrants*	51	11	62

*All took the MCAT; 68% had baccalaureate degrees.

CHAPTER

11

University of Puerto Rico School of Medicine

San Juan, Puerto Rico

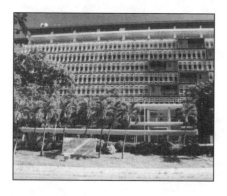

Dr. Francisco Joglar, *Dean*
Margarita Rivera, *Admissions Officer*
Zoraida Cruz, *Director, Financial Aid Office*
Dr. Gladys Gonzalez-Navarrete, *Assistant Dean for Student Affairs*

ADDRESS INQUIRIES TO:

Central Admissions Office
School of Medicine
Medical Sciences Campus
University of Puerto Rico
P.O. Box 365067
San Juan, Puerto Rico 00936-5067
(787) 758-2525, Ext. 5215; 282-7117 (FAX)
Web site: http://medweb.rcm.upr.edu

MISSION STATEMENT – PUBLIC INSTITUTION

The mission of the University of Puerto Rico School of Medicine is to transmit, enrich, and increase knowledge in the medical sciences through teaching, research, and clinical service. The school is committed to achieve the ideals of personal and academic excellence through the interdisciplinary model for providing education and health services, especially at the primary level. An academic and institutional environment conducive to personal and professional development of both students and faculty will be provided by the school.

GENERAL INFORMATION

The University of Puerto Rico School of Medicine was established in 1949. The affiliated hospitals of the Puerto Rico Medical Center and the Hospital Consortium, which include the main health care facilities in other cities, serve the medical school for teaching purposes. On the Medical Sciences Campus, the School of Medicine works in close relation with the School of Dentistry, the College of Allied Health Professions, the Faculty of Biosocial Sciences and Graduate School of Public Health, the School of Nursing, and the School of Pharmacy in an interdisciplinary team approach. Its location, adjacent to the University District Hospital, permits integration of basic and clinical departments and an improved utilization of all Medical Sciences Campus resources.

CURRICULUM

The new curriculum has been designed to last four academic years. The first two years include the fundamentals of biological, behavioral, and clinical sciences and are mostly handled by the basic sciences departments. Part of the sophomore year is dedicated to pathophysiology, physical diagnosis, and basic clerkship, which are offered by a multidisciplinary faculty. Small-group sessions utilizing the problem-based learning approach are introduced at the beginning of the medical studies. Human behavior, environmental factors, and public health concepts are integrated into the curriculum. The third and fourth years are dedicated to required clinical experiences and elective courses. The use of diverse educational strategies, increased use of educational technology, and diversification of teaching exercises are emphasized. Through the Hispanic Center of Excellence, the curriculum has been focused toward community-oriented primary care exposure. Support services, counseling, tutorials, and other services are provided to students to assist in retention. Students are graded on a letter grade system during all four years.

REQUIREMENTS FOR ENTRANCE

Applicants are required to take the MCAT not later than August of the year before admission, and complete a minimum of 90 semester hours of accredited college work with no less than 2.50 overall and science GPA, which must be completed no later than the academic year (not summer session) preceding admission. Since our curriculum is conducted in English and Spanish, demonstrated fluency in speaking, reading, and writing both languages is required. College work must include the following courses.

	Sem. hrs.
Biology	8
General Chemistry (with lab)	8
Organic Chemistry (with lab)	8
Physics (with lab)	8
English	12
Spanish	12
Behavioral and Social Sciences*	12

*Coursework must be in sociology, psychology, political sciences, economics, or anthropology.

In addition to the above requirements, coursework in biochemistry, anatomy, cell biology, liberal arts, and humanities are strongly recommended. Working knowledge in computers and their application is required, given the integration of computer technology in the medical curriculum.

The School of Medicine accepts CLEP and Advanced Placement examinations toward the fulfillment of admission requirements if credits are officially granted and clearly indicated on the college transcript as having been accepted by that college.

Since the preclinical courses in the School of Medicine are largely scientific in nature, it is to the student's advantage to obtain a well-rounded undergraduate education.

SELECTION FACTORS

Since the University of Puerto Rico School of Medicine is a state-supported institution, preference will be given to qualified applicants who are legal residents of Puerto Rico. Highly qualified non-Puerto Rico residents must demonstrate strong ties to Puerto Rico. To determine strong residential ties to Puerto Rico, the Admissions Committee will review the applicant's birthplace, high school attended, college attended, and parent's legal residence. Only those applicants who meet three out of the four categories demonstrate strong ties to Puerto Rico and will be forwarded secondary applications. Foreign national applicants with an established residence in Puerto Rico will be considered only if, at the time of application, they are either U.S. citizens or have been granted a permanent resident visa in the United States.

In selecting students the Admissions Committee considers the candidate's academic performance, MCAT scores, recommendations of instructors, attitudinal and other personality factors assessed in personal interviews, extracurricular activities, and any other pertinent information. Personal interviews are conducted only by invitation from the Admissions Committee for those students with high numerical ranks according to the admission formula. Interviews are conducted only on the site of the medical school or the affiliated hospitals at the Puerto Rico Medical Center. The admission formula gives equal weight to academic indices and MCAT scores, with somewhat less weight given to ratings derived from evaluations by premedical committees and interviewers. Rejected applicants are given the opportunity to reapply for admission. Applicants, without exception, must submit all application material and supporting documents by December 1 of the year preceding the school year for which they request admission.

The School of Medicine has the policy of giving equal opportunity for education and training in the practice of the health professions without regard to race, creed, sex, national origin, age, or handicap

The school accepts transfer applications into the third-year class from residents of Puerto Rico who are presently enrolled and have satisfactorily completed the first two years of the medical curriculum at an LCME-accredited medical school. Promotion into the third year must be recommended by the original school. In addition to completing the same requirements for admission into the first-year class, they must pass Step 1 of the USMLE. Deadline to submit application and supporting documents is May 1 of the same year of admission.

Accepted students for the 2003 class had the following credentials: *mean GPA,* 3.68 (range 2.83–4.00; 99 percent above 3.00); *mean science GPA,* 3.57 (range 2.58–4.00; 93 percent above 3.00); *mean and range of MCAT scores,* VR-7 (4–12), PS-8 (5–13), WS-L-N (J–T), BS-8 (4–11); *sex,* 49 percent women; *residence,* 100 percent from Puerto Rico; *overall*

acceptance rate, 726 applications were received, and 120 offers of acceptance were made to obtain a first-year class of 115 students.

FINANCIAL AID

Financial aid is available to students. Awards are made on the basis of confidential applications submitted by students. Financial need is the major criterion. Applicants who require scholarship assistance may make application in conjunction with the application for admission or before April 30. Financial need will not influence the selection process. Forms are available from the Financial Aid Office upon request. We do not offer financial assistance to foreign students.

Institution Type: *Public*
Application Process: *AMCAS, see chapter 4.*

APPLICATION AND ACCEPTANCE POLICIES FOR 2005–2006 FIRST-YEAR CLASS

Filing of AMCAS application
  Earliest date: June 1, 2004
  Latest date: Dec. 1, 2004
School application fee to all applicants: $15
Oldest MCAT scores considered: 2002
Does not have Early Decision Program
Acceptance notice to regular applicants
  Earliest date: Dec. 2004
  Latest date: March 15, 2005
Applicant's response to acceptance offer
  Maximum time: 2 weeks
Requests for deferred entrance considered: No
Deposit to hold place in class (applied to tuition):
  $100, due with response to acceptance offer;
  nonrefundable
Estimated number of new entrants: 115
Starting date: Aug. 2005

TUITION AND STUDENT FEES PER YEAR FOR 2003–2004 FIRST-YEAR CLASS

Tuition   Student fees: $2,392
  Resident: $5,000
  Nonresident: $10,000; Pays according to a
    standardized fee scale (U.S. mainland and
    foreign residents)

INFORMATION ON 2003–2004 FIRST-YEAR CLASS

Number of	In-State	Out-of-State	Total
Applicants	309	417	726
Applicants Interviewed	141	0	141
New Entrants*	115	0	115

*All took the MCAT; 92% had baccalaureate degrees.

CHAPTER

11

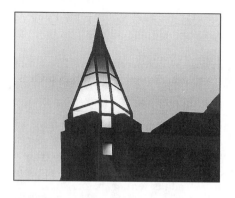

Brown Medical School

Providence, Rhode Island

Dr. Richard W. Besdine, *Interim Dean of Medicine and Biological Sciences*
Kathleen A. Baer, *Director of Admissions and Financial Aid*
Dr. Stephen R. Smith, *Associate Dean for Medical Education*
Dr. Alicia D. Monroe, *Associate Dean of Medicine, Minority Affairs*

ADDRESS INQUIRIES TO:

Office of Admissions and Financial Aid
Brown Medical School
97 Waterman St., Box G-A212
Providence, Rhode Island 02912-9706
(401) 863-2149; 863-3801 (FAX)
E-mail: MedSchool_Admissions@brown.edu
Web site: http://bms.brown.edu

MISSION STATEMENT

The medical program at Brown Medical School has two major goals for its graduates: that they be broadly and liberally educated men and women, and that they view medicine as a socially responsible human service profession.

GENERAL INFORMATION

Brown University, founded in 1764, is the seventh oldest college in America and the third oldest in New England. In 1963 a Master of Medical Science program, a six-year course of study emphasizing the basic sciences and encompassing the four years of premedical education and the first two years of medical school, was inaugurated. A program in medicine leading to the M.D. degree was accredited in 1975 as a four-year medical school. In 1981 the trustees of Dartmouth College and the Corporation of Brown Medical School approved the Brown-Dartmouth Medical Program to which 15 medical students are admitted jointly. Students spend the first two years at Dartmouth Medical School and transfer to Brown Medical School for the last two years.

Entry into the first year of Brown Medical School is possible through several admission routes. Brown offers an eight-year, undergraduate/M.D. continuum (the Program in Liberal Medical Education), which admits students as high school seniors. (See Chapter 10.) Individuals also may apply through the standard AMCAS admissions process, as well as to the M.D./Ph.D. Program.

Additionally, entry into the first year is available to students enrolled in the premedical, post-baccalaureate programs at Bryn Mawr College, Goucher College and Columbia University; to students enrolled in the Early Identification Program in conjunction with Providence College, Tougaloo College, Rhode Island College or the University of Rhode Island; and to graduates of Brown University or students currently enrolled in an undergraduate or graduate program at Brown.

Individuals also may apply to the Brown-Dartmouth Program. Additional information regarding this program can be obtained by contacting Dartmouth Medical School directly.

Students attending any U.S. or Canadian medical school accredited by the Liaison Committee on Medical Education and Rhode Island residents attending foreign medical schools accredited by the W.H.O. may apply for advanced standing admission into the medical school.

CURRICULUM

The Medical School is based on Brown's campus and in the university's affiliated hospitals (Bradley, Butler, Memorial, Miriam, Rhode Island [including Hasbro Children's Hospital], Women and Infants, and Veterans Affairs hospitals).

The first year is devoted to courses in human morphology, mammalian physiology, human histology, medical microbiology, general pathology, molecular and regulatory biochemistry, human neurobiology, medical interviewing, and an integrated approach to psychiatry.

The second-year curriculum consists of pathophysiology, systemic pathology, integrated pathophysiology/pharmacology, neurologic pathophysiology, epidemiology, clinical psychiatry and clinical medicine, including physical diagnosis.

Students in the third and fourth years are required to satisfactorily complete 50 weeks of clinical clerkships and 30 weeks of electives. The clinical clerkships include internal medicine (12 weeks), surgery (8 weeks), psychiatry (6 weeks), obstetrics and gynecology (6 weeks), pediatrics (6 weeks), family medicine (6 weeks), and community health (6 weeks). Additional requirements include a four-week advanced clinical clerkship in medicine, surgery or pediatrics, an ambulatory longitudinal clerkship (one-half day per week for six months), an eight-week selective clerkship, and four weeks of surgical electives.

The graduate programs offered to M.D./Ph.D. candidates are artificial organs, biomaterials, and cellular technology; ecology and evolutionary biology; epidemiology, biostatistics and health services research; molecular biology, cell biology and biochemistry; molecular pharmacology and physiology; neuroscience; pathobiology; and biomedical engineering.

REQUIREMENTS FOR ENTRANCE

Students admitted to Brown Medical School must attain competence in the sciences basic to medicine and sufficient to provide adequate preparation for medical school. Applicants are expected to demonstrate competence by successfully completing courses in the following areas of study:

Semesters

Biology 2
Biochemistry 1
Calculus 1
Probability and Statistics 1
General Chemistry 2
Organic Chemistry 1
Physics 2
Social and Behavioral Sciences 2

SELECTION FACTORS

All applicants are selected on the basis of academic achievement, faculty evaluations, evidence of maturity, motivation, leadership, integrity, and compassion. Applicants to the M.D./Ph.D. program also are evaluated on the basis of their research accomplishment and potential. In order to be eligible for consideration, candidates generally must present a minimum cumulative grade point average of 3.00 (on a 4.00 scale) in courses taken as a matriculated student at an undergraduate college. Applicants who have attended graduate school generally must achieve a cumulative grade point average of 3.00 (on a 4.00 scale) in courses taken in graduate school. In addition, applicants must have completed the requirements for a baccalaureate degree prior to matriculation into medical school. All applicants must be capable of meeting the competency requirements expected of all graduates, with reasonable accommodation, as described in the document *An Educational Blueprint for the Brown Medical School*. This information is included with the letter of acceptance.

Brown University adheres to a policy of equal opportunity in medical education and therefore considers applicants without regard to sex, race, religion, age, disability, status as a veteran, national or ethnic origin, sexual orientation, gender identity or gender expression. A strong affirmative action program is maintained in all admission entry routes. Applications from Rhode Island residents and from members of groups underrepresented in medicine are especially encouraged.

FINANCIAL AID

Brown Medical School makes every effort to assist students in meeting the cost of their medical education through a combination of low-interest loans and scholarships. Approximately 66 percent of our students receive some type of financial assistance. Employment during the school year is discouraged. Financial aid may be awarded to foreign national students on an extremely limited basis. M.D./Ph.D. students are eligible for a graduate fellowship (tuition and stipend) during the Ph.D. portion of their studies and a full tuition scholarship during the last two years of medical school following successful completion of Ph.D. work.

INFORMATION ABOUT DIVERSITY PROGRAMS

Brown Medical School particularly invites applications from individuals who are members of ethnic and racial groups traditionally underrepresented in American medicine. Established in 1981, the Office of Minority Affairs (OMA) has as its primary objective the recruitment, retention, and graduation of students from groups underrepresented in medicine. The OMA provides academic and personal counseling, workshops on test-taking approaches, information and guidance on special prizes and scholarship awards, and a program that links students from groups underrepresented in medicine with alumni/ae from such groups.

Institution Type: *Private*
Application Process: *AMCAS, see chapter 4.*

APPLICATION AND ACCEPTANCE POLICIES FOR 2005–2006 FIRST-YEAR CLASS

Filing of application
    Earliest date: July 1, 2004
    Latest date: Dec. 15, 2004
School application fee to all applicants: $80
Oldest MCAT scores considered: 2001
Does not have Early Decision Program
Acceptance notice to regular applicants
    Earliest date: Jan. 1, 2005
    Latest date: Varies
Applicant's response to acceptance offer
    Maximum time: 3 weeks
Requests for deferred entrance considered: Yes
Deposit to hold place in class: None
Estimated number of new entrants: 68
Starting date: Sept. 2005

TUITION AND STUDENT FEES PER YEAR FOR 2003–2004 FIRST-YEAR CLASS

Tuition: $31,872   Student fees: $2,138

INFORMATION ON 2003–2004 FIRST-YEAR CLASS

Number of	In-State	Out-of-State	Total
Applicants	56	1,655	1,711
Applicants Interviewed*	13*	41	57
New Entrants†	12	57	69

*Excludes PLME students.

†All had baccalaureate degrees; 16% took the MCAT.

CHAPTER
11

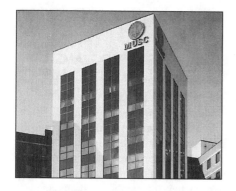

Medical University of South Carolina College of Medicine

Charleston, South Carolina

Dr. Joseph G. Reves, *Dean*
Dr. Paul B. Underwood, *Associate Dean for Admissions*
Dr. Deborah Deas, *Associate Dean for Admissions*
Wanda L. Taylor, *Director of Admissions*

ADDRESS INQUIRIES TO:

Office of Enrollment Services
Medical University of South Carolina
41 Bee Street, PO Box 250203
Charleston, South Carolina 29425
(843) 792-3283; (843) 792-3764 (FAX)
E-mail: taylorwl@musc.edu
Web site: www.musc.edu

MISSION STATEMENT

The college is committed to maintaining an educational environment for all students which prepares them for a career of excellence in the practice of medicine and service to their communities. It is concerned with ensuring optimal opportunities for all students, faculty, and administration, including all backgrounds and levels of diversity, to achieve full potential.

GENERAL INFORMATION

The College of Medicine of the Medical University of South Carolina (MUSC) is a public institution that was founded in Charleston in 1824 and is the South's oldest medical school. Its major clinical facilities comprise the MUSC Medical Center, which consists of the Medical University Hospital, the Children's Hospital, the Storm Eye Institute, the Psychiatric Institute, the Hollings Cancer Center, and the Gazes Cardiac Research Institute-Thurmond Biomedical Research Building. The adjacent Veterans Administration Hospital and Charleston Memorial Hospital, along with consortium and community hospitals in Greenville, Spartanburg, Columbia, and Florence, supply additional facilities for clinical teaching.

In addition to the classical basic science and clinical departments, there is a Department of Family Medicine, which conducts a model program in the clinical area.

CURRICULUM

The goal of the College of Medicine is to produce a caring and competent physician capable of choosing any postgraduate career. The curriculum during the first two years addresses four major objectives: provision of basic science concepts; acquisition of problem-solving strategies; development of skills which permit the performance of an adequate history and physical examination; and an introduction to the role of the physician in society. During these years emphasis is placed on small-group instruction. The curriculum was changed in fall 1999, to expand and improve opportunities for independent self-directed learning. Students are being exposed earlier to certain clinical skills and approaches.

The junior year consists of seven core clerkships. The clinical core consists of eight weeks each of internal medicine, obstetrics-gynecology, pediatrics, and surgery, as well as four weeks each of family medicine, psychiatry, and neurology. In addition, all students take a block of 40 hours of clinical nutrition. During these experiences, emphasis is placed on the development of clinical, interpersonal, and professional competence.

During the senior year, students take a minimum of seven 4-week rotations. The student is required to take a clinical externship (in general medicine, pediatrics, or surgery) and one month each of ambulatory surgery and internal medicine. The remaining four blocks are elective and, depending on previous academic performance, can be taken at approved sites throughout the state and country.

The College of Graduate Studies and the College of Medicine offer a combined program leading to both the M.D. and Ph.D. degrees. The purpose of this combined program is to provide competence in medicine plus detailed knowledge and research training in one of the related sciences without sacrificing the customary requirements for either degree. A student interested in the combined program must apply simultaneously to the College of Medicine and the College of Graduate Studies.

REQUIREMENTS FOR ENTRANCE

The MCAT and a minimum of three years of college (90 semester hours) are required. Preference is given to applicants who have completed four years of college and earned a baccalaureate degree. Only those applicants with extremely unusual circumstances are admitted after 90 semester hours. There are no specific course requirements. Students are advised to construct courses of study that are intellectually interesting and challenging for them individually. Any education that engenders curiosity and enthusiasm for learning is desirable. Students who choose to major in a science should select a broad range of studies outside the sciences as well.

SELECTION FACTORS

Selection is based on a total evaluation of the student. Objectively derived data allow the College of Medicine to set a minimum level for academic performance, above which students can do the work of medical school without academic difficulty. These data are based on the cumulative GPA and total MCAT scores. Students who pass this academic level are invited for interviews. Acceptance into medical school from the selection pool is then based on evaluation of noncognitive traits as well as previous accomplishments that are desirable in future physicians. These noncognitive traits include emotional stability, integrity, reasoning skills, enthusiasm, brightness, and genuine concern for others. The accomplishments that are rated include letters of recommendation, leadership experiences, volunteer/work experiences, and shadowing/clinical exposure valuable to becoming a physician. Application through the Early Decision Program is encouraged for those applicants from S.C. who have competitive grades and MCAT scores.

South Carolina residency is a primary admission consideration. Nonresident applicants are considered; however, due to limited facilities, few are selected and superior credentials are necessary for acceptance. Foreign students without a permanent residence visa are not considered.

FINANCIAL AID

Scholarship funds, including some state scholarships, are available to entering students. The James B. Edwards Scholars Program provides full tuition, fees, and living expenses for the entire medical education of a few select entering students. The Dean's Awards provide free tuition and fees annually for the entire medical education of two entering freshmen. Loan programs are also available. Additional information regarding scholarships can be found on the following Web site: www.musc.edu/com/student_resources2.html

INFORMATION ABOUT DIVERSITY PROGRAMS

Students from groups underrepresented in medicine are strongly encouraged to apply, and there is an active recruitment program in place. The Postbaccalaureate Reapplication Education Program (PREP) is an integrative, individually tailored course of undergraduate study prescribed for underprepared but promising South Carolina students who seek admission to MUSC. The full-time, 12-month curriculum may include undergraduate courses in the areas of biology, physics, chemistry, and mathematics, a learning strategies course, human gross anatomy, and a course in critical thinking/reasoning skills. Applicants from groups underrepresented in medicine who apply to the College of Medicine, but do not meet the minimum academic requirements for interview, automatically will be considered for the PREP. Two students are usually chosen for PREP each year.

There is not a separate application for PREP. Nonaccepted students, who have filed AMCAS applications, are those considered by the Admission Committee for this program.

There is also a summer program for selected students from the South Carolina HBCUs (Historical Black Colleges and Universities).

The Office of Diversity and the Center for Academic Excellence provide counseling and support services. Academic assistance is provided to students through tutorial programs, test-taking skills, training, and the like.

TRANSFER

Because of limited space, the College of Medicine does not routinely accept transfer students from U.S. or foreign medical schools. The only students considered are those with spouses who are accepted into one of MUSC's residency programs.

Institution Type: *Public*
Application Process: *AMCAS, see chapter 4.*

APPLICATION AND ACCEPTANCE POLICIES FOR 2005–2006 FIRST-YEAR CLASS

Filing of AMCAS application
 Earliest date: June 1, 2004
 Latest date: Dec. 15, 2004
School application fee to all applicants:
 $55 *for on-line filing* subject to change
Oldest MCAT scores considered: 2000
Does have Early Decision Program (EDP)
 For South Carolina residents only.
 EDP application period: June 1–Aug. 2004
 EDP applicants notified by: Oct. 1, 2004
Acceptance notice to regular applicants
 Earliest date: Oct. 15, 2004
 Latest date: March 15, 2005 or until class is filled
Applicant's response to acceptance offer
 Maximum time: 4 weeks
Requests for deferred entrance considered: Yes
Deposit to hold place in class: $225, due with response to acceptance offer
Deposit refundable prior to: May 16, 2005
Estimated number of new entrants: 135 (25 EDP)
Starting date: August 2005

TUITION AND STUDENT FEES PER YEAR FOR 2003–2004 FIRST-YEAR CLASS

Tuition
 Resident: $4,544
 Nonresident: $14,604

Student fees:
 Resident: $11,170
 Nonresident: $28,472

INFORMATION ON 2003–2004 FIRST-YEAR CLASS

Number of	In-State	Out-of-State	Total
Applicants	415	1,079	1,494
Applicants Interviewed	303	28	331
New Entrants*	138	6	144†

*99% had baccalaureate degrees; 100% took the MCAT.
† Includes 9 M.D.-Ph.D. students.

University of South Carolina School of Medicine

Columbia, South Carolina

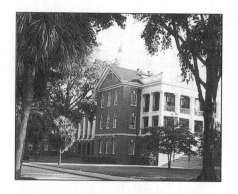

Dr. Larry R. Faulkner, *Vice President for Medical Affairs and Dean*
Dr. Richard A. Hoppmann, *Associate Dean for Medical Education and Academic Affairs*
Peggy Lynch, *Assistant Director of Student Services/Financial Aid*
Dr. Carol L. McMahon, *Assistant Dean for Minority Affairs*

ADDRESS INQUIRIES TO:

Associate Dean for Medical Education and Academic Affairs
University of South Carolina
School of Medicine
Columbia, South Carolina 29208
(803) 733-3325; 733-3328 (FAX)
Web site: www.med.sc.edu

MISSION STATEMENT

The mission of the University of South Carolina School of Medicine is to improve the health of the people of the state of South Carolina through the development and implementation of programs for medical education, research, and the delivery of health care. Programs will be developed in collaboration with affiliated institutions, and allocation of resources will be based upon the physician manpower and health care needs of South Carolina, the effectiveness and efficiency of specific programs, and the accreditation requirements of all appropriate organizations. Medical education and graduate education at all levels are conducted in a highly personal atmosphere that emphasizes a balance among scientific disciplines, humanistic concerns, and societal needs.

GENERAL INFORMATION

The University of South Carolina School of Medicine was established in 1974 by the South Carolina General Assembly in conjunction with the Veterans Administration. The charter class matriculated in 1977 and graduated in 1981. Initially housed on the main campus of the University of South Carolina, the School of Medicine moved its administrative and faculty offices, teaching and research laboratories, and first- and second-year educational facilities in 1983 to completely renovated historic buildings on a 93-acre campus adjacent to the Dorn Veterans Hospital. The 90,000-volume medical library is accessible to medical students on a 24-hour-a-day basis.

Clinical instruction takes place in a variety of area hospitals that provide an ample number of teaching beds and extensive outpatient facilities. These include the 649-bed Palmetto Richland Memorial Hospital, the major regional medical center; the 270-bed William S. Hall Psychiatric Institute, the teaching and research division of the South Carolina Department of Mental Health; the 447-bed Dorn Veterans Affairs Medical Center; and the 60-bed Moncrief Army Hospital, a short-term general hospital located at Fort Jackson, the regional army training center. In addition, core clinical training can be pursued at the Greenville Memorial Hospital, while elective opportunities are available throughout South Carolina at community hospitals affiliated with the Area Health Education Consortium (AHEC), at other medical centers in the United States, and abroad.

CURRICULUM

The School of Medicine offers a program of study designed to provide education and training in the art and science of medicine and to prepare students for a wide variety of medical career choices. Each of the first two years of the regular four-year medical program consists of two academic semesters composed of both basic science and clinically relevant coursework in which students are exposed to patients in various inpatient, outpatient, community, and rural settings. The correlation between basic and clinical science information in the first two years is emphasized by means of an interdisciplinary, four-semester Introduction to Clinical Practice course continuum.

The third year consists of required clinical clerkships in medicine, surgery, pediatrics, obstetrics-gynecology, family medicine, and psychiatry. The fourth year is devoted to advanced clinical work, including 20 weeks each of required and elective rotations, during which students have the opportunity to strengthen their clinical skills and pursue individual academic interests and career goals in preparation for the lifelong study of medicine.

A six- to seven-year combined M.D.-Ph.D. program in biomedical sciences is available to students interested in careers in academic medicine and medical research. A five-year combined M.D.-M.P.H. program is also available.

REQUIREMENTS FOR ENTRANCE

The MCAT and the equivalent of three years of undergraduate work are required. Strong preference is given to those applicants who will have earned their baccalaureate degrees prior to matriculation. Specific minimum coursework requirements are:

Sem. hrs.

General Biology or Zoology (with lab) 8
Inorganic Chemistry (with lab) 8
Organic Chemistry (with lab). 8

General Physics (with lab) 8
College Mathematics 6
    A minimum of college algebra is
    required; calculus is recommended.
English Composition and Literature 6

The science and mathematics requirements must be acceptable for continued study by departmental majors. Courses in biochemistry and histology are strongly recommended.

With the exception of these specific courses, applicants are encouraged to pursue their personal educational interests without regard to any specific field of study. Quality of coursework rather than the field in which it is taken is the most important consideration.

Applicants are required to take the MCAT by the fall of the year of application.

SELECTION FACTORS

The selection process involves the comparative evaluation and review of all available application data, including MCAT scores, undergraduate academic performance, comments contained in letters of evaluation, and the results of personal interviews with members of the Admissions Committee. The opportunity for admission is greatest for legal residents of South Carolina. Competitive nonresidents must have superior credentials. The ultimate selection of a student is based upon a total and comparative appraisal of the applicant's suitability for the successful practice of medicine.

The AMCAS application is used for preliminary screening. After this initial review, the Admissions Committee may request the applicant to submit additional material for the final application, such as letters of evaluation and a photograph, as well as extend an invitation for personal interviews at the medical campus in Columbia. Each applicant is evaluated on the basis of individual qualifications without regard to age, race, creed, national origin, sex, or handicap.

The School of Medicine can accept an application for transfer from any student who is currently enrolled, and in good standing, in a medical school accredited by the Liaison Committee on Medical Education and who meets the prerequisite requirements.

FINANCIAL AID

The School of Medicine participates in all federally funded loan and scholarship programs. Additionally, there is a School of Medicine-sponsored low-interest loan program available to students with proven need. Over 92 percent of enrolled students receive financial assistance in the form of scholarships, loans, and/or grants. The Office of Student Services makes every effort to provide information and assistance to help students meet their financial obligations. Ultimate responsibility for arranging the financing of his/her medical education must rest with the student. Students seeking part-time employment

during medical school should have the prior approval of the director of student services.

INFORMATION ABOUT DIVERSITY PROGRAMS

The School of Medicine actively encourages applications from members of groups underrepresented in the medical profession. There is diverse membership on the Admissions Committee. For additional information, contact the assistant dean for minority affairs at (803) 733-3319.

Institution Type: *Public*
Application Process: *AMCAS, see chapter 4.*

APPLICATION AND ACCEPTANCE POLICIES FOR 2005–2006 FIRST-YEAR CLASS

Filing of AMCAS application
  Earliest date: June 1, 2004
  Latest date: Dec. 1, 2004
School application fee after screening: $45
Oldest MCAT scores considered: 2000
Does have Early Decision Program (EDP)
  EDP for South Carolina residents only
  EDP application period: June 1–Aug. 1, 2004
  EDP applicants notified by: Oct. 1, 2004
Acceptance notice to regular applicants
  Earliest date: Oct. 15, 2004
  Latest date: Until class is filled
Applicant's response to acceptance offer
  Maximum time: 2 weeks
Requests for deferred entrance considered: Yes
Deposit to hold place in class (applied to tuition):
  $100, due with response to acceptance offer
Deposit refundable prior to: May 16, 2005
Estimated number of new entrants: 85 (5 EDP)
Starting date: Aug. 2005

TUITION AND STUDENT FEES PER YEAR FOR 2003–2004 FIRST-YEAR CLASS

Tuition   Student fees: $50
  Resident: $16,900
  Nonresident: $48,870

INFORMATION ON 2003–2004 FIRST-YEAR CLASS

Number of	In-State	Out-of-State	Total
Applicants	332	715	1,047
Applicants Interviewed	215	72	287
New Entrants*	73	10	83

*All took the MCAT and had baccalaureate or higher degrees.

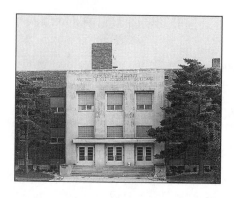

University of South Dakota School of Medicine

Vermillion, South Dakota

Dr. Robert C. Talley, *Dean*
Dr. Paul C. Bunger, *Dean, Medical Student Affairs*
Carol Hemmingson, *Financial Aid Assistant*
Dr. Gerald J. Yutrzenka, *Director, Minority Affairs*

ADDRESS INQUIRIES TO:

Medical School Admissions
University of South Dakota
School of Medicine
414 East Clark Street
Vermillion, South Dakota 57069
(605) 677-6886; 677-5109 (FAX)
E-mail: usdsmsa@usd.edu
Web site: http://med.usd.edu/md

MISSION STATEMENT

The mission of the University of South Dakota School of Medicine is to provide the opportunity for South Dakota residents to receive a quality, broad-based medical education with an emphasis on family practice. The curriculum is to be established to encourage graduates to serve people living in medically underserved areas of South Dakota and to require excellence in the basic sciences and in all clinical disciplines. The School of Medicine is to provide to its students and to the people of South Dakota excellence in education, research, and service. To these ends, the school provides educational pathways leading to the Doctor of Medicine and the Doctor of Philosophy degrees. Quality health care for the people of South Dakota is addressed by undergraduate, graduate, and continuing education programs, as well as by basic and applied medical research. The School of Medicine serves as a technical resource in the development of health care policy in the state and provides extension and research initiatives to improve the health care of the citizens of South Dakota.

GENERAL INFORMATION

The School of Medicine was established in 1907 as a two-year school for the basic medical sciences and has been in continuous operation since that time. The school was physically expanded in 1960 and again in 1969 and is scheduled for new construction beginning in 2004.

In 1974, a degree-granting program began with the first third-year class beginning in 1975 at two clinical training sites, one in Yankton and one in Sioux Falls. A West River clinical training site in Rapid City was later added. The primary objective of the medical school is the training of family practice physicians for South Dakota.

In 1994, the School of Medicine opened the USDSM Health Science Center on the Sioux Falls campus. The Health Science Center houses the School of Medicine's clinical departments and administrative offices, and provides teaching space for the Sioux Falls campus. The South Dakota Health Research Foundation's Cardiovascular Research Institute is also located in Sioux Falls. In 1998, the Karl and Mary Jo Wegner Health Science Information Center was opened as a regional biomedical information library.

CURRICULUM

A thorough knowledge of the basic biomedical medical sciences is emphasized during the first two years. An understanding of these basic concepts provides fundamental knowledge of the human body and hence a rational approach to the diagnosis and treatment of disease. Students are also introduced to patients in the affiliated hospitals. At the end of year two, each student spends four weeks with a physician in a primary care setting in a South Dakota community. For the Sioux Falls and West River sites, the third year is hospital based and consists of six major clerkships: Family Medicine, Internal Medicine, Pediatrics, Obstetrics/Gynecology, Psychiatry, and Surgery. Each site also has significant ambulatory clinic experience throughout the year. For the Yankton site, the third year is a clinic based program with students rotating through all six of the clerkships throughout the year and following patients during hospitalizations. During year four, students have required clerkships in Rural Family Medicine, Emergency Medicine, and Surgical subspecialties as well as having elective clerkships available both within and outside South Dakota. Primary care medicine is emphasized throughout all four years.

Student progress is recorded each semester using the conventional letter grading system (A, B, C, D, F). Students must pass Step 1 of the USMLE to advance through year three, a Step 2-CK to graduate, and must take Step 2-CS before graduation. They must also pass a school administered OSCE to graduate.

REQUIREMENTS FOR ENTRANCE

The MCAT and at least three years of college are required. Each applicant must have completed at least 64 semester hours from an accredited college to be considered for admission and have completed at least 90 semester hours to matriculate. At matriculation, a baccalaureate degree from an accredited undergraduate institution is preferred. The following courses are required, although specific courses may be waived under certain conditions:

	Years
General Biology or Zoology (with lab)	1
General Chemistry (with lab)	1
Organic Chemistry (with lab) or second-semester biochemistry	1
General Physics (with lab)	1
College Mathematics	1

Analytical geometry and calculus are preferred.

All science courses should involve lab work. Chemistry courses should include qualitative analysis and the study of aliphatic and aromatic compounds.

Additional courses in genetics, cell biology, biochemistry, statistics, behavioral sciences, and computer science are recommended.

All required courses should be the same courses taken by majors in each area. Students are encouraged to obtain a broad background in the natural and social sciences and in the humanities, and they should develop good oral and written communication skills. If AP or CLEP credits are on the college transcript, these may be accepted as a fullfilment of a prerequisite providing that there is evidence of proficiency in the subject; examples of proficiency may be successful completion of a more advanced course in that field or a strong MCAT score.

The MCAT is required and must be taken within three years of application and no later than August of the year of application. No application is reviewed by the Admissions Committee until the AMCAS application, letters of recommendation, and supplementary application have been received, and the interviews have been completed.

SELECTION FACTORS

Applicants are chosen on the basis of intellect, character, and motivation. Information about the applicant considered by the Committee on Admissions includes: academic achievement as indicated by the student's scholastic records; retentiveness and ability to perform under pressure as reflected by MCAT scores; curiosity, learning habits, and fitness for a career in medicine as viewed by the applicant's former instructors; and assessments of personal factors of the applicant as determined by interviews conducted by the Admissions Committee. Applicants invited to interview must meet in person with at least two members of the Admissions Committee. Interviews are conducted at the office or clinic of the interviewer or at the Vermillion Campus.

Accepted applicants for the 2003 entering class had the following credentials: *science GPA,* 3.55; *nonscience GPA,* 3.73; *total/overall GPA,* 3.62; *gender,* 46 percent women; *undergraduate major,* 86 percent in science and 14 percent in nonscience. *MCAT scores* (mean): *VR*-9.2; *PS*-8.6; WS-O; *BS*-8.8.

The school does not discriminate on the basis of race, gender, creed, national origin, age, or disability. Priority for supplemental applications is shown to legal residents of South Dakota, nonresidents with strong ties to South Dakota, and Native Americans affiliated with federally recognized tribes in the region. The School of Medicine does not participate in an

Early Assurance Program. An Alumni Student Scholars Program (ASSP) offers a limited number of provisional acceptances to South Dakota high school seniors who meet strict criteria.

The School of Medicine will consider applications for transfer only into Year 2 or Year 3 and only from students who are currently in good standing at an LCME-accredited medical school. Transfer opportunities are very limited, and priority is given to South Dakota residents.

FINANCIAL AID

Economic status plays no role in the admissions process. Low-interest loans are available to matriculated students on the basis of demonstrated financial need. Approximately 98 percent of the student body receive financial aid.

Institution Type: *Public*
Application Process: *AMCAS, see chapter 4.*

APPLICATION AND ACCEPTANCE POLICIES FOR 2005–2006 FIRST-YEAR CLASS

Filing of AMCAS application
  Earliest date: June 1, 2004
  Latest date: Nov. 15, 2004
School application fee after screening: $35
Oldest MCAT scores considered: 2002
Does not have Early Decision Program
Acceptance notice to regular applicants
  Earliest date: Dec. 10, 2004
  Latest date: Until class is filled
Applicant's response to acceptance offer
  Maximum time: 2 weeks
Requests for deferred entrance considered: Yes
Deposit to hold place in class (applied to tuition):
  $100, due with response to acceptance offer
Deposit refundable prior to: June 1, 2005
Estimated number of new entrants: 50
Starting date: Aug. 2005

TUITION AND STUDENT FEES PER YEAR FOR 2003–2004 FIRST-YEAR CLASS

Tuition   Student fees: $5,119**
  Resident: $12,498
  Nonresident: $29,937

INFORMATION ON 2003–2004 FIRST-YEAR CLASS

Number of	In-State	Out-of-State	Total
Applicants	106	315	421
Applicants Interviewed	97	20	117
New Entrants*	44	6	50

* 92% took the MCAT due to Alumni Student Scholars Program and 100% had baccalaureate degrees.

**Includes required insurance fees.

CHAPTER

11

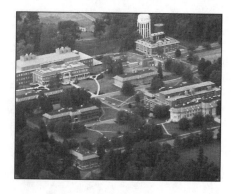

East Tennessee State University
James H. Quillen College of Medicine

Johnson City, Tennessee

Dr. Ronald D. Franks, *Dean of Medicine and*
    Vice President for Health Affairs
Edwin D. Taylor, *Assistant Dean for Admissions and Records*
Ruth Angle, *Director, Office of Financial Services*
Dr. Stephanie Leeper, *Associate Dean for Student Affairs*

ADDRESS INQUIRIES TO:

Assistant Dean for Admissions and Records
East Tennessee State University
James H. Quillen College of Medicine
P.O. Box 70580
Johnson City, Tennessee 37614-1708
(423) 439-2033; 439-2110 (FAX)
E-mail: sacom@etsu.edu
Web site: http://qcom.etsu.edu

MISSION STATEMENT

The primary mission of the Quillen College of Medicine is to educate future physicians, especially those with an interest in primary care, to practice in underserved rural communities. In addition, the college is committed to excellence in biomedical research and is dedicated to the improvement of health care in Northeast Tennessee and the surrounding Appalachian Region.

GENERAL INFORMATION

Since its beginning in 1978 the ETSU Quillen College of Medicine has established itself as a national leader in its programs in primary care and especially rural medicine. Our students enjoy an exceptional success rate in the national residency match and over 60% of graduates choose a career in primary care. Our Community Partnerships Program is nationally recognized and our Rural Primary Care Track has both exceeded our expectations and has taught us much. Student input and participation are encouraged in all facets of their medical education. A collegial atmosphere is encouraged at all levels. Our campus is unified on the grounds of the VA Medical Center pictured above.

The school is located in Tennessee's fourth largest metropolitan area (population 1.2 million) and on the campus of the state's fourth largest university (enrollment 12,000 plus). It is supported by modern and convenient medical centers and clinics throughout the Tri-Cities, as well as hospitals and clinics located in small, rural communities like Rogersville and Mountain City.

The school enrolls one class of 60 new students in August of each year. Residency training programs are available in family medicine, internal medicine, surgery, psychiatry, pediatrics, pathology, and obstetrics-gynecology. An accelerated residency training program in family medicine is also available.

CURRICULUM

The Quillen College of Medicine has always enjoyed a dynamic and ever-changing curriculum. A major curriculum revision is currently underway with expected implementation for the 2003 and 2004 entering classes. The new model is being drawn up by faculty and students and is changing our curriculum to one that maximizes the use of modem technology in teaching while increasing direct clinical exposure for students. Drawing on lessons learned from our own Rural Primary Care Track, successful models in use at other schools, and imaginative input from faculty and students, our new curriculum includes a mix of traditional, systems-based and case-based learning.

The curriculum includes a wide range of educational experiences, varied patient populations and hospitals, a small class size, and a highly diversified faculty who consider students as colleagues. Patient contact comes early in the curriculum and continues throughout. Flexibility is allowed for students to decelerate a portion of curriculum for elective courses including research and advanced clinical studies.

Student input is a key component in curricular change, along with the rapidly changing body of knowledge and the needs of the profession. The goals of the curriculum are to prepare students to be well grounded in the sciences and art of medicine, capable practitioners of their profession, and self-directed, lifelong learners.

Computers are an essential part of the learning process. Due to their increasing importance, a working knowledge of computers and Web-based resources will prove very beneficial to the student while at the Quillen College of Medicine. The campus provides the largest open-access computer lab in the Tennessee Board of Regents System, the seventh largest system in the nation.

REQUIREMENTS FOR ENTRANCE

Applicants must be U.S. or Canadian citizens or possess a U.S. permanent resident visa. The MCAT and a minimum of 90 semester hours of credit, applicable toward a B.A. or B.S. degree at a regionally accredited institution, make up the minimum requirement, although most selected students complete the entire four years. Specific required courses are:

320

	Sem. hrs.
Biology (with lab)	8
General or Inorganic Chemistry (with lab)	8
Organic Chemistry (with lab)	8
Physics (with lab)	8
Communications skills courses	9

Undergraduate preparation in Biochemistry is strongly suggested. Applicants are urged to follow their personal interests in developing their premedical courses of study with the exception of the courses noted above. Preference is not given to any undergraduate major, but a broadly based education that prepares the student to be a self-directed, lifelong learner is suggested. CLEP credit in any of the required premedical courses is acceptable, provided that one or more advanced courses in the same area are successfully completed later.

The acquisition of important skills is further suggested, such as the ability to read with speed, comprehension, and retention; the ability to understand concepts and draw logical conclusions; the ability to adapt; the ability to communicate effectively; and the ability to apply knowledge effectively.

Most courses and clerkships are graded on the standard A, B, C system with P/F grades used where appropriate.

Flexibility in the curriculum is allowed for those with research interest or those seeking the masters or Ph.D. in biomedical science or other programs.

SELECTION FACTORS

Admission to the College of Medicine is based upon a competitive selection process involving those applicants who meet the minimum requirements for admission consideration. The responsibility of the Admissions Committee is to select those students who give the promise of being not merely satisfactory medical students but also capable, responsible physicians of high ethical standards. The Admissions Committee screens applicants on the basis of academic achievement, MCAT scores, letters of recommendation, pertinent extracurricular research and work experiences, and evidence of nonscholastic accomplishments.

After a general screening, the Admissions Committee may request supplementary information and a personal interview with the applicant. Interviews are held only on the campus and are at the applicant's expense.

Admission preferences are for residents of the state of Tennessee who are U.S. citizens, veterans of U.S. military service, and students with baccalaureate degrees prior to enrollment. Marginally qualified nonresidents should not apply.

Some characteristics of the students accepted for the 2003 entering class were: *mean GPA,* 3.5; *mean MCAT score,* (*VR*–9.5, *PS*–8.9, *BS*–9.3); *sex,* 45 percent women; *students from groups underrepresented in medicine,* 13 percent.

FINANCIAL AID

The need for student financial assistance is not a consideration in the selection process. Scholarships, grants, and loans are available for students who demonstrate need as defined by a federal needs analysis and who meet the specific criteria set forth by the various agencies.

Further information may be obtained by writing directly to the medical school director for financial aid. Practice-related scholarships may be available through the Financial Aid Office.

INFORMATION ABOUT DIVERSITY PROGRAMS

The College of Medicine actively seeks applicants of both sexes and members of groups underrepresented in medicine. African-American matriculants may be eligible for financial awards from the state of Tennessee. Support services are available to matriculants to assist in the timely completion of the medical curriculum. ETSU does not discriminate on the basis of race, sex, creed, national origin, age, or disability. The university is an equal opportunity/affirmative action employer.

Institution Type: *Public*
Application Process: *AMCAS, see chapter 4.*

APPLICATION AND ACCEPTANCE POLICIES FOR 2005–2006 FIRST-YEAR CLASS

Filing of AMCAS application
  Earliest date: June 1, 2004
  Latest date: Dec. 1, 2004
School application fee after screening: $50
Oldest MCAT scores considered: 2002
Does have Early Decision Program (EDP)
  EDP application period: June 1–Aug. 1, 2004
  EDP applicants notified by: Oct. 1, 2004
Acceptance notice to regular applicants
  Earliest date: Oct. 15, 2004
  Latest date: Until class is filled
Applicant's response to acceptance offer
  Maximum time: 2 weeks
Requests for deferred entrance considered: Yes
Deposit to hold place in class (applied to tuition):
  $100, due with response to acceptance offer
Deposit refundable prior to: May 16, 2005
Estimated number of new entrants: 60 (4 EDP)
Starting date: Aug. 2005

TUITION AND STUDENT FEES PER YEAR FOR 2003–2004 FIRST-YEAR CLASS

Tuition	Student fees (include
Resident: $15,110	microscope rental): $1,640**
Nonresident: $30,800	

INFORMATION ON 2003–2004 FIRST-YEAR CLASS

Number of	In-State	Out-of-State	Total
Applicants	422	611	1,033
Applicants Interviewed	148	38	186
New Entrants*	57	3	60

*All took the MCAT; and had baccalaureate degrees.
**Includes student health insurance fee of $895.

321

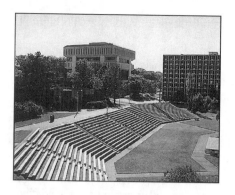

Meharry Medical College
School of Medicine

Nashville, Tennessee

Dr. PonJola Coney, *Dean and Senior Vice President for Health Affairs*
Allen D. Mosley, *Director, Admissions and Records*
Vickie L. Johnson, *Director, Student Financial Aid*
Dr. Pamela Williams, *Vice Dean, School of Medicine*

ADDRESS INQUIRIES TO:

Director, Admissions and Records
Meharry Medical College
1005 D. B. Todd Boulevard
Nashville, Tennessee 37208
(615) 327-6223; 327-6228 (FAX)
E-mail: admissions@mmc.edu
Web site: www.mmc.edu

MISSION STATEMENT

Meharry Medical College exists to provide excellent education and training in the health sciences, while placing special emphasis on providing opportunities for African Americans and individuals from disadvantaged backgrounds.

Meharry is also committed to the delivery of high quality patient care services to the people of middle Tennessee and the development of national models of health care delivery.

Further, Meharry is dedicated to the conduct of basic and patient oriented research on diseases and conditions that contribute to disparities in health status.

GENERAL INFORMATION

In October 1876, Meharry Medical College was founded and established as the Meharry Medical Department of Central Tennessee College by the Freedmen's Aid Society of the Methodist Episcopal Church. Meharry's inception was part of the society's continuing effort to educate freed slaves and to provide health care services for the poor and underserved. Today, the School of Medicine continues to provide excellent educational opportunities to promising African Americans and other ethnic students from groups underrepresented in medicine.

Clinical teaching facilities include the Metropolitan Nashville General Hospital, York Veterans Affairs Medical Center, Blanchfield Army Community Hospital, and the Elam Community Mental Health Center. In addition, clinical instruction is carried out at the Nashville Veterans Affairs hospital, Vanderbilt University Medical Center, Childrens Hospital, and a number of affiliated hospitals and clinics.

The provision of primary care, particularly in medically underserved areas, is a special emphasis, as is health disparities research.

CURRICULUM

There are two programs leading to the M.D. degree, a traditional four-year program and a five-year program. Both programs are divided into the preclinical and clinical years.

The preclinical years begin with gross anatomy, microanatomy, neuroscience, biochemistry, introduction to clinical medicine I, and physiology during the first-year; they conclude with behavioral sciences, microbiology, pharmacology, pathology, introduction to clinical medicine II (includes pathophysiology, clinical correlations, and physical diagnosis), and medical genetics during the sophomore year.

The five-year curricular program differs from the four-year program in that the freshman year is split into two segments, which span a two-year period. The first segment (Freshman I) consists of a summer prematriculation program known as the Mini Academic Program for Success (MAPS), which prepares students for the rigors of medical school and provides an introduction to first-year coursework. This is followed in the fall and spring semesters by gross anatomy, microanatomy, neuroscience, and introduction to clinical medicine. The Freshman II segment consists of biochemistry, introduction to clinical medicine, and physiology. The sophomore year is the same as that of the four-year program.

The clinical years consist of two 4-week blocks of family medicine, and psychiatry; two 8-week blocks of obstetrics and gynecology and pediatrics; and two 12-week blocks of internal medicine and surgery during the junior year that spans 48 weeks. The 32-week senior year consists of five 4-week blocks of preventive medicine, psychiatry, internal medicine, Area Health Education Center exposure (ambulatory rotation, served in an urban or rural underserved area), and radiology; and three 4-week blocks of guided electives.

Internal and external examinations are used in the assessment of student performance in addition to standardized patients. Passage of USMLE Steps 1 and 2 is required for graduation. A letter grading system (A, B, C, F) is used in all segments of the curriculum to report student achievement.

REQUIREMENTS FOR ENTRANCE

The MCAT is required. The baccalaureate degree is desirable; however, three years of college work is acceptable. Premedical work must include:

	Sem./Qtr. hrs
General Biology or Zoology (with lab)	8/12
General Chemistry (with lab)	8/12
Organic Chemistry (with lab)	8/12
General Physics (with lab)	8/12
English Composition and Literature	6/9

All premedical education must be taken at an approved college in the United States, including the courses listed as requirements for admission.

Applicants are urged to take the MCAT in the spring of the year in which they apply, to permit earlier consideration of their applications.

SELECTION FACTORS

Applicants are selected on a competitive basis with regard to cognitive and noncognitive skills that denote probable success in medical school. Performance in the basic science prerequisite subjects (general biology, inorganic chemistry, organic chemistry, and physics) and MCAT scores form the basis for screening for the interview process in which the noncognitive aspects of the applicant are assessed. Meharry accepts students from all parts of the country, with preferential consideration given to equally qualified applicants from states that contract to subsidize the education of their citizens at Meharry. While special empathy is held for minority and disadvantaged applicants of all origins, Meharry Medical College seeks to attract a wide demographic, cultural, and educational population to reflect the caliber of social interchange in which the eventual practice of medicine will occur.

Early Decision Program applicants must have their complete application on file by August 1 for consideration.

Meharry Medical College does not discriminate on the basis of race, sex, creed, national origin, age, or handicap.

FINANCIAL AID

Financial aid awards are based on analyses of student needs and academic achievement. The limited financial aid program includes scholarships, grants-in-aid, and loans.

Because of fluctuation in federal and private support for financial aid programs, the types and amounts of awards are revised and adjusted on a continuing basis. Therefore, it is necessary for applicants to plan their financial program as carefully as their academic program.

INFORMATION ABOUT DIVERSITY PROGRAMS

For over 125 years, Meharry has produced a large percentage of the minority health professionals in the United States and abroad. Of the 2002 entering class, 56 percent were women and 86 percent were students from groups underrepresented in medicine or disadvantaged students.

Institution Type: *Private*
Application Process: *AMCAS, see chapter 4.*

APPLICATION AND ACCEPTANCE POLICIES FOR 2005–2006 FIRST-YEAR CLASS

Filing of AMCAS application
  Earliest date: June 1, 2004
  Latest date: Dec. 15, 2004
School application fee to all applicants: $60
Oldest MCAT scores considered: 2002
Does have Early Decision Program (EDP)
  EDP application period: June 1–Aug. 1, 2004
  EDP applicants notified by: Oct. 1, 2004
Acceptance notice to regular applicants
  Earliest date: Oct. 15, 2004
  Latest date: Until class is filled
Applicant's response to acceptance offer
  Maximum time: 3 weeks
Requests for deferred entrance considered: Yes
Deposit to hold place in class (applied to tuition):
  $300, due with response to acceptance offer;
  nonrefundable
Estimated number of new entrants: 80
Starting date: July 2005

TUITION AND STUDENT FEES PER YEAR FOR 2003–2004 FIRST-YEAR CLASS

Tuition: $26,352   Student fees: $5,260***

INFORMATION ON 2003–2004 FIRST-YEAR CLASS

Number of	*In-State*	*Out-of-State*	*Total*
Applicants	**	**	**
Applicants Interviewed	**	**	**
New Entrants*	16	64	80

*All took the MCAT; and had baccalaureate degrees.
**Data not available.
***Includes $2427.50 (optional laptop fee)

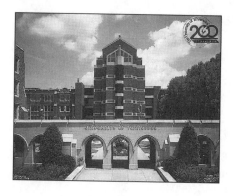

University of Tennessee, Health Science Center College of Medicine

Memphis, Tennessee

Dr. Henry G. Herrod, *Dean*
Dr. Hershel P. Wall, *Associate Dean for Admissions and Student Affairs*
E. Nelson Strother, Jr., *Assistant Dean for Admissions and Student Affairs*

ADDRESS INQUIRIES TO:

University of Tennessee, Health Science Center
College of Medicine
910 Madison Avenue, Suite 500
Memphis, Tennessee 38163
(901) 448-5561; 448-1740 (FAX)
Web site: www.utmem.edu/Medicine

MISSION STATEMENT

The Faculty of the College of Medicine is committed to the education of a health professional whose primary responsibility will be the prevention, evaluation, and treatment of disease in the public. As such, the educational programs of the college are designed to help young men and women to become knowledgeable, skillful and compassionate physicians who seek to understand as well as learn. Students are imbued with the ideal that the study of medicine is a lifelong process and with the moral concept of a physician's deep commitment to high moral and ethical standard regarding patients, colleagues, the profession and society as a whole.

GENERAL INFORMATION

The University of Tennessee College of Medicine traces its origin to 1851 as the Medical Department of the University of Nashville. Today the Health Science Center consists of the Colleges of Allied Health Sciences, Dentistry, Graduate Health Sciences, Health Science Engineering, Medicine, Nursing, and Pharmacy, and the School of Social Work. The College utilizes over 20 facilities statewide for its training programs to include, within Memphis, the Boston-Baskin Cancer Group, Bowld Hospital, Campbell Clinic, LeBonheur-Children's Medical Center, Methodist University Hospital, Regional Medical Center, Semmes-Murphy Clinic, St, Jude Children's Research Hospital, UT Medical Group and Veterans Affairs Medical Center and, outside Memphis, the UT Knoxville Medical Center and Erlanger Medical Center in Chattanooga.

CURRICULUM

The biomedical sciences portion of the curriculum is approximately 72 weeks in duration. The first year begins in August and is devoted to the courses of Gross Anatomy; Prevention, Community and Culture (PCC); Doctoring: Recognizing Signs and Symptoms (DRS); and Molecular Basis of Disease and Physiology until the end of March. Thereafter, some concepts in Hemotology and Immunology in the courses of Pathophysiology and Microbiology, respectively, and in Pathology and Pharmacology are presented in the months of April and May. The second year begins in August and includes courses in Pharmacology, Microbiology, and Pathology. An interdisciplinary Pathophysiology course is coordinated closely with Pathology. Other multi-disciplinary courses in the second year are Neurosciences, PCC, and DRS.

Students are introduced to clinical medicine beginning their first semester through PCC and DRS which are presented in each year. These courses expose students to the real life practice of medicine by placing them in a community physician's office and emphasizing professionalism.

Students proceed directly into the third year clinical clerkships upon 1) successful completion of the Biomedical Sciences and 2) obtaining a passing score on the United States Medical Licensing Examination (USMLE), Step 1. During the clerkships, the students focus their attention and efforts on patient problem-solving and experience an increasing level of responsibility throughout the rotations. The fourth year is composed of six 4-week clerkships, one week of PCC and four 4-week electives. Clerkships and electives allow for increased responsibility in patient care as well as the opportunity to pursue areas of individual interest.

REQUIREMENTS FOR ENTRANCE

A minimum of 90 semester hours and the MCAT are required. However, with rare exception, the completion of an undergraduate degree will be necessary in order to meet educational expectations. The Committee on Admissions is particularly impressed by students whose education has provided a broad range of intellectual experience, including opportunities for analytical thinking and independent study. Furthermore, prospective candidates are strongly encouraged to major in their area of greatest interest; there is no requirement that a student major in the sciences. Regardless of choice of major, applicants are encouraged to pursue a course of study that achieves balance between both science and nonscience coursework. The required courses are:

Sem. hrs.

Biology (with lab) 8
Inorganic Chemistry (with lab) 8
Organic Chemistry (with lab) 8
General Physics (with lab) 8
English Composition and Literature 6
Electives 52

SELECTION FACTORS

The criteria the Committee on Admissions uses in the selection process are the academic record, MCAT scores, preprofessional evaluations, and personal interviews. The required personal interviews by members of the Committee on Admissions provide the candidates with an opportunity to review their curricular and extracurricular activities. More important, the interviewers gain insights into the character of the applicants as well as how they have formulated individual plans for the study and practice of medicine.

Applicants must be citizens or permanent residents of the United States at the time of application. Applications are considered from a nine-state region consisting of Tennessee and its contiguous states (Mississippi, Arkansas, Missouri, Kentucky, Virginia, North Carolina, Georgia, and Alabama). In addition, children of University of Tennessee alumni may be considered regardless of their state of residence. Since priority is given to qualified Tennesseans, out-of-state applicants must possess superior qualifications to be considered by the Committee on Admissions. Currently, only 10 percent of the entering class may be non-resident students. Upon initial review of the AMCAS application, a supplemental application will be forwarded to applicants considered competitive for further review by the Committee on Admissions.

Transfer or advanced standing applications will be considered for the third year only. Applicants must be residents of Tennessee at the time of admission to the medical school in which the student has been enrolled, must be enrolled in an LCME-accredited institution, and must pass the United States Medical Licensing Examination, Step 1. In addition, the applicant must provide evidence of circumstances necessitating a transfer. Deadline for application is April 1.

Some characteristics of the 2003 entering class were the following: *mean GPA,* 3.61; *mean MCAT scores, VR*-9, *PS*-9, *WS*-0, *BS*-10; *women,* 42 percent; *students from groups underrepresented in medicine,* 12 percent.

FINANCIAL AID

Approximately 80% of medical students receive some form of assistance to cover educational costs. Both need-based and merit aid programs are available. The three basic types of aid include grant/scholarships, loans, and part-time employment. Given the rigor of the academic program, medical students are awarded part-time employment only if requested. While the majority of aid awarded to medical students across the U.S., as well as at the UT Health Science Center, consists of loan programs, it should be noted that substantial scholarship awards are available to highly qualified medical students. We are especially fortunate to offer five annual merit awards of $20,000 each for four years. Selection is made by the College of Medicine Admissions Committee.

The Free Application for Federal Student Aid (FAFSA) is the only application required to apply for financial aid at the University of Tennessee Health Science Center. Applicants who complete the FAFSA prior to the last day of February each year and who also provide parent information are considered for all types of financial aid.

INFORMATION ABOUT DIVERSITY PROGRAMS

The University of Tennessee College of Medicine actively encourages applicants from members of groups underrepresented in medicine. The Committee on Admissions evaluates nonacademic, as well as academic factors, in the selection process, with consideration being given to the unique backgrounds and challenges of these applicants. Among American medical schools, the University of Tennessee Health Science Center College of Medicine is a national leader in the admission, matriculation, and graduation of these students from groups underrepresented in medicine.

Institution Type: *Public*
Application Process: *AMCAS, see chapter 4.*

APPLICATION AND ACCEPTANCE POLICIES FOR 2005–2006 FIRST-YEAR CLASS

Filing of AMCAS application
  Earliest date: June 1, 2004
  Latest date: Nov. 15, 2004
School application fee after screening: $50
Oldest MCAT scores considered: 2000
Does not have Early Decision Program
Acceptance notice to regular applicants:
  Earliest date: Oct. 15, 2004
  Latest date: April 1, 2005
Applicant's response to acceptance offer:
  Maximum time: 2 weeks
Requests for deferred entrance considered: Yes
Deposit to hold place in class (applied to tuition):
  $100, due with response to acceptance offer
Deposit refundable prior to: May 16, 2005
Estimated number of new entrants: 150
Starting date: Aug. 2005

TUITION AND STUDENT FEES PER YEAR FOR 2003–2004 FIRST-YEAR CLASS

Tuition   Student fees: $1,373
  Resident: $16,048
  Nonresident: $31,962

INFORMATION ON 2003–2004 FIRST-YEAR CLASS

Number of	In-State	Out-of-State	Total
Applicants	503	851	1,354
Applicants Interviewed	290	53	343
New Entrants*	143	7	150

*All took the MCAT; 98% had baccalaureate degrees.

CHAPTER

11

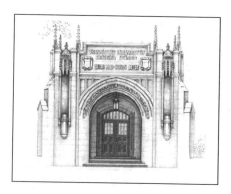

Vanderbilt University School of Medicine

Nashville, Tennessee

Dr. Steven G. Gabbe, *Dean*
Dr. J. Harold Helderman, *Assistant Dean for Admissions*
Vicky L. Cagle, *Director of Financial Aid*
Dr. George C. Hill, *Associate Dean for Diversity in Medical Education*

ADDRESS INQUIRIES TO:

Office of Admissions
215 Light Hall
Vanderbilt University
School of Medicine
Nashville, Tennessee 37232-0685
(615) 322-2145; 343-8397 (FAX)
Web site: www.mc.vanderbilt.edu/medschool/

MISSION STATEMENT

Vanderbilt University School of Medicine's mission is to educate physicians at all levels of their professional experience: medical school; postgraduate education, including basic science and clinical training; and continuing education for the practicing physician. The faculty seeks to provide students with the attitudes and background, based on sound biomedical science, to continue their education lifelong. At Vanderbilt, every medical student has access to examples of the highest standards of biomedical investigation and clinical practice. The desired end is a graduate who has been challenged and stimulated in as many areas of medicine as are feasible within the limits of a four-year course of study.

GENERAL INFORMATION

Vanderbilt University School of Medicine is a private medical school located on the campus of Vanderbilt University. The Vanderbilt University Medical Center and affiliated hospitals provide a total of over 5,000 beds for diversified, comprehensive clinical experience. These hospitals share common goals of education, research, patient care, and community service. Participation in fundamental and clinical research is encouraged.

CURRICULUM

Medical education at Vanderbilt is oriented toward promoting the intellectual development of students and equipping them with the disciplined approach, knowledge, and skills required of both a physician and scientist. The curriculum provides the student with a fundamental knowledge of basic medical principles, but flexibility is stressed. Changes in curriculum content and teaching methods continually evolve from Vanderbilt's focus upon new ways to assist students in their preparation for a lifetime of learning. While sufficient structure is maintained for adequate guidance, the curriculum offers a productive blend of required and elective courses throughout all four years of the program.

Vanderbilt encourages students to develop their full intellectual talents and places great emphasis upon acquiring a sympathetic understanding of the behavior of the human being in health and sickness. The school's education is comprehensive, encompassing the entire span of medicine. In addition to providing a thorough basic education, the curriculum is designed to emphasize the relationship of emotional, social, and environmental factors to medical disorders.

To provide well-balanced exposure to both clinical and research experiences, Vanderbilt allows students wide latitude in their learning process and encourages self-motivation. Research experience is part of the required curriculum for first-year students and is also available during the elective and summer periods. The Vanderbilt Medical Scientist Training Program in the Biomedical Sciences allows the student to engage in research and study in a basic discipline while pursuing studies toward the M.D. degree. For interested select students, this combined M.D.-Ph.D. program broadens the scope of training so that graduates may choose to assume positions of responsibility and leadership as investigators and medical educators.

The School of Medicine is organized to ensure opportunity for excellence by providing unusual opportunities for close association with the faculty.

REQUIREMENTS FOR ENTRANCE

The MCAT is required. A bachelor's degree is recommended, and most successful candidates have earned the bachelor's degree by the time they enroll in the medical school. Required courses are:

	Sem. hrs.
Biology and/or Zoology (with 2 hrs. of lab)	8
Not more than half may be in botany.	
Inorganic Chemistry (with 2 hrs. of lab)	8
Organic Chemistry (with 2 hrs. of lab)	8
Must cover aliphatic and aromatic compounds.	
Physics (with 2 hrs. of lab)	8
English and Composition	6

No preference is given to any one college major. Besides meeting the specific requirements, students should devote their time to strengthening their educational foundation of fundamental knowledge and broadening their cultural background.

AP, CLEP, and pass/fail credits will not be accepted as ful-filling required pre-requisite coursework unless supplemented by advanced work in the same area. The English requirement can be satisfied by reading/writing courses outside the English department if so designated on the AMCAS Academic Record.

SELECTION FACTORS

Applications are invited without regard to race, sex, creed, national origin, or state of residence. Applicants must possess sufficient intellectual ability, emotional stability, and sensory and motor functions to meet the academic requirements of the school of medicine, without fundamental alteration in the nature of this program. Applications are reviewed in two stages. The initial review is made from material provided through AMCAS. Competitive strength of credentials reflect-ing preparation for medical studies, motivation, personal qual-ities, and educational background, as these relate to career promise in medicine are evaluated by the Admissions Committee and determine the recipients of secondary applica-tions. Applicants receiving favorable initial review are invited to file a secondary application, which requires a $50 applica-tion fee, except in demonstrated circumstances of serious financial hardship. Those who are sent a secondary application also are invited for an interview. In evaluating candidates, no specific categories of applicants are identified; there is no point system for any categories. Rather, there is a holistic review of the academic performance and non-academic factors such as patient care experience, research experience, extracur-ricular involvement, leadership roles, sports activities, rela-tionship to the medical school, applicants from underserved populations, and applicants that would enhance the diversity of the class toward improved education in the broadest sense. Interviews are held at Vanderbilt.

The 104 members of the 2003 first-year class graduated from 56 different colleges and universities. They hail from 32 states. Nine are enrolled in the Medical Scientist Training Program. The *mean GPA* for the class is 3.77 and the *mean MCAT score* is 10.76.

Vanderbilt undergraduates, with at least a 3.5 GPA, are eli-gible to apply for early acceptance during the spring of the sophomore year. Those accepted are encouraged to broaden their curricular experiences. The number of early acceptance candidates in the school's current classes ranges from 4 to 12. Beginning with the 2004 first year class, the Early Acceptance Program will be a binding decision program.

Acceptance for transfer is limited to the third year, filling places made by attrition only. Opportunities for transfer are rarely available because of the low attrition rate. Those students who have completed the second year in good standing at LCME-accredited U.S. or Canadian medical schools are eligible to apply. The deadline for applying for transfer is March 1.

FINANCIAL AID

Approximately 80% of the student body receive financial aid. Every effort is made to see that each student that applies has sufficient funds to meet the total estimated cost of atten-dance by utilizing a variety of loans and scholarships. International students are eligible to be considered for need-based institutional scholarships and loans; however, because students are ineligible for federal financial aid programs, Student Financial Services is not able to offer the same level of financial assistance that is available to other students.

For further information, contact Student Financial Services at (615) 343-6310.

INFORMATION ABOUT DIVERSITY PROGRAMS

Vanderbilt invites applicants from a broad spectrum of student backgrounds to submit an application for admission. Applications are sought from members of groups presently not adequately represented in medicine who feel a commitment to helping resolve the special problems of health care delivery to underserved groups.

Institution Type: *Private*
Application Process: *AMCAS, see chapter 4.*

APPLICATION AND ACCEPTANCE POLICIES FOR 2005–2006 FIRST-YEAR CLASS

Filing of AMCAS application
    Earliest date: June 1, 2004
    Latest date: Nov. 15, 2004
School application fee after screening: $50
Oldest MCAT scores considered: 2001
Does have Early Decision Program (EDP)
    EDP application period: June 1–Aug. 1, 2004
    EDP applicants notified by: Oct. 1, 2004
Acceptance notice to regular applicants
    Earliest date: Oct. 15, 2004
    Latest date: Until class is filled
Applicant's response to acceptance offer
    Maximum time: 2 weeks
Requests for deferred entrance considered: Yes
This is a binding referral. Applicant cannot apply to other schools.
Deposit to hold place in class: None
Estimated number of new entrants: 104 (5 EDP)
Starting date: Aug. 2005

TUITION AND STUDENT FEES PER YEAR FOR 2003–2004 FIRST-YEAR CLASS

Tuition: $30,100   Student fees: $2,057

INFORMATION ON 2003–2004 FIRST-YEAR CLASS

Number of	In-State	Out-of-State	Total
Applicants	240	3,267	3,507
Applicants Interviewed	52	843	895
New Entrants*	16	88	104

*All had baccalaureate degrees; 97% took the MCAT.

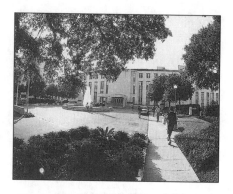

Baylor College of Medicine

Houston, Texas

Dr. Peter G. Traber, *President*
Dr. Major Bradshaw, *Dean of Education*
Dr. L. Leighton Hill, *Senior Associate Dean, Admissions*
Dr. Lloyd H. Michael, *Sr. Associate Dean, Admissions*

ADDRESS INQUIRIES TO:

Office of Admissions
Baylor College of Medicine
One Baylor Plaza
Houston, Texas 77030
(713) 798-4842
E-mail: melodym@bcm.tmc.edu
Web site: http://public.bcm.tmc.edu/admissions/

MISSION STATEMENT

The mission of Baylor College of Medicine is to promote health for all people through education, research, and public service.

The college pursues this mission by sustaining excellence in educating medical and graduate students, primary care and specialty physicians, biomedical scientists and allied health professionals; by advancing basic and clinical biomedical research; by fostering public awareness of health and the prevention of disease; and by promoting patient care of the highest standard.

GENERAL INFORMATION

Baylor College of Medicine is a private, nonsectarian institution governed by an independent Board of Trustees of community leaders. Baylor College of Medicine is the academic center around which the 675-acre Texas Medical Center was developed. The Baylor faculty currently is composed of 1,732 full-time members and another 1,791 on a part-time and voluntary basis. Facilities include teaching and research buildings and seven affiliated teaching hospitals (including private, county, and Veterans Affairs hospitals), which together have approximately 5,000 beds. The Texas Medical Center is located in a university, residential, and park area in the southwest section of Houston.

CURRICULUM

The goal of the educational program at Baylor College of Medicine is to provide the highest-quality educational experience in the art and science of medicine, fostering a drive for excellence among all students. The curriculum is structured to prepare graduates to pursue careers as primary care physicians, specialists, research scientists, academic physicians, or physicians involved in public health policy. The Baylor curriculum integrates basic and clinical sciences throughout the four-year program. This integration includes direct patient-care experiences early in the first year and a focus on core

basic science topics prior to graduation. This integration also includes special courses featuring integrated problem-solving and clinical skills training that encourage application of content learned in lectures and labs.

The Baylor curriculum is unique in that the basic sciences are taught in slightly less than 1½ years, giving students more time to take advantage of a wealth of clinical experiences. During the preclinical curriculum, study periods are scheduled prior to exams generally at the end of each block, followed by a short vacation. During the clinical curriculum, students have flexibility in organizing their schedules to complete 56 weeks of required clinical clerkships, 4 weeks of selectives, and 20 weeks of elective experiences. Approximately 225 discrete electives are available at Baylor and throughout the Texas Medical Center. Interested students are given opportunity to do research or to apply for a combined M.D./Ph.D. program. Students with an interest in ethics, research, or international health or geriatrics may participate in tracks designed for the specific topic. Additional tracks being considered are the underserved, women's health and medical economics.

The Baylor/Rice program in Health Sciences Management consists of a dual-degree program of M.D./M.B.A. with a health care focus. The program is sponsored jointly by the Jones School of Management at Rice University and by Baylor College of Medicine. It is possible for a student to obtain a masters degree in education from the University of Houston. A combined M.D./J.D. program with the U of H Law Center has been developed and only awaits board approval. It is a six year program and the anticipated start date is August 2005.

REQUIREMENTS FOR ENTRANCE

The MCAT is required. Applicants are strongly advised to take the MCAT in the spring of the year of application and to have their science course requirements completed at the time of application.

The baccalaureate degree is highly desirable. In recent years very few students matriculated without a baccalaureate degree. Applicants must have satisfactorily completed a minimum of 90 undergraduate semester hours (or an equivalent number of quarter hours) at a fully accredited college or university in the United States prior to enrollment. Courses must include:

	Years
General Biology (with lab)	1
General Chemistry (with lab)	1

Organic Chemistry (with lab). 1
English 1

SELECTION FACTORS

All applicants offered places in the class are interviewed on the Baylor College of Medicine campus. The Admissions Committee selects for interview applicants whose files are complete and who are considered to be competitive for admission. All information available is utilized in the selection process. In evaluating the applicant's academic record, attention is paid to course selections, academic challenge imposed by the student's curriculum, and the extent to which extracurricular activities and employment may have broadened a student's experiences or limited the applicant's opportunity for high academic achievement.

Intellectual ability and academic achievement alone are not sufficient to support the development of the ideal physician. To work effectively in a profession dependent upon interpersonal relationships, physicians should possess those traits of personality and character which permit them to communicate effectively with warmth and compassion.

There are 168 students in each first-year class; approximately 70–75 percent are residents of Texas.

Requests for deferred entrance (delayed matriculation) from accepted students will be considered but are not encouraged. Such requests must be in writing and will be reviewed on an individual basis.

Students matriculating in 2003 had the following credentials: *mean GPA,* 3.76; *average total MCAT score,* 34.3; *sex,* 49; percent women; *undergraduate major,* 65 percent in sciences, with the remainder from a variety of fields.

Baylor College of Medicine does not discriminate on the basis of race, sex, creed, national origin, age, or disability.

FINANCIAL AID

Financial need is not a factor in the selection of students. Aid funds are provided by private donors, the Board of Trustees, and various state and federal loan, scholarship, and work-study programs. Employment for spouses and part-time employment for students is available. Financial aid information and application materials are sent to all accepted applicants and a financial aid officer is available for consultation with students and parents.

INFORMATION ABOUT DIVERSITY PROGRAMS

Baylor College of Medicine encourages applications from members of groups underrepresented in medicine.

Students from these groups comprise a substantial portion of the student body, and the Admissions Committee has members from these groups as well. For additional information contact Dr. James L. Phillips, Senior Associate Dean, at 713-798-8646.

Institution Type: *Private*
Application Process: *AMCAS, see chapter 4.*

APPLICATION AND ACCEPTANCE POLICIES FOR 2005–2006 FIRST-YEAR CLASS

Filing of AMCAS Application
  Earliest date: June 1, 2004
  Latest date: Nov. 1, 2004
Secondary application fee to all applicants: $50
Oldest MCAT scores considered: 2000
Does have Early Decision Program (EDP)
  EDP application period: June 1–Aug. 1, 2004
  EDP applicants notified by: Oct. 1, 2004
Acceptance notice to regular applicants
  Earliest date: Oct. 15, 2004
  Latest date: Until class is filled
Requests for deferred entrance considered: Yes
Deposit to hold place in class (applied to tuition):
  $300, due May 16, 2005; nonrefundable
Estimated number of new entrants: 168 (5 EDP)
Starting date: July 2005

TUITION AND STUDENT FEES PER YEAR FOR 2003–2004 FIRST-YEAR CLASS

Tuition   Student fees: $3,008
  Resident: $6,550
  Nonresident: $19,650

INFORMATION ON 2003–2004 FIRST-YEAR CLASS

Number of	In-State	Out-of-State	Total
Applicants	1,160	2,937	4,097
Applicants Interviewed	394	247	641
New Entrants	131	37	168

*All had baccalaureate degrees; 99% took the MCAT.

CHAPTER
11

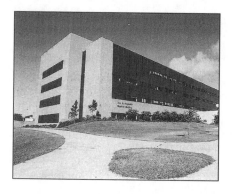

Texas A&M University System Health Science Center College of Medicine

College Station, Texas

Dr. Christopher C. Colenda, *Dean*
Dr. Kathleen F. Fallon, *Associate Dean for Student Affairs and Admissions*
Filomeno G. Maldonado, *Assistant Dean for Admissions*
Wanda J. Watson, *Director of Recruitment and Special Programs*

ADDRESS INQUIRIES TO:

Office of Student Affairs and Admissions
Texas A&M University System Health Science Center
College of Medicine
159 Joe Reynolds Medical Bldg.
College Station, Texas 77843-1114
(979) 845-7743; 845-5533 (FAX)
E-mail: admissions@medicine.tamu.edu
Web site: http://medicine.tamu.edu

MISSION STATEMENT

The Texas A&M University System Health Science Center College of Medicine is dedicated to the education of humane and highly skilled physicians and to the development of knowledge in the biomedical and clinical sciences. To achieve its mission, the College of Medicine utilizes the varied resources of the Texas A&M University System HSC, The Scott & White Clinic and Hospital, the Olin E. Teague Veterans Center, and physicians in private practice. In order to improve the quality and efficacy of health and medical care through its programs of medical education and research, the College of Medicine will continue:

- To maintain a small, high quality medical education program, which graduates physicians prepared to enter graduate study in any medical specialty, including primary care. The medical education program includes a strong emphasis on the humanistic and ethical aspects of medicine.
- To develop a program of research in selected areas of biomedical and clinical science and to join in collaborative programs with other elements of the HSC, through which the knowledge and skills can be utilized to improve the health and medical care of specific segments of the population.
- To educate a small number of biomedical scientists to conduct research in areas that will form the foundation for advances in the prevention, diagnosis, and treatment of disease.

GENERAL INFORMATION

Established in 1973, Texas A&M University College of Medicine is part of the Texas A&M University System Health Science Center, a public institution. The College of Medicine's administrative offices and basic science campus are located in College Station on the campus of Texas A&M University. Texas A&M University, whose research budget is among the top five in the nation, is a comprehensive land, sea, and space grant university with a total enrollment of 36,082 undergraduate students and 6,861 graduate and professional students. The clinical campus consists of the Central Texas Veterans Health Care System, a consortium of four (4) Veterans Affairs hospitals and outpatient clinics that serves veterans in a 35-county-wide primary care service area of central Texas; the Olin E. Teague Veterans Center in Temple, Texas; the Scott and White Clinic and Hospital in Temple, Texas; Darnall Army Community Hospital at nearby Fort Hood in Killeen, Texas; and Driscoll Children's Hospital in Corpus Christi, Texas. These comprehensive facilities provide 1,976 teaching beds and aggregate annual outpatient visits in excess of 2 million.

The College of Medicine is chartered to grant the degree of doctor of medicine.

CURRICULUM

The primary goal of the curriculum is to produce undifferentiated physicians of the highest caliber. A second principal mission is the systematic utilization of the vast intellectual and technological resources available within other disciplines of the parent university in collaborative research and instructional programs.

The College of Medicine offers a four-year program leading to the M.D. degree. The first two years are taught on the Texas A&M University campus in College Station and include an organ systems curriculum which integrates the traditional basic sciences along with instruction in behavioral science, working with patients, physical diagnosis, humanities in medicine, community medicine, leadership in medicine, and epidemiology and bio-statistics. Although the faculty is organized along disciplinary lines, courses are scheduled to assure a high degree of integration of subject matter across disciplines. Correlation of the basic sciences with clinical medicine is achieved from the start, with clinical correlation experiences in all courses and regularly scheduled sessions for clinical instruction and practice in both years 1 and 2.

The third- and fourth-year clinical programs, conducted predominantly on the Temple campus at the Scott and White Clinic and Hospital and the Olin E. Teague Veterans Center, consist of traditional clerkships and a mixed rotation of ambulatory care experiences. In addition, each student spends a minimum of six weeks in an approved family medicine clerkship in a nonurban location.

Electives are available in both basic and clinical sciences. A standardized letter grading system (A, B, C, F) is utilized.

Selected students may participate in the combined M.D.-Ph.D. program.

REQUIREMENTS FOR ENTRANCE

The MCAT and 90 semester hours of appropriate undergraduate study from an accredited U.S. institution are required. Required courses are:

Credit Hrs./Years
General Biology (with lab) 8/1
Additional advanced Biological Science 6/1
Inorganic Chemistry (with lab) 8/1
Organic Chemistry (with lab) 8/1
General Physics (with lab) 8/1
Calculus or Math-based Statistics 3½
English 6/1

Applicants are urged to take the MCAT in the spring of the year of application. Early application is encouraged.

SELECTION FACTORS

Academic ability, as evidenced by grades in college courses and performance on the MCAT, is an important selection criterion. Equally important are personal traits such as interpersonal and communication skills, maturity, motivation, and compassion. In addition, it is critical for members of the Admissions Committee to understand the circumstances of applicants and give careful consideration to other factors such as dedication to service, circumstances indicative of some hardship, need to work, support from faculty and mentors, evidence of interest in primary care, or service in a rural or underserved area, and knowledge of cultural factors as they may impact health care. It is also important for applicants to have some knowledge and experience of the profession of medicine. However, it must be understood that not all of the applicants under review will be either interviewed or offered admission. Competitive applicants are invited for personal interviews, which are conducted between the College Station and Temple campuses on Thursdays. Each applicant is scheduled for two 30-minute individual interviews with some combination of faculty Admissions Committee members, Medical student's Admissions Committee members, and faculty guest interviewers. Admission to the College of Medicine is open to qualified individuals regardless of race, color, religion, gender, age, national origin, or disability.

The College of Medicine received 2,233 applications for the 74 places in the 2003 entering class. Five hundred and twenty-eight were interviewed. The class is comprised of 90% *Texas residents*, 59% *women*, and 16% *students from groups underrepresented medicine*. Among the students enrolled, 86% received baccalaureate degrees, 11% had graduate degrees, and 3% was admitted without degrees. The choice of major varied among the students, but 80% chose majors in the sciences. Thirty-two colleges and universities throughout the state and nation are represented among the members of the entering class. The class is distinguished by a *mean college GPA* of 3.65 and *average MCAT scores* for the individual sections of 9.0 (or 27 total).

FINANCIAL AID

Scholarship and loan funds are available to students with financial need from local, state, and national sources. In addition, three full-tuition scholarships, which pay for resident tuition over four years, may be awarded to the year's top-ranked applicants and outstanding students with financial need. Financial needs of the applicant are not a consideration in the admission process, and after acceptance, every effort is made to assist students in meeting their financial requirements.

Approximately 90 percent of the students currently in the program are receiving some form of financial aid. For further information, contact the director of student financial aid at ☞ http://medicine.tamu.edu/StudentAffairs/finaid01.htm.

INFORMATION ABOUT DIVERSITY PROGRAMS

The College of Medicine is committed to identifying and recruiting qualified students from disadvantaged backgrounds and groups underrepresented in medicine. As part of its commitment to this effort, the College of Medicine administers several programs for disadvantaged students. The Joint Admissions Medical Program (JAMP) is open to students from disadvantaged backgrounds. In addition, the Office of Student Affairs facilitates the adjustment and the retention of students through established student organizations and a chapter of the SNMA.

Institution Type: *Public*
Application Process: *Texas Medical and Dental Schools Application Service*

APPLICATION AND ACCEPTANCE POLICIES FOR 2005–2006 FIRST-YEAR CLASS

Application must be made through the Texas Medical and Dental Schools Application Service, Suite 6.400, 702 Colorado, Austin, Texas 78701.
via: www.utsystem.edu/tmdsas/
Filing of Application:
  Earliest date: May 1, 2004
  Latest date: Nov. 1, 2004
School application fee to all applicants:
Resident: $55 for application to one school plus $10 for each additional school
Non-resident: $100 for application to one school plus $10 for each additional school
School secondary application fee: $45
  (required, non-refundable)
Oldest MCAT scores considered: 2000
Does not have Early Decision Program
Acceptance notice to regular applicants
  Earliest date: Feb. 1, 2005
  Latest date: Until class is filled
Applicant's response to acceptance offer
  Maximum time: 2 weeks
Requests for deferred entrance considered: Yes
Deposit to hold place in class: None
Estimated number of new entrants: 80
Starting date: Aug. 2005

TUITION AND STUDENT FEES PER YEAR FOR 2003–2004 FIRST-YEAR CLASS

Tuition	Student fees: $1,559
Resident: $6,550	
Nonresident: $19,650	

INFORMATION ON 2003–2004 FIRST-YEAR CLASS

Number of	In-State	Out-of-State	Total
Applicants	2,029	204	2,233
Applicants Interviewed	507	21	528
New Entrants*	69	5	74

*80% took the MCAT; 97% had baccalaureate degrees.

CHAPTER
11

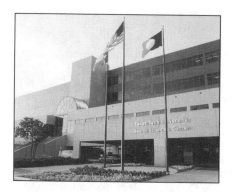

Texas Tech University Health Sciences Center School of Medicine

Lubbock, Texas

Dr. Richard V. Homan, *Vice President for Clinical Affairs and*
  Dean for School of Medicine
Dr. Bernell K. Dalley, *Associate Dean, Admissions and Student Affairs*
E. Marcus Wilson, *Director, Financial Aid*

ADDRESS INQUIRIES TO:

Texas Tech University Health Sciences Center
School of Medicine
Office of Admissions, Room 2B116
3601 4th Street, Lubbock, Texas 79430
(806) 743-2297; 743-2725 (FAX)
Web site: www.ttuhsc.edu/SOM/admissions

MISSION STATEMENT

Texas Tech University Health Sciences Center School of Medicine provides the highest standard of excellence in higher education, while pursuing continuous quality improvement. The medical school is committed to medical education and health care delivery for its 135,000 square mile serving area of West Texas via regional academic health centers in Lubbock, Amarillo, El Paso, and Odessa and to prepare graduates of the institution for real world medicine. At the same time and as part of improvement of health care, its efforts include support of meaningful academic research for the betterment of future health care.

GENERAL INFORMATION

Texas Tech University School of Medicine, established in 1969, is part of the Texas Tech University Health Sciences Center. The School of Medicine is adjacent to Texas Tech University, which has an enrollment of 27,569 students. All medical students spend the first two years at the Lubbock campus; third and fourth year students receive their clinical training in Lubbock, Amarillo, or El Paso. At each academic health center the primary teaching hospital is located in close proximity to the medical school facility. Affiliations with the primary teaching hospital and other community hospitals provide over 2,900 beds for clinical teaching. The medical school has 431 full-time and 9 part-time faculty members and more than 902 volunteer clinical faculty members.

CURRICULUM

The four-year curriculum provides a broad introduction to medical knowledge while developing the student's analytical, problem-solving skills. The first two years are divided into four terms, with an emphasis on basic sciences. Introduction to clinical material begins in the first year with preceptorial experiences, including shadowing of community physicians and training in patient history and interviewing. These experiences may be augmented by doing summer preceptorships following the first

year of medical school. It continues in the second year with the introduction to clinical medicine course, which integrates pathophysiology and physical diagnosis. Small group discussions of clinical cases – problem-based learning – also takes place in the first and second years. The clinical curriculum includes clerkships in family medicine, internal medicine, neurology, obstetrics-gynecology, pediatrics, psychiatry, and surgery. It also includes experience with family medicine in the community setting. The electives program consists of five electives chosen by the students in consultation with their advisors.

Research opportunities are available in the summer following the first year. In addition, there is a Research Honors Program in which the student devotes a full year to research between the second and third years. An integrated M.D.-Ph.D. program providing stipends and tuition scholarships to especially qualified candidates is also available.

A dually accredited joint M.B.A.–M.D. program is offered in which qualified students may earn both degrees within a four-year period beginning the summer before entry to medical school. Students will complete a 54-hour M.B.A. in Health Organization Management in addition to the M.D.

Students are graded using a categorical grading system: Honors, High Pass, Pass, Low Pass and Fail.

REQUIREMENTS FOR ENTRANCE

At least three years of study (90 semester hours) with recorded grades in a U.S.- or Canadian-accredited college or university are required. All prerequisite courses must be taken in a U.S. or Canadian school. The completion of four years of college and a B.S. or B.A. degree is *highly desirable* before entrance into medical school.

Specific course requirements have been kept at a minimum to permit maximum flexibility in the selection of well-rounded students. Graded prerequisite courses require a grade of "C" or better.

Sem. hrs. or AP credit

Biology or Zoology 12
Biology lab (minimum) 2
Inorganic Chemistry (with lab) 8
Organic Chemistry (with lab). 8
Physics (with lab) 8
Calculus (or Math-based Statistics) 3
English 6

The MCAT is also a requirement for admission. It is recommended that students take the MCAT in the spring of the year in which application will be made.

SELECTION FACTORS

Applications are invited from qualified residents of the state of Texas and service area counties of New Mexico and Oklahoma. Only U.S. citizens or applicants with permanent resident visas are considered. Application forms and procedural information may be obtained from the Texas Medical and Dental Schools Application Service (www.utsystem.edu/tmdsas). A secondary application to Texas Tech University Health Sciences Center School of Medicine is also required and is linked to the main application *or* via www.ttuhsc.edu/som/admissions.

The Admissions Committee carefully reviews the applications of all individuals meeting the entrance requirements. Although evidence of high intellectual ability and a record of strong academic achievement are essential for success in the study of medicine, the committee also looks for such qualities as compassion, motivation, the ability to communicate with people, maturity, and personal integrity. There is no discrimination on the basis of race, sex, creed, national origin, age, or disability.

Personal interviews are offered to those candidates deemed competitive for admission. Interviews are conducted at the Lubbock and El Paso campuses.

Students in the 2003 entering class had the following credentials: *mean GPA,* 3.63; 41 percent *women;* 8 percent *Hispanic/Mexican American,* 2 percent *Black/African American* and 25 percent *Asian;* 67 percent *science majors;* 93 percent Texas *residents.*

FINANCIAL AID

Financial aid is available for students who demonstrate need. Applications for financial assistance are processed after an applicant has been accepted. Detailed information on available programs can be obtained from the Office of Student Financial Aid. Over 93 percent of the student body receive some type of financial assistance. Employment, other than during the summer, is discouraged.

INFORMATION FOR DISADVANTAGED STUDENTS

The School of Medicine takes disadvantaged status into account in evaluation of an applicant's overall status. Qualified students from educationally and/or socioeconomically disadvantaged backgrounds are encouraged to apply.

SPECIAL PROGRAMS

Agreements have been developed with Texas Tech University Health Sciences Center School of Medicine, Texas Tech University, West Texas A&M University, University of Texas at El Paso and Austin College to provide early acceptance of qualified students into TTUHSC School of Medicine. In order to qualify for an interview in the third semester of college, applicants must meet entrance requirements, including an established performance on the SAT/ACT, and maintenance of a high grade point average (GPA), including a specified number of prerequisite courses. All coursework must be taken at the college/university through which the applicant is

applying. The applicant will then be invited to the Lubbock campus for an interview. If the Admissions Committee recommends acceptance of the applicant, and provided the applicant maintains the required GPA for the remainder of their undergraduate education, candidates are guaranteed admission to Texas Tech School of Medicine in the fall following graduation with a Bachelor's degree. The Medical College Admissions Test (MCAT) is waived for these applicants.

Institution Type: *Public*
Application Process: *Texas Medical and Dental Schools Application Service*

APPLICATION AND ACCEPTANCE POLICIES FOR 2005–2006 FIRST-YEAR CLASS

Filing of application
    Earliest date: May 1, 2004
    Latest date: Nov. 1, 2004
Main application fee to all applicants: $55 plus $10 for each additional school. (Nonresidents–$100 plus $10 for each additional school.)
Secondary application fee to TTUHSC School of Medicine–$40 (required – *subject to change*)
Oldest MCAT scores considered: 2001
Does have Early Decision Program (EDP)
    For Texas residents only
    EDP application period: May 1–August 1, 2004
    EDP applicants notified by: Oct. 1, 2004
Acceptance notice to regular applicants
    Earliest date: Feb. 1, 2005
    Latest date: Until class is filled
Applicant's response to acceptance offer
    Maximum time: 2 weeks
Requests for deferred entrance considered: Yes
Placement guarantee fee to hold place in class:
    $100, due April 1, 2005 (nonrefundable)
Estimated number of new entrants: 140 (1 EDP)
Starting date: Aug. 2005

TUITION AND STUDENT FEES PER YEAR FOR 2003–2004 FIRST-YEAR CLASS

Tuition   Student fees: $1,181
    Resident: $7,654
    Nonresident: $20,754

INFORMATION ON 2003–2004 FIRST-YEAR CLASS

Number of	In-State	Out-of-State	Total
Applicants	2,036	166	2,202
Applicants Interviewed	633	18	651
New Entrants†	124	6	130

*Includes $701 general use fee.
†100% took the MCAT and had baccalaureate degrees.

CHAPTER

11

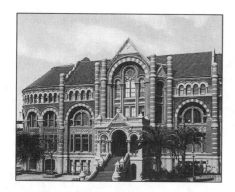

University of Texas
Medical School at Galveston

Galveston, Texas

Dr. Stanley M. Lemon, *Dean*
Dr. Lauree Thomas, *Associate Dean for Student Affairs and Admissions*
Betty Hazelbaker, *Director, Student Financial Aid*

ADDRESS INQUIRIES TO:

Office of Medical School Admissions
University of Texas Medical Branch at Galveston
301 University Boulevard
Galveston, Texas 77555-1317
(409) 772-3517; 747-2909 (FAX)
E-mail: tsilva@utmb.edu
Web site: www.utmb.edu

GENERAL INFORMATION

The University of Texas Medical Branch (UTMB) at Galveston was established in 1891 and graduated its first class in 1892. It is a state-owned medical center with the Medical Branch hospitals under direct supervision of the UTMB administration. The Medical Branch has 8 hospitals with 923 open beds, 75 hospital clinics, and 93 outpatient clinics. The Shriners Burn Institute, the Marine Biomedical Institute, and the Institute for the Medical Humanities also serve as teaching and research facilities.

CURRICULUM

The University of Texas Medical Branch School of Medicine has as its mission to provide innovative teaching, scholarly scientific investigation, and state of the art patient care in a learning environment to better the health of Texas. The Integrated Medical Curriculum (IMC) is a four-year program that emphasizes continuous integration of basic medical sciences with clinical medicine, early clinical skills and clinical experiences, and professionalism. In this student-centered curriculum, which utilizes small group problem based learning, computer assisted instruction, lectures, and labs, the basic medical sciences are learned in clinical contexts. Beyond knowledge acquisition, the IMC emphasizes the development of skills in problem solving, clinical data-gathering and decision-making, independent study, and lifelong learning. Its organ system based approach and clinical science contexts promote basic science integration across disciplines.

Through all four years of the IMC, there is a heavy emphasis on the acquisition and refinement of clinical skills through working with standardized patients beginning the first week of medical school. The 3rd and 4th years of the IMC, revised in 2003, are centered on ambulatory and inpatient experiences in Emergency Medicine, Family Medicine, Internal Medicine, Neurology, Obstetrics & Gynecology, Pediatrics, Psychiatry,

and Surgery. A unique feature of the 3rd year curriculum is an elective month, which allows students to expand their experience in a primary care field or to explore potential career interests in a medical specialty. The 4th year also includes an acting internship, community-based ambulatory medicine, and a scholarly project in which a basic science or medical humanities topic is explored in depth. The twenty weeks of electives, depending upon previous academic performance, may be taken at approved US or international sites. UTMB employs a grading system of Honors, High Pass, Pass, and Fail for the required core courses and Pass/Fail for the elective courses.

REQUIREMENTS FOR ENTRANCE

The MCAT and a minimum of 90 semester hours of college work including specific courses are required. The baccalaureate degree is highly desirable. Coursework is acceptable only if completed at U.S. colleges and universities with accreditation from one of the regional accrediting agencies.

Applicants are encouraged to take the MCAT in the spring of the year of application. MCAT taken in the fall of the year of anticipated matriculation may be received too late for consideration. Applicants are encouraged to complete the required courses and/or take the MCAT by the time they submit an application.

The required courses are: *Years*
Biology 2
  One year must include lab.
Inorganic Chemistry (with lab) 1
Organic Chemistry (with lab). 1
General Physics (with lab) 1
Calculus or Math-based Statistics . . . . ½
English 1

Science courses should be equivalent to coursework required for college science majors. A broad background in the humanities is encouraged.

SELECTION FACTORS

All information available is utilized in the selection process. The most significant factors are intellect, achievement, character, interpersonal skills, and motivation. In evaluating candidates, consideration is given to the total academic record, the results of aptitude and achievement tests, college preprofessional committee evaluations, and the personal interview. Only those applicants whose personal qualifications, academic records, aptitude, achievement test scores, and preprofessional evaluations are considered sufficiently competitive are invited for personal interviews. Only U.S. citizens or applicants with permanent visas are considered. Preference is given to legal residents of Texas. Up to 10 percent of the class may be filled with residents of other states.

Accepted applicants for the 2002 entering class had the following credentials: *average GPA,* 3.64; *average total MCAT score* 27: *residence,* 98 percent from Texas.

FINANCIAL AID

Long-term, low-interest loans and short-term loans of varying interest rates are available to students with financial need. A number of scholarships funded by private donors are available. Most of these are based on need; some are based on academic achievement. A number of scholarships are available to disadvantaged students. Students must provide parents' information on the Free Application for Federal Student Aid (FAFSA) in order to be considered for certain individual scholarships and grants. Considerable individual attention is provided to students to help them with their fiscal planning, debt management, and exploration of various funding options. Applications for financial assistance are provided to students who have been accepted for admission and have indicated that they will attend the University of Texas Medical School at Galveston. There are no fixed deadlines. Inquiries must be directed to the Office of Enrollment Services.

INFORMATION FOR ECONOMICALLY AND DISADVANTAGED STUDENTS

The University of Texas Medical Branch at Galveston is committed to increasing the number of disadvantaged students in medicine. Each applicant is reviewed by experienced members of the Committee on Admissions with particular emphasis on the applicant's potential. Both cognitive and noncognitive qualifications are considered. All applicants are considered on the basis of individual achievement and promise. Following admission, a broad range of support services are available to assist students in completing the medical curriculum. Specific information about the services provided to applicants can be obtained by contacting the Office of Student Affairs. The University of Texas Medical Branch does not discriminate on the basis of race, sex, creed, national origin, age, or handicap.

Institution Type: *Public*
Application Process: *Texas Medical and Dental Schools Application Service*

APPLICATION AND ACCEPTANCE POLICIES FOR 2005–2006 FIRST-YEAR CLASS

Filing of application
  Earliest date: May 1, 2004
  Latest date: Nov. 1, 2004
School application fee: None
Application center fees
  Resident: $55 for application to one school plus
    $10 for each additional school applied to in the
    University of Texas System
  Nonresident: $100 for application to one school plus
    $10 for each additional school applied to in the
    University of Texas System
Oldest MCAT scores considered: April 2000
Does not have Early Decision Program
Acceptance notice to regular applicants
  Earliest date: Feb. 1, 2005
  Latest date: Until class is filled
Applicant's response to acceptance offer
  Maximum time: 2 weeks
Requests for deferred entrance considered: Yes
Deposit to hold place in class: None
Estimated number of new entrants: 200
Starting date: Aug. 2005

TUITION AND STUDENT FEES PER YEAR FOR 2003–2004 FIRST-YEAR CLASS

Tuition   Student fees: $627
  Resident: $7,450
  Nonresident: $20,550

INFORMATION ON 2003–2004 FIRST-YEAR CLASS

Number of	In-State	Out-of-State	Total
Applicants	2,378	329	2,707
Applicants Interviewed	876	105	981
New Entrants*	195	10	205

*All took the MCAT; 99% had baccalaureate degrees.

CHAPTER

11

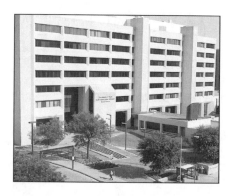

University of Texas
Medical School at Houston

Houston, Texas

Dr. Stanley G. Shultz, *Interim Dean*
Dr. Albert E. Gunn, *Associate Dean for Admissions*
Cristina R. Mendez, *Coordinator of Admissions*

ADDRESS INQUIRIES TO:

Office of Admissions-Room 1.126
University of Texas
Medical School at Houston
6431 Fannin, Suite 1.126
Houston, Texas 77030
(713) 500-5116; 500-0604 (FAX)
Web site: www.med.uth.tmc.edu

MISSION STATEMENT

The mission of the University of Texas Medical School at Houston is to provide the highest quality of education and training of future physicians for the state of Texas, in harmony with the state's diverse population, and to conduct the highest caliber of research in the biomedical and health sciences.

GENERAL INFORMATION

The University of Texas Medical School at Houston was authorized in May 1969 by the Texas Legislature. The Medical school is part of the University of Texas System.

The medical school is located in the Texas Medical Center in Houston in order to take advantage of the many other medical institutions in the area. The major teaching hospital is Memorial Hermann Hospital, a 650-bed general medical and surgical hospital. Other major teaching hospitals include the University of Texas M.D. Anderson Cancer Center, St. Joseph Hospital, San Jose Clinic, Southwest Memorial Hospital, and the Lyndon Baines Johnson Hospital, a facility of the Harris County Hospital District.

CURRICULUM

In September 1977 a four-year educational program began. The first two academic years are divided into four semesters. Three months of vacation time are provided for first-year students between the first and second academic years. The initial four semesters are devoted to preparing the student for the specific clerkship experiences that constitute the clinical years. During the first two academic years the student becomes familiar with the basic and applied biomedical sciences. As the student progresses from a study of the morphology of the human body and the fundamentals of molecular and cellular biology to that of the normal and abnormal structure and function of the various organ systems, the techniques of interviewing, history

taking, and performance of physical and mental status examinations are introduced. Appropriate material from the behavioral sciences is presented concomitantly, as are opportunities to become familiar with the realities and problems of human medicine and family practice.

After completion of this educational sequence, the student progresses through a series of clinical clerkships in the major clinical disciplines for the next 12 months. In the remaining year, there are four months of required clerkships, four periods of electives, and one period reserved for additional instruction in medical jurisprudence, clinical epidemiology, medical ethics, and technical skills. In consultation with faculty, each student devises an educational sequence that relates specifically to ultimate career goals and postgraduate educational plans.

Problem-based learning is extensively employed in achieving the school's educational objectives.

REQUIREMENTS FOR ENTRANCE

Students must take the MCAT and complete at least 90 undergraduate credit hours at a U.S. or Canadian university. A baccalaureate degree is highly desirable and recommended. The specific premedical credits listed below are required.

	Sem. hrs.
Biology	14
One year must include lab.	
Inorganic Chemistry (with lab)	8
Organic Chemistry (with lab).	8
Physics (with lab)	8
Calculus.	3
English	6

While the applicant should demonstrate aptitude for and achievement in the basic sciences, it is essential that an in-depth experience in some area of the humanities be obtained. Liberal arts majors are encouraged.

Applicants should take the MCAT in the spring of the year of application.

SELECTION FACTORS

Applicants are selected on the basis of motivation and potential for service, especially in the state of Texas. Academic ability is evaluated to ensure those who are accepted can complete medical studies. Emphasis is given to students who have a broad education and who display intellectual interest. A command of the language with ability to write and speak well is essential. The applicant's academic record is evaluated with special attention to the subjects taken and the demonstration of a broadly based comprehensive educational experience. The overall philosophy is that knowledge is an end in itself; while vocational-type curricula are not ruled out, liberal arts are preferred. Universities with core curricula generally provide the type of diversity sought in subject distribution. Significant attention is given to humanitarian endeavors, achievement in a nonacademic field of activity, and specific interest by the applicant in the University of Texas Medical School at Houston. Applicants are invited for personal interviews based on the admissions criteria available on our Web site. In the interview, which is an important element in the selection process, applicants are expected to cogently discuss their motivation and the experiences that led them to a medical career. It is also anticipated they will discuss their intellectual interests and generally demonstrate their suitability to enter a learned profession. Admission decisions are made in light of the school's mission, with preference given to Texas residents and those who will practice in shortage areas and specialties in the state. Veterans status is also considered. The University of Texas Medical School at Houston does not discriminate on the basis of race, sex, creed, national origin, age, or handicap.

Accepted students for the 2003 entering class had the following credentials: *mean GPA,* 3.64; *residence,* 96.0 percent from Texas; *mean MCAT,* BS-9.7, PS-9.5, VR-9.2, WS-P. For additional information concerning admissions criteria for the University of Texas Medical School at Houston, go to www.med.uth.tmc.edu/.

FINANCIAL AID

Scholarship and loan funds are available to students with financial need from local, state, federal, and national sources. Financial independence is not a criterion for admission as indicated by the fact that 88 percent of the students enrolled at present have received financial aid.

Institution Type: *Public*
Application Process: *Texas Medical and Dental Schools Application Service*

APPLICATION AND ACCEPTANCE POLICIES FOR 2005–2006 FIRST-YEAR CLASS

Filing of application
    Earliest date: May 1, 2004
    Latest date: Nov. 1, 2004
School application fee: None
Application center fees
    Resident: $55 for application to one school plus
        $10 for each additional school applied to of those
        participating
    Nonresident: $100 for application to one school plus
        $10 for each additional school applied to of those
        participating
Oldest MCAT scores considered: 2000
Does not have Early Decision Program
Acceptance notice to regular applicants
    Earliest date: Feb. 1, 2005
    Latest date: Until class is filled
Applicant's response to acceptance offer
    Maximum time: 2 weeks
Requests for deferred entrance considered: No
Deposit to hold place in class: None
Estimated number of new entrants: 200
Starting date: August 2005

TUITION AND STUDENT FEES PER YEAR FOR 2003–2004 FIRST-YEAR CLASS

Tuition   Student fees: $1,587
  Resident: $8,275
  Nonresident: $21,375

INFORMATION ON 2003–2004 FIRST-YEAR CLASS

Number of	In-State	Out-of-State	Total
Applicants	2,378	378	2,756
Applicants Interviewed	1,090	50	1,140
New Entrants*	194	8	202

*All took the MCAT; 100% had baccalaureate degrees.

CHAPTER

11

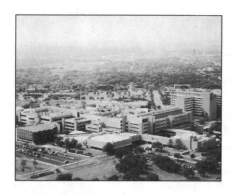

University of Texas
Medical School at San Antonio

San Antonio, Texas

Dr. Steven A. Wartman, *Dean*
Dr. David J. Jones, *Associate Dean for Admissions*
Dr. Leonard E. Lawrence, *Associate Dean for Student Affairs*

ADDRESS INQUIRIES TO:

Medical School Admissions
Registrar's Office - MSC 7702
University of Texas Health Science Center at San Antonio
7703 Floyd Curl Drive
San Antonio, Texas 78229-3900
(210) 567-2665; 567-2645 (FAX)
E-mail: msprospect@uthscsa.edu
Web site: http://som.uthscsa.edu

MISSION STATEMENT

The mission of the UTHSCSA Medical School is to serve the needs of the citizens of Texas by: providing medical education and training to medical students and physicians at all career levels with special commitment to the preparation of physicians for careers in the practice of primary health care; conducting biomedical and other health-related research; delivering exemplary quality health care; and providing a responsive resource in health-related affairs for the nation and the state, with particular emphasis on South Texas.

GENERAL INFORMATION

The University of Texas Medical School at San Antonio was created by the Texas Legislature in 1959 as a four-year school of medicine and graduated its first class in 1970. In late 1972 the medical school and its fellow institutions, the Dental School, and the Graduate School of Biomedical Sciences were designated the University of Texas Health Science Center at San Antonio. Clinical instruction is carried out at the University Hospital, University Health Center, Audie Murphy Veterans Hospital, and affiliated hospitals, which include Santa Rosa Medical Center, Wilford Hall USAF Hospital, Brooke Army Hospital, the Aerospace Medical Division of USAF, and Baptist Memorial Hospital System.

The Regional Academic Health Center located in the Rio Grande Valley in Harlingen, Texas, is a second clinical education campus. At the end of their second year, twenty four students will move to Harlingen to complete their third and fourth years of medical school. The third year students will rotate through all of the clinical clerkships at the Harlingen campus: internal medicine, surgery, Obstetrics and Gynecology, pediatrics, psychiatry, and family practice. Fourth year students will participate in the same didactic and externship opportunities available at the San Antonio campus. Clinical training facilities include Valley Baptist Hospital and Su Clinica Familiar, both of which are located in Harlingen, Texas.

CURRICULUM

A four-year curriculum is offered. The first month is devoted to an introduction to patient care, and throughout the first two years one-half day per week is devoted to clinical integration activities. In the first year, the traditional basic science courses are taught. The second year is anchored by the pathology course, and it incorporates pharmacology, medicine, pediatrics, obstetrics and gynecology, and surgery coordinated by organ systems. Behavioral sciences and an introduction to psychiatry are also included. The third academic year is spent entirely in the clinical setting in eight consecutive assignments of six weeks each in family practice, medicine, the medical specialties, surgery, the surgical specialties, obstetrics and gynecology, psychiatry, and pediatrics. The senior year includes a didactic period of two months, with the rest of the academic year consisting of elective courses. Some time is also available to the students for interviews for postgraduate training or for vacation. A letter grading system is used.

REQUIREMENTS FOR ENTRANCE

The MCAT and the equivalent of three academic years (90 semester hours) are required for admission. Courses specifically required (with a grade of C or better) are:

	Sem. Hrs.
Biology	14
One year must include lab.	
Inorganic Chemistry (with lab)	8
Organic Chemistry (with lab)	8
General Physics (with lab)	8
Calculus or Math-based Statistics	3
English	6

Science courses should be equivalent to coursework as required for college science majors. Candidates are desired who have a broad humanities background.

SELECTION FACTORS

Ranking of applicants is done with consideration for: GPA; separate MCAT component scores; evaluation by premedical advisors; the candidate's potential relative to society's health care needs; and judgment by the Committee on Admissions of the candidate's nonacademic achievements and personal qualifications such as responsibility, integrity, maturity, and motivation. In addition, bilingual language ability, hometown or county of residence that has been designated a medically underserved area, socioeconomic history, positions of leadership held, communication skills and clinical/volunteer experiences are considered. No person shall be excluded from participation in, denied the benefits of, or subject to discrimination under any program or activity sponsored or conducted by the University of Texas System on the basis of age, race, national origin, religion, or sex. Although legal residents of Texas are preferred, up to 10 percent of entrants may be nonresidents if their credentials are especially outstanding.

Accepted students for the 2003 entering class had the following credentials: *mean GPA,* 3.50 (range 2.7–4.0); *mean total MCAT score* 28 (range 20–35); *sex,* 60 percent women; *residence,* 5 percent nonresidents; *overall acceptance rate,* 235 acceptances were offered to obtain a class of 200 first-year students.

All procedural information including electronic submission of applications is available through the Texas Medical and Dental Schools Application Service.

Questions related to completeness of an application or other information should be directed to the Office of Student Services, Medical Admissions at the Health Science Center (msprospect@uthscsa.edu).

Further information is available at ✏ http://student services.uthscsa.edu/.

FINANCIAL AID

Financial assistance for students in need is available in the form of loans and a limited number of scholarships. Student employment, though not encouraged, is permissible provided a satisfactory level of achievement is maintained. Part-time student employment opportunities are available at the Health Science Center as well as in the hospitals located in close proximity. Financial considerations do not influence admission decisions, although the school recognizes that many families are unable to bear the full cost of medical education. Accepted applicants can obtain complete information regarding financial assistance from the financial aid administrator in the Office of Student Services (✏ http://studentservices.uthsca.edu).

Institution Type: *Public*
Application Process: *Texas Medical and Dental Schools Application Service*

APPLICATION AND ACCEPTANCE POLICIES FOR 2005–2006 FIRST-YEAR CLASS

Filing of application
    Earliest date: May 1, 2004
    Latest date: Nov. 1, 2004
School application fee: None
Application center fees
    Resident: $55 for application to one school plus
        $10 for each additional school
    Nonresident: $100 for application to one school plus
        $10 for each additional school
Oldest MCAT scores considered: 2001
Does not have Early Decision Program
Acceptance notice to regular applicants
    Earliest date: Feb. 1, 2005
    Latest date: Until class is filled
Applicant's response to acceptance offer
    Maximum time: 2 weeks
Requests for deferred entrance considered: Yes
Deposit to hold place in class: None
Estimated number of new entrants: 200
Starting date: July 2005

TUITION AND STUDENT FEES PER YEAR FOR 2003–2004 FIRST-YEAR CLASS

Tuition   Student fees: $3,475
    Resident: $6,550
    Nonresident: $19,650

INFORMATION ON 2003–2004 FIRST-YEAR CLASS

Number of	In-State	Out-of-State	Total
Applicants	2,387	321	2,708
Applicants Interviewed	879	71	950
New Entrants*	196	8	204

*All took the MCAT; 98% had baccalaureate degrees.

CHAPTER
11

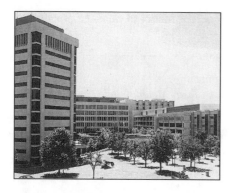

University of Texas Southwestern Medical Center at Dallas Southwestern Medical School

Dallas, Texas

Dr. Robert J. Alpern, *Dean*
Dr. Susanna Parker, *Associate Dean for Student Affairs*
Dr. James Wagner, *Associate Dean for Student Affairs*
Dr. J. Scott Wright, *Director of Admissions*
Dr. Byron Cryer, *Associate Dean for Minority Student Affairs*

ADDRESS INQUIRIES TO:

University of Texas
Southwestern Medical Center at Dallas
5323 Harry Hines Boulevard
Dallas, Texas 75390-9162
(214) 648-5617; 648-3289 (FAX)
Web site: www.utsouthwestern.edu/medapp
E-mail: admissions@utsouthwestern.edu

MISSION STATEMENT

Southwestern Medical School's mission is to produce physicians who will care for patients in a responsible and humanistic manner and maintain lifelong medical scholarship. An important focus of UT Southwestern's educational efforts is training primary care physicians and preparing doctors who will practice in under-served areas of Texas. Additionally, the medical school seeks to prepare students seeking careers in academic medicine and research.

GENERAL INFORMATION

Southwestern Medical School, founded in 1943, is a part of the University of Texas Southwestern Medical Center at Dallas, a multifaceted academic institution nationally recognized for its excellence in educating physicians, biomedical scientists, and health care professionals. Located just north of downtown Dallas, the 100-acre campus includes modern classrooms and laboratories and an extensive medical library, as well as a recreation center, tennis and indoor and outdoor basketball courts, jogging paths, and a six-acre wooded bird sanctuary. Clinical training takes place at university sites and affiliated institutions including Parkland Memorial Hospital, the James Aston Ambulatory Care Center, Zale Lipshy University Hospital, Children's Medical Center, Dallas Veterans Affairs Medical Center, Southwestern Institute of Forensic Sciences, Baylor University Medical Center, Presbyterian Hospital of Dallas, Methodist Hospitals of Dallas, St. Paul Medical Center, Texas Scottish Rite Hospital for Children, and John Peter Smith Hospital in Fort Worth.

CURRICULUM

Southwestern Medical School offers a four-year curriculum based on departmental as well as interdisciplinary teaching. The purpose of the first two years is to provide a strong background in the basic sciences as well as an introduction to clinical medicine.

The first-year curriculum is designed to begin the study of the normal human body and its processes at the molecular and cellular levels. Biochemistry, anatomy, and genetics are presented concurrently for the first portion of the year, building together the concepts of macromolecular and cellular interactions within tissues. A problem-based course, Clinical Ethics in Medicine, introduces first-year students to taking histories from standardized patients along with content in ethics, human behavior, and prevention. The spring term is composed of courses in physiology and neurosciences, cell biology, and human behavior and psychopathology. At the completion of the first year, a vertical course in human reproduction and endocrinology provides an overall synthesis, based on the previous coursework.

The second year is an organ-system-based curriculum that integrates pharmacology, microbiology, pathology, and clinical medicine. It begins a study of core principles and then proceeds through each organ system, where these integrated topics are discussed. Contact with patients begins early in the second year with history taking and physical examination as well as visits to outpatient clinics.

The third and fourth years provide intense clinical experiences involving the student in direct inpatient and outpatient care. The junior year is composed of 12 weeks of internal medicine, 6 weeks each of psychiatry and obstetrics/gynecology, 8 weeks each of surgery and pediatrics, and 4 weeks of family practice. The fourth year provides a series of one-month clinical rotations; required months in neurology, subinternship in internal medicine on a ward or an intensive care unit, an ambulatory care rotation, and an acute care rotation. In addition, there are four months of electives.

Every year the curriculum becomes more computer based. Learning material in multimedia format is presently provided by direct network connection as well as CD-ROM. Therefore, UT Southwestern requires each student to own a personal computer for use during the first two years of medical school. Purchase and support of student computers are facilitated by the medical school. Additionally, several computer labs dedicated exclusively to student use are available on campus.

REQUIREMENTS FOR ENTRANCE

The MCAT (taken within the last five years) and at least three years (90 semester hours) of accredited college work are required. Preference is given to applicants who have or will have earned a bachelor's degree. Minimum course requirements are:

340

	Years
Biology	2

One year must include lab.

Inorganic Chemistry (with lab)	1
Organic Chemistry (with lab)	1
Physics (with lab)	1
Calculus or Statistics	½
English	1

We strongly encourage applicants to take one semester of biochemistry. Sound preparation in basic science is essential, but a broad background in the humanities and an understanding of people and their problems are equally necessary. Applicants are urged to take the MCAT in the spring of the year of application and to complete required coursework before applying, if possible.

SELECTION FACTORS

The Admissions Committee considers all of the following in evaluating each applicant's acceptability: scores from the MCAT; academic performance in college as reflected in the GPA; the rigor of the undergraduate curriculum; recommendations from the college premedical committee or college faculty; extracurricular activities; socioeconomic background; time spent in outside employment; personal integrity and compassion for others; the ability to communicate; other personal qualities and individual factors such as leadership, social/family support, self-appraisal, maturity/coping skills, and determination; and motivation for a career in medicine. In addition, applicants are evaluated with regard to the mission of Southwestern Medical School. State law requires that at least 90 percent of the class be residents of Texas. Therefore, the minimum credentials for nonresidents are more stringent than those for Texas residents.

Early application is strongly advised. A personal on-campus interview is required and is initiated by invitation from the Admissions Committee. Interviews are held on Saturdays from early September until mid-December.

FINANCIAL AID

UT Southwestern works directly with students to obtain funding for their medical education. Most of the financial aid available is obtained through federal and state loan programs. However, a limited number of scholarships from private sources are available. Nonresidents are eligible to pay resident tuition on receipt of a competitive academic scholarship. Students rarely discontinue school for financial reasons.

INFORMATION ABOUT DIVERSITY PROGRAMS

The Admissions Committee at Southwestern Medical School recognizes the need for increased numbers of physicians from groups underrepresented in medicine and encourages applications from Texas residents who are members of these groups.

COMBINED DEGREE PROGRAMS

Southwestern Medical School offers the combined M.D.-Ph.D. Program for those qualified individuals who intend to pursue careers as physician-scientists. The medical school also offers a program leading to the degree M.D. with Research Distinction to recognize students who distinguish themselves in the conduct of meaningful clinical or basic research activities and to encourage them to develop their capabilities and enlarge their research experience during medical school. Additionally, UT Southwestern offers five-year programs leading to the M.D.-M.B.A. degrees (with the School of Management at the University of Texas at Dallas) and the M.D./M.P.H. degrees (with the University of Texas at Houston School of Public Health).

Institution Type: *Public*
Application Process: *Texas Medical and Dental Schools Application Service* and AMCAS***

*M.D. program (www.utsystem.edu/tmdsas)
**M.D./Ph.D. applications
Contact the admission office for more information.

APPLICATION AND ACCEPTANCE POLICIES FOR 2005–2006 FIRST-YEAR CLASS

Filing of application
  Earliest date: May 1, 2004
  Latest date: Nov. 1, 2004
School application fee to all applicants: none
Oldest MCAT scores considered: 2000
Does not have Early Decision Program
Acceptance notice to regular applicants
  Earliest date: Feb. 1, 2005
  Latest date: Varies
Applicant's response to acceptance offer
  Maximum time: 3 weeks
Requests for deferred entrance considered: Yes
Deposit to hold place in class: None
Estimated number of new entrants: 220
Starting date: Aug. 2005

TUITION AND STUDENT FEES PER YEAR FOR 2003–2004 FIRST-YEAR CLASS

Tuition   Student fees: $1,272
  Resident: $7,660
  Nonresident*: $20,760

INFORMATION ON 2003–2004 FIRST-YEAR CLASS

Number of	In-State	Out-of-State	Total
Applicants	2,231	399	2,630
Applicants Interviewed	574	69	643
New Entrants†	195	23	218

*Nonresidents are eligible to pay resident tuition on receipt of a competitive academic scholarship.

†All took the MCAT; 98% had baccalaureate degrees.

CHAPTER **11**

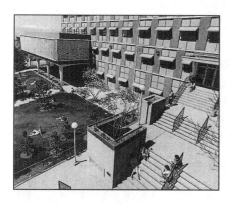

University of Utah School of Medicine

Salt Lake City, Utah

Dr. Lorris Betz, *Senior Vice President for Health Sciences*
Dr. David J. Bjorkman, *Interim Dean*
Dr. Wayne M. Samuelson, *Associate Dean*
Dr. Ronald M. Harris, *Assistant Dean*

ADDRESS INQUIRIES TO:

Kathy Z. Doulis
Director of Admissions
University of Utah School of Medicine
30 North 1900 East Room 1C029
Salt Lake City, Utah 84132-2101
(801) 581-8546; FAX (801) 581-2931
E-mail: kathy.doulis@hsc.utah.edu
Web site: http://uuhsc.utah.edu/som

CURRICULUM

In the first two years of medical school, students will receive a solid foundation in the sciences basic to medicine, including gross anatomy, embryology, histology, biochemistry, pharmacology, immunology, microbiology, genetics, physiology, pathology, and organ system pathophysiology. Courses cover such topics as health-care financing and delivery, community and public health, research methodology and medical literature analysis, biostatistics, and epidemiology. The critical skills of communicating with, examining, and diagnosing patients are also covered in depth.

The third year of the curriculum centers on clinical clerkships in internal medicine, surgery, obstetrics and gynecology, pediatrics, family practice, psychiatry, and neurology.

During the fourth year a sub-internship, which serves as a transition to residency, and a 2-week medical ethics course, are also required.

REQUIREMENTS FOR ENTRANCE

The Admissions Committee is eager to admit students with a broad perspective of life. The school believes that the true physician not only is skilled in medicine and the allied sciences but also is a person of culture and broad intelligence.

The MCAT is required and must be taken within three years of application.

A bachelor's degree and undergraduate transcript is required before entering the School of Medicine. Only applicants who have completed most of their schooling in an accredited U.S. or Canadian college or university will be considered. In addition to a bachelor's degree, the applicant must have subject matter competence in the following courses:

Chemistry: Two (2) years that should include both a general chemistry series including a laboratory (incorporating both quantitative and qualitative analysis) and an organic series that includes a laboratory: Advanced Placement credit earned with a score of 4 or 5 is acceptable toward fulfillment of this requirement.

Physics: One (1) year with a laboratory.

Writing/Speech: One (1) year of courses that emphasize written and/or verbal communication.

Biology: Two (2) courses. One (1) course must be in cellular biology or biochemistry.

Social Science: One (1) course. (history, economics, anthropology, psychology)

Humanities: One (1) course. (e.g., art, music, drama, literature, etc.)

Diversity: One (1) course that focuses on the culture, history and/or current circumstances of one or more non-dominant groups in the United States. (e.g., Ethnic Minorities in the United States, Introduction to Gender Studies, Gender and Social Change, Racial and Ethnic Politics.) Diversity course(s) taken to fulfill requirements of the degree granting undergraduate institution are acceptable.

All required prerequisites must be completed prior to medical school matriculation.

Advanced Placement, CLEP, independent study, online, or correspondence courses will not be accepted for these requirements (except for general chemistry as noted above). All premedical coursework must be completed at an accredited college or university in the United States or Canada.

Letters of Recommendation (6):

• Academic letters (3 letters): One must be from a science professor. letters must clearly indicate the professor who taught the applicant in a classroom setting.

• Supervisor letter (3 letters): Letters documenting research, community service and medical experience (patient exposure of M.D. shadowing) are required. The letters must clearly indicate the applicant's relationship with the letter writer.

SELECTION FACTORS

The School of Medicine carefully considers both the cognitive and noncognitive credentials of an applicant. Cognitive credentials include science, non-science, and overall GPA. MCAT scores, breadth and difficulty of academic coursework, and other criteria. Noncognitive credentials include a sincere and appropriate motivation for attending medical school, a realistic self-appraisal, adequate awareness of the medical profession, leadership ability, demonstrated ability to handle the demands of medical school and the medical profession, commitment to community service, and the ability to communicate and interact with patients compassionately, ethically and effectively and demonstration of professional behavior in all interactions.

The majority of positions (approximately 75) are offered to established Utah residents. Eight positions are reserved for residents of Idaho (under contractual arrangements) and approximately 19 are available to nonresidents. For consideration, nonresidents must apply to the M.D./Ph.D. program (applications are available for U.S. citizens and permanent U.S. residents only), be specifically recognized as a member of a population group underrepresented in the physician workforce, or have significant ties to Utah (i.e. lived in, own property in, or have family member who live in Utah).

All offers of acceptance are conditional upon satisfactory results of a criminal background check. The Student Handbook sets students guidelines and discusses the School of Medicine's disciplinary process and associated due process procedures. Students are provided a copy during the first week of orientation and are expected to follow its guidelines.

Students entering in the fall of 2003 had a *mean* GPA of 3.6 and *mean* MCAT score of 30.

Application may be made no more than three consecutive times. Transfer positions to the medical school are available only if the spouse of the transferring student is a member of our medical school faculty or is accepted into one of our postgraduate residency-training programs. Medical students in their third year who have successfully completed USMLE Step 1 and are enrolled in a fully LCME-accredited United States or Canadian medical school in good standing may be considered for transfer if a position is available.

The Admissions Committee will not consider applicants who have been dismissed, are on probation, or have been suspended from another medical school. If reinstated they may be eligible for transfer under the current transfer policy.

The School of Medicine has specific policies against discrimination with respect to an applicant's age, gender, sexual orientation, race, national origin, religion, disability and status as a Vietnam or disabled veteran. The University of Utah provides reasonable accommodations to the known disabilities of applicants. Detailed information is available at our Web site ✑ www.med.utah.edu/som.

FINANCIAL AID

In addition to the federal subsidized and unsubsidized Stafford Loans and Federal Perkins Loan, a limited number of institutional loans and scholarships are awarded each year. All awards are based on the student's need as determined by the University of Utah Financial Aid Office. Financial aid is supplementary to the contribution that can be made by the student and/or family, who are expected to provide the maximum assistance possible.

THE OFFICE OF DIVERSITY AND COMMUNITY OUTREACH

Under the direction of the assistant dean of diversity and community outreach, this office assists the School of Medicine in fulfilling its commitment to recruiting, admitting, and graduating a diverse student body, working closely with applicants from varied backgrounds, including applicants from rural Utah communities and those who are educationally, socially or financially disadvantaged and applicants from those groups underrepresented among the physician work force in the United States. The office provides academic advising and assistance to these applicants in their preparation for and application to medical school, and presents a series of pre-college and premedical educational outreach programs throughout the state. The office also seeks to assure retention of matriculated students through academic and personal counseling and support services.

Institution Type: *Public*
Application Process: *AMCAS, see chapter 4.*

APPLICATION AND ACCEPTANCE POLICIES FOR 2005–2006 FIRST-YEAR CLASS

Filing of AMCAS application
    Earliest date: June 1, 2004
    Latest date: Nov. 1, 2004
School application fee after screening: $100
Oldest MCAT scores considered: 2002
Does not have Early Decision Program (EDP)
Acceptance notice to regular applicants
    Earliest date: Oct. 15, 2004
    Latest date: Until class is filled
Applicant's response to acceptance offer
    Maximum time: 2 weeks
Requests for deferred entrance considered: No
Deposit to hold place in class (applied to tuition):
    $100, due with response to acceptance offer
Deposit refundable prior to: May 16, 2005
Estimated number of new entrants: 102
Starting date: Aug. 2005

TUITION AND STUDENT FEES PER YEAR FOR 2003–2004 FIRST-YEAR CLASS

Tuition   Student fees: $622
    Resident: $13,297
    Nonresident: $25,172

INFORMATION ON 2003–2004 FIRST-YEAR CLASS

Number of	In-State	Out-of-State	Total
Applicants	388	729	1,117
Applicants Interviewed	265	98	363
New Entrants*	77	25	102

*All took the MCAT and had baccalaureate degrees.

CHAPTER
11

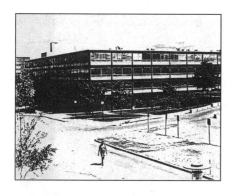

University of Vermont
College of Medicine

Burlington, Vermont

Dr. John N. Evans, *Acting Dean*
Dr. Cathleen J. Gleeson, *Associate Dean for Admissions and
    Minority Affairs Officer*
Shelley Corrigan, *Financial Aid Officer*

ADDRESS INQUIRIES TO:

The University of Vermont
College of Medicine
Office of Admissions
E215 Given Building
89 Beaumont Avenue
Burlington, VT 05405
(802) 656-2154
E-mail: MedAdmissions@uvm.edu
Web site: www.med.uvm.edu

GENERAL INFORMATION

The University of Vermont College of Medicine is located on the eastern shore of Lake Champlain in the city of Burlington, Vermont, a community of about 38,000 people. Established in 1822, it is the seventh oldest medical school in the United States. The College of Medicine recognizes the need for primary care physicians, clinical specialists, and research scientists. Our curriculum provides a general professional education in both basic and clinical sciences, followed by a period structured to meet each student's individual goals.

Our principal teaching hospital is Fletcher Allen Health Care's Medical Center Hospital of Vermont Campus, a 500-bed hospital adjacent to the College of Medicine. The hospital provides community care for Burlington and the surrounding communities and tertiary referral care for patients from the entire state of Vermont and from the northern Adirondack region of New York State.

CURRICULUM

The College of Medicine is committed to preparing each student to become an excellent practicing physician, teacher, scientist and public citizen.

February 2002 marked the implementation of the University of Vermont College of Medicine's new Vermont Integrated Curriculum (VIC) — the result of over four years of collaborative work by faculty, students, community members, and educational consultants. Its areas of focus include progressive skill development, health care systems, preventive care such as nutrition, and a greater understanding of applied sciences, particularly genetics, ethics and epidemiology. VIC also places emphasis on the areas of professionalism, cultural competency, scholarly research, teaching skills, and community service for each student.

The full Vermont Integrated Curriculum progresses through three levels of increasing competency. Block courses in Level I/Foundations provide students with a fundamental understanding of the basic biology of health and illness within systems ranging from genes to organs to individuals to populations. A comprehensive assessment of integrated knowledge and skills occurs at the end of the first year and again at the completion of the level mid-way through the second year of school. Level II/Clinical Clerkships focuses on the student's development of clinical skills, decision-making skills, and application of foundational sciences. It consists of seven clerkships with a longitudinal "bridge" curriculum of advanced sciences and clinical skills over a period of 13 months. Students advance to Level III/ Advanced Integration after successful achievement on a clinical competency exam. During the final 15 months of Advanced Integration, the student gains an understanding of the impact of economic, social, and political systems on the health care environment. This level includes acting internships, an emergency medicine rotation, and a teaching practicum.

Throughout the college's curriculum, complementary curricular themes aim to teach student's to take an integrated approach to patient care and responsibility for their own professional development. Student Leadership groups provide student's with an opportunity to collaborate with classmates, a faculty facilitator and various members from the community. These groups, which span foundations, support professional development and research projects.

A combined M.D./Ph.D. program is available for qualified applicants with a strong motivation toward a career in academic medicine and the biomedical sciences. Students receive tuition and financial support during all years of the program. Details about the M.D./Ph.D program can be found at www.med.uvm.edu/mdphd.

REQUIREMENTS FOR ENTRANCE

Applicants must have completed at least three years of undergraduate study in an accredited college or university in the United States or Canada. The MCAT is required and applicants are urged to take it in the spring of the year of application and also to have their basic premedical requirements completed by the time of application. The undergraduate program must include the following coursework:

	Years/Credit Hours
Biology (with lab)	1/8
General Chemistry (with lab)	1/8
Organic Chemistry (with lab)	1/8
General Physics (with lab)	1/8

In addition, we recommend that one course in biochemistry or molecular genetics be taken. Recommended areas of study also include literature, mathematics, behavioral sciences, history, philosophy, and the arts. Secondary school Advanced Placement courses will be recognized only if credit for them appears on the college transcript.

SELECTION FACTORS

The Committee on Admissions seeks a heterogeneous student body. We look for evidence of the promise of excellence accompanied by genuine concern for the welfare of others. Effective interpersonal skills are considered especially important and successful applicants often have a history of service to community. Selection of an applicant for admission is based upon the past pattern of academic performance plus an assessment of the applicant's fitness for the study and practice of medicine in terms of aptitude, interests, experience, motivation, leadership abilities, attitudes and maturity.

Letters of recommendation and a personal interview are required and form an important part of the application process. Approximate 550 applicants are invited to interview at the college. Approximately one third of our student body comes from Vermont with the remaining seats filled with students from other states, including 10 students from the Maine Access Program. Students from groups underrepresented in medicine are encouraged to apply for admission. The University of Vermont does not discriminate on the basis of race, color, sex, sexual orientation, religion, age, handicap, national origin, or Vietnam veteran status.

The unique structure of the curriculum, and the minimal student attrition, generally precludes accepting transfer students. However, after January 1, students wishing to explore the possibility of transferring may request an application that outlines requirements for transfer. Students who transfer generally complete two years of school elsewhere and then enroll during the middle of the second year at the University of Vermont. Decisions may be delayed until August.

The 2002 entering class had the following characteristics: *mean GPA,* 3.5; *mean MCAT,* 9.39 (Verbal Reasoning), 9.25 (Biological Sciences), 9.67 (Physical Sciences); *residence,* 27 from Vermont, 9 from Maine, 61 from other states; *undergraduate major,* 76 percent in the natural or biological sciences; 4,655 applications received, and 194 acceptances offered to obtain a class of 97 students.

Because of the November 1 deadline, early application is recommended. Extensions are not granted.

FINANCIAL AID

Financial aid funds are limited and are primarily in the form of loans. Funds are distributed according to relative need. Entering students are considered for awards on the same basis as those already enrolled. An applicant's financial status has no bearing on admission determination.

Thanks to a generous gift from the Freeman Foundation, all instate students with financial need, and a limited number of out of state students, are eligible for a $10,000 per year scholarship designed to encourage UVM medical students to practice in Vermont. Students who sign an annual intent indicating so are eligible for $10,000 for each academic year.

Institution Type: *Public*
Application Process: *AMCAS, see chapter 4.*

APPLICATION AND ACCEPTANCE POLICIES FOR 2005–2006 FIRST-YEAR CLASS

Filing of AMCAS application
  Earliest date: June 1, 2004
  Latest date: Nov. 1, 2004
School application fee to all applicants: $80
Oldest MCAT scores considered: 2001
Does have Early Decision Program (EDP)
  EDP application period: June 1–Aug. 1, 2004
  EDP applicants notified by: Oct. 1, 2004
Acceptance notice to regular applicants
  Earliest date: Oct. 15, 2004
  Latest date: Until class is filled
Applicant's response to acceptance offer
  Maximum time: 2 weeks
Requests for deferred entrance considered: Yes
Deposit to hold place in class (applied to tuition):
  $100, due with response to acceptance offer
Deposit refundable prior to: May 16, 2005
Estimated number of new entrants: 100 (4 EDP)
Starting date: Aug. 2005

TUITION AND STUDENT FEES PER YEAR FOR 2003–2004 FIRST-YEAR CLASS

Tuition   Student fees: $981
  Resident: $22,300
  Nonresident: $39,020

INFORMATION ON 2003–2004 FIRST-YEAR CLASS

Number of	In-State	Out-of-State	Total
Applicants	68	4,800	4,868
Applicants Interviewed	36	468	504
New Entrants*	28	72	100

*All took the MCAT and had baccalaureate degrees.

CHAPTER

11

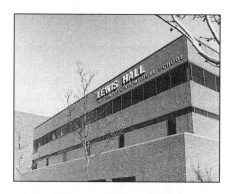

Eastern Virginia Medical School

Norfolk, Virginia

Dr. Evan R. Farmer, *Dean and Provost*
Dr. Robert M. McCombs, *Associate Dean for Admissions*
Susan L. Castora, *Director of Admissions*
Gail C. Williams, *Assistant Dean for Student Affairs and
    Director of Minority Affairs*

ADDRESS INQUIRIES TO:

Office of Admissions
Eastern Virginia Medical School
721 Fairfax Avenue
Norfolk, Virginia 23507-2000
(757) 446-5812; 446-5896 (FAX)
Web site: www.evms.edu

MISSION STATEMENT

The Eastern Virginia Medical School is a private community-based academic institution dedicated to medical and health education, biomedical research, and the enhancement of health care in the Commonwealth of Virginia.

GENERAL INFORMATION

The Eastern Virginia Medical School (EVMS) was established in 1973 in response to the desire of the Hampton Roads community to enhance the quality and diversity of health care throughout the region. Because of its history, the mission of EVMS is deeply rooted in the education and training of primary care physicians. This mission has been recently revitalized through a series of innovative programs established through the Center for Generalist Medicine. The additional benefit achieved by the creation of an academic health center has been the promotion and expansion of medical research and the development of several centers of excellence such as the Jones Institute for Reproductive Medicine, the Center for Pediatric Research, the Strelitz Diabetes Institute, and the Glennan Center for Geriatric Medicine.

Through its affiliation with over 33 health care facilities, including Sentara Norfolk General Hospital, the Children's Hospital of the Kings Daughters, the U.S. Naval Medical Center in Portsmouth, and the Veterans Affairs Hospital in Hampton, EVMS provides health care for more than one quarter of Virginia's population as well as neighboring regions of North Carolina. EVMS provides a community-based educational program arming students with the requisite scientific, academic, and humanistic skills most relevant to practicing medicine into the twenty-first century. Three hundred seventy six full-time and part-time faculty and over one thousand community faculty provide students with exposure to a broad range of clinical experiences and to the diversity of medical care delivery systems.

CURRICULUM

The curriculum has been designed to educate students in both the science of human biology and art of the practice of medicine. Throughout the first two years, students are introduced to clinical medicine through two vehicles: the nationally recognized Theresa A. Thomas Professional Skills Teaching and Assessment Center, utilizing standardized patients, and a Longitudinal Mentorship with a generalist physician in community practice.

Careful coordination between basic sciences and generalist disciplines permits an integrated curriculum, so that students can appreciate the clinical correlation to their scientific studies. Weekly small-group sessions, facilitated by basic scientists and clinical scholars, introduce students to clinical problem solving. Areas covered relate to clinical skills development, including medical interviewing, doctor-patient relationships, and medical ethics. In sum, through this early introduction to clinical medicine, students learn the art of medical history taking and physical examination along with the application of basic science knowledge to patient care.

The third year clinical clerkships focus on ambulatory care in community-based sites in balance with inpatient care experiences. In addition to the required clerkships in family medicine, internal medicine, pediatrics, obstetrics and gynecology, psychiatry, and surgery are rotations in substance abuse, geriatrics, and surgical subspecialties. For those students interested in generalist medicine, electives are offered in special populations and rural health care, and an elective honors track in generalist medicine. For those interested in research or subspecialty care, at least six months are available in elective opportunities. The Jones Institute for Women's Health, the Diabetes Center, and the Center for Pediatric Research are but a few of the excellent resources to enhance skills in research.

Overall, students are graded as honors, high pass, pass, or fail. Evaluation of clinical skills is a central component of the education process through the use of standardized patients.

EVMS offers combined programs (B.S.-M.D.) with several colleges and universities within the state allowing outstanding undergraduate students the opportunity to explore varied educational and life experiences as they prepare for a career in medicine.

REQUIREMENTS FOR ENTRANCE

The MCAT and a minimum of 100 college semester hours at an accredited American or Canadian college or university are required. Coursework must include the following subjects:

	Years
Biology (with lab)	1
General Chemistry (with lab)	1
Organic Chemistry (with lab)	1
Physics (with lab)	1

Applicants are expected to have grades of C or better in all required courses. Credits earned through Advanced Placement programs or CLEP are acceptable. Applicants may enhance their chances of acceptance by taking graduate coursework in a natural science. In recent years, students matriculating at EVMS have had a *mean GPA* of 3.41 and have averaged 10 in each section of the MCAT.

SELECTION FACTORS

EVMS does not discriminate on the basis of sex, race, creed, age, national origin, marital status, or handicap. After obtaining a completed AMCAS application, a supplementary application packet is sent to those applicants receiving a favorable initial screening, based on both objective and subjective factors, including grades, MCAT scores, medical exposure, and life experience.

For each applicant, the Admissions Committee considers the entire academic record, including science and overall GPA, MCAT scores, exposure to the medical field, maturity, character, and motivation. The application fee will be waived if a fee waiver is granted by AMCAS.

Preference is given to legal residents of Virginia. In addition, recognizing the goals set by the Virginia legislature, EVMS is seeking persons with personal and background traits that indicate a high potential for becoming a family physician, general pediatrician, general internist, or general obstetrician.

Applicants who have completed one or more years in a medical school accredited by the Liaison Committee on Medical Education can be considered for transfer into the second or third year of our curriculum only to fill vacancies that may arise with the withdrawal of previously enrolled students. All transfers must meet the requirements stated for general admission.

FINANCIAL AID

The ability of a student to provide for the costs of education is not a factor in the admissions selection process. Over 90 percent of the student body receives financial assistance. Scholarships are limited, and loans constitute the majority of aid received. Students may fully meet the costs of medical school at EVMS, providing they meet all federal criteria, meet citizenship requirements, are creditworthy, and maintain satisfactory academic progress. For those interested in a primary care obligation, there are numerous federal and state scholarships available. Virginia residents also benefit from the state-funded Tuition Assistance Grant Program (TAGP), which provides annual grants of approximately $1,700.

Applicants for financial assistance must file the cost-free FAFSA and other additional required forms. For additional details and assistance in financial planning, please contact the Office of Financial Aid at (757) 446-5813.

INFORMATION ABOUT DIVERSITY PROGRAMS

Eastern Virginia Medical School is committed to producing a diverse physician workforce to help meet the health care needs of the region. Applicants from rural or other underserved regions and those who have been disadvantaged or underrepresented for economic, racial, or social reasons, and who possess the motivation and aptitude required for the study of medicine, are strongly encouraged to apply.

Institution Type: *Private*
Application Process: *AMCAS, see chapter 4.*

APPLICATION AND ACCEPTANCE POLICIES FOR 2005–2006 FIRST-YEAR CLASS

Filing of AMCAS application
  Earliest date: June 1, 2004
  Latest date: Nov. 15, 2004
School application fee after screening: $90
Oldest MCAT scores considered: 2002
Does have Early Decision Program (EDP)
  EDP application period: June 1–Aug. 1, 2004
  EDP applicants notified by: Oct. 1, 2004
Acceptance notice to regular applicants
  Earliest date: Oct. 15, 2004
  Latest date: Until class is filled
Applicant's response to acceptance offer
  Maximum time: 2 weeks
Requests for deferred entrance considered: Yes
Deposit to hold place in class (applied to tuition):
  $200, due with response to acceptance offer
Deposit refundable prior to: May 16, 2005
Estimated number of new entrants: 110 (2 EDP)
Starting date: August 2005

TUITION AND STUDENT FEES PER YEAR FOR 2003–2004 FIRST-YEAR CLASS

Tuition	Student fees: $2,966**
Resident: $18,975	
Nonresident: $35,075	

INFORMATION ON 2003–2004 FIRST-YEAR CLASS

Number of	*In-State*	*Out-of-State*	*Total*
Applicants	719	1,846	2,565
Applicants Interviewed	303	330	633
New Entrants*	60	50	110

*All had baccalaureate degrees; 94% took the MCAT.
**Includes health insurance $1,676: w/o health insurance.

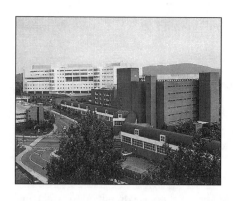

University of Virginia
School of Medicine

Charlottesville, Virginia

Dr. Arthur T. Garson, *Vice President and Dean, School of Medicine*
Dr. R. J. Canterbury, *Associate Dean for Admissions*
Dr. Beth A. Bailey, *Assistant Dean for Admissions*
Dr. Norm Oliver, *Associate Dean for Diversity*

ADDRESS INQUIRIES TO:

Medical School Admissions Office
PO Box 800725
University of Virginia
School of Medicine
Charlottesville, Virginia 22908
(434) 924-5571; 982-2586 (FAX)
E-mail: medsch-adm@virginia.edu
Web site: www.healthsystem.virginia.edu/internet/admissions/

MISSION STATEMENT

The mission of the University of Virginia School of Medicine is:

- To educate students in the health sciences in order to fulfill the need for practitioners and scientists;
- To provide cost-effective, high-quality patient care at primary, secondary, and tertiary levels as needed by the citizens of the region and nation;
- To produce new knowledge required to advance health by conducting research in the basic, clinical, and social sciences; and,
- To provide public service as needed by citizens or by public jurisdictions.

GENERAL INFORMATION

Authorized by Thomas Jefferson, the University of Virginia School of Medicine was opened for instruction in 1825, making it one of the oldest medical schools in the South.

Both the School of Medicine and the University of Virginia Hospital are located on the grounds of the University of Virginia in Charlottesville. The University of Virginia Medical Center cares for 27,000 inpatients and 400,000 outpatients annually. The University Hospital staffs 552 beds, 61 infant bassinets, and 7 separate intensive care units.

CURRICULUM

Starting with the entering class of 2000, the School of Medicine has introduced a new curriculum designed to prepare medical students for the practice of medicine in the 21st century. The new curriculum integrates scientific knowledge, clinical care, and research throughout the entire four years of medical school. It draws from a rich tradition of excellence in basic science and clinical training, and integrates new ways to focus on the patient and the physician-patient relationship. This new curriculum also alters the methods of instruction. Classroom lecture time is decreased by nearly half. Most scheduled classes are held in the morning and students have three or four afternoons free each week in years 1 and 2 for productive self-study or elective activities. Small group activities and individual teaching have been increased to maximize interactions between students and faculty. Basic science concepts are presented in the context of clinical cases. The new curriculum also introduces students to patients and clinical cases from the first day of medical school. A new first year course, The Practice of Medicine, teaches professionalism, interviewing skills, physical diagnosis, and ethics in small groups. All other courses are correlated with these clinical experiences.

The elective program of the fourth year offers students the opportunity to pursue their own interests and to sample diverse training experiences in medical centers from Alaska to South America. Students may choose from a wide variety of electives, including clinical experience, graduate courses, and research activities.

Students selected for the Generalist Scholars Program receive enhanced training in disease prevention, health promotion, substance abuse, family therapy, clinical epidemiology, and office procedural skills.

Many opportunities exist for students who are interested in medical research. Prominent among these opportunities is the Medical Scientist Training Program. This accelerated program leads to both M.D. and Ph.D. degrees and utilizes the facilities of both the School of Medicine and the Graduate School of Arts and Sciences. It is designed specifically to prepare a limited number of highly qualified men and women for careers in both research and clinical medicine. Medical students may also elect to extend their education to include a year of basic science or clinical research. Medical students may also elect to pursue one of three Master's programs: MS in Health Evaluation Sciences, MA in Bioethics and MS in Public Health.

REQUIREMENTS FOR ENTRANCE

The MCAT is required and must be taken no later than the fall of the year of application and no earlier than spring of 2002. The minimum undergraduate college requirement for admission is 90 semester hours of graded coursework in a U.S. or Canadian school; however, it is unusual to accept students who will not have received the baccalaureate degree by the time of enrollment. Without exception the following courses are required:

	Years
Biology (with lab)	1
General Chemistry (with lab)	1
Organic Chemistry (with lab)	1
General Physics (with lab)	1

Other than these courses, the college curriculum for the premedical student should be planned in accord with individual interests and aptitudes to gain as broad an educational background as possible.

Advanced Placement credit is acceptable if such credit is indicated on the undergraduate college transcripts as having been accepted by the college toward fulfillment of requirements for the bachelor's degree. Students are expected to pursue advanced courses if Advanced Placement credit was awarded for any of the required science courses (including laboratory work).

SELECTION FACTORS

Preference is given to residents of Virginia. Applications from well-qualified nonresidents are welcomed, but early application is advised. Foreign nationals should have baccalaureate degrees from American or Canadian colleges or universities; reapplicants should show significant improvement in their applications. The Committee on Admissions does not discriminate on the basis of race, gender, sexual preference, creed, national origin, age, or disability.

Numerical criteria, work and volunteer experience, interpersonal and communication skills, letters of recommendations, and the interview influence committee decisions. The Admissions Committee does not grant regional interviews or interviews by applicant request.

The class entering in 2003 had a *mean overall GPA* of 3.70 and a *mean MCAT score* of 10.7.

FINANCIAL AID

In addition to Federal Stafford Loans, the University of Virginia School of Medicine provides school-funded scholarships and loans to students who demonstrate need via the Free Application for Federal Student Aid. Parental financial information is required for all applicants who wish to receive aid from school funds. Approximately 85 percent of the student body receive financial aid. Student employment is not encouraged. Financial aid applications are available online at www.healthsystem.virginia.edu/financialaid on January 1 or immediately after acceptance. For more information, contact Ms. Nancy Zimmer, financial aid director, at (434) 924-0033.

INFORMATION ABOUT DIVERSITY PROGRAMS

This institution is committed to increasing the representation in medicine of persons from groups underrepresented in medicine. To this end, we welcome applications from qualified out-of-state and in-state students from groups underrepresented in medicine. Structures in place to facilitate preparation and success of students include: (1) content-based MCAT summer program; (2) extensive tutorial and other academic support programs upon admission; and (3) need-based financial assistance. Early completion of application for admission is strongly recommended. The Admissions Committee has diverse members, and a team of committed faculty and administrators provides support at all levels for students from groups underrepresented in medicine. For more information, please contact Dr. Norm Oliver, Associate Dean for Diversity at mno3p@virginia.edu.

Institution Type: *Public*
Application Process: *AMCAS, see chapter 4.*

APPLICATION AND ACCEPTANCE POLICIES FOR 2005–2006 FIRST-YEAR CLASS

Filing of AMCAS application
  Earliest date: June 1, 2004
  Latest date: Nov. 1, 2004
School application fee to all applicants: $75
Oldest MCAT scores considered: 2002
Does not have Early Decision Program
Acceptance notice to regular applicants
  Earliest date: Oct. 15, 2004
  Latest date: Until class is filled
Applicant's response to acceptance offer
  Maximum time: 3 weeks
Requests for deferred entrance considered: Yes
Deposit to hold place in class: None
Estimated number of new entrants: 142
Starting date: Aug. 2005

TUITION AND STUDENT FEES PER YEAR FOR 2003–2004 FIRST-YEAR CLASS

Tuition
  Resident: $21,000   Resident fees: $1,486
  Nonresident: $33,000   NonResident fees: $1,536

INFORMATION ON 2003–2004 FIRST-YEAR CLASS

Number of	In-State	Out-of-State	Total
Applicants	711	2,866	3,577
Applicants Interviewed	205	297	502
New Entrants*	92	48	140

*All took the MCAT and had baccalaureate degrees.

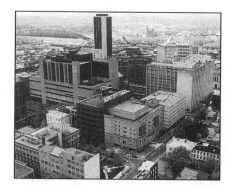

Virginia Commonwealth University School of Medicine

Richmond, Virginia

Dr. H. H. Newsome, *Dean*
Dr. Cynthia M. Heldberg, *Associate Dean for Admissions*
Judith Cramer, *Assistant Director for Financial Aid*
Agnes L. Mack, *Director of Admissions*
Donna Jackson, *Director of Student Outreach Programs*

ADDRESS INQUIRIES TO:

Virginia Commonwealth University
School of Medicine
P.O. Box 980565
Richmond, Virginia 23298-0565
(804) 828-9629; 828-1246 (FAX)
Web site: www.medschool.vcu.edu

MISSION STATEMENT

The mission of Virginia Commonwealth University's School of Medicine is constant improvement of the quality of health care for citizens of Virginia, using innovative, scholarly activity to create new knowledge, to provide better systems of medical education, and to develop more effective health care methods. The primary aim of the School of Medicine is to provide an academic environment appropriate for the education of its students and continuing education directed towards the needs of practicing physicians.

GENERAL INFORMATION

The School of Medicine, which has been in continuous operation since 1838, is the founding institution of the Medical College of Virginia Campus of Virginia Commonwealth University. The health science campus includes not only the school of medicine but also the only school of dentistry in the state plus schools of nursing, pharmacy, and allied health professions. The vitality of Virginia Commonwealth University's campus research programs is reflected in the caliber of its faculty, the success of its patient care programs, and the level of research funding generated. With 750 hospital beds at the main campus, the largest emergency room, and the largest neonatal intensive care unit in the state, plus 800 beds at one of the newest VA hospitals in the South, the Medical College of Virginia campus is one of the largest university-owned medical centers in the United States and affords its students an unparalleled clinical experience. The campus is located near the financial and governmental areas of downtown Richmond, the capital of Virginia and one of the South's most historic and cosmopolitan cities.

CURRICULUM

The first year is spent studying normal structure and function in a traditional discipline format. The second year emphasizes pathogenesis of disease and its manifestations and is taught in an organ system manner. Pathogenesis, pathology, pharmacology, and the major manifestations and principles of management are discussed in each of the major body systems.

There is a longitudinal experience in clinical medicine for first- and second-year students. Students spend two afternoons per month in a small group learning the fundamentals of clinical medicine. This is supplemented by a clinical experience in the office of a primary care physician two afternoons per month. This unique clinical experience is integrated with the basic science curriculum in a way that enhances and enriches the student's learning. There is a computer lab with over 40 workstations and a full array of commercial and in-house, faculty-developed educational software.

In the third year, the clinical rotations are at the University and Veterans Affairs Hospitals, with ambulatory care rotations at nonuniversity primary care sites. Computer educational workstations, distributed throughout the hospitals and clinics, give students access to the university library databases, expert decision support systems, and educational software programs.

During the fourth year, the student may choose from a wide variety of electives both at the university and throughout the United States. Additionally there are elective programs serving the first and second years.

REQUIREMENTS FOR ENTRANCE

The MCAT is required. A demonstrated competence in basic science is essential, although a science major is not required. Each matriculant must have at least 90 semester hours or equivalent in an accredited college. Courses must include:

	Semesters
Biology (with lab)	2
General Chemistry (with lab)	2
Organic Chemistry (with lab)	2
General Physics (with lab)	2
College Mathematics	2
English	2

Applicants are urged to take the MCAT in the spring of the year of application and no later than the fall of that year. Early Decision Program applicants must have MCAT scores available when applying. The school has a guaranteed admissions program with Virginia Commonwealth University's undergraduate honors program. High school seniors who have 1270 or better on their SATs and a GPA of 3.5 may apply. They must complete the usual premed requirements all honors program requirements, and maintain a 3.5 GPA throughout their undergraduate years.

SELECTION FACTORS

Applicants are selected on the basis of their potential as prospective physicians as well as students of medicine. Attributes of character, personality factors, academic skills, and exposure to medicine are considered along with academic performance, GPA, MCAT scores, letters of recommendation, and personal interviews at the School of Medicine.

The school gives preference to bona fide residents of the Commonwealth of Virginia and does not discriminate on the basis of age, race, sex, creed, national origin, or handicap. Foreign nationals must be permanent residents at the time of application.

The 2003 entering class of 184 students had the following credentials: *undergraduate major,* 25 percent in arts or humanities, 72 percent in sciences; *degrees,* 41 with graduate degrees, including 2 doctorate degrees; *residence,* 55 percent Virginia residents; *students from groups underrepresented in medicine,* 7.6 percent black; *sex,* 47 percent women; *mean overall undergraduate GPA,* 3.46; *MCAT average score,* 9.5.

The uniform acceptance date is October 15 with additional selections in December, January, and February. Applicants who have been rejected in previous years should demonstrate significant improvement in their academic credentials before reapplying.

FINANCIAL AID

Assistance to students in meeting the cost of their medical education is available in the form of loans and scholarships, and financial counseling is offered by the Financial Aid Office of the School of Medicine. The Free Application for Federal Student Aid (FAFSA) is used in awarding need-based aid. Parent information should be included on this form to be considered for the Department of Health and Human Services programs.

The School of Medicine's Financial Aid Office administers all major federal aid programs and coordinates with the School of Medicine in the administration of state, private, and institutional scholarships and loans. The Financial Aid Office responds to requests for information within 24 hours. Application forms and aid fact sheets are available in mid-January of each year. Applications for aid may be made prior to notification of acceptance by the School of Medicine. The Federal Identification number for VCU is 003735. This must appear on the FAFSA. Applicants are encouraged to seek all

resources available to them and apply as early as feasible to maximize the possibility of obtaining funding. Over 90% of the medical students receive some form of financial aid. Financial assistance is not available to students who are not U.S. citizens or permanent residents.

Information may be obtained from the following address: Financial Aid Office, VCU School of Medicine, P.O. Box 980565, Richmond, Virginia 23298; the location is 11th and Broad Streets in Richmond.

Institution Type: *Public*
Application Process: *AMCAS, see chapter 4.*

APPLICATION AND ACCEPTANCE POLICIES FOR 2005–2006 FIRST-YEAR CLASS

Filing of AMCAS application
    Earliest date: June 1, 2004
    Latest date: Nov. 15, 2004
School application fee after screening: $80
Oldest MCAT scores considered: 2001 (August)
Does have Early Decision Program (EDP)
    EDP application period: June 1–Aug. 1, 2004
    EDP applicants notified by: Oct. 1, 2004
Acceptance notice to regular applicants
    Earliest date: Oct. 15, 2004
    Latest date: Until class is filled
Applicant's response to acceptance offer
    Maximum time: 2 weeks
Requests for deferred entrance considered: Yes
Deposit to hold place in class (applied to tuition):
    $100, due with response to acceptance offer
Deposit refundable prior to: May 16, 2005
Estimated number of new entrants: 184 (5 EDP)
Starting date: August 2005

TUITION AND STUDENT FEES PER YEAR FOR 2003–2004 FIRST-YEAR CLASS

Tuition   Student fees: $1,523
    Resident: $18,500
    Nonresident: $34,328

INFORMATION ON 2003–2004 FIRST-YEAR CLASS

Number of	In-State	Out-of-State	Total
Applicants	790	3,119	3,909
Applicants Interviewed	296	333	629
New Entrants*	100	84	184

*All had baccalaureate degrees; 95% took the MCAT.

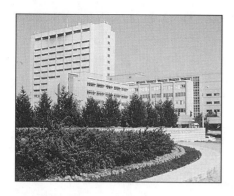

University of Washington
School of Medicine

Seattle, Washington

Dr. Paul G. Ramsey, *Dean*
Dr. Werner E. Samson, *Assistant Dean for Admissions*
Patricia T. Fero, *Admissions Officer*

ADDRESS INQUIRIES TO:

Admissions Office
Health Sciences Center A-300, Box 356340
University of Washington
Seattle, Washington 98195-6340
(206) 543-7212
E-mail: askuwsom@u.washington.edu
Web site: www.washington.edu/medicine/som/index.html

MISSION STATEMENT

The School has a dual mission reflecting a commitment to maintain a balance between:
• Meeting the health-care needs of the region, especially by recognizing the importance of primary care and providing service to underserved populations, and
• Advancing knowledge and assuming leadership in the biomedical sciences and in academic medicine.

GENERAL INFORMATION

The University of Washington School of Medicine was established in 1945. For complete information about policies, procedures, and programs, candidates are referred to the current University of Washington General Catalog available from the University Bookstore at (206) 634-3400 or on-line at www.washington.edu/students/crscat/index.html.

CURRICULUM

The first two years of the curriculum are identified as the basic science curriculum. It consists of three phases or groups of courses: discipline-based courses; organ systems taught by basic and clinical disciplines; and introduction to clinical medicine and health care. The academic demands of the basic curriculum are scaled so that most students will be able to take elective courses.

The clinical curriculum is pursued predominantly in the third and fourth years. It includes clerkships in internal medicine, family medicine, obstetrics-gynecology, pediatrics, psychiatry, and surgery; additional clinical selectives in neurology, surgery (including subspecialties), rehabilitation medicine/chronic care and emergency medicine/trauma; and clinical electives chosen by the student.

The required Independent Investigative Inquiry requirement enables students to do a research project and study an area of medicine of their choice in depth.

The UWSOM has a College system which has as its primary goals overseeing a four-year curriculum of clinical skills and professionalism, teaching the second-year Introduction to Clinical Medicine course, and providing a consistent faculty mentor to each student throughout her/his medical school career. Students are randomly assigned upon matriculation to one of five Colleges and to one College faculty mentor.

A unique aspect of the curriculum is the WWAMI program of decentralized medical education (see Chapter 5). All students enrolled at the University of Washington School of Medicine are encouraged to take a portion of training at sites away from the University of Washington Seattle campus. Offers of acceptance, therefore, are conditional upon agreement to participate in the WWAMI program.

REQUIREMENTS FOR ENTRANCE

The MCAT taken in the spring of 2002 or thereafter is required. This exam must be taken no later than the autumn of the year before possible matriculation. Under exceptional circumstances, the GRE taken since 2002, may be considered during the admissions process; however, if accepted, the applicant will be required to take the MCAT prior to matriculation. The following course requirements must be completed before matriculation:

Sem. hrs.

Biology 8
Chemistry 12
    (May be satisfied by taking any combination of
    inorganic, organic, biochemistry, or molecular
    biology courses.)

A biochemistry course is strongly recommended. The UWSOM first year biochemistry course is taught with the presumption that the fundamentals such as molecular genetics and the structure and activity of proteins and metabolism are already mastered.

Physics 4
Other science 8
    (May be satisfied by taking other courses in any
    of the above categories.)

Proficiency in English, basic mathematics, and information technologies is also essential. Entering students are required to have a personal computer.

Under exceptional circumstances, certain course requirements may be waived for individuals with unusual achievements and academic promise.

All entrants in recent years have fulfilled requirements for a bachelor's degree. No major is preferred, but a broad educational background is encouraged.

Applicants who are seriously considered will be requested to submit supplemental information, one part of which will be a premedical committee evaluation or three individual letters submitted from instructors who have taught the candidate in a collegiate course (a mixture of evaluations from the sciences and humanities is recommended). In addition, signed documentation indicating the student's ability to meet our essential requirements (with or without reasonable accommodations) for graduation, as well as authorization for a criminal background check (necessitated by Washington state law) is required.

All supplemental materials must be submitted by January 15, 2005. Early submission of application and supplemental materials is encouraged.

Candidates who wish to be considered for the M.D.-Ph.D. program must submit the Medical Scientist Training Program (MSTP) application. This application is sent to all eligible candidates along with the acknowledgment of receipt of the medical school application. All candidates considered eligible for this program after initial review of the MSTP application will be requested to send further supplementary materials.

SELECTION FACTORS

Candidates for admission are considered comparatively on the basis of academic performance, motivation, maturity, personal integrity, and demonstrated humanitarian qualities. Research experience, community service, disadvantaged background, and interest in serving the underserved are other important considerations. A knowledge of the needs of individuals and society and an awareness of health care delivery systems are essential. Extenuating circumstances in an applicant's background are evaluated as they relate to these selection factors.

Students entering in the fall of 2003 had a *mean total GPA* of 3.69. *Mean scores on the MCAT* were as follows: *VR*-10.0, *PS*-10.3, *BS*-10.8, *WS*-P.

Residents of the states of Washington, Wyoming, Alaska, Montana, or Idaho are eligible to apply. Individuals with a demonstrated interest in research may apply for the M.D.-Ph.D. program (MSTP) regardless of residency. Applicants from outside this five-state region who come from disadvantaged backgrounds or who have demonstrated a commitment to serving underserved populations will be considered. Foreign applicants, in addition to the above requirements, must also have a permanent resident visa.

After the completed applications are screened, applicants considered to be competitive will be invited to Seattle for an interview.

FINANCIAL AID

Financial status has no bearing on chances for admission. All applicants for aid must submit data for an analysis of need through the FAFSA. The application receipt deadline of February 28 must be met, regardless of admission date, in order to receive highest priority for aid; applicants should apply on line (www.fafsa.ed.gov) or mail the FAFSA form mid-February or earlier. Approximately 83 percent of the student body receives some form of aid, most of which is in the form of loans. Financial aid applications are available in January. Contact the School of Medicine's Financial Aid Office at (206) 685-2520.

Institution Type: *Public*
Application Process: *AMCAS, see chapter 4.*

APPLICATION AND ACCEPTANCE POLICIES FOR 2005–2006 FIRST-YEAR CLASS

Filing of AMCAS application
  Earliest date: June 1, 2004
  Latest date: Nov. 1, 2004
School application fee after screening: $35
Oldest MCAT scores considered: 2002
Does not have Early Decision Program
Acceptance notice to regular applicants
  Earliest date: Nov. 1, 2004
  Latest date: Until class is filled
Applicant's response to acceptance offer
  Maximum time: 2 weeks before May 15;
  1 week thereafter
Requests for deferred entrance considered: Yes
Deposit to hold place in class (applied to tuition):
  $100, due with firm response to acceptance offer;
  nonrefundable
Estimated number of new entrants: 178
Starting date: Sept. 2005

TUITION AND STUDENT FEES PER YEAR FOR 2003–2004 FIRST-YEAR CLASS

Tuition: Student fees: $400
  Resident: $12,448
  Nonresident: $29,388

INFORMATION ON 2003–2004 FIRST-YEAR CLASS

Number of	In-State*	Out-of-State	Total
Applicants	963	1,942	2,905
Applicants Interviewed	671	79	750
New Entrants	165	13	178†

*In-state figures include Washington, Wyoming, Alaska, Montana, and Idaho residents.
†All took the MCAT and had baccalaureate degrees.

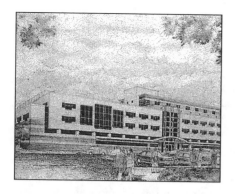

Marshall University
Joan C. Edwards School of Medicine

Huntington, West Virginia

Dr. Charles H. McKown, Jr., *Vice President and Dean*
Cynthia A. Warren, *Assistant Dean for Admissions and Student Affairs*
Jack L. Toney, *Director of Student Financial Aid*
Dr. Marie C. Veitia, *Associate Dean for Student Affairs*

ADDRESS INQUIRIES TO:

Admissions Office
Marshall University
Joan C. Edwards School of Medicine
1600 Medical Center Drive
Huntington, West Virginia 25701-3655
(304) 691-1738; (800) 544-8514; (304) 691-1744 (FAX)
Web site: musom.marshall.edu

MISSION STATEMENT

The Marshall University School of Medicine has a special mission to respond to the health care needs of West Virginians. We emphasize training in the primary care specialties and encourage graduates to practice in the state's underserved rural areas. Marshall now ranks second in the nation in the percentage of graduates who choose to enter a primary care specialty.

GENERAL INFORMATION

The Marshall University School of Medicine was developed under the Veterans Administration Medical Assistance and Health Training Act passed by Congress in 1972. The School of Medicine was granted full accreditation and graduated its first class in 1981.

The School of Medicine is a community-based program. The school's many affiliations provide the opportunity to experience medical practice in varied settings: a $32 million ambulatory care center, the Veterans Affairs Medical Center, successful rural clinics, highly specialized tertiary-care services in community hospitals, offices of private physicians, and others.

CURRICULUM

In the first year, the basic sciences courses of anatomy, physiology, neurosciences, medical cell and molecular biology, and biochemistry are supplemented by medical ethics and a clinical interdepartmental course entitled Introduction to Patient Care, which features students' supervised exposure to direct patient care and covers physical diagnosis and behavioral medicine. Ample unscheduled time during the first year allows students opportunities for independent problem-based and small group learning. The second year includes pharmacology, pathology, microbiology, genetics, psychopathology, community medicine, physical diagnosis, immunology, medical ethics, and introduction to clinical medicine. Clinical integration of basic concepts occurs in all courses. During the third and fourth years, students are rotated through clerkships at participating community hospitals and other locations in the clinical fields of medicine, surgery, pediatrics, psychiatry, family practice, and obstetrics-gynecology. Three months of rural health care at approved sites are required by all students. Twenty-seven weeks are devoted to electives in the senior year. A standard letter grading system (A, B, C, D, F) is utilized.

REQUIREMENTS FOR ENTRANCE

The MCAT is required. The baccalaureate degree is preferred. However, exceptionally well qualified students with three years of college education or the equivalent may be considered for admission. All required courses must be passed with a grade of C or better by June 1 of the year of matriculation. Required science courses cannot be taken through correspondence programs. Minimum course requirements are:

	Sem. hrs.
General Biology or Zoology (with lab)	8
Inorganic Chemistry (with lab)	8
Organic Chemistry (with lab)	8
Physics (with lab)	8
English Composition and Rhetoric	6
Behavioral or Social Sciences	6

With the exception of these specific courses, applicants are encouraged to pursue their personal educational interests. Quality of coursework rather than the field in which it is taken is the more important consideration.

It is urged that applicants take the MCAT in the spring of the year of application but no later than the fall of that year.

SELECTION FACTORS

There is no discrimination because of race, sex, religion, age, handicap, sexual orientation, or national origin. Qualified members of groups who are underrepresented in medicine are especially encouraged to apply.

Applicants are evaluated on the basis of their academic records, MCAT scores, recommendations from instructors, and personal qualifications as judged through interviews. Interviews are arranged only by invitation of the Admissions Committee.

Academic achievement alone is not a sufficient foundation for success in the profession of medicine. Applicants must exhibit excellence in character, motivation, and ideals. Behavioral qualities deemed essential for a career in medicine include, but are not limited to, good judgment, integrity, responsibility, and sensitivity.

As a state-assisted institution, the School of Medicine gives preference in selection of students to West Virginia residents. A limited number of positions will be available to well-qualified nonresidents from states contiguous to West Virginia or to non-residents who have strong ties to West Virginia. Other nonresidents are not considered. Only applicants who are U.S. citizens or who have permanent resident visas are eligible for admission.

The August 2003 entering class had the following profile: *resident,* 89 percent West Virginia residents; *mean overall GPA,* 3.5; *gender,* 49 percent women; *undergraduate major,* 87 percent in biological sciences, chemistry, or preprofessional curriculum; *degrees,* 47 bachelor's degrees, 3 master's degrees, 1 law degree, and 2 without degrees; *undergraduate schools,* 35 students attended West Virginia schools.

The School of Medicine considers for transfer admission those applicants who are currently in good standing at an allopathic medical school. Positions are limited by attrition and are rarely available. The residency policy for regular admissions also applies to transfer admissions with the exception that only U.S. citizens are considered.

FINANCIAL AID

The financial needs of the applicant are not a consideration in the admissions process. There are a variety of resources for financial assistance available to medical students. Currently 90 percent of the students are receiving financial assistance. Further information and applications for financial aid may be obtained from Marshall at the following address: Office of Financial Aid, Marshall University, Huntington, West Virginia 25755.

Because of the rigorous nature of the medical program, students are advised not to attempt outside employment during the academic year.

The supplemental application fee will be waived for individuals who have been granted an AMCAS fee waiver.

Institution Type: *Public*
Application Process: *AMCAS, see chapter 4.*

APPLICATION AND ACCEPTANCE POLICIES FOR 2005–2006 FIRST-YEAR CLASS

Filing of AMCAS application
    Earliest date: June 1, 2004
    Latest date: Dec. 1, 2004
School application fee to all applicants:
    Residents: $50
    Nonresidents: $80
Oldest MCAT scores considered: 2002
Does not have Early Decision Program (EDP)
Acceptance notice to regular applicants
    Earliest date: Oct. 15, 2004
    Latest date: Until class is filled
Applicant's response to acceptance offer
    Maximum time: 2 weeks
Requests for deferred entrance considered: Yes
Deposit to hold place in class: None
Estimated number of new entrants: 50
Starting date: Aug. 2005

TUITION AND STUDENT FEES PER YEAR FOR 2003–2004 FIRST-YEAR CLASS

Tuition   Student fees: $514
    Resident: $12,190
    Nonresident: $32,020

INFORMATION ON 2003–2004 FIRST-YEAR CLASS

Number of	In-State	Out-of-State	Total
Applicants	207	502	709
Applicants Interviewed	159	25	184
New Entrants*	47	6	53

*All took the MCAT; 96% had baccalaureate degrees.

CHAPTER

11

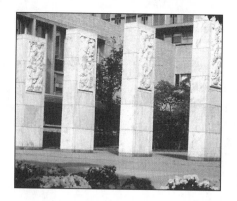

West Virginia University School of Medicine

Morgantown, West Virginia

Dr. Robert D'Alessandri, *Vice President/Dean*
Dr. G. Anne Cather, *Associate Dean for Student Services
and Professional Development, Minority Affairs Representative*
Dr. David M. Morgan, *Chair, Admissions Committee*
Candace Frazier, *Financial Aid Officer*

ADDRESS INQUIRIES TO:

Office of Student Services
West Virginia University School of Medicine
Health Sciences Center
P.O. Box 9111
Morgantown, West Virginia 26506
(304) 293-2408; 293-7814 (FAX)
Web site: www.hsc.wvu.edu/som/

MISSION STATEMENT

The mission of the West Virginia University School of Medicine is to improve the health of West Virginians through the education of health professionals, through basic/clinical scientific research and research in rural health care delivery, through the provision of continuing professional education, and through participation in the provision of direct and supportive health care.

GENERAL INFORMATION

West Virginia University, a public institution, has offered the first two years of the medical curriculum continuously since 1902. Four decades ago the Health Sciences Center was established, including the School of Medicine and the schools of dentistry, nursing, and pharmacy. A modern physical plant provides facilities for the schools, including three hospitals—the 400-bed Ruby Memorial Hospital with a Level 1 trauma center, the 80-bed Chestnut Ridge Psychiatric Hospital, and the 80-bed Health South Mountainview Regional Rehabilitation Hospital, as well as the Mary Babb Randolph Cancer Center and the WVU Eye Institute. Clinical instruction is also provided in the Charleston Division of the Health Sciences Center, and the Eastern Panhandle Division.

CURRICULUM

The educational program of the School of Medicine is designed to provide students with a foundation upon which they can base further preparation for any branch of medicine, specifically primary care, other specialty practice, teaching, research, or a combination of these career objectives.

In the first and second years the plan of study is directed toward the principles and methodology of the basic medical sciences. However, the basic courses are designed so that the student begins to synthesize concepts of patient care. The first-year basic science courses are integrated through lectures, common test methods, and problem-based learning clinical applications. Clinical experiences are introduced the first semester of the first year. Summer externships are available in most primary care fields. Additional early exposure to patient-oriented instruction is through the introduction to clinical medicine, community medicine, and other behavioral medicine courses during the second basic science year.

A traditional third-year curriculum gives the student a foundation in history taking, examination, patient relations, laboratory aids, diagnosis, treatment, and use of medical literature in the major clinical disciplines.

The fourth year is composed of requirements (60 percent) and electives (40 percent). Requirements include critical care medicine; anesthesia; surgical subspecialties; and a medicine, family practice, or pediatrics subinternship. Three months of rural rotations during the third and fourth years are also required.

Students with exceptional interest in research will be considered for the Medical Scientist M.D.-Ph.D. program. The Ph.D. is offered in over eight disciplines. An M.D.-M.P.H. program is also offered.

An honors/satisfactory/unsatisfactory plus narrative grading system is used in the School of Medicine. 100 hours of community service are required for graduation. Students are expected to demonstrate professionalism at all times.

REQUIREMENTS FOR ENTRANCE

The MCAT and a minimum of three years of college in an accredited US or Canadian school (minimum of 90 semester hours or equivalent) are required. All required courses must be passed with a grade of C or better by January 1 of the matriculation year. College work must include:

	Sem. hrs.
Biology or Zoology (with lab)	8
Inorganic Chemistry (with lab)	8
Organic Chemistry (with lab)	8
General Physics (with lab)	8
English	6
Behavioral or Social Sciences	6

We highly recommend that applicants complete courses in biochemistry and cellular/molecular biology. Fundamental competence in communication skills is emphasized as a great need.

Additional coursework should be designed to provide breadth leading toward a bachelor's degree in a major field of the applicant's own choosing, not necessarily in the natural sciences or in a premedical curriculum. Computer literacy is required.

Applicants are strongly encouraged to (and Early Decision Program applicants <u>must</u>) take the MCAT no later than April of the year before they hope to enter medical school. Applicants may apply as early as June 1 and usually should apply no later than mid-August. Interviews are held only on-site beginning in September. No applicant is admitted without an interview. Acceptances will be issued periodically throughout the interview period.

Occasional transfer applications are accepted from medical students in LCME-accredited schools who are in good academic and professional standing with compelling circumstances to transfer. Students from other doctoral-level programs (dental, podiatric, graduate, etc.) are ineligible for advanced standing. West Virginia residents receive priority consideration.

SELECTION FACTORS

As a state-supported school, the School of Medicine gives preference in selection of students to West Virginia residents, but places are available each year to well-qualified non-residents, especially those who have strong ties to the state of West Virginia. Choice of students is based upon scholarship, MCAT scores, community service, leadership, medical experience, personal qualifications as judged by interviews, and recommendations from qualified persons. Although most students present a bachelor's degree at matriculation, occasionally carefully selected individuals may be admitted at the end of three years (90 semester hours) of college work.

The School of Medicine does not discriminate on the basis of race, sex, creed, national origin, age, or handicap. Qualified members of groups underrepresented in medicine are encouraged to apply. The Health Careers Opportunity Program is available for disadvantaged students or those from groups underrepresented in medicine.

Approximately one-third of the students will be required to spend their clinical years at the Charleston Division of the West Virginia University School of Medicine. Additionally, a small number of students will spend their clinical years at our new Eastern Panhandle campus.

The 2002 entering class had the following profile: *residence,* 90 percent West Virginia residents; *mean overall GPA,* 3.69; *mean MCAT scores,* VR-8.8, PS-8.9, WS-N, BS-9.4; *gender,* 40 percent women; *undergraduate major,* 90 percent in biological sciences, chemistry, or preprofessional curriculum;

degrees, 96 bachelor's degrees, 6 graduate degrees; *undergraduate schools,* 60 students attended West Virginia schools.

FINANCIAL AID

Approximately 90 percent of the school's medical students receive financial aid. A limited number of scholarship awards are available to well-qualified students based on financial need and merit. In addition, multiple loan funds are also available. Students' spouses with reasonable training and experience ordinarily have little difficulty in finding work near the medical school, the University, or Morgantown. Medical students are discouraged from seeking outside employment

Institution Type: *Public*
Application Process: *AMCAS, see chapter 4.*

APPLICATION AND ACCEPTANCE POLICIES FOR 2005–2006 FIRST-YEAR CLASS

Filing of AMCAS application
  Earliest date: June 1, 2004
  Latest date: Dec. 1, 2004
School application fee to all applicants: $100
Oldest MCAT scores considered: 2003
Does have Early Decision Program (EDP)
  For West Virginia residents only
  EDP application period: June 1–Aug. 1, 2004
  EDP applicants notified by: Oct. 1, 2004
Acceptance notice to regular applicants
  Earliest date: Oct. 15, 2004
  Latest date: Until class is filled
Applicant's response to acceptance offer
  Maximum time: 2 weeks
Requests for deferred entrance considered: Yes
Deposit to hold place in class (applied to tuition):
  $200 for resident, $400 for nonresident
Deposit refundable prior to: May 1, 2005
Estimated number of new entrants: 110 (10 EDP)
Starting date: August 2005

TUITION AND STUDENT FEES PER YEAR FOR 2003–2004 FIRST-YEAR CLASS

Tuition   Student fees: $2,048
  Resident: $12,366
  Nonresident: $30,106

INFORMATION ON 2003–2004 FIRST-YEAR CLASS

Number of	In-State	Out-of-State	Total
Applicants	231	627	858
Applicants Interviewed	149	107	256
New Entrants*	80	28	108

*All took the MCAT; 99% had baccalaureate degrees.

CHAPTER **11**

Medical College of Wisconsin

Milwaukee, Wisconsin

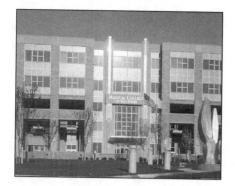

Dr. Michael J. Dunn, *Dean and Executive Vice President*
Michael T. Istwan, *Director of Admissions*
Linda L. Pascal, *Director of Student Financial Services*
Dr. Earnestine Willis, *Associate Dean for Multicultural Affairs*

ADDRESS INQUIRIES TO:

Office of Admissions
Medical College of Wisconsin
8701 Watertown Plank Road
Milwaukee, Wisconsin 53226
(414) 456-8246; 456-6506 (FAX)
Web site: www.mcw.edu/acad/admission

MISSION STATEMENT

The Medical College of Wisconsin is a private, academic medical center dedicated to leadership and excellence in:
Education – Teaching the physicians and scientists of tomorrow, while embracing the skills of today's health professionals.
Research – creating new knowledge in basic and clinical science through biomedical, behavioral and health services research.
Patient Care – caring humanely and expertly for patients and providing leadership in health services.
Community Service – forging regional, national and global partnerships in education, health care and research for the betterment of human health.

GENERAL INFORMATION

With roots going back to the last century, the Medical College of Wisconsin became an independent, freestanding school of medicine in 1967. Located on the campus of the Milwaukee Regional Medical Center, it is a private medical school with a public mission of education, research, patient care, and community service. Strong relationships and special educational programs are maintained with other educational institutions throughout Wisconsin. Major affiliated teaching hospitals include the Froedtert Hospital, Clement J. Zablocki Veterans Affairs Medical Center, and the Children's Hospital of Wisconsin. Additional affiliations with both private and community hospitals bring the number of teaching beds available for clinical education to over 7,000.

CURRICULUM

The curriculum is designed to provide a solid foundation for a career in any discipline of medicine. In the first two years, students acquire a thorough knowledge of the basic medical sciences. Courses in anatomy, neuroscience, biochemistry, physiology, biostatistics, and psychiatry comprise the first year. The second-year courses include microbiology, pathology, pharmacology, and psychiatry. The clinical continuum provides first- and second-year students with integrated early generalist experiences, the fundamental skills and attitudes of professional development, and knowledge in the following disciplines: human behavior, bioethics and care of the terminally ill, information management, physical diagnosis, and health care systems.

The third year consists of required clinical clerkships during which students gain experience in the major disciplines of medicine. Clerkships include two month rotations in Internal Medicine, Surgery, and Pediatrics, and a one and a half month clerkships in Obstetrics and Gynecology and Psychiatry and Neurology. Students will also participate in a one month clerkship in family medicine and a one month clerkship incorporating training in advanced life and training support and Anesthesiology clinical experiences. Students may also select a two-week, non-graded elective experience or a four-week graded experience.

During the fourth year, students complete three one-month rotations in surgery; a medical selective and a subinternship (internal medicine, pediatrics, or family medicine); and six one-month electives.

Students with a particular interest in research can pursue a variety of options, including the Honors in Research program or joint M.S.-M.D. or M.D.-Ph.D. degree programs. Four students are selected annually for the Medical Scientist Training Program, which culminates with the awarding of both the M.D. and Ph.D. degrees at the end of a seven-year period of study. A five-year extended curriculum is available to students who wish to carry out their studies in the M.D. program over a longer period of time.

REQUIREMENTS FOR ENTRANCE

The MCAT is required and must be taken no more than three years prior to matriculation. A minimum of three years of undergraduate work (90 semester hours) at an accredited college or university in the United States or Canada is required; however, students are strongly encouraged to complete a baccalaureate degree before entering the Medical College of Wisconsin. Because the school accepts students from a variety of major fields of study, students are encouraged to determine their fields of major study according to their personal interest. Each prospective medical student must take the following courses for *graded credit* at an accredited college or university in the United States or Canada:

	Graded Credit
Biology (with lab)	8
General Chemistry (with lab)	8

Organic Chemistry (with lab) 8
Physics (with lab) 8
English (should stress composition) 6
Mathematics

Completion of a course in algebra in high school or college.

Officially granted Advanced Placement (AP) credit will <u>only</u> be accepted to fulfill 3 graded credits of English.

Applicants to the Medical College of Wisconsin who attend undergraduate colleges/universities that do not give graded credit for coursework will not be considered for admission.

Students must be capable of expressing themselves effectively, both orally and in writing.

SELECTION FACTORS

The college seeks students who are well suited to the competent and ethical practice of medicine. Successful applicants will have a mature sense of values, sound motivation, demonstrated academic achievement, willingness and ability to assume responsibility, and be of high moral and ethical character.

The selection of students is based on a careful analysis of each candidate's suitability for the profession of medicine. Undergraduate achievement and MCAT scores are carefully evaluated, but academic excellence alone does not assure acceptance. Subjective factors, including the candidate's statement on the AMCAS application, academic recommendations, and personal interviews are also important.

Interviews are an integral part of the admissions process, and all applicants being seriously considered are interviewed before being offered an acceptance. Interviews are scheduled only at the request of the Admissions Committee, following a review of the application, and are done only at the College. Applications are reviewed based upon completion date, and interviews and offers are made on a rolling basis until the class is filled. Applicants are encouraged to complete their file as early as possible.

The Medical College of Wisconsin accepts about forty percent of its entering class from Wisconsin, with the remainder coming from other states. Women represented 46 percent of the 2003 entering class. The Medical College of Wisconsin does not discriminate on the basis of race, gender, creed, disability, age, national origin, or sexual orientation.

FINANCIAL AID

Most financial assistance available through the college, including federal and institutional scholarships and loans, is awarded solely on the basis of need. The Financial Aid Office develops a financial aid package for each student, based upon individual needs. The office helps direct students to additional sources of support. Applicants are strongly encouraged to initiate their financial aid application as soon as they have been interviewed. *A stipulation of acceptance for all applicants includes documentation of a current clean credit report, and compliance with the medical college's credit guidelines.* Because of restrictions placed on loan and scholarship funds, foreign citizens are not eligible for financial aid. All foreign applicants must file proof of financial support before they are eligible for acceptance.

INFORMATION FOR MULTICULTURAL STUDENTS

The Medical College of Wisconsin actively seeks applications from talented students from groups underrepresented in medicine, inclusive of out of state residents. In addition to academic achievement, MCAT scores, letters of recommendation, and personal interviews, the Admissions Committee carefully considers the student's motivation and cultural and educational background. Through the Office of Multicultural Student Affairs, a variety of programs exist to assist these students, demonstrating the college's strong commitment to their recruitment, retention, and graduation. Further information concerning programs for students from groups underrepresented in medicine may be obtained from the associate dean for the Office of Multicultural Student Affairs.

Institution Type: *Private*
Application Process: *AMCAS, see chapter 4.*

APPLICATION AND ACCEPTANCE POLICIES FOR 2005–2006 FIRST-YEAR CLASS

Filing of AMCAS application
  Earliest date: June 1, 2004
  Latest date: Nov. 1, 2004
School application fee to all applicants: $60
Oldest MCAT scores considered: 2002
Does have Early Decision Program (EDP)
  EDP application period: June 1–Aug. 1, 2004
  EDP applicants notified by: Oct. 1, 2004
Acceptance notice to regular applicants
  Earliest date: Oct. 15, 2004
  Latest date: Until class is filled
Applicant's response to acceptance offer
  Maximum time: 4 weeks
Requests for deferred entrance considered: Yes
Deposit to hold place in class (applied to tuition):
  $100, due with response to acceptance offer
Deposit refundable prior to: May 16, 2005
Estimated number of new entrants: 204 (10 EDP)
Starting date: August 2005

TUITION AND STUDENT FEES PER YEAR FOR 2003–2004 FIRST-YEAR CLASS

Tuition   Student fees: $106
  Resident: $26,094
  Nonresident: $31,150

INFORMATION ON 2003–2004 FIRST-YEAR CLASS

Number of	In-State	Out-of-State	Total
Applicants	493	3,201	3,694
Applicants Interviewed	206	373	579
New Entrants*	99	106	205

*All took the MCAT; 99% had baccalaureate degrees.

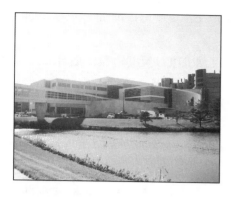

University of Wisconsin Medical School

Madison, Wisconsin

Dr. Philip M. Farrell, *Dean*
Lucy J. Wall, *Assistant Dean for Admissions*
Dr. Gloria V. Hawkins, *Assistant Dean for Minority Affairs*

ADDRESS INQUIRIES TO:

Admissions Committee
Health Sciences Learning Center
University of Wisconsin Medical School
750 Highland Avenue
Madison, Wisconsin 53705-2221
(608) 263-4925; 262-2327 (FAX)
Web site: www.med.wisc.edu

MISSION STATEMENT

The University of Wisconsin Medical School is committed to meeting the health needs of Wisconsin and beyond through excellence in education, research, patient care, and service. The UW Medical School seeks to be one of the preeminent medical schools by excelling in the creation, integration, and transfer of knowledge through a combination of basic, transla-tional, and clinical research; a greater emphasis on active learning; and consistently outstanding patient care.

GENERAL INFORMATION

The University of Wisconsin Medical School initiated a two-year medical education program in 1907 and expanded to a full four-year program in 1924. The present University of Wisconsin Center for Health Sciences—which includes the Medical School and University Hospital and Clinics—is located on the university campus in Madison. The new Health Sciences Learning Center houses the first and second year teaching facilities and administrative offices. The medical school basic science departments are located in the Medical Sciences Center. The Clinical Science Center houses the clin-ical departments, University Hospital and Clinics, School of Nursing, and Wisconsin Clinical Cancer Center. In addition to the University Hospital and Clinics, other clinical sites in Madison and throughout the state are utilized in the educational program.

CURRICULUM

The educational and research programs have been developed to educate students to become qualified to undertake any career in medicine. Our curriculum introduces students to the general-ist practice of medicine by exposing students to community-based settings in the first and second years. The curriculum emphasizes: active learning; case-based problem-solving;

interdisciplinary teaching by the basic science and clinical faculty throughout the first and second years; a four-year curriculum that prepares students for either a primary care or specialty career; diverse clinical clerkship experiences around the state, including inner-city and rural sites; and an eight-week one-on-one preceptorship with an experienced clinician in Year 4. The senior year provides elective opportunities for study at other institutions and abroad.

Opportunities for research are available to medical students in individually arranged programs leading to the M.S. and Ph.D. degrees or by nondegree arrangements. Competitive support is offered to resident and nonresident students entering as M.D.-Ph.D. candidates. Letter grades are used to evaluate students' academic performance throughout the four-year curriculum.

REQUIREMENTS FOR ENTRANCE

The MCAT is required. Applicants are strongly encouraged to take the MCAT in the spring before application. Consideration of applicants who indicate they are taking the fall MCAT will be delayed, without detriment, until receipt of those scores.

Applicants must have a minimum of three years (90 semester hours) of college work by the time of matriculation. However, applicants are encouraged to obtain a baccalaureate degree before matriculation. Courses in English, Biochemistry, Quantitative Analysis, Calculus, and electives in the humanities and social sciences are recommended. College work must include:

	Semesters
General Zoology or Biology (with lab)	1
Advanced Zoology or Biology (with lab)	1
Inorganic/General Chemistry (with lab)	2
Organic Chemistry (with lab)	2
General Physics (with lab)	2
Mathematics	2

SELECTION FACTORS

Breadth of academic and nonacademic interests and expe-riences, ability to communicate with others, motivation for medicine, personal characteristics, and intellectual ability are some of the factors considered by the Admissions Committee. The Admissions Committee seeks students with diverse backgrounds and interests, which are of value in training professionals for good health care delivery. A preprofessional committee evaluation or three academic letters of recommendation plus one nonacademic letter of recommendation are required and must be submitted no later than December 1. Following the initial screening process, applicants will be invited for personal interviews to complete the application process.

The University of Wisconsin Medical School does not discriminate on the basis of race, sex, creed, national origin, age, or handicap. Women, disadvantaged students, and students from rural areas and groups underrepresented in medicine are encouraged to apply. Preference is given to residents of Wisconsin. Nonresident applicants are competing for relatively few places. Secondary applications are sent only to eligible applicants who are academically qualified, following a screening of the AMCAS application. Applications are accepted from foreign nationals who have a permanent resident visa in the United States. The 2003 entering class had an *average GPA* of 3.74; *average MCAT* scores were VR–10.0, PS–10.2, WS–P, BS–10.6.

FINANCIAL AID

All financial aid allocated by the University of Wisconsin Medical School is awarded on the basis of proven need. Need is calculated as the necessary expenses incurred while attending medical school minus the resources provided to the student by outside agencies, personal resources, and available parental resources. Priority for financial aid, especially grant awards, will be given to students with the greatest need. The major proportion of total financial aid is available in the form of loans. Approximately 90 percent of the students receive financial assistance.

INFORMATION ABOUT DIVERSITY PROGRAMS

The University of Wisconsin Medical School is committed to increasing the number of physicians from groups underrepresented in medicine and those showing evidence of socioeconomically- and educationally-disadvantaged backgrounds. Applications are encouraged from persons with socioeconomic disadvantages and from groups underrepresented in medicine.

Institution Type: *Public*
Application Process: *AMCAS, see chapter 4.*

APPLICATION AND ACCEPTANCE POLICIES FOR 2005–2006 FIRST-YEAR CLASS

Filing of AMCAS application
   Earliest date: June 1, 2004
   Latest date: Nov. 1, 2004
School application fee after screening: $45
Oldest MCAT scores considered: 2000
Does have Early Decision Program (EDP)
   For Wisconsin residents only
   EDP application period: June 1–Aug. 1, 2004
   EDP applicants notified by: Oct. 1, 2004
Acceptance notice to regular applicants
   Earliest date: Oct. 15, 2004
   Latest date: until class is filled
Applicant's response to acceptance offer
   Maximum time: 2 weeks
Requests for deferred entrance considered: Yes
   (for Wisconsin residents only)
Deposit to hold place in class: None
Estimated number of new entrants: 150 (10 EDP)
Starting date: August 2005

TUITION AND STUDENT FEES PER YEAR FOR 2003–2004 FIRST-YEAR CLASS

Tuition: Student Fees: $585
   Resident: $21,153
   Nonresident: $32,277

INFORMATION ON 2003–2004 FIRST-YEAR CLASS

Number of	In-State	Out-of-State	Total
Applicants	518	1,384	1,902
Applicants Interviewed	**	**	466
New Entrants*	130	20	150

*100% had baccalaureate degrees; 82% took the MCAT.
**Data not available.

CHAPTER

Information About Canadian Medical Schools
Accredited by the LCME and by the CACMS

The 16 medical schools in Canada are affiliate institutional members of the AAMC and participate in the Association's activities. The Canadian medical schools are accredited jointly by the LCME and the Committee on Accreditation of Canadian Medical Schools (CACMS) of the Association of Canadian Medical Colleges. All are M.D. degree-granting schools with high-quality educational programs.

Admission policies and procedures of Canadian schools are similar in many respects to those followed in U.S. schools; thus, many of the suggestions for applicants in chapters 1 through 9 will also apply. Differences exist, however, in the relative importance given by schools to various factors in the selection process. Applicants should refer to the individual school entries for details on these differences.

Fourteen Canadian medical schools offer four-year programs; two, McMaster and Calgary, are three-year programs. The University of Montreal converted from a five- to a four-year curriculum in 1992. With the introduction of the four-year curriculum there, some students are now admitted into a one-year preparatory program prior to commencing the M.D. curriculum.

Selection Criteria

Pre-university education differs in Canada from the 12-year elementary and secondary system in the United States. Significant differences also exist from province to province in Canada. As reflected in the individual school entries, these differences affect the number of years of undergraduate instruction required of applicants to various Canadian medical schools. In addition to differences due to the educational system, individual schools may also have their own additional requirements. Table 12-A shows that physics, inorganic and organic chemistry, biology, humanities, and English are the most common subjects required in undergraduate education by the Canadian schools.

Language of Instruction

Three Canadian medical schools—Laval, Montreal and Sherbrooke, all located in the province of Quebec—require students to be fluent in French as all instruction is in that language. Instruction in the other 13 schools is in English, although the University of Ottawa offers the M.D. curriculum in both French and English.

Residency Requirements

Because universities are a provincial responsibility in Canada, most medical schools give preference to Canadian citizens and permanent residents residing in the province where the medical school is located. Individual schools may prefer to select students from specific regions within the province. Prospective applicants should be aware of these preferences to maximize their chances of being admitted.

A number of foreign students are accepted into Canadian medical schools each year. In this context, "foreign" refers to persons who are neither citizens of Canada nor permanent residents in Canada at the time of application. Two medical schools, Memorial University in St. John's, Newfoundland, and McGill University in Montreal, Quebec, have a specific number of places reserved for applicants from the United States. Other faculties of medicine in Canada either have or are considering the introduction quotas for both U.S. and other foreign applicants. Foreign students, including U.S. students, pay substantially higher tuition fees. Applicants from outside Canada should consult a particular school to ascertain whether that school considers applications from non-Canadian citizens or non-immigrants.

Academic Record/Suitability

Although an excellent academic record is a very important factor in gaining admission to a Canadian medical school, a great deal of effort goes into assessing applicants' suitability for a medical career based on other factors. Personal suitability is assessed in a variety of ways by the schools; applicants who can demonstrate that they possess the qualities considered important in the practice of medicine may sometimes be admitted even if their academic record is not outstanding. Conversely, applicants with outstanding records who do not possess these qualities may not gain a place in medical school.

Most applicants to Canadian medical schools are interviewed prior to acceptance, so the interview information in Chapter 7 will be useful.

MCAT

Eleven Canadian medical schools require applicants to take the MCAT: Alberta, British Columbia, Calgary, Dalhousie, Manitoba, McGill, Memorial, Queen's, Saskatchewan, Toronto, and Western Ontario.

Other Considerations

Applicants and entrants to Canadian schools today are often older than their counterparts in past years. Most medical schools no longer have age-related admissions policies, although older applicants are not quite as successful in gaining admission as younger ones. Prospective candidates should check school statistics regarding the age range of new entrants.

Canadian faculties of medicine do not discriminate on the basis of race, religion, or gender in admitting new students. The admission of native Canadian (Indian and Inuit) students is encouraged in several Canadian medical schools.

The number of female applicants has risen dramatically in recent years, with correspondingly larger proportions of entering classes consisting of women. Women comprised 57.4 percent of the 2002-2003 applicant pool, and the success rate for women was slightly higher than that for men. The first-year classes at Canadian medical schools was 59 percent female in 2002-2003. Overall, 28 percent of applicants received at least one offer of admission.

Expenses/Financial Aid

Tuition and student fees for Canadian and non-Canadian students in the 2003-2004 entering class are provided in Table 12-B and in individual school entries. Expenses vary from school to school and from student to student. Tuition at several Canadian schools is slightly higher for the first year than for successive years. Tuition and fees at all Canadian universities are expected to increase substantially in the next several years.

Some financial aid information is provided in the individual school entries. Eligible Canadian students may apply for a Canadian Student Loan, or may apply to the Department of Education in their province for a provincial student loan.

TABLE 12-A
Subjects Required by Three or More Canadian Medical Schools, 2005–2006 Entering Class

Required Subject	No. of Schools (n=12)
Physics	6
Inorganic Chemistry	10
Organic Chemistry	9
Biology	10
English	6
BioChemistry	5
Humanities	7

NOTE: Figures based on data provided fall 2003. Four of the 16 medical schools (Calgary, Dalhousie, McMaster, and Toronto) did not indicate specific course requirements and are not included in the tabulations.

TABLE 12-B

Tuition and Student Fees for 2003–2004 First-Year Students at Canadian Medical Schools (In Canadian Dollars)

Categories of Students	Range	Median	Average
Canadian	3,250 - 16,207	9,853	9,895*
Non-Canadian, Regular*	11,969-30,440	20,160	22,663*
Non-Canadian, Contract*	28,979 - 39,473	31,000	32,775*

NOTE: Figures based on data provided fall 2003.

* Average residents were derived from all 16 Canadian schools. Average nonresidents (regular) data were derived from 9 Canadian schools reporting (7 schools to not accept nonresidents into regular quota positions). Average nonresidents (contract) data were derived from 8 schools which accept foreign students into above-quota positions on a cost-recovery, contract basis.

Source: Association of Canadian Medical Colleges

Ontario Medical School Application Service (OMSAS)

The Ontario Medical School Application Service (OMSAS) is a non-profit, centralized application service for applicants to the six medical schools in Ontario. OMSAS provides only the application processing service; each medical school is autonomous in reaching its admission decisions. All applications to the Ontario medical schools must be made through OMSAS.

The on-line application, COMPASS.OMSAS is available in early July. Completed applications must be received at OMSAS by October 1. Applicants will be required to register their intention to apply by directly entering the COMPASS.OMSAS on-line application system by September 15. Register at ✑ www.ouac.on.ca/omsas/. Official transcripts and references must be received at OMSAS by October 1. Applicants are advised to submit their application and supporting documents in advance of the deadline.

For the instruction booklet containing information about application procedures and admission requirements, visit ✑ www.ouac.on.ca/omsas/

Information Sources

Further information about admission requirements, curricula of Canadian medical schools, and medical education in Canada is provided in catalogs available from each school, and downloaded free of charge from the ACMC Web site. A printed version of *Admission Requirements of Canadian Faculties of Medicine* (edited 2003 for admission in 2004/05) can also be ordered, priced at CDN$20 for distribution in Canada, CDN$25 for US residents, and CDN$35 for overseas requests. Order from:

The Association of Canadian Medical Colleges
774 Echo Drive
Ottawa, Ontario
Canada K1S 5P2
(613) 730-0687
Information is also available at their Web site: ✑ www.acmc.ca.

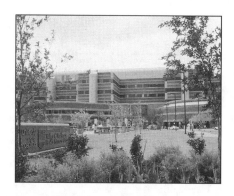

University of Alberta
Faculty of Medicine and Dentistry

Edmonton, Alberta

Dr. D. L. J. Tyrrell, *Dean*
Dr. Marc Moreau, *Assistant Dean, Admissions*
M. Healey, *Admissions Officer*

ADDRESS INQUIRIES TO:

Admissions Officer, Admissions
2-45 Medical Sciences Building
University of Alberta
Faculty of Medicine and Dentistry
Edmonton, Alberta
Canada, T6G 2H7
(780) 492-9524; 492-9531 (FAX)
E-mail: admissions@med.ualberta.ca
Web site: www.med.ualberta.ca

MISSION STATEMENT

Dedicated to the optimizations of health through scholarship and leadership in our education programs, in fundamental and applied research and in the prevention and treatment of illness in conjunction with the Capital Health Authority and other partners.

Vision: To be nationally and internationally recognized leaders investing in education, research and service, making important contributions to Health.

GENERAL INFORMATION

The Faculty of Medicine at the University of Alberta was founded in 1913.

The Medical Sciences Building, the Clinical Sciences Building, the Walter C. Mackenzie Health Sciences Centre, and the University of Alberta Hospitals are located on the university campus. Clinical instruction is also given at the Royal Alexandra Hospital, Edmonton General Hospital, Misericordia Hospital, Alberta Hospital, Glenrose Hospital, Cross Cancer Institute, and Grey Nuns Hospital.

Student counseling services and student health services are available to all University of Alberta students.

CURRICULUM

The Faculty of Medicine conducts a fully accredited, four-year program leading to the degree of doctor of medicine. Each of the first two years consists of 33 weeks of instruction, from early September until mid-May. The final two years are conducted as a continuum, during which each student has a four-week holiday period.

The first two years of the curriculum are an integrated systems-based program covering the basic and clinical sciences. It is primarily case based and uses a mixture of lectures and small-group sessions with some problem-based learning. The last two years are composed of a student internship of at least 56 weeks, during which the student is assigned to hospitals affiliated with the faculty for clinical study and experience, a selective program in medicine and surgery, and an elective program that allows students to develop their own curriculum and spend a minimum of 12 weeks in one or more subject areas of their choice.

Throughout the program, emphasis is on self-education; much instruction is on a small-group basis.

A graduate training program leading to eligibility for specialist qualifications by the Royal College of Physicians and Surgeons of Canada is offered in most clinical specialties. Programs leading to the degree of master of science or doctor of philosophy in any of the basic medical sciences and in most of the clinical medical sciences are conducted under the direction of the Faculty of Graduate Studies and Research of the university.

Opportunity for research in the basic medical sciences is available to those students interested in spending a year or more in this type of work and obtaining a bachelor of science in medicine degree.

REQUIREMENTS FOR ENTRANCE

The MCAT is compulsory. All students considering medicine must register in a degree program and maintain good standing in that program. Regardless of the degree program, the student must take courses in the following subjects:

Biological Sciences: General Biology
Biochemistry
Chemistry: Inorganic and Organic Chemistry
General Physics
Statistics
English

These courses must be full-year courses (equivalent to six-credit courses at the University of Alberta) or two single-term courses (equivalent to three-credit courses at the University of Alberta) with the exception of statistics and biochemistry, in which a single three-credit course is acceptable.

Students are encouraged to obtain a baccalaureate degree prior to admission but may apply after two or three years in a degree program. To be considered for early selection, a student must have all the prerequisites as well as exceptional academic (minimum GPA of 3.7 on a 4.0 scale) and personal qualifications. Mature applicants may be given special consideration.

SELECTION FACTORS

Selection is based upon quality of scholastic achievement, personal suitability, and performance on the MCAT. Alberta residents are preferred, although each year out-of-province applicants are considered for 15 percent of first-year places. An interview and letter(s) of reference are required. All information on each candidate is considered by the Admissions Committee, and the quota is filled by the best candidates available.

ABORIGINAL APPLICANTS

The Faculty of Medicine and Dentistry may provide up to three positions over the regular quota of 125 for the M.D. program to Aboriginal applicants. For clarification, it is noted that students who are Aboriginal ancestry within the meaning of the Constitution Act of 1982, Section 35. (2) will be considered in this category.

Candidates will be subject to normal minimum admission requirements and approval by the Faculty of Medicine and Dentistry Admissions Committee. If there are no qualified Aboriginal students in any given year, these positions will not be allocated to other applicants.

Aboriginal student applicants and prospective premedical students are encouraged to contact the Coordinator, Native Health Care Careers, Faculty of Medicine and Dentistry, for individual counseling and career planning.

M.D.–PH.D. PROGRAM

Highly qualified students motivated toward a career in medical research may wish to consider the M.D.-Ph.D. program.

FINANCIAL AID

Loans are available under the Canada Student Loan Plan or the Province of Alberta Loan Plan to Canadian citizens or permanent residents who have been in Canada and in Alberta for 12 months prior to the beginning of the academic term.

Institution Type: *Public*

APPLICATION AND ACCEPTANCE POLICIES FOR 2005-2006 FIRST-YEAR CLASS

Fees and expenses are in Canadian dollars.

Filing of application
   Earliest date: July 2, 2004
   Latest date: Nov. 1, 2004
School application fee to all applicants: $60
Oldest MCAT scores considered: 1991
Does not have Early Decision Program
   Acceptance notice to regular applicants
   Earliest date: March-June 2005
   Latest date: until class is filled
Applicant's response to acceptance offer
   Maximum time: 2 weeks
Requests for deferred entrance considered: Yes
Deposit to hold place in class (applied to tuition):
   $175, due with response to acceptance offer;
   nonrefundable
Estimated number of new entrants: 125
Starting date: September 2005

TUITION AND STUDENT FEES PER YEAR FOR 2003-2004 FIRST-YEAR CLASS

Tuition*   Student fees: $463.34
   Canadian: $10,066.24
   Non-Canadian: N/A

INFORMATION ON 2003-2004 FIRST-YEAR CLASS

Number of	In-Province	Out-of-Province	Total
Applicants	427	540	967
Applicants Interviewed	234	65	299
New Entrants†	108	17	125

*Includes student fees; no longer broken down into tuition and fees.
†All took the MCAT; 85% had baccalaureate degrees.

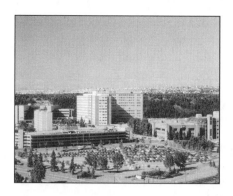

University of Calgary Faculty of Medicine

Calgary, Alberta

Dr. Grant Gall, *Dean of Medicine*
Adele Meyers, *Admissions Officer*
Linda Sharma, *Director, Awards and Financial Aid*

ADDRESS INQUIRIES TO:

Office of Admissions
University of Calgary
Faculty of Medicine
3330 Hospital Drive, N.W.
Calgary, Alberta
Canada T2N 4N1
(403) 220-4262
E-mail: staylor@ucalgary.ca
Web site: www.med.ucalgary.ca/admissions

MISSION STATEMENT

What kind of medical school do we wish to be?

- A medical school responsive to community and societal needs—not only of the present but of the future.
- A medical school determined to shape the future of society, i.e., a medical school that leads with vision, developing new ideas, resources, technology, health care, and scientific professionals that will ensure that the preferred or desired future will become a reality.
- A medical school rooted in basic research and discovery, the creation of new knowledge, and the transfer of that knowledge and discovery to benefit society.
- A medical school committed to excellence and pursuit of excellence, to high quality and standards, to continuous evaluation of status quo, to assurance of quality, to effective and efficient outcomes, and to continuous improvement in all endeavours.
- A medical school committed to innovation and creativity in education, research, clinical service, administration and management, and development of human resources and technology.
- A medical school with a sense of values, principles, and priorities.

GENERAL INFORMATION

The Faculty of Medicine at the University of Calgary accepted its first students in September 1970. In 1972 the Faculty of Medicine moved into its permanent facilities in the Calgary Health Sciences Centre. The centre has been designed to complement the objectives of the faculty's integrated teaching program.

CURRICULUM

The curriculum is based on clinical presentations the way patients present to physicians. One hundred twenty clinical presentations have been defined ranging from simple to complex and are grouped by body system and human development. The first course offered is principles for medicine, which serves to introduce the different modes of solving clinical problems and the basic concepts essential to an understanding of human structure, function, and growth as well as provision of comprehensive medical care to the individual, the family, and society. Introductory clinical skills of communication and physical examination also commence in the first weeks of the curriculum. Following principles of medicine is the first of the interdisciplinary body systems courses. Approximately two-thirds of the student's time is allocated to these regularly scheduled courses. The remaining period is available for elective study and the independent study or tutorial program. Each academic year lasts about 11 months. The problem-solving approach, combined with the curriculum design, is intended to facilitate the integration between the conventional basic and clinical sciences. As well, students have the opportunity to reinforce in a clinical setting what they have learned in the body systems as they progress through each of the systems. The curriculum also focuses on the relevance of the family and the community in health and disease.

The school employs a pass/fail grading system. Interested students may apply for the combined M.D.-M.Sc. or M.D.-Ph.D. program. At the end of the three years, students will be granted the M.D. degree. The school's philosophy is to produce generalist physicians who can proceed to further training in specialty, family medicine, or research.

REQUIREMENTS FOR ENTRANCE

All students are required to take the MCAT by the fall of the year before anticipated enrollment. Most students have a B.A. or B.Sc. degree before entering the Faculty of Medicine, although a few extremely well qualified students have been admitted after two years in an arts or science program. There is some advantage to majoring in a science area, but the student who has excelled in behavioral science or any other undergraduate area may be accepted.

The following undergraduate courses are recommended: a full year of general biology, mammalian physiology, organic and inorganic chemistry, biochemistry, English, physics, calculus, and one semester of psychology, sociology, or anthropology.

SELECTION FACTORS

The Admissions Committee selects applicants without discrimination to gender, race, religion, or age and attempts to apply six criteria: undergraduate academic achievement, employment history, extracurricular activities, an essay, letters of recommendation, and the MCAT. Final applicants will be required to attend an interview at the University of Calgary at their own expense. Final applicants will also be required to write an on-site essay on a topic assigned by the Admissions Committee. Preference is given to Alberta residents. We do not accept applications from individual international students. Presently, seats for international students are limited to those students who come from institutions/countries with whom the Faculty of Medicine has a formal, contractual agreement. Rejected applicants are given the opportunity to reapply for admission. Applicants who have been asked to withdraw or who have been suspended or expelled from any medical school will not usually be considered.

ADMISSION OF STUDENTS BY TRANSFER

The University of Calgary Faculty of Medicine will consider application by students for transfer only from other LCME-accredited medical schools and only under special circumstances. Approval of transfer will be based on evaluation of the candidate and his/her past performance and on the availability of positions. Because the first and second years of the three-year M.D. program at the University of Calgary are regarded as a continuum of coursework, transfers will only be considered in the final or clerkship year.

FINANCIAL AID

The majority of students obtain financial aid through student loans. Because the students attend school 11 months each year, summer employment is unlikely, and, therefore, financial support must be sufficient to meet their requirements over the subsequent three years. The student awards officer will provide information about student loans, bursaries, and awards. The financial status of the applicant does not affect acceptance into the program.

Students receive a total stipend of $3,420 for the third (final) year.

Institution Type: *Public*

APPLICATION AND ACCEPTANCE POLICIES FOR 2005-2006 FIRST-YEAR CLASS

Fees and expenses are in Canadian dollars.

Filing of application
    Earliest date: July 15, 2004
    Latest date: Nov. 15, 2004
School application fee to all applicants: $85
Oldest MCAT scores considered: 1991
Does not have Early Decision Program
Acceptance notice to regular applicants
    Earliest date: May 15, 2005
    Latest date: Varies
Applicant's response to acceptance offer
    Maximum time: 15 days
Requests for deferred entrance considered: Yes
Deposit to hold place in class (applied to tuition):
    $100, due with response to acceptance offer
Deposit refundable prior to: June 15, 2005
Estimated number of new entrants: 100
Starting date: August 2005

TUITION AND STUDENT FEES PER YEAR FOR 2003-2004 FIRST-YEAR CLASS

Tuition   Student fees: $487
    Canadian: $9,932
    Non-Canadian: $35,000

INFORMATION ON 2003-2004 FIRST-YEAR CLASS

Number of	In-Province	Out-of-Province	Total
Applicants	604	797	1,401
Applicants Interviewed	191	86	277
New Entrants†	85	15	100

†All took the MCAT; 88% had baccalaureate degrees.
‡15 Canadian; 7 International

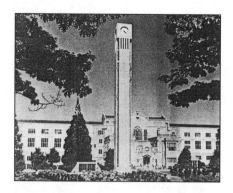

University of British Columbia
Faculty of Medicine

Vancouver, British Columbia

Dr. Gavin C.E. Stuart, *Dean, Faculty of Medicine*
Dr. Vera Frinton, *Associate Dean, Admissions*
Dr. Rosemary McCutcheon, *Student Financial Assistant Office*

ADDRESS INQUIRIES TO:

Faculty of Medicine, Deans Office Admissions
University of British Columbia
317-2194 Health Sciences Mall
Vancouver, British Columbia
Canada V6T 1Z3
(604) 822-4482; 822-6061 (FAX)
E-mail: admissions@md.ubc.ca
Web site: www.admissions.med.ubc.ca

MISSION STATEMENT

Our mission is to advance the knowledge, understanding, and health of our society through education, scholarship, and health care with excellence as the most important criterion. We create knowledge and advance learning to improve the health of individuals and our communities.

GENERAL INFORMATION

On March 15, 2002, the government of British Columbia announced funding for the expansion of the UBC Faculty of Medicine Undergraduate program.

The plan is to create a partnership in medical education with the University of Northern British Columbia, the University of Victoria and the regional Health Authorities.

The goal is to expand first-year enrollment from the current 128 students to 256 students by 2010. The first increase is planned in fall 2004 with the addition of 72 students in total, comprising 24 new seats in each of the three medical program sites. A further increase of 24 in the Vancouver-Fraser Medical Program will occur in 2005 with a final increase across all three programs taking place in 2010. By 2010, BC will have one of the largest medical schools in Canada.

In addition to increasing the supply of physicians across BC, the planned expansion will also: provide an education model for other Canadian jurisdictions, contribute to meeting federal health care recommendations, and advance BC's economic and educational capacity.

CURRICULUM

The MD Undergraduate Program is built on principles of student self-directed learning, integration of biomedical and social sciences, early clinical contact, information management, professional development and social responsibility.

The curriculum encourages students to develop attitudes and skills for lifelong learning so they are able to keep up to date with changes in the practice of medicine. The current UBC curriculum will be enhanced by contributions from our partnerships with medical and educational specialists from across British Columbia.

The first two years of the four-year program teach the foundations of medicine through a mixture of small group tutorials, lectures, laboratories, interaction with patients, community-based assignments and self-study. All students in the expanded program will be together in Vancouver for the first term after which they will be distributed to the three sites. In the third and fourth years students are learning in clinical settings and will be based in teaching hospitals and clinical settings throughout the province.

REQUIREMENTS FOR ENTRANCE

The MCAT, a minimum of three years (90 semester hours) of accredited college coursework, and a minimum of a B average or second class standing (70 percent) are required. The faculty recommends that students take courses in behavioral sciences, biometrics and statistics, and physics. A baccalaureate degree is not a prerequisite.

The minimum subject requirements are:

Years

General Biology . . . . full year
General Biochemistry . . . . full year, 2nd year or higher
General Chemistry . . . . full year
Organic Chemistry . . . . full year
English Literature and Composition . . . . full year

SELECTION FACTORS

The selection of candidates for admission to UBC's medical school is governed by guidelines established by the Senate of UBC, and is the responsibility of the Faculty of Medicine Admissions Selection Committee.

The selection process reflects the values of the UBC Faculty of Medicine and all university partners in BC's medical school. The process is designed to choose well-rounded students who meet the goals of the expanded, distributed program; who can be expected to perform well in the rigorous curriculum and problem-based learning format; and who can balance and enrich their academic experience with strong non-academic skills and interests. Similarly, selection processes of other Canadian medical schools reflect their own individual values, and are designed to select candidates who would most likely be successful in their respective programs.

The UBC Faculty of Medicine's Associate Dean of Equity oversees the selection process to ensure that all applicants are given careful consideration without regard to age, gender, race, religion, or marital and economic status.

FINANCIAL AID

UBC and the Faculty of Medicine are committed to ensuring that financial circumstances are not a barrier to qualified domestic students. For the 2003/04 academic year, approximately $350,000 is available in scholarships for students in the Faculty of Medicine MD program. Students may also qualify for bursary amounts of up to $3,000 per term for single students and $5,000 for students with dependents. Emergency loan funds are also available from both the Student Financial Assistance Office and the Faculty of Medicine.

Graduates who practice in rural areas are eligible for a number of financial incentives.

Please see the following for more details:

Forgiveness of up to 20% of student loans per year:

☞ www.aved.gov.bc.ca/studentservices/student/finish/debt_red/bc_nurse.htm

Recruitment and retention bonuses:

☞ www.healthservices.gov.bc.ca/cpa/publications/rural_programs.pdf

For more information regarding financial aid and awards, please contact Rosemary McCutcheon, Student Financial Assistance Officer for the Faculty of Medicine, at rosemary.mccutcheon@ubc.ca or (604) 875-4500, or visit ☞ www.admissions.med.ubc.ca or http://students.ubc.ca/finance.

Institution Type: *Public*

APPLICATION AND ACCEPTANCE POLICIES FOR 2005-2006 FIRST-YEAR CLASS

Fees and expenses are in Canadian dollars.

Filing of application
    Earliest date: June 15, 2004
    Latest date: Oct. 1, 2004
School application fee: $105 British Columbia
    applicants; $155 out-of-province applicants;
    additional $30 to evaluate out-of-province transcripts
Oldest MCAT scores considered: April 2000
Does not have Early Decision Program
Acceptance notice to regular applicants
    Earliest date: May 23, 2005
    Latest date: August 29, 2005
Applicant's response to acceptance offer
    Maximum time: 3 weeks
Requests for deferred entrance considered: Yes
Deposit to hold place in class (applied to tuition):
    $300, due with response to acceptance offer;
    nonrefundable
Estimated number of new entrants: 224
Starting date: Sept. 2005

TUITION AND STUDENT FEES PER YEAR FOR 2003-2004 FIRST-YEAR CLASS

Tuition: $10,272   Student fees: $651

INFORMATION ON 2003-2004 FIRST-YEAR CLASS

Number of	In-Province	Out-of-Province	Total
Applicants	703	226	929
Applicants Interviewed	366	23	389
New Entrants*	124	4	128

*All took the MCAT; 94.5% had baccalaureate degrees.

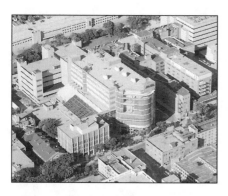

University of Manitoba
Faculty of Medicine

Winnipeg, Manitoba

Dr. B. Hennen, *Dean*
Dr. Fred Aoki, *Assistant Dean, Admissions*
Ms. Beth Jennings, *Manager Admissions & Student Affairs*

ADDRESS INQUIRIES TO:

Chair, Admissions Committee
Faculty of Medicine
University of Manitoba
270-727 McDermot Avenue
Winnipeg, Manitoba
Canada R3E 3P5
(204) 789-3494; 789-3929 (FAX)
E-mail: registrar_med@umanitoba.ca
Web site: www.umanitoba.ca/faculties/medicine/admissions/index.html

MISSION STATEMENT

The advancement of learning through teaching, scholarship and service to society by offering to outstanding undergraduate and graduate students the best education available; by carrying out scholarly activities judged to be excellent when measured against the highest international standards; and by providing service to society in those ways for which we are well-suited by virtue of our academic strengths.

GENERAL INFORMATION

The Manitoba Medical College was established in 1883 and from its beginning was affiliated with the University of Manitoba. The first class of six graduated in 1886. In 1918 the Manitoba Medical College became the Faculty of Medicine of the University of Manitoba. In 1924 it received approval as a Class A medical school. The medical buildings are adjacent to the Health Sciences Centre in Winnipeg, which is some distance from the main university campus.

Teaching hospitals affiliated with the Faculty of Medicine are the Health Sciences Centre (Children's, Adults', Women's, and Respiratory and Rehabilitation hospitals—1,064 beds); St. Boniface General Hospital (900 beds); Deer Lodge Veterans Hospital (500 beds); Grace Hospital (306 beds); Seven Oaks Hospital (336 beds); Victoria Hospital (254 beds); and Misericordia Hospital (409 beds).

CURRICULUM

Medicine is a four-year course at the University of Manitoba. In the first and second years there are, on the average, thirty hours of formal instruction per week for forty weeks. The first- and second-year curriculum covers the basic and clinical sciences, clinical and communication skills, and professional attitudes and behavior pertinent to the practice of medicine. It is composed of six instructional blocks that address the core concepts of health and medicine, human growth and development, and four organ systems-based blocks. The third and fourth years are devoted to preclerkship (nine weeks); clerkships (eight clerkships of seven weeks duration each); electives (thirteen weeks); and basic science review. A pass/fail system of evaluating student performance has been adopted, and, consequently, no rank in class or grades is given.

REQUIREMENTS FOR ENTRANCE

Applicants must have, or be eligible to receive, their bachelor's degree by June 2004 from a university recognized by the University of Manitoba. In addition, all applicants must write the MCAT by August, 2004.

The following subjects must be included in the course of study:

	Credit hrs.
Biochemistry	6
English or French Literature	6

In other respects, the content of the coursework must satisfy either the university's B.A. or B.Sc. degree requirements. Applicants must write the MCAT no later than August of the year preceding entry.

SELECTION FACTORS

Selection by the Committee on Admissions is made on the basis of a composite score, calculated as follows: (i) adjusted grade-point score: maximum, 10 percent; (ii) MCAT score: maximum, 50 percent; and (iii) personal assessment score: maximum, 40 percent. The personal assessment score is based on an autobiographical essay of approximately 1,200 words, a standardized questionnaire sent to references named by the applicant, and the results of an interview with a panel of three interviewers. Ninety percent of the 85 places available in the entering class are usually filled in this way. However, about 10 percent of successful applicants with acceptable but noncompetitive undergraduate performance may be selected on the basis of special premedical experience (educational or occupational) of relevance to the study and practice of medicine. Preference is given to undergraduates and graduates of the universities in Manitoba who are Canadian citizens or permanent residents of Canada. At the discretion of the committee, a limited number of places may be made available to undergraduates of other Canadian universities. Special consideration will be given to the Native populations of Manitoba, consistent with efforts made to recruit and retain applicants from the aboriginal populations, rural and inner-city areas.

Applicants for the 2002 entering class with a minimum GPA of 3.6 were interviewed, and 29 percent of those interviewed were enrolled.

Advanced standing consideration is given to candidates in Medicine I and II attending schools formally accredited by the joint LCME/CACMS accreditation committee to bring a class up to its first-year enrollment limit.

FINANCIAL AID

Under the Canadian Students Loan Act, Canadians can obtain interest-free loans during their undergraduate course in medicine. Bursaries from the university and from the provincial government are available to deserving students. Students may also obtain assistance from the W. K. Kellogg Student Loan Program and from the Gordon Bell/College of Physicians and Surgeons (Manitoba) Loan Fund. Several entrance scholarships are also available.

OTHER PROGRAMS

Most graduates of the University of Manitoba Faculty of Medicine gain licensure by completing the two-part Medical Council of Canada Qualifying Examination (MCCQE), plus earning certification by either the Royal College of Physicians and Surgeons of Canada or the College of Family Physicians of Canada.

Specialty training is approved by the Royal College of Physicians and Surgeons of Canada and is conducted in the Affiliated Teaching Hospitals of the University of Manitoba. The University of Manitoba currently holds Royal College approval for 45 specialty training programs.

The Family Medicine Program is a two-year integrated training program leading to certification by the College of Family Physicians of Canada. The program is conducted in the affiliated teaching hospitals as well as in rural settings.

Continuing Medical Education is provided for practicing physicians. The Faculty of Medicine also provides opportunities for graduate studies in all the basic science departments as well as in selected clinical departments. Vibrant research activities are conducted by dedicated basic science and clinical staff.

A formal Bachelor of Science in the Medicine Research Program is offered to selected medical students in the summers following first- and second-year medicine. Summer opportunities are also available for rural medicine placements as well as placements with the Northern Medical Unit. The faculty offers M.Sc. and Ph.D. programs in all of its major departments, as well as a joint M.D.-Ph.D. program.

Institution Type: *Public*

APPLICATION AND ACCEPTANCE POLICIES FOR 2005-2006 FIRST-YEAR CLASS

Fees and expenses are in Canadian dollars.

Filing of application
  Earliest date: Aug. 1, 2005
  Latest date: TBD – Check Web site
School application fee to all applicants: $60
Oldest MCAT scores considered: 2001
Does not have Early Decision Program
Acceptance notice to regular applicants
  Earliest date: April 18, 2005
  Latest date: Until class is filled
Applicant's response to acceptance offer
  Maximum time: 2 weeks
Requests for deferred entrance considered: Yes
Deposit to hold place in class (applied to tuition):
  $500, due with response to acceptance offer
Estimated number of new entrants: 85
Starting date: Aug. 2005

TUITION AND STUDENT FEES PER YEAR FOR 2003-2004 FIRST-YEAR CLASS

Tuition: $7,595   Student fees: $200

INFORMATION ON 2003-2004 FIRST-YEAR CLASS

Number of	In-Province	Out-of-Province	Total
Applicants	259	266	525
Applicants Interviewed	205	49	254
New Entrants*	80	9	89

*All took the MCAT and had baccalaureate degrees.

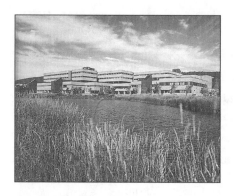

Memorial University of Newfoundland Faculty of Medicine

St. John's, Newfoundland

Dr. J. Rourke, *Dean of Medicine*
Dr. J. Barter, *Assistant Dean for Admissions*
Janet McHugh, *Admissions Officer*

ADDRESS INQUIRIES TO:

Janet McHugh, Admissions Officer
Memorial University of Newfoundland
Faculty of Medicine
St. John's, Newfoundland
Canada A1B 3V6
(709) 777-6615; 777-8422 (FAX)
E-mail: munmed@mun.ca
Web site: www.med.mun.ca/admissions

MISSION STATEMENT

Our purpose is to enhance the health of people by educating physicians and health scientists, by conducting research in clinical and basic medical sciences and applied health sciences and by promoting the skills and attitudes of lifelong learning.

GENERAL INFORMATION

Memorial is the only university in the province of Newfoundland. The university was established as Memorial College in 1925 and incorporated as a university in 1949. In 1959 campus buildings were erected on a 1,000-acre site. There are some 12,000 undergraduates and a faculty of about 1,000 (including visiting professors) working on the campus, which is situated on the periphery of St. John's. The medical school is housed in the Health Sciences Centre with General Hospital (531 beds) and a biomedical library. The medical school is fully accredited by the Committee on Accreditation of Canadian Medical Schools (CACMS) of the Association of Canadian Medical Colleges and the Canadian Medical Association, the Liaison Committee on Medical Education (LCME) of the Association of American Medical Colleges, and the American Medical Association. These accreditations mean that the medical school is equivalent in every respect to other medical schools in Canada and the United States.

Approved teaching programs for interns and residents are under the direction of the medical school. These programs are based at associate hospitals in St. John's and other provincial centers with a total bed complement of 3,116 covering inpatient and outpatient services in virtually all branches of medicine. Research work is being conducted both in the hospitals and in the Health Sciences Centre.

Residences for single and married students are provided on the campus, and the university maintains a list of approved off-campus accommodations. A health service is open to all students.

CURRICULUM

The curriculum, the physical structure, and the administrative organization of the school were planned to allow for maximum cooperation among the various basic science and clinical disciplines. The M.D. degree is granted upon completion of the fourth year. Canadian students write the LMCC (Medical Council of Canada) Examinations and US students write the USMLE (United States Medical Licensing Examination).

During the first year of the medical program, students take introductory courses in cell structure and functions, biochemistry, physiology, molecular genetics, pharmacology, microbiology, anatomy, behavioral science, ethics, interviewing skills, and community medicine. These opportunities are provided in a wide range of medical settings—family practice, general hospital, rural hospital, and public health programs.

In the second half of the first year and the second year, teaching has a systems approach; material from anatomy, physiology, pathology, and clinical medicine is presented in an integrated manner. The third year is a structured clinical clerkship that includes eight weeks of electives, and the fourth year is made up of electives and selectives. Rotations for Rural Medicine take place in the first, third, and fourth years.

A pass/fail system is used for grading.

The opportunity exist for medical students to pursue both a clinical and research training programme (i.e. M.D./Ph.D.). Medical students may apply through the Offices of Undergraduate Medical Education and Research/Graduate Studies for this programme.

REQUIREMENTS FOR ENTRANCE

A bachelor's degree is required. In exceptional circumstances, an application may be considered from someone who does not hold a bachelor's degree; such an applicant will have completed at least 20 one-semester courses and be a student who has work-related or other experience acceptable to the admissions committee. The course of study must include two courses in English. All applicants must take the MCAT prior to the application deadline.

Because of the limited number of places available and the intense competition for entry, applicants are advised to pursue a degree program of their choice and prepare for the MCAT.

Although science courses are not required, a basic knowledge of the physical and life sciences may be helpful in writing the MCAT and in the medical program.

SELECTION FACTORS

The school admits students on the basis of residency priority as follows: bona fide residents of Newfoundland and Labrador, of New Brunswick, of Prince Edward Island, of other Canadian provinces and non-Canadians. In every case a high academic standard is required. Memorial University does not discriminate on the basis of race, marital status, sex, creed, national origin, or disability. Age by itself is not used as a basis for selection or rejection. However, both age and length of time away from full-time academic studies may be taken into consideration.

Normally, the medical school does not accept transfer students from other medical schools. In rare circumstances, a transfer may be considered if there is space available.

FINANCIAL AID

Financial assistance is available to medical students through government student loan programs. Information can be obtained by contacting the Student Affairs Office at: Student Affairs Office, Faculty of Medicine, Memorial University of Newfoundland, St. John's, NF, A1B 3VC; telephone (709) 777-6690; or E-mail mdray@mun.ca.

INFORMATION FOR MINORITIES, DISADVANTAGED, AND/OR NONTRADITIONAL APPLICANTS

Although there is no formal affirmative action process at this medical school, the Admissions Committee does take into consideration the background of applicants in making its decisions.

Institution Type: *Public*

APPLICATION AND ACCEPTANCE POLICIES FOR 2005-2006 FIRST-YEAR CLASS

Fees and expenses are in Canadian dollars.

Filing of application
  Earliest date: July 2, 2004
  Latest date: October 15, 2004
School application fee to all applicants: $75
Oldest MCAT scores considered: 1999
Does not have Early Decision Program
Acceptance notice to regular applicants
  Earliest date: March 1, 2005
  Latest date: Until class is filled
Applicant's response to acceptance offer
  Maximum time: 14 days
Requests for deferred entrance considered: Yes
Deposit to hold place in class (applied to tuition):
  $200, due with response to acceptance offer;
  nonrefundable
Estimated number of new entrants: 60
Starting date: Sept. 2005

TUITION AND STUDENT FEES PER YEAR FOR 2003-2004 FIRST-YEAR CLASS

Tuition
  Resident: $6,250   Resident fees: $511
  Non Canadian: $30,000   Non Canadian fees: $801

INFORMATION ON 2003-2004 FIRST-YEAR CLASS

Number of	In-Province	Out-of-Province	Total
Applicants	179	445	624
Applicants Interviewed	123	102	225
New Entrants*	44	16	60

*All took the MCAT and 98% had baccalaureate degrees.

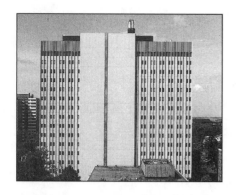

Dalhousie University
Faculty of Medicine

Halifax, Nova Scotia

Dr. Harold Cook, *Interim Dean*
Dr. Dan Hughes, *Assistant Dean, Admissions and Student Affairs*

ADDRESS INQUIRIES TO:

Admissions & Student Affairs
Room C-132, Lower Level, Clinical Research Centre
Dalhousie University
Halifax, Nova Scotia
Canada B3H 4H7
(902) 494-6369 (FAX)
E-mail: medicine.admissions@dal.ca
Web site: www.med.dal.ca/

GENERAL INFORMATION

Dalhousie University, a privately endowed institution founded in 1838, established the Faculty of Medicine in 1868. The main responsibility of the Faculty of Medicine is to the three Maritime Provinces of Canada (Nova Scotia, New Brunswick, and Prince Edward Island), which have a population of some 1.7 million.

The teaching hospitals located in the immediate vicinity of the medical school have a total of 2,300 beds covering inpatient and outpatient services in all branches of medicine.

University housing and a comprehensive Student Health Service are available.

CURRICULUM

The aim of the four-year course of study in medicine is to provide a basic education that would permit a graduate to enter any branch of postgraduate training.

The academic year for Medicine One and Medicine Two begins in early September and extends to the end of May. Medicine Three begins in late August/early September and ends in the following September. Medicine Four begins in late September and extends until May of the following year. The M.D. degree is granted upon successful completion of the fourth year.

During the first two years of the curriculum, students will learn predominantly in small groups, working with a tutor. The curriculum is organized around clinical problems to provide an integrated context for students to learn both basic and clinical science, and to begin the development of clinical reasoning skills. The third and fourth years are predominantly clinical, with 3rd year comprised of 12 week units in the major disciplines. The 4th year is arranged beginning with blocks of elective time and then students finish with a unit in Continuing and Preventive Care. The years being broken into a series of rotations within the various clinical disciplines. Starting in the first year, Dalhousie students have extensive patient contact hours, as the school places great emphasis on the development of clinical skills. In addition to small-group teaching, which emphasizes independent learning, teaching methods include lectures, laboratories, and bedside teaching.

In addition to the basic M.D. program, Dalhousie offers a bachelor of science in medicine program.

Dalhousie University through its Faculty of Medicine offers university-arranged and university-supervised clinical training, which meets national accreditation standards, for postgraduate medical trainees.

In all provinces with the exception of Quebec, the basis for licensure for the majority of trainees in a postgraduate training program affiliated with a CACMS/LCME medical school is successful completion of the two-part Medical Council of Canada Qualifying Examination (MCCQE), plus certification by either the College of Family Physicians of Canada or the Royal College of Physicians and Surgeons of Canada. There is great competition for entry into all programs.

The family medicine program at Dalhousie is a two-year integrated training experience following the M.D. leading to certification by the College of Family Physicians of Canada.

Specialty training is approved by the Royal College of Physicians and Surgeons of Canada and is conducted in affiliated teaching hospitals in both Halifax and Saint John. Dalhousie University currently holds Royal College approval for 41 specialty training programs.

The Faculty of Medicine maintains an active program of continuing medical education for practicing physicians in the Maritime Provinces. Research and graduate education are in all the basic science departments and in most of the clinical departments.

REQUIREMENTS FOR ENTRANCE

A university degree and the writing of the MCAT are absolute requirements. Students applying in the fall of 2004 for admission in September 2005 must have written either the April 2000 or subsequent MCAT. The April writing of the MCAT will not be considered for entry in September of the same year. There are no absolute prerequisite courses required. The major objective is that premedical education encompasses broad study in the physical, life, and social sciences and the humanities. The minimum requirement for entry, however, is a baccalaureate degree.

All applicants must meet the following minimum academic requirements:

Maritime Applicants: A minimum academic average of B+ (77 percent or higher) or a GPA of 3.30 based on a full course load of 5 full courses in the last two undergraduate years, or three out of four years plus MCAT scores of 8 and above, with a minimum score of 24.

Non-Maritime Applicants: A minimum academic average of A– (80 percent or higher) or a GPA of 3.70 based on a full course load of 5 full courses in the last two undergraduate years, or three out of four years plus MCAT scores of 10 and above, with a minimum score of 30.

Background in the physical and life sciences will help a student deal with the considerable load of scientific information involved in undergraduate medical study. Courses in the social sciences and humanities will be helpful in understanding human behavior in health and illness. The ability to communicate effectively, both orally and in writing, is essential. The committee believes that attracting students with a rich variety of educational backgrounds is in the interest of all students. Such preparation supports the training of outstanding physicians.

The medical undergraduate student has to deal with a great deal more information per unit of time than is usually the case in university undergraduate programs in arts and science. Therefore, the Admissions Committee will consider not only the academic grades of applicants but the type and degree of difficulty of university courses completed.

SELECTION FACTORS

Sources of information and factors considered by the Admissions Committee include academic requirements, ability as judged on university records and on the MCAT, confidential assessments received from referees of the applicant's choice and from any others the committee may wish to consult, interviews (selected applicants only), and place of residence. Detailed comments and explanations on these selection factors may be obtained in the Faculty of Medicine Calendar.

Dalhousie does not discriminate on the basis of race, sex, creed, national origin, age, or handicap.

FINANCIAL AID

A few entrance scholarships and entrance bursaries are awarded to students in the first year who are residents of the Maritime Provinces. The Dalhousie Medical Alumni Association Entrance Scholarship, the Dr. E. James Gordon Scholarship, and the Halifax Medical Society Entrance Scholarship are available to anyone regardless of residency. A number of bursaries and prizes are available in each year. The university maintains a loan fund, which is interest-free

until graduation. Applicants are advised not to plan to earn money in time-consuming work, which may jeopardize their academic standing.

INFORMATION ABOUT DIVERSITY PROGRAMS

Students from groups underrepresented in medicine will be considered on their individual merits.

Dalhousie University is an affirmative action and equal-opportunity educational institution.

Institution Type: *Public*

APPLICATION AND ACCEPTANCE POLICIES FOR 2005-2006 FIRST-YEAR CLASS

Fees and expenses are in Canadian dollars.

Filing of application
    Earliest date: Sept. 1, 2004
    Latest date: Oct. 31, 2004
School application fee to all applicants: $70
Oldest MCAT scores considered: 2000
Does not have Early Decision Program
Acceptance notice to regular applicants
    Earliest date: Feb. 1, 2005
    Latest date: June 30, 2005
Applicant's response to acceptance offer
    Maximum time: 4 weeks
Requests for deferred entrance considered: Yes
Deposit to hold place in class (applied to tuition):
    $200, due with response to acceptance offer;
    nonrefundable
Estimated number of new entrants: 90
Starting date: August 2005

TUITION AND STUDENT FEES PER YEAR FOR 2003-2004 FIRST-YEAR CLASS

Tuition   Student fees: $519
    Canadian: $10,460
    Non-Canadian: $15,460

INFORMATION ON 2003-2004 FIRST-YEAR CLASS

Number of	Maritime	Non-Maritime	Total
Applicants	241	115	356
Applicants Interviewed	240	40	280
New Entrants*	81	9	90

*All took the MCAT and had baccalaureate degrees.

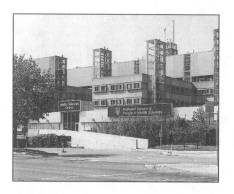

McMaster University
Undergraduate Medical Programme
School of Medicine

Hamilton, Ontario
Dr. John Kelton, *Vice President and Dean (Health Sciences)*
Dr. Alan Neville, *Assistant Dean M.D. Programme*
Dr. Harold Reiter, *Chair, M.D. Admissions*
Cathy Oudshoorn, *M.D. Programme Administrator*

ADDRESS INQUIRIES TO:

Admissions and Records
HSC 1M7-Health Sciences Centre
McMaster University
1200 Main Street West
Hamilton, Ontario
Canada L8N 3Z5
(905) 525-9140, Ext. 22235; 546-0349 (FAX)
E-mail: mdadmit@mcmaster.ca
Web site: www.fhs.mcmaster.ca/mdprog

GENERAL INFORMATION

The Faculty of Health Sciences at McMaster University offers programs in health sciences education, including undergraduate and postgraduate medical education, and in health sciences research. The clinical programs use the teaching hospital and extensive ambulatory facilities of the McMaster Division of the Hamilton Health Sciences Corporation, but also involve clinical teaching units at the major Hamilton hospitals and community health care centers. The Undergraduate Medical Programme was initiated in 1969, and the first class of students graduated in May 1972.

CURRICULUM

The three-year program (130 weeks of instruction) in medicine at McMaster uses an approach to learning that will apply throughout the physician's career. The components have been organized in a relevant and logical manner with early exposure to patients. Flexibility is ensured to allow for the variety of student backgrounds and career goals.

The graduates of McMaster's Undergraduate Medical Programme will have developed the knowledge, ability, and attitudes necessary to qualify for further education in any medical career. The general goals for students in the program include the following: the development of competency in problem-based learning and in problem solving, the development of the personal characteristics and attitudes compatible with effective health care, the development of clinical and communication skills, and the development of the skills to be a lifelong, self-directed learner.

To achieve the objectives of the Undergraduate Medical Programme, students are introduced to patients and their problems within the first unit. They are presented with a series of health care problems and questions requiring the understanding of principles and data collection. Much of the students' learning occurs within the setting of the small-group tutorial. Faculty members serve as tutors/facilitators or as sources of expert knowledge.

The Undergraduate Medical Programme is arranged as a four-unit preclerkship sequence followed by a clerkship; there are additional elective opportunities, both in block periods (totaling 26 weeks) and horizontal electives taken concurrently with ongoing units. Unit 1 is a 12-week introduction to concepts and information from three knowledge perspectives: population, behavior, and biology. In addition, a major theme of the entire curriculum, the life cycle, is developed as a perspective and anchors the three subunits of Unit 1: Early Development, Maturation, and Aging. Units 2, 3, and 4 are 14-week units organized on the basis of organ systems, where biomedical and health care problems are analyzed in depth. The clerkship emphasizes the clinical application of concepts learned in the earlier units and consists of experience in inpatient and ambulatory settings. These include internal medicine, family medicine, surgery, psychiatry, obstetrics-gynecology, anesthesia, and pediatrics. Unit 6, which follows the clerkship, is an interactive unit in which students will tackle issues derived from societal expectations of a practicing physician.

REQUIREMENTS FOR ENTRANCE

Completion of a minimum of three full years at an accredited university with at least an overall second class (B) average is required. There are no course prerequisites. The MCAT is not required.

Applicants who are not Canadian citizens or landed immigrants in Canada will be invited to interview only when they are considered to be clearly more suitable on all criteria than Canadian candidates.

Both academic achievement and personal qualities are considered. Academic achievement is assessed on the basis of course grades. Personal qualities and attributes are assessed on the basis of a submission written by the applicant, an autobiographical sketch, three references, and performance in a Multiple Mini Interview (MMI). The Faculty does not accept applications for transfer into the programme.

SELECTION FACTORS

Students and members of the community and faculty are involved in the assessment of applicants. The aim is to select students who not only have the necessary academic standards but also display characteristics that are deemed to be important for the study and practice of medicine. These include characteristics that suggest sensitivity to the needs of the community; sensitivity to the emotional, psychological, and physical aspects of patients; the ability to detect and solve problems; the ability to learn independently; the ability to function as a member of a small group; and the ability to plan one's career in a way that reflects the needs of the community.

Applicants rating highest in academic achievement and in personal qualities will be invited to the MMI. Some weighting according to bona fide residence may be applied according to the following priorities: Ontario or outside Ontario. From these applicants, 138 students will be selected to fill the entering class.

FINANCIAL AID

Medical students at McMaster, in addition to facing the general scarcity of financial assistance, are unable to rely on summer employment as a source of funds. In this situation, it is incumbent on students admitted to the Undergraduate Medical Programme to clarify immediately their fiscal situations and to secure or identify sufficient support to meet their financial obligations over the subsequent three years.

There are some government programs (available only to Canadians) and private agencies that offer financial assistance to medical students. The M.D. Programme and the central University Financial Aid Program offer quite a large bursary program to supplement financial resources of students in financial need. As well, the M.D. Programme administers a small loans program for students in need.

Institution Type: *Public*
Application Process: *OMSAS, see chapter 11.*

APPLICATION AND ACCEPTANCE POLICIES FOR 2005-2006 FIRST-YEAR CLASS

Fees and expenses are in Canadian dollars.

Filing of OMSAS application
    Earliest date: July 1, 2004
    Latest date: Oct. 1, 2004 (4:30 p.m. E.S.T.)
OMSAS fee: $175 for one school applied to in
    Ontario; $75 for each additional school
Oldest MCAT scores considered: None
Does not have Early Decision Program
Acceptance notice to regular applicants
    Earliest date: May 31, 2005
    Latest date: Until class is filled
Applicant's response to acceptance offer
    Maximum time: 2 weeks
Requests for deferred entrance considered: Yes
Deposit to hold place in class (applied to tuition):
    $1,000; nonrefundable
Estimated number of new entrants: 138
Starting date: September 2005

TUITION AND STUDENT FEES PER YEAR FOR 2003-2004 FIRST-YEAR CLASS

Tuition:	Student fees: $553
Resident: $14,445	
Non-resident: $41,697.90	

INFORMATION ON 2003-2004 FIRST-YEAR CLASS

Number of	In-Province	Out-of-Province	Total
Applicants	2,752	928	3,680
Applicants Interviewed	338	37	375
New Entrants	125	13	138

CHAPTER

12

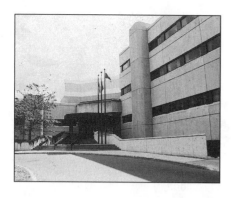

University of Ottawa
Faculty of Medicine

Ottawa, Ontario

Dr. Peter Walker, *Dean*
Dr. Richard L. Hébert, *Assistant Dean, Admissions*
Dr. Arlington Dungy, *Associate Dean, Alumni and Student Affairs*
Nicole Racine, *Admissions Officer*

ADDRESS INQUIRIES TO:

Admissions
University of Ottawa
Faculty of Medicine
451 Smyth Road
Ottawa, Ontario
Canada K1H 8M5
(613) 562-5409; 562-5651 (FAX)
E-mail: admissmd@uottawa.ca
Web site: www.medicine.uottawa.ca/eng/undergraduate.html

MISSION STATEMENT

The Faculty of Medicine is committed to the advancement of health through education, research and exemplary patient care for the well-being of the society we serve.

To fulfill these responsibilities, the Faculty of Medicine seeks to prepare a sufficient number of students to function professionally in both official languages.

The physician graduates of the faculty will be well prepared to address the present and future health needs of the Canadian population and to function as part of a multidisciplinary team, dedicated to the promotion of health and the management of illness. They will adhere to the highest standards of ethical and professional conduct consistent with the code developed by the faculty. Our graduates will be technically competent, adept at problem solving and committed to lifelong learning. They will exhibit compassion toward patients and their families, respect toward their peers and an inquiring attitude. They will be committed to maintaining their professional competence and will strive for appropriate use of health care resources.

GENERAL INFORMATION

The University of Ottawa received its charter from the province of Ontario in 1866. It was founded by the Missionary Oblates of Mary Immaculate, who were its administrators until 1965, when important structural reforms were introduced through an act of the legislative assembly of the province of Ontario. The management of the university is now under the Board of Governors consisting of members from various sectors of the community. The management, discipline, and control of the university are free from the restrictions and control of any outside body, whether lay or religious. The Faculty of Medicine was established in 1945. In 1978 the health sciences were regrouped into the Faculty of Health Sciences comprising the School of Medicine, the School of Nursing, and the School of Human Kinetics. In 1989, however, the Faculty of Medicine regained its status as a separate academic unit.

CURRICULUM

During their undergraduate training, students acquire the knowledge, skills, and attitudes necessary to recognize, understand, and apply effective, efficient strategies for the prevention and treatment of common and important health problems. The program integrates the basic and clinical sciences throughout the four years of study. Emphasis is placed on self-learning principles, and facts are assimilated in a multidisciplinary fashion, within the context of clinical problems. Lectures and seminars are used to discuss basic concepts, explore new developments, and provide overviews of the biomedical sciences fundamental to the practice of medicine. Training occurs in ambulatory, primary, secondary, and tertiary settings, with students functioning as members of the medical team in collaboration with other health professionals. The program emphasizes health promotion and disease prevention and is responsive to individual needs and abilities and to the changes occurring in society and the health care system.

The program fosters the qualities of trust and compassion, communication skills, ethical professional conduct, and patient advocacy.

The program is scheduled over four calendar years and is divided into two stages. The first stage includes 70 weeks of study of essential biomedical principles and consists of 13 multidisciplinary blocks. The students learn communication and clinical skills in an integrated fashion with the study of body systems. The second stage, of two years duration, is devoted to clinical clerkships; an extended period of 16 weeks is available for elective study.

REQUIREMENTS FOR ENTRANCE

Applicants are not required to write the MCAT to be eligible to apply.

Students in the following categories are eligible to apply for admission to the first year of the four-year program in the Faculty of Medicine:

(1) Students who have completed successfully in a university three years (full-time studies) of a bachelor's degree program. Required coursework must include:

Years
Biochemistry* (without laboratory) 1
General Chemistry* (with laboratory) 1
Organic Chemistry* (with laboratory) 1
General Biology or Zoology (with laboratory). 1
Humanities 1

Two of the three chemistries are required.

(2) Students of other universities who have completed studies equivalent to those listed above. (Equivalence is determined by the University of Ottawa Faculty of Medicine.)

SELECTION FACTORS

Academic excellence, assessment of the detailed autobiographical sketch and interview rating are the main selection criteria used by the Admissions Committee. Academics are measured by an assessment of marks and by a comparison of the applicant's academic record in relationship with those of the other applicants.

Due to the limited class size, it is to be noted that meeting the above minimum standard does not guarantee admission. No preference is given to academic achievement in one program over another as long as the prerequisites for eligibility have been met. Furthermore, in selecting the students, the Admissions Committee reserves the right to assess, in the applicant's program, the level of difficulty of the courses and/or their pertinence for future medical studies at the University of Ottawa and the performance achieved by the candidate in these courses. No quota is predetermined before the selection is made; each file meeting the requirements is studied individually.

No candidate will be admitted without an interview, and the rating of the interview and of other nonacademic data will be taken into account in the admission process.

It is highly desirable that the candidate who has a broad exposure to biology and physical sciences also have a broad exposure to the arts, humanities, and social sciences.

In view of the limited number of places available, a candidate whose GPA is below 3.4 (scale of 4.0) has considerably less chance of being admitted, depending on the year's competition.

Sex, race, age, religion, and socioeconomic status play no part in the selection process. Only applications from Canadian citizens or permanent residents or applications from children of alumni of the University of Ottawa can be considered.

Knowledge of both official languages of the university will be an asset (but not a prerequisite).

Applicants who are in the third year of a program at the time they apply must, before June 1, submit an official transcript.

FINANCIAL AID

Students may apply to the Student Financial Aid Office of the university and to their respective provincial governments for loan assistance. The Ontario Medical Association Bursaries and Loan Fund, the Kellogg Foundation Loan Fund, and a special bursaries fund are administered by the Awards Committee of the Faculty of Medicine. The Association of Professors of the University also provides a limited number of bursaries. Most of these awards are made on the basis of demonstrable financial need and good academic standing.

Institution Type: *Public*
Application Process: *OMSAS, see chapter 11.*

APPLICATION AND ACCEPTANCE POLICIES FOR 2005-2006 FIRST-YEAR CLASS

Fees and expenses are in Canadian dollars.

Filing of OMSAS application
 Earliest date: July 1, 2004
 Latest date: Oct. 1, 2004
OMSAS fee: $175
School application fee: $75
Oldest MCAT scores considered: None required
Does not have Early Decision Program
Acceptance notice to regular applicants
 Earliest date: End of May 2005
 Latest date: Until class is filled
Applicant's response to acceptance offer
 Maximum time: 2 weeks
Requests for deferred entrance considered: Yes
Deposit to hold place in class (applied to tuition)
 $1,000; nonrefundable
Estimated number of new entrants: 123
Starting date: September 2005

TUITION AND STUDENT FEES PER YEAR FOR 2003-2004 FIRST-YEAR CLASS

Tuition: $14,000   Student fees: $539

INFORMATION ON 2003-2004 FIRST-YEAR CLASS

Number of	In-Province	Out-of-Province	Total
Applicants	1,754	693	2,447
Applicants Interviewed	*	*	489
New Entrants†	108	15	123

*Data not available.
96.7% of 123 registrants had baccalaureate degrees.

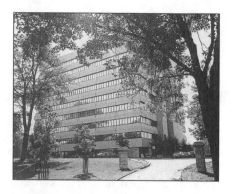

Queen's University
Faculty of Health Sciences
School of Medicine

Kingston, Ontario

Dr. D.C. Holland, *Assistant Dean, Undergraduate Medical Education*
Thelma C. Rikley, *Manager, Undergraduate Medical Education*
Anne Cumpson, *Admissions Officer*

ADDRESS INQUIRIES TO:

Admissions Office
Queen's University
Faculty of Health Sciences
School of Medicine
Kingston, Ontario
Canada K7L 3N6
(613) 533-2542; 533-3190 (FAX)
Web site: http://meds.queensu.ca/medicine/

MISSION STATEMENT

Our mission is to educate health professionals and students in the biomedical sciences by conducting research, by generating a spirit of enquiry, and by serving the health needs of the people of southeastern Ontario, drawing on Queen's learning environment to enable our graduates to become the leading clinicians of Canada's rural, northern, and urban communities and the researchers and educators of the nation's future.

GENERAL INFORMATION

Queen's University School of Medicine, established in 1854, is an integral part of a university of more than 10,000 full-time students. The campus is situated within the city of Kingston, which is located on Lake Ontario at the origin of the St. Lawrence River and has a population of 135,000.

The provision of health care services in Kingston is presently being restructured and will change over the next two years. The Kingston General Hospital will provide most in-patient care for the region. There will be a site for ambulatory care, which, at the present, is centered at the Hotel Dieu Hospital. Chronic care, geriatrics, palliative care, and rehabilitation services are currently provided at St. Mary's of the Lake Hospital.

CURRICULUM

The curriculum is integrated throughout with faculty from different departments contributing to each course. The program is a four-year curriculum with three sequential phases:

Phase I—Introduction to the Sciences Relevant
to Medicine . . . . 16 weeks
Phase II—System-Oriented Clinically-Based
Learning . . . . 63 weeks
Phase III—Clinical Clerkship . . . . 68 weeks

The Medicine in Society Phase extends throughout the four years and includes information literacy, medical ethics, law in medicine, psychosocial aspects of medicine, and history of medicine as well as topics in family medicine, rehabilitation medicine, growth and development, geriatrics, and community health and epidemiology. These subjects have been chosen to relate to, and enhance, the material that the students will learn in the respective Phases I-III.

Students are introduced in their first year to communication and physical examination. Clinical Skills runs throughout the curriculum to provide the students with opportunities to learn and practice interviewing, history taking, physical examination, clinical reasoning, medical record keeping, and approaches to diagnosis and management. There is an eight-week Critical Enquiry Elective at the end of the second year. This time provides an opportunity for students to investigate a medical question in depth and may involve data collection and analysis. Self-directed learning is emphasized in the curriculum, and learning formats include whole class lectures, tutorials, seminars, symposia, and problem-based learning. Assessment is done using criterion-referenced examinations, small-group evaluation, and objective structured clinical examinations (OSCE) for clinical skills. Evaluation is honors/pass/fail.

REQUIREMENTS FOR ENTRANCE

The minimum academic requirement for admission is three years of study in any university program (a minimum of 15 full courses).

Candidates are required to successfully complete the equivalent of a full-year (2 semesters) university-level course in each of the following:

	Years
Biological Sciences	1
Physical Sciences	1
Humanities or Social Sciences	1

As a requirement for admission, the student must have completed Hepatitis B immunization, and documentation of Hepatitis B serological status must be provided to the School's Undergraduate Office. A student seeking admission will be required to provide documentation of serological status for Hepatitis B, and to undergo further testing as required, after being offered a place. The offer of a place will only be confirmed after this documentation is presented, but the presence of *Hepatitis B Antigen positivity* will not influence the student's acceptance for admission.

All applicants are required to write the MCAT prior to the deadline date for submission of applications to OMSAS.

To be eligible for admission, candidates must be Canadian citizens, Canadian permanent residents (landed immigrants) by February 1 following submission of the OMSAS application, or the children of Queen's University alumni who are residents outside Canada. Verification must be sent to the Admissions Office at the time of application.

SELECTION FACTORS

One hundred students are admitted annually into the first medical year and are selected on the basis of a strong academic record and assessment of personal characteristics considered to be most appropriate for the study of medicine at Queen's University and for the subsequent practice of medicine. The following steps are used to identify the group to be invited for interview and for assessment of personal qualities: the cumulative converted GPA based on all years of undergraduate study and the results of the MCAT. Applications of those below the cutoff will be reviewed by members of the Admissions Committee, who will utilize specific guidelines to identify any unusual circumstances.

Candidates who do not make the academic cut based on their undergraduate grade-point average but who have completed graduate work are considered in this group. The cutoff is based on the median grade-point average of all candidates for the given year.

Given that it is practicable to interview approximately 400 candidates for 100 positions, the Admissions Committee attempts to include as many highly qualified candidates as it can while taking into consideration as many anomalous situations as possible in attempting to give maximum benefit to the applicant population without discriminating against any sector. Unfortunately, it is not possible to interview all of the many highly qualified candidates that apply to our program.

The personal assessment score for those candidates who meet the criteria for steps 1 and 2 is determined from the assessment of the confidential letters of reference, the personal information form, the autobiographic sketch (50 percent), and the personal interview (50 percent), from which candidates will be ranked for offers and placement on the waiting list.

The Admissions Committee does not give preference to applicants who have studied in any particular university program. Applicants are encouraged to consider all of the undergraduate programs available to them and to embark on the course of studies in which they have the greatest interest and that would prepare them for an alternate career should they not gain a place in medicine.

No preference is shown to applicants at any particular level of training.

Place of residence and location of the university where studies have been undertaken are not criteria in selection. Age, gender, race, and religion are not factors considered in the selection process.

Because of the unique structure of the medical curriculum, candidates are not usually considered for admission with advanced standing or transfer.

INFORMATION ABOUT DIVERSITY PROGRAMS

There is an alternate admissions process available to Aboriginal candidates.

Institution Type: *Public*
Application Process: *OMSAS, see chapter 11.*

APPLICATION AND ACCEPTANCE POLICIES FOR 2005-2006 FIRST-YEAR CLASS

Fees and expenses are in Canadian dollars.

Filing of OMSAS application
  Earliest date: July 1, 2004
  Latest date: Oct. 1, 2004
OMSAS fee: $175 plus an institutional levy of $75 for
  each medical school selection
Oldest MCAT scores considered: 1991
Does not have Early Decision Program
Acceptance notice to regular applicants
  Earliest date: May 31, 2005
  Latest date: Until class is filled
Applicant's response to acceptance offer
  Maximum time: 2 weeks
Requests for deferred entrance considered: Yes
Deposit to hold place in class: $1,000, applied to tuition,
  due with response to acceptance offer; nonrefundable
Estimated number of new entrants: 100
Starting date: September 2005

TUITION AND STUDENT FEES PER YEAR FOR 2003-2004 FIRST-YEAR CLASS

Tuition   Student fees: $771.86
  Canadian: $13,500
  Non-Canadian: $20,160

INFORMATION ON 2003-2004 FIRST-YEAR CLASS

Number of	In-Province	Out-of-Province	Total
Applicants	920	468	1,388
Applicants Interviewed	N/A	N/A	474
New Entrants*	75	25	100

*All took the MCAT; 98% had baccalaureate degrees.

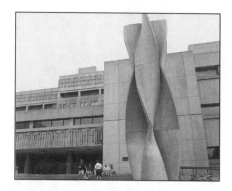

University of Toronto
Faculty of Medicine

Toronto, Ontario

Dr. C. David Naylor, *Dean*
Dr. M. Shandling, *Director, Admissions and Awards*
Bill Gregg, *Coordinator, Admissions and Awards*

ADDRESS INQUIRIES TO:

University of Toronto
Faculty of Medicine
Toronto, Ontario
Canada M5S 1A8
(416) 978-2717; 971-2163 (FAX)
Web site: www.library.utoronto.ca/medicine/
    educational_programs/undergrad.html

MISSION STATEMENT

The faculty of medicine has been educating medical students and conducting internationally recognized research for more than 100 years. The school has grown into one of the largest health sciences complex in North America with more than 4,500 students in undergraduate and graduate medical education programs, rehabilitation sciences and graduate study.

GENERAL INFORMATION

The medical school was founded in 1843 as part of King's College, which later became the University of Toronto. The school is a faculty of the university and, as such, receives support from the government of Ontario.

CURRICULUM

The four-year curriculum is focused on student-centered learning. The preclerkship phase (approximately 82 weeks) consists of six multidisciplinary courses, each of which is built upon a series of patient-based cases. Selected lectures, seminars, and laboratory exercises will complement small-group, problem-based learning sessions. Themes for the courses will include the following: the determinants of health; structure and function; the brain, behavior, and communication; metabolism and nutrition; pathobiology of disease; and the foundations of medical practice. Students are required to fulfill specific learning objectives for each course and will be assessed both within and at the completion of each course. In addition, longitudinal clinical and community experiences—beginning in Year 1—are intended to provide students with the opportunity to acquire knowledge and skills through direct interaction with patients.

Following the preclerkship, students spend approximately 78 weeks as clinical clerks. This phase of medical education enables the student to participate in the study and care of patients as a member of a clinical team, which includes residents and the attending staff physician or surgeon. As clerks, medical students rotate for defined periods through hospital services, including medicine, surgery, obstetrics, paediatrics, family medicine, and psychiatry. Each rotation includes community experiences as well as elements of problem-based learning and basic science.

As part of the clerkship, students spend a total of 18 weeks in elective rotations to allow them to explore areas of medicine of particular interest. Clerks may choose to participate in the most technically sophisticated medical units or medical research, work with family physicians in a rural setting, or spend part of their elective working in another country.

During the clerkship, students apply to the Canadian Resident Matching Service to select the program with which they wish to do their postgraduate training. Applications must be submitted in the fall, and students are notified in March as to the program to which they have been matched.

A joint M.D.-Ph.D. program is offered in the Faculty of Medicine and the School of Graduate Studies for individuals wishing to make a commitment to research in addition to the practice of clinical medicine. Students accepted into the combined program may pursue the dual degrees via either a sequential or an integrated route. Interested individuals must apply to the M.D. program at the Faculty of Medicine in the usual manner and request an application from the coordinator of the M.D.-Ph.D. program. Entry into the M.D.-Ph.D. program is dependent upon acceptance into the M.D. program.

REQUIREMENTS FOR ENTRANCE

All applicants are required to write the MCAT prior to the deadline date for submission of applications to OMSAS. A minimum of three years in a degree program at a Canadian university or, for applicants enrolled at a non-Canadian university, an honours bachelor's degree is required.

The faculty does not accept applications for transfer into the program.

Enrollment in the first-year class is currently 198 students.

All applicants are required to have satisfactorily completed the following courses: two full-course equivalents in life sciences plus one full-course equivalent in social sciences or humanities or languages.

It is recommended, although not required, that applicants complete a university-level course in biometrics or statistics.

SELECTION FACTORS

Applicants are judged initially upon their academic and nonacademic records. In addition, attention is paid to the results of the MCAT, statements of referees, and an autobiographical essay. Applicants are also required to appear for an interview in Toronto. Definite preference is given to Canadian residents. A maximum of seven places will be offered to applicants with student visas. Sex, race, and religion are not considered in determining those applicants to whom places are offered.

Successful candidates must be deemed by the Admissions Committee to be acceptable in all aspects of the admissions process. This may include cumulative grade-point average, MCAT scores, published papers, supervisor's letters, nonacademic factors, English proficiency, performance on interview, and any other criteria put forward by the faculty.

FINANCIAL AID

Financial aid is available under the Province of Ontario Student Assistance Program and the Canada Student Loan Program. Applicants are referred to the publications of the Department of University Affairs for details of the regulations governing these awards. Applicants are advised not to plan to earn money in time-consuming work that may jeopardize their standing during the academic year.

Institution Type: *Public*
Application Process: *OMSAS, see chapter 11.*

APPLICATION AND ACCEPTANCE POLICIES FOR 2005-2006 FIRST-YEAR CLASS

Fees and expenses are in Canadian dollars.

Filing of OMSAS application
  Earliest date: July 1, 2004
  Latest date: Oct. 1, 2004
OMSAS fee: $175
School application fee to all applicants: $75
Oldest MCAT scores considered: 1999
Does not have Early Decision Program
Acceptance notice to regular applicants
  Earliest date: May 31, 2005
  Latest date: Until class is filled
Applicant's response to acceptance offer
  Maximum time: 14 days
Requests for deferred entrance considered: Yes
Deposit to hold place in class: $1,000 applied to tuition; nonrefundable
Estimated number of new entrants: 198
Starting date: Sept. 2005

TUITION AND STUDENT FEES PER YEAR FOR 2003-2004 FIRST-YEAR CLASS

Tuition
  Canadian: $16,207
  Non-Canadian: $28,957

Student fees:
  Canadian: $1,080.50
  Non-Canadian: $1,692.97

INFORMATION ON 2003-2004 FIRST-YEAR CLASS

Number of	In-Province	Out-of-Province	Total
Applicants	1128	477	1,605
Applicants Interviewed	291	122	413
New Entrants†	173	22	195

†All took the MCAT; 87% had baccalaureate degrees.

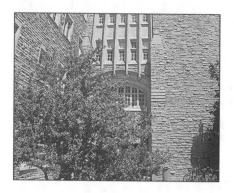

University of Western Ontario
Faculty of Medicine & Dentistry
Health Sciences Addition

London, Ontario

Dr. Carol P. Herbert, *Dean*
Dr. J.A. Silcox, *Associate Dean, Admissions/Student & Equity Affairs*
Darla McNeil, *Manager, Medicine Admissions Office*
Dr. Francis Chan, *Assistant Dean for Equity and Gender*

ADDRESS INQUIRIES TO:

Admissions/Student & Equity Affairs
Faculty of Medicine & Dentistry
The University of Western Ontario
London, Ontario
Canada N6A 5C1
(519) 661-3744; 661-3797 (FAX)
E-mail: Admissions@med.uwo.ca
Web site: www.med.uwo.ca

MISSION STATEMENT

The University of Western Ontario Faculty of Medicine & Dentistry will be internationally recognized for leadership in patient-centered and community-oriented medical and dental education and for excellence and innovation in specific areas of research. To do this: 1) We will promote a learning environment focussed on building knowledge to improve human and ecosystem health. 2) We will collaborate with our institute and hospital partners to excel as a research community. 3) We will graduate physicians and dentists who will respond to community needs. 4) We will work in partnership with health organizations and communities in Southwestern Ontario to develop a regional academic health sciences network. 5) We will lead in development, assessment and maintenance of innovative models of medical and dental education and health care. 6) We will value diversity, collegiality, caring, and interdependence of students, faculty, and staff. 7) We will be accountable to our students, our community, and one another as faculty and staff members.

GENERAL INFORMATION

The Faculty of Medicine of the University of Western Ontario had its origin in 1882 and came under the direct control of the university in 1912. The University of Western Ontario (U.W.O.) is a private university but in receipt of government grants in common with other universities of Ontario having faculties of medicine.

CURRICULUM

The undergraduate medical curriculum is a four-year program that is patient centered in its content, and student centered in its delivery. It is designed to provide each student with an opportunity to acquire the knowledge, skills, and attitudes required to advance to postgraduate training leading to clinical practice, research, or other medical careers. The educational format is a blend of lectures, laboratory experience, small group problem-based learning sessions, and supervised clinical experiences.

Years One and Two: The first two years of the curriculum provide the student with a solid grounding in the basic and clinical sciences. These two years are each divided into a series of blocks: Introduction to Medicine, The Thorax, The Abdomen, Head and Neck, Back and Limbs, and Systems. Within each block, various subject areas are presented, which integrate the basic and clinical sciences.

The weekly timetable is structured around a presenting case, which is introduced at the beginning of each week. The case provides the stimulus for instruction, and is designed to highlight a number of objectives of the M.D. program. Throughout the week, the student is exposed to a variety of teaching methods including small group tutorials, problem-based learning, lectures and large group discussions, self-instructional materials, and laboratories.

Students participate in early patient contact that emphasizes a patient-centered approach to medicine, beginning in year one. Part of being a good physician is understanding the community in which patients live, and the first two years of the program provide a variety of opportunities for student involvement in the community.

Years Three and Four: The third and fourth years of medicine include a 52-week integrated clerkship, clinical electives, and advanced basic science electives.

During the third-year clerkship, the student becomes an active member of clinical care teams in the following medical disciplines: family medicine, medicine, obstetrics and gynecology, pediatrics, psychiatry, and surgery. Under the supervision of faculty and more senior house staff, clerks are given graded responsibility in the diagnosis, investigation, and management of patients in hospital, clinic, and outpatient settings.

Beginning in year four, clinical electives are arranged entirely by the student in any area of medicine, at Western or in other centers. After completion of the clinical electives, students return to Western in February for the transition period, which includes: Advanced Basic Sciences (e.g., surgical anatomy, medical physiology), Advanced Communication Skills, General Review, Health Care Systems, etc. This permits students to further integrate the basic and clinical aspects of medicine in light of their clinical experience.

REQUIREMENTS FOR ENTRANCE

All applicants must submit results of the MCAT. MCAT test results will be accepted provided the test was written no more than five years prior to the October application deadline.

To be eligible to apply students must have completed or be currently enrolled in a program leading to an undergraduate degree at a recognized university. Students must have completed a minimum of 15 full or equivalent courses by the end of the academic year (September – April) in which application is being made. In addition, students must have registered in courses in such a way that there have been *at least* two full academic years (taken during September - April) in which a minimum of five full or equivalent courses (30 credit hours) have been taken concurrently.

Only those terms in which at least five full or equivalent courses (30 credit hours) are taken will be used in the calculation of GPA admission cutoffs.

When students are required to take more than five full courses during any September – April academic year because of program requirements, the five *best* courses will be used in the calculation of GPA admission cutoffs.

Three full or equivalent senior courses (second year and above) must be included in each of the two undergraduate years being used to determine compliance with established GPA cutoffs.

Applicants who have earned a degree from a recognized university, may elect to continue in full time undergraduate studies, so that academic standing may be improved for application to medical school, for a one year period only. The special year must contain five full or equivalent courses (30 credit hours) with a minimum of four full or equivalent courses at the honors level (numbered 200 or higher at Western). Honors level courses at Western numbered 200 are equivalent to third year courses at all other universities; first year courses are not acceptable in the "special year".

Graduate students are required to have complete all requirements for their graduate degrees *and their theses (if required) must be submitted for defense by the examination committee* prior to registration in the Faculty of Medicine and Dentistry MD Program.

Prior to being permitted to register in the MD Program, all applicants who are granted admission will be required to have completed successfully the following university-level courses:

- one full or equivalent course in Biology with a laboratory component,
- one full or equivalent course in Organic Chemistry with a laboratory component, **or**
- two half courses in Organic Chemistry, at least one of which shall have a laboratory component, **or**
- two half courses one in *each* of Organic Chemistry (with a lab component) and Biochemistry (with or without a lab component),
- one other full or equivalent science course from a discipline unrelated to Biology and Chemistry.
- A total of three full, or equivalent, non-science courses, at least one of which must be an essay course (validity of essay course will be audited).

SELECTION FACTORS

Enrollment is limited. Admission to the Doctor of Medicine Program is competitive, and the possession of the minimum requirements does not assure acceptance. Admission consideration is based on academic achievement, MCAT scores, and a personal interview score. Only those applicants deemed competitive will be selected for an interview.

Institution Type: *Public*
Application Process: *OMSAS, see chapter 11.*

APPLICATION AND ACCEPTANCE POLICIES FOR 2005-2006 FIRST-YEAR CLASS

Fees and expenses are in Canadian dollars.

Filing of OMSAS application
    Earliest date: June 1, 2004
    Latest date: early Oct. 2004
OMSAS fee: $175, plus $75 for each school
    (subject to change)
Oldest MCAT scores considered: no more than
    5 years prior to October deadline
Does not have Early Decision Program
Acceptance notice to regular applicants
    Earliest date: last working day in May 2005
    Latest date: Until class is filled
Applicant's response to acceptance offer
    Maximum time: 2 weeks
Requests for deferred entrance considered: No
Deposit to hold place in class: $1,000
Number of new entrants: 133
Starting date: Sept. 2005

TUITION AND STUDENT FEES PER YEAR FOR 2003-2004 FIRST-YEAR CLASS

Tuition: $14,566*   Student fees: $827*

INFORMATION ON 2003-2004 FIRST-YEAR CLASS

Number of	In-Province	Out-of-Province	Total
Applicants	†	†	1,550
Applicants Interviewed	†	†	375
New Entrants‡	†	†	133

*Subject to change
†Data not available.
‡All took the MCAT.

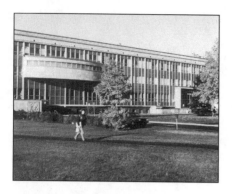

Université Laval
Faculty of Medicine

Ste-Foy, Quebec

Dr. Pierre J. Durand, *Dean*
Dr. Guy Pomerleau, *Chair, Admission Committee*
Denis Verret, *Admission Officer*

ADDRESS INQUIRIES TO:

Secretary, Admissions Committee
Université Laval
Faculty of Medicine
Ste-Foy, Quebec
Canada G1K 7P4
(418) 656-2131, ext. 2492; 656-2733 (FAX)
E-mail: admission@fmed.ulaval.ca
Web site: www.fmed.ulaval.ca

MISSION STATEMENT

The overall goal of the program is to assure a formation which prepares students for practicing medicine competently in a contemporary health system, with emphasis on an approach which is scientific, global and humanistic. In addition, the program strives to prepare students for a lifetime of continued learning.

GENERAL INFORMATION

Université Laval was established in 1852 by a Royal Charter granted by Queen Victoria. It was named after Monseigneur de Laval, first bishop of Quebec.

Research opportunities are provided in all the basic sciences and in many fields of clinical investigation. The clinical teaching is provided through a network of affiliated health institutions. Residence accommodations are provided for many students. There is a University Health Service for students as well as vocational guidance and counseling services.

CURRICULUM

The curriculum aims to prepare students to undertake any career in medicine. During the first two years, the program provides early introduction to clinical problems and interdepartmental teaching by both basic science and clinical faculty. This part of the curriculum is designed to be flexible and can be spread over three calendar years. The basic clinical clerkships are given in the third and fourth years and provide a basic exposure to each major clinical discipline, including family medicine. The curriculum is monitored by both faculty and students.

REQUIREMENTS FOR ENTRANCE

Since all instruction is in French, fluency in the French language is an essential prerequisite.

Under the present Quebec educational system, the minimum requirements are two years of college (Health Sciences Program) and the diploma of collegial studies of the Ministry of Education (D.E.C.).

For other applicants, a degree in biological or health science is required.

Specific course requirements are:

Sem. hrs.

General Biology (with lab) 8
General or Inorganic Chemistry (with lab) 8
Organic Chemistry 8
General Physics (with lab) 2
Mathematics through Calculus 2
    Must include analytical geometry, college
    algebra, and trigonometry.
French
Humanities
Behavioral and Social Sciences

The MCAT is not required, although the scores are considered when available.

SELECTION FACTORS

Preference is given to applicants from the province of Quebec. Admission requirements for application from Quebec colleges (CEGEP) and universities include a standardized autobiographical note and a three-hour group session called Assessment by Simulation (APS). This test evaluates different personal characteristics of the candidates. A few outstanding French-speaking candidates are admitted from other Canadian provinces and the United States. These candidates are selected on the basis of different parameters: scholastic achievement, interview, and curriculum vitae. Sex, race, religion, age, and socioeconomic status are not considered in the selection process.

FINANCIAL AID

Financial aid is available to Quebec residents through the Bursaries Division of the Provincial Ministry of Education. Summer scholarships of $2,000 are also available to students who wish to devote their vacation period to research. There is no financial assistance for foreign applicants.

Institution Type: *Public*

APPLICATION AND ACCEPTANCE POLICIES FOR 2005-2006 FIRST-YEAR CLASS

Fees and expenses are in Canadian dollars.

Filing of application
　Earliest date: Nov. 15, 2004
　Latest date:　March 1, 2005 (for Quebec colleges)
　　　　　　　　Jan. 15, 2005 (for others)

School application fee to all applicants: $30
Oldest MCAT scores considered: 2001
Does not have Early Decision Program
Acceptance notice to regular applicants
　Earliest date: May 15, 2005
　Latest date: Until class is filled
Applicant's response to acceptance offer
　Maximum time: 10 days
Requests for deferred entrance considered: No
Deposit to hold place in class: None
Estimated number of new entrants: 189
Starting date: September 2005

TUITION AND STUDENT FEES PER YEAR FOR 2003-2004 FIRST-YEAR CLASS

Tuition　　　　　　　　　Student fees: $1,500
　Resident: $3,000
　Nonresident: $15,000

INFORMATION ON 2003-2004 FIRST-YEAR CLASS

Number of	In-Province	Out-of-Province	Total
Applicants	1,443	148	1,591
Applicants Interviewed	409	23	432
New Entrants*	179	7	186

*41% had baccalaureate degrees.

McGill University
Faculty of Medicine

Montreal, Quebec

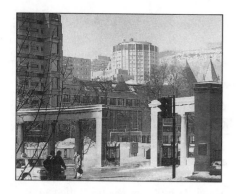

Dr. Abraham Fuks, *Dean*
Dr. Philip R. Beck, *Associate Dean, Admissions*
Judy Stymest, *Director of Student Aid*

ADDRESS INQUIRIES TO:

Admissions Office
McGill University
Faculty of Medicine
3655 Promenade Sir William Osler
Montreal, Quebec
Canada H3G 1Y6
(514) 398-3517; 398-4631 (FAX)
Web site: www.med.mcgill.ca/admissions/

MISSION STATEMENT

The advancement of learning through teaching, scholarship, and service to society: by offering to outstanding undergraduate and graduate students the best education available; by carrying out scholarly activities judged to be excellent when measured against the highest international standards; and by providing service to society in those ways for which we are well-suited by virtue of our academic strengths.

Within this context, the mission of the Faculty of Medicine is to pursue internationally significant scholarship and to provide undergraduate, graduate and professional programmes of the highest academic quality so that we may contribute to the well being of mankind.

GENERAL INFORMATION

The Faculty of Medicine was established in 1829. It selects students from a variety of cultural and academic backgrounds and provides them with a medical education that places emphasis upon both basic medical sciences and clinical medicine. There are seven university teaching hospitals, seven specialty teaching hospitals, and nine special research centers and units. The Quebec (Canadian) health care system has only one category of patient. All patients are available for the teaching of medical students. This gives McGill graduates the clinical skills for which they are renowned throughout the world. Research opportunities, available at the undergraduate and graduate levels, are provided in all of the basic medical sciences and in many fields of clinical medicine. The university offers residential facilities and provides student services, including a health service.

The language of instruction is English.

The Faculty of Medicine offers a four-year undergraduate medical curriculum (M.D./C.M. program). It also offers an M.D./M.B.A. program in response to the increasing need for doctors to acquire management skills that are unique to health care.

Similarly, a seven-year combined MD/PhD program is offered for students interested in a research career in academic medicine.

The Faculty of Medicine is accredited by the Liaison Committee on Medical Education of the AAMC and the AMA. Studying at McGill is identical to studying medicine in a U.S. medical school. U.S. students studying at McGill write the USMLE exams in the same way and at the same time as U.S. students studying in U.S. medical schools. These students return automatically to the United States for residency.

U.S. program directors recognize the high caliber of McGill graduates, and McGill students are very competitive in U.S. residency applications.

CURRICULUM

The curriculum recognizes the importance of a solid database and a multidisciplinary approach to medical education with integration of clinical and basic science. It permits a variety of teaching and evaluation methods, emphasizing small-group teaching. Approximately 50 percent of the sessions are lectures. The other 50 percent include small-group teaching, computer-based instruction, and laboratories.

The curriculum is composed of four components entitled Basis of Medicine (BOM), Introduction to Clinical Medicine (ICM), Practice of Medicine (POM), and Back to Basics (BTB). The BOM component, occupying the first 18 months, introduces the fundamental pillars of medicine, such as anatomy and physiology. The students have extensive opportunities for "hands on" laboratory sessions and have patient contact sessions. The bulk of forms are available in electronic format (CD-Rom and the Web).

The clinical component is two phased. The initial portion, ICM, is of a six-month duration. The student learns the techniques of physical examination and develops clinical reasoning strategies. Included are bedside teaching in the university hospitals, visits to community centers, exposure to family physicians in private offices, and the use of standardized patients for the teaching of specific skills.

The third component, POM, starts in the middle of the third year and provides exposure to the core disciplines of Medicine: Internal Medicine, Pediatrics, Surgery, Obstetrics and Gynecology, Psychiatry, Family Medicine and Geriatric Medicine. This component provides extensive clinical contact, under supervision by faculty members. The curriculum has been structured so as to ensure that all core clerkship rotations are completed in time for the residency application process. Specific attention is placed on professionalism.

The ICM and POM components of the curriculum offer several opportunities for elective rotations, each of a four-weeks duration.

The last component is Back to Basics. It occupies the remainder of the fourth year. It is designed to reinforce the importance of the basic sciences in clinical practice.

The evaluation system at this faculty is multifaceted and includes small-group assessments, written examinations, oral clinical examinations, assessment of written case reports, and others. The grading system is pass/fail.

McGill offers an M.D./M.B.A. program in response to the increasing need for doctors to acquire management skills that are unique to health care.

Similarly, a seven-year combined M.D./Ph.D. program is offered for students interested in a research career in academic medicine.

EARLY DECISION

Well-rounded students with a strong academic record and high MCAT scores may apply for the early decision program. Successful candidates who accept our offer of admission to the Faculty of Medicine at McGill must withdraw their application(s) to, or acceptance(s) from, other medical schools in order to maintain their accepted status at McGill.

REQUIREMENTS FOR ENTRANCE

Applicants to the M.D./C.M. program must have received, or be in the final year of a course of study leading to, a bachelor's degree. Specific requirements include the MCAT and university-level courses in each of the following:

	Credit hrs.
General Biology (with lab)	6
General Chemistry (with lab)	6
Organic Chemistry (with lab)	6
Physics (with lab)	6

Prerequisite courses completed more than eight years ago must be repeated. Exceptions may be made for applicants with advanced degrees in the material concerned.

University-level courses in biochemistry or cell biology and molecular biology are strongly recommended.

A Med-P program is restricted to residents of the province of Quebec who are attending the provincial colleges of general and professional education.

No places for transfer are available.

SELECTION FACTORS

Selection of students by the admissions committee is based upon academic achievement and an assessment of personal characteristics and accomplishments. Academic achievement is determined from the academic record in undergraduate studies and the result of the Medical College Admission Test. While completed graduate degrees are taken into consideration, applicants should know that the undergraduate CGPA is the major consideration in measuring academic performance. Applicants to the M.D./C.M. program must have undergraduate overall GPAs of 3.5 or better and a total of 30 or more in the MCAT scores.

The initial assessment of personal qualities and achievements is made from a study of the autobiographical letter and the letters of reference. Those applicants who are considered the most competitive will be invited for interviews. The files of candidates who are not invited for interviews are not considered further.

Following the interview the components of the application process overall—GPAs and MCAT scores for applicants to the M.D./C.M. program, CRC scores for applicants to the Med-P program, the autobiographical letter, and interview performance

scores are aggregated. Places in the entering class are offered to those whose aggregated scores are most competitive.

The decisions are final and are not subject to appeal.

Students accepted into the 2003 entering class had the following academic profile: *mean overall GPA,* 3.77; *mean MCAT scores VR*-9.74, *PS*-10.30, *BS*-11.35.

Institution Type: *Public*
Application Process: *www.med.mcgill.ca/admissions/*

APPLICATION AND ACCEPTANCE POLICIES FOR 2005-2006 FIRST-YEAR CLASS

Fees and expenses are in Canadian dollars.
Filing of application
  Earliest date: Sept. 1, 2004
  Latest date: Nov. 15, 2004 (out-of-province applicants applying to the regular M.D., C.M. program and the M.D.-Ph.D. program); Nov. 15, 2004 (applicants to the M.D.-M.B.A. program); Jan. 15, 2005 (Quebec resident applicants to the M.D.C.M. program); March 1, 2005 (Quebec resident applicants to the Med-P program)
School application fee to all applicants: $60
Oldest MCAT scores considered: 2001
Does have Early Decision Program
  EDP application period: June 1–Sept. 30, 2004
  EDP applicants notified by: Oct. 1, 2004
Acceptance notice to regular applicants
  Earliest date: Feb. 15, 2005
  Latest date: Varies
Applicant's response to acceptance offer
  Maximum time: 2 weeks
Requests for deferred entrance considered: Yes
Deposit to hold place in class (applied to tuition):
  $500, due with response to acceptance offer
Deposit refundable prior to: May 16, 2005
Estimated number of new entrants: 160 (3 EDP)
Starting date: August 2005

TUITION AND STUDENT FEES PER YEAR FOR 2003-2004 FIRST-YEAR CLASS

First-year Tuition   Student fees: $2,454.65
  Resident: $3,559.04
  Non-Quebec Canadian: $8,903.04
  U.S. & International: $22,439.04, CDN

INFORMATION ON 2003-2004 FIRST-YEAR CLASS

Number of	In-Province	Out-of-Province	Total
Applicants	582	398	980
Applicants Interviewed	241	102	343
New Entrants*	128	32†	160

*All new entrants into the four-year program took the MCAT and had baccalaureate degrees.

†Of this total 16 were U.S. citizens and 6 were citizens of foreign countries. Two additional students (1 non-Quebec Canadian student and 1 Quebec student) have been accepted into the first year of the M.D.-M.B.A. program. The first year of this program is spent in the Faculty of Management.

CHAPTER

12

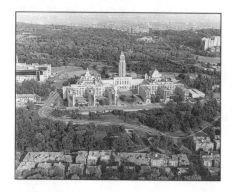

Université de Montréal
School of Medicine

Montreal, Quebec

Dr. Jean-Lucien Rouleau, *Dean of Faculty of Medicine*
Dr. Pierre Rousseau, *President of Admission Committee*
Dr. Raymond Lalande, *Vice Dean, Undergraduate Studies*

ADDRESS INQUIRIES TO:

Committee on Admission
Université de Montréal
School of Medicine
P.O. Box 6128, Station Centre-Ville
Montreal, Quebec
Canada H3C 3J7
(514) 343-6265; 343-6629 (FAX)
E-mail: admmed@ere.umontreal.ca
Web site: http://www.med.umontreal.ca

MISSION STATEMENT

The Faculty of Medicine of the Universite de Montreal seeks through its undergraduate medical program to provide a general preparation so that students will be able to enter postgraduate training in either family medicine or a medical specialization or fields related to research, teaching or health care management.

GENERAL INFORMATION

The Faculty of Medicine of the University of Montreal can be traced back to a school first established in Montreal in 1843 and incorporated in 1845 under the name of Ecole de Médecine et de Chirurgie de Montréal. In 1891 the school merged with the Faculty of Medicine of the Montreal Branch of Laval University, which had been founded in 1877. In 1920, by an act of the Quebec legislature, the Montreal branch of Laval University was granted its independence, and the school of medicine became known by its present name.

All instruction is in French, and clinical instruction is carried out at 14 affiliated teaching hospitals and research centers.

CURRICULUM

In September 1993 a new four-year curriculum came into effect. The first year is devoted to basic biological and behavioral sciences. Clinical exposure begins with Year 1. It consists of two years (70 weeks) of problem-based learning during which students are exposed to biomedical and psychosocial sciences basic to medicine. Courses are interdisciplinary and system based. Introduction to clinical skills takes place in a continuous fashion throughout those two preclinical years. Ninety hours of electives are mandatory during the first two years. The third and fourth years consist of an 80-week clerkship.

In the new curriculum, formal lecturing is reduced to a minimum and replaced by active methods, especially problem-based learning and small-group discussion.

A premedical year is restricted to students having just graduated from the provincial colleges of general and professional education. Students who have completed one to three years at the university level in humanities are also eligible for the premedical year. Opportunities exist to pursue a combined M.D.-M.Sc. and M.D.-Ph.D. curriculum.

Residency training in the teaching hospitals is under the responsibility of the Faculty of Medicine. Various courses and symposia are organized by the continuing medical education division.

REQUIREMENTS FOR ENTRANCE

A thorough knowledge of the French language is a prerequisite. Under the present Quebec educational system, the minimum requirement is two years of college (Health Sciences Program) and the diploma of collegial studies of the Department of Education (D.E.C.).

The college curriculum should provide a wide cultural background. Coursework must include: philosophy, behavioral and social sciences, French, English, mathematics (analytical geometry, calculus, college algebra, and trigonometry), and sciences (biology, inorganic and organic chemistry, and physics).

SELECTION FACTORS

Candidates accepted must be either Canadian citizens or landed immigrants, but due consideration will be given to French-speaking applicants from other provinces of Canada and from the United States. Selection of candidates is competitive and based on a global score derived from scholastic records and an interview. Interviews, conducted on the site of the medical school, are granted to about one-quarter of the applicants selected from their scholastic records. This interview can be eliminatory. For candidates holding a Ph.D. degree, performance in research may constitute an important selection factor. No consideration is given to race, sex, creed, or age.

FINANCIAL AID

Financial aid is available to students through the Bursaries Division of the Department of Education, the Kellogg Foundation Loan Fund, the Scholarships and Loan Committee of the university, and the Jean Frappier Fund. Summer scholarships are also available.

Institution Type: *Public*

APPLICATION AND ACCEPTANCE POLICIES FOR 2005-2006 FIRST-YEAR CLASS

Fees and expenses are in Canadian dollars.

Filing of application
    Latest date: January 15, 2005
School application fee to all applicants:
    $50 paper, $30 electronic
Does not have Early Decision Program
Acceptance notice to regular applicants
    Earliest date: May 15, 2004
    Latest date: Until class is filled
Applicant's response to acceptance offer
    Maximum time: two weeks
Requests for deferred entrance considered: No
Deposit to hold place in class: None
Estimated number of new entrants: 227
Starting date: August 2005

TUITION AND STUDENT FEES PER YEAR FOR 2003-2004 FIRST-YEAR CLASS

Tuition   Student fees: $437
    Resident: $2,225
    Nonresident: $13,585

INFORMATION ON 2003-2004 FIRST-YEAR CLASS

Number of	In-Province	Out-of-Province	Total
Applicants	1,717	314	2,031
Applicants Interviewed	699	13	712
New Entrants	231	5	236

University of Sherbrooke
Faculty of Medicine

Sherbrooke, Quebec

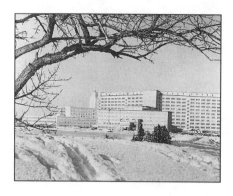

Dr. Réjean Hébert, *Dean*
Dr. Paul Grand Maison, *Vice Dean*
Dr. Claude Cyr, *Chair, Admissions Committee*

ADDRESS INQUIRIES TO:

Admission Office
University of Sherbrooke
Faculty of Medicine
3001, 12e Avenue Nord
Sherbrooke, Quebec
Canada J1H 5N4
(819) 564-5208; 564-5378 (FAX)
E-mail: Admission-Med@USherbrooke.ca
Web site: www.usherbrooke.ca

MISSION STATEMENT

As required by modern medical teaching, the Faculty of Medicine is integrated into a developing Health Sciences Center to serve all members of the health team. This Center includes a modern 700-bed teaching hospital. A Department of Nursing offers several programs of study at university level. The Faculty of Medicine offers residential facilities on campus. Twelve hospitals, many health centers, and CLSC are affiliated with the Faculty of Medicine.

GENERAL INFORMATION

Officially founded in February 1961, the Faculty of Medicine at the University of Sherbrooke is a French-speaking institution. It admitted its first students in September 1966.

CURRICULUM

Since 1987, a new four-year curriculum has begun. The form of teaching is now a problem-based learning program. Formal lecturing has been reduced to a minimum. Audiovisual facilities, seminars, small-group discussions, panels, field work, and case studies are used extensively. Most learning sessions integrate many disciplines representing various departments.

The M.D. degree is granted after successful completion of a four-year course. Students work in the hospital network from the beginning of their first year. The clerkship is a 16-month clinical training starting with the winter trimester of the third year.

Postgraduate programs are available in most departments leading to the M.Sc. or Ph.D. degree, and a diploma can be obtained in community health. Residency training is offered in all major specialties.

A joint M.D.-M.Sc. program is offered to students who are enrolled in an M.D. program with outstanding academic records. The medical student must have completed two years of the four-year M.D. program. The main objective of the joint program is to form doctors who will have achieved a scientific approach of medicine and who will also be able to pursue scientific activities among a team.

REQUIREMENTS FOR ENTRANCE

The minimum requirement for admission is two years of college under the present Quebec educational system—Collège d'enseignement général et professionnel (C.E.G.E.P.). B.A. or B.Sc. degrees are fully acceptable. The minimum science curriculum is as follows:
Candidates with a B.A. or B.Sc. degree:

Semesters

General Biology (with lab) 2
General Chemistry (with lab). 2
Organic Chemistry (with lab). 2
General Physics (with lab) 3
Mathematics through Calculus. 3

Must include analytical geometry, college algebra, and trigonometry.

C.E.G.E.P. candidates:

College diploma (D.E.C.) with major in sciences.

The college curriculum should also provide a wide cultural background in the humanities (including philosophy and literature) and in the social and behavioral sciences (including history, psychology, and sociology). Since all instruction is in French, fluency and reading ability in the French language are essential prerequisites.

The MCAT is not required.

SELECTION FACTORS

Admission to the Faculty of Medicine is based primarily on ability and premedical achievement, as demonstrated by scholastic records. A learning skills test is included in the selection.

One hundred-twelve places are reserved for applicants from the province of Quebec. Fifteen additional places are reserved for applicants from New Brunswick for admission. There is also one place available for an applicant from Prince Edward Island, plus one from Nova Scotia. Two places are available for qualified foreign applicants with a student visa. Applicants must be fluent in both written and spoken French.

FINANCIAL AID

Financial aid is available to resident students through the Bursaries Division of the Provincial Ministry of Education, the Scholarships and Loans Committee of the university, and a few private foundations.

Institution Type: *Public*

APPLICATION AND ACCEPTANCE POLICIES FOR 2005-2006 FIRST-YEAR CLASS

Fees and expenses are in Canadian dollars.

Filing of application
  Earliest date: Nov. 2004
  Latest date: March 1, 2005
School application fee to all applicants: $30
Oldest MCAT scores considered: Not required
Does not have Early Decision Program
Acceptance notice to regular applicants
  Earliest date: May 2005
  Latest date: Aug. 8, 2005
Applicant's response to acceptance offer
  Maximum time: June 1, 2005
Requests for deferred entrance considered: No
Deposit to hold place in class (applied to tuition):
  $200, due with response to acceptance offer;
  nonrefundable
Estimated number of new entrants: 150
Starting date: August 2005

TUITION AND STUDENT FEES PER YEAR FOR 2003-2004 FIRST-YEAR CLASS

Tuition and student fees:
  Canadian: $3,054.66
  Non-Canadian: $16,769.58

INFORMATION ON 2003-2004 FIRST-YEAR CLASS

Number of	In-Province	Out-of-Province	Total
Applicants	1,420	164	1,584
Applicants Interviewed	453	47	500
New Entrants*	124	26	150

*20% had baccalaureate degrees, 80% had post-secondary degrees.
Non-Canadian, 2

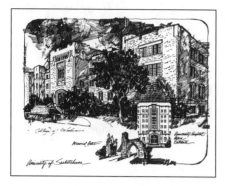

University of Saskatchewan College of Medicine

Saskatoon, Saskatchewan

W. L. Albritton, *Dean*
J. T. Sibley, *Director of Admissions and Student Affairs*

ADDRESS INQUIRIES TO:

Secretary, Admissions
University of Saskatchewan
College of Medicine
B103 Health Sciences Building, 107 Wiggins Road
Saskatoon, Saskatchewan
Canada S7N 5E5
(306) 966-8554; 966-6164 (FAX)
E-mail: med.admissions@usask.ca
Web site: www.usask.ca/medicine

GENERAL INFORMATION

The University of Saskatchewan began teaching medical students in a two-year medical sciences program in 1926. The present college was introduced in 1953 with a four-year curriculum leading to the M.D. degree. In 1968 the curriculum changed to five years with a one-year premedical university requirement. The curriculum reverted to a four-year program in 1988 with a minimum two-year premedical requirement.

Clinical teaching is based at the Royal University Hospital, St. Paul's and Pasqua City hospitals in Saskatoon, and the Plains Health Centre and General Hospital in Regina. Students also complete rotations in Saskatchewan Health Districts.

The maximum size of each entering class is 60 students.

CURRICULUM

The College of Medicine provides a curriculum leading to the general professional education of the physician; graduates may select careers in family medicine, specialty practice, public health, research, or teaching. During the course of the undergraduate M.D. curriculum, students may obtain a B.Sc. (Med.) degree in the basic medical sciences.

The current curriculum was launched in the fall of 1997.

Phase A (31 weeks) provides students with an overview of the basic science disciplines appropriate to the study of medicine, as well as an introduction to professional skills (including primary clinical skills) within the context of developing the patient–doctor relationship. This phase includes a two-week clinical experience done in one of the Saskatchewan Health Districts. Phase B (35 weeks) enables students to acquire specific knowledge in those subjects bridging the basic and clinical

sciences and to enhance basic clinical skills. Phase C (16 weeks), enables learning of the principles and methods in core clinical knowledge and linking courses. Phase D (67 weeks) of clinical clerkships provides an opportunity to apply the knowledge, skills, and attitudes students have acquired to the management of patients. Provision is made for clinical electives.

Learning in the basic and clinical sciences has been organized by body systems with a problem-solving emphasis.

REQUIREMENTS FOR ENTRANCE

Two full years of university study are required after graduation from secondary school. The following courses or their equivalent are required:

	Credit hrs.
Biochemistry	6
General Biology (with lab)	6
General Chemistry (with lab)	3
General Physics (with lab)	6
Organic Chemistry (with lab)	3
English (Literature and Composition)	6
Social Sciences or Humanities (full course)	6

Standard First Aid Certificate.

The MCAT is required, and scores must be available at time of application. A minimal score of 8 will be required in the sciences and Verbal Reasoning sections, and N in Writing Sample; however, either one 7 or an M will be accepted.

The applicant must be a Canadian citizen or landed immigrant of at least three years at the time of application.

SELECTION FACTORS

The Admissions Committee considers academic ability and personal qualities assessed through scholastic records, letters of recommendation, and results of a personal interview by a team of four persons. All eligible candidates are interviewed during a weekend in March. At the time of selection, academic ability and personal qualities are weighted approximately 3 to 1. For the 2003 entering class, the average GPA was 87.7 percent, and the average interview score was 20 of a possible 24 points.

FINANCIAL AID

Various loan funds and scholarships are available. A limited number of bursaries enable students to engage in research between the end of one academic year and the beginning of another.

INFORMATION ABOUT DIVERSITY PROGRAMS

There is an Aboriginal Access Program for Saskatchewan residents.

Institution Type: *Public*

APPLICATION AND ACCEPTANCE POLICIES FOR 2005-2006 FIRST-YEAR CLASS

Fees and expenses are in Canadian dollars.

Filing of application
  Earliest date: Aug. 1, 2004
  Latest dates
      In-province: Dec. 1, 2004
      Out-of-province: Dec. 1, 2004
School application fee:
  Saskatchewan residents: $40
  Non-Saskatchewan residents: $75 plus transcript fee*
Oldest MCAT scores considered: 2000
Does not have Early Decision Program
Acceptance notice to regular applicants
  Earliest date: April 30, 2005
  Latest date: Varies
Applicant's response to acceptance offer
  Maximum time: 2 weeks
Requests for deferred entrance considered: Yes
Deposit to hold place in class (applied to tuition):
  $200, due with response to acceptance offer;
  nonrefundable
Estimated number of new entrants: 60
Starting date: August 2005

TUITION AND STUDENT FEES PER YEAR FOR 2003-2004 FIRST-YEAR CLASS

Tuition: $10,168   Student fees: $150

INFORMATION ON 2003-2004 FIRST-YEAR CLASS

Number of	In-Province	Out-of-Province	Total
Applicants	118	225	343
Applicants Interviewed	111	39	150
New Entrants†	56	4	60

*Transcript fees are $25 for Canadian universities and $50 for non-Canadian universities.

100% entrants took the MCAT; 17% of those admitted had baccalaureate degrees.

Resources for Other Health Careers

1. American Association of Colleges of Osteopathic Medicine
   Suite 310, 500 Friendship Boulevard, Chevy Chase, MD 20815
   (301) 968-4100; www.aacom.org

2. American Association of Colleges of Pharmacy
   1426 Prince Street, Alexandria, VA 22314-2841
   (703) 739-2330; www.aacp.org

3. American Association of Colleges of Podiatric Medicine
   Suite 322, 1350 Piccard Drive, Rockville, MD 20850-4307
   1 (800) 922-9266; www.aacpm.org

4. American Association of Dental Schools
   1625 Massachusetts Avenue, N.W., Suite 600 Washington, D.C. 20036-2212
   www.adea.org

5. Association of American Veterinary Medical Colleges
   Suite 710, 1101 Vermont Avenue, N.W., Washington, D.C. 20005-3521
   (202) 371-9195; (202) 842-0773 (fax); http://aavmc.org

6. Association of Schools and Colleges of Optometry
   Suite 510, 6110 Executive Boulevard, Rockville, MD 20852
   (301) 231-5944; www.opted.org; email: admin@opted.org

7. Association of Schools of Public Health
   Suite 910, 1101 15th Street, N.W., Washington, D.C., 20005
   (202) 296-1099; info@asph.org; www.asph.org

Publications for the Health Professions

1. *270 Ways to Put Your Talent to Work in the Health Field*
   Single copy, $15.00 (National Health Council, 1730 M Street, N.W., Suite 500, Washington, D.C. 20036)

2. Autsin, L., *What's Holding You Back? 8 Critical Choices for Women's Success*
   Basic Books, 2000

3. Bickel, J., *Women in Medicine: Getting In, Growing & Advancing*
   Thousand Oaks, CA: Sage, 2000 (805-499-9774; www.sagepub.com)

4. Bickel, J., Ruffin, A. *Gender-association Differences in Matriculating and Graduating Medical Students.*
   Academic Medicine, 70:552-559, June 1994 (www.academicmedicine.org)

5. *Educational Survival Skills Study Guide*
   Free (Office of Statewide Health Planning and Development, Health Professions Career Opportunity Program, 1600 Ninth Street, Room 441, Sacramento, CA 95814)

6. *Financial Advice and Health Careers Resources Directory for Minority Students*
   Free (Office of Statewide Health Planning and Development, Health Professions Careers Opportunity Program, 1600 Ninth Street, Room 441, Sacramento, CA 95814)

7. *Health Pathways Quarterly Newsletter*
   Free (Office of Statewide Health Planning and Development, Health Professions Careers Opportunity Program, 1600 Ninth Street, Room 441, Sacramento, CA 95814)

8. *Informed Decisions-Making: Part I, Financial Planning and Management for Medical Students;*
   Part II, Sources of Financial Assistance for Medical School. National Medical Fellowships, Inc. 1993,
   $15.00 per set (National Medical Fellowships, Inc., 5 Hanover Square, 15th Floor, New York, NY 10004; (212) 483-8880; www.nwfonline.org)

9. *The Journal for Minority Medical Students*
   Published quarterly. $10.00 annually (Spectrum Unlimited, 4203 Canal Street, New Orleans, LA 70119; 1(800) 661-3319 or (504) 488-5100; (504) 488-7072 [fax])

10. Kaltreider, Nancy B., *Dilemmas of a Double Life, Women Balancing Careers and Relationship.*
    Jason Aronson, Inc., 1997

11. *Minorities in Medicine: A Guide for Premedical Students*
    Free (Office of Statewide Health Planning and Development, Health Professions Career Opportunity Program, 1600 Ninth Street, Room 441, Sacramento, CA 95814

12. *Minority Student Opportunities in United States Medical Schools, 2002*
    16th Edition (Association of American Medical Colleges, Department 66, Washington, D.C. 20055; (202) 828-0416)

13. More, S.E., *Restoring the Balance: Women Physicians and the Profession of Medicine, 1850-1995.*
    Harvard U. Press, 2000

14. *Need a Lift? College Financial Aid Handbook*
    $3.00 prepaid, plus .95 shipping (The American Legion; P.O. Box 1050, Indianapolis, Indiana 46206; www.legion.org)

15. *The Student Guide 2000-2001*
    Free (U.S. Department of Education. Federal Student Aid Information Center, P.O. Box 84, Washington, D.C. 20044-0084; 1-800-4-FED-AID, 1-800-433-3243; www.ed.gov/studentaid)

16. *Time Management for Students*
    Free (Office of Statewide Health Planning and Development, Health Professions Career Opportunity Program, 1600 Ninth Street, Room 441, Sacramento, CA 95814)

17. Wear, D. (ed), *Women in Medical Education: An Anthology of Experience*
    Albany, NY: SUNY Press, 1996

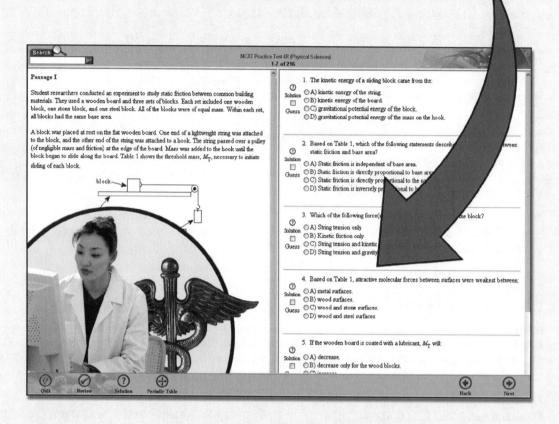
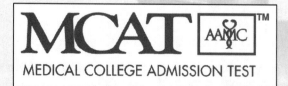

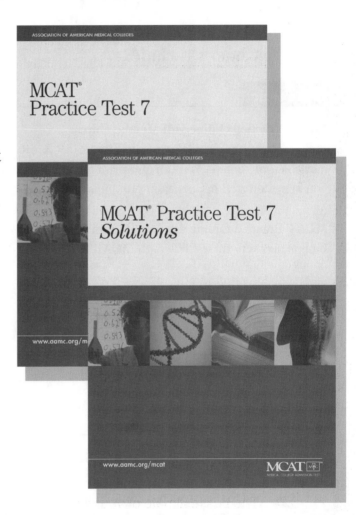
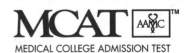

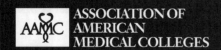
Order MCAT Practice Tests online!

For a complete, up-to-date listing of MCAT Practice Tests or to place your order, please visit www.aamc.org/publications.

Popular Choices Include:

Web Format

MCAT Practice Online Full Membership
Full membership includes access to 3R, 4R, 5R & 6R - all with Solutions, plus the additional features available only online. You can also print out the tests, but not the Solutions. This is the best value if you are interested in purchasing multiple practice tests.

MCAT Practice Online 4R, 5R, 6R, and 7
Online access to these full-length MCAT Practice Tests is also sold separately.

MCAT Practice Online 3R
This special offer provides free access to one full-length MCAT. This is a great option if you are uncertain whether to purchase paper or Web versions.

* Requires an e-mail account and IE V5.0 or greater, AOL V6.0, Netscape 7.0, or Mozilla 1.0. Purchase entitles single-user access from the time of purchase through two administratiosn of the MCAT.

Paper Format

MCAT Practice Tests 5R, 6R, and 7 with Solutions
These MCAT Practice Tests are available in printed booklets, with Solutions printed separately. This format is identical to the paper test administration format, and offers the best print quality. These tests are used in some commercial review courses and by pre-health professions advisors in "mock" MCAT administrations.

> **MCAT Practice Tests are the only authentic MCAT tests available. They provide the most realistic example of a real MCAT test and your scores are generated by the same methods as a real MCAT. Our online practice tests include solutions with detailed explanations of each answer. Always up-to-date, MCAT Practice Tests are your best choice for preparation.**